THE U.S. HEALTHCARE SYSTEM

Published by JB - Jossey-Bass
Published simultaneously in Canada.

For general information on our other products and services, please contact our Customer Care Department within the U.S. at 800-956-7739, outside the U.S. at 317-572-3986, or fax 317-572-4002.

Wiley publishes in a variety of print and electronic formats and by print-on-demand. Some material included with standard print versions of this book may not be included in e-books or in print-on-demand. If this book refers to media such as a CD or DVD that is not included in the version you purchased, you may download this material at http://booksupport.wiley.com. For more information about Wiley products, visit www.wiley.com.

Library of Congress Cataloging-in-Publication Data is Available:

ISBN 9780470631522 (paperback)
ISBN 9781118418345 (ePDF)
ISBN 9781118415399 (ePub)

Cover Design: Wiley
Cover Image: ©Katty2016/Shutterstock

Printed in the United States of America

FIRST EDITION

PB Printing   C10012681_080119

THE U.S. HEALTHCARE SYSTEM

Origins, Organization and Opportunities

JOEL I. SHALOWITZ, MD, MBA

JB JOSSEY-BASS™
A Wiley Brand

To Mervin Shalowitz, MD: father, teacher, colleague, and friend

CONTENTS

LIST OF EXHIBITS

FOREWORD

I have been teaching a survey course on the American healthcare system in MBA and MPH programs for more than 30 years. During this time, students have constantly expressed frustration at the system's incredible complexity, leading to inefficiencies and wastefulness. In fact, calling it *a* system is really a misnomer—it is more like a cluster of variably interrelated subsystems. One needs only to look at the financing systems for proof of this fragmentation: Medicare, Medicaid, the Children's Health Insurance Program (CHIP), employer-based health insurance, Health Insurance Exchange–based coverage, Veterans Administration care, and TRICARE for families of active military. These mechanisms are just the major ways healthcare is paid in our country. Add to this disarray the complexities of different types of provider organizations, technology companies, and other healthcare entities and a person is likely to offer one of three solutions to our problems: throw up one's hands and walk away, offer incremental changes, or blow up the system and start over by, for example, instituting a single payer system.

In order to make sense of the complexity of these problems and solutions, this textbook takes a very different approach from others textbooks on this subject. For each topic, I present a detailed, relevant history as background for understanding its current status. I take this approach for two reasons. First, before we can make plans for improvements, we need to fully understand where we are now. To understand where we are now, we must understand how we got here. Second, with the exception of innovative technologies, *nothing in healthcare is new*. For example, Western society has tried many types of financing, organizational structures, and regulations. Each of these attempts has created its own set of problems. Since the problems are also not new, it is necessary to understand what was tried in the past to fix them, the contexts in which the solutions were attempted, and why these attempts succeeded or failed.

With this approach, it also becomes easier to deliver three overarching goals for this book.

First, provide *frameworks* for understanding problems. When one is faced with a difficulty in the healthcare system, it is useful to understand the *type* of problem it is. For examples: Is it a quality issue? Is it an issue of a trade-off between quality and access? Is it a pricing issue? Once the problem is properly framed, it can be placed in the context of the entire system, and rational solutions can begin to form. Consider a medical analogy. A patient presents with symptoms. If a physician can identify them as belonging to problems in a particular organ system, investigation is then much easier and can lead to a more rapid diagnosis and treatment plan.

Second, provide *facts*. A working knowledge of the subject is always necessary to begin framing a problem. For example, understanding the structure and funding streams of Medicare is essential to identifying key issues and solutions.

Third, healthcare is changing so rapidly that it is difficult to keep up with regulations, organizational changes, and technological innovations, to name a few. I have, therefore, provided *extensive resources* so that one can get updates more easily. This last item would seem easy in the internet age. However, in writing this book, I have been struck by the fragmentation of information and, occasionally, the errors in what has been accepted as "common knowledge." For example, I found it interesting that HIPAA issues (the federal program that deals with patient privacy and security) are handled by the Office of Civil Rights.

As you read this book, I hope you will gain an appreciation not only of the complexities and problems of our healthcare system but also of the opportunities to implement truly effective and meaningful changes.

ACKNOWLEDGMENTS

While this work is a single-author text, the professional career encouragement and support I have received have been invaluable to its conceptualization and execution. Unfortunately, the three mentors I wish to thank are no longer with us: Professor Morton Kamien, Dean Emeritus Donald Jacobs, and my father, Mervin Shalowitz, MD, to whom this book is dedicated.

The personal encouragement and patience of my wife, Madeleine Shalowitz, MD, MBA, has been priceless. My children also deserve a note of appreciation for their gentle nudges: "So how's the book going, Dad?" Thanks to David Shalowitz, MD, MS, Kira Spivack, and Ilana Shalowitz. Finally, a special acknowledgment to the late Murphy Shalowitz, who was my constant companion throughout the writing of this book.

INTRODUCTION TO THE U.S. HEALTH CARE SYSTEM

CHAPTER

1

UNDERSTANDING AND MANAGING COMPLEX HEALTHCARE SYSTEMS

DEFINITIONS

JULIET.

> *... What's in a name? That which we call a rose*
> *By any other word would smell as sweet ...*

—William Shakespeare, *Romeo and Juliet*, Act 2, Scene 2

> *Anyone who can set the terms of a debate can win it.*

—Attributed to George Edward Reedy, White House press secretary
under U.S. President Lyndon B. Johnson

Before we try to understand how healthcare systems are structured and function, we need to consider some definitions. First, how do we define the word "health"? The answer is important because it frames such decisions as our population focus for care, how we design facilities, how we train our professionals and ancillary personnel, how we develop new technologies, and how we structure insurance products. Unfortunately, many societies (including the United States) define health in terms of the absence of disease and focus on acute care as their model of what society should provide.[1] This view about the meaning of health is strikingly obvious if one compares self-reported health status to objective measures, such as life expectancy. For example, in a survey of 37 countries, Japan's ranking for self-reported health is 36th and the United States is first. However, Japan's life expectancy ranks first while the United States ranks 27th.[2]

Since health is often viewed as an absence of some type of bodily derangement, we first need to define three terms: illness, disease, and sickness. Dictionaries often provide circular definitions for these three terms, but it is useful to distinguish among them for purposes of addressing the healthcare issues just mentioned. The most helpful explanations were written by Marinker[3] more than 40 years ago:

> [Disease is] a pathological process, most often physical as in throat infection, or cancer of the bronchus, sometimes undetermined in origin, as in schizophrenia. The quality which identifies disease is some deviation from a biological norm. There is an objectivity about disease which doctors are able to see, touch, measure, smell.

> [Illness is] a feeling, an experience of unhealth which is entirely personal, interior to the person of the patient. Often it accompanies disease, but the disease may be undeclared, as in the early stages of cancer or tuberculosis or diabetes. Sometimes illness exists where no disease can be found. Traditional medical education has made the deafening silence of

---

[1]Fox, E. (1997). Predominance of the curative model of medical care: A residual problem. *JAMA, 278*, 761–763.
[2]OECD Better Life Index. Retrieved March 28, 2018 from http://www.oecdbetterlifeindex.org/topics/health.
[3]Marinker, M. (1975). Why make people patients? *Journal of Medical Ethics, 1*(2), 81–84.

illness-in-the-absence-of-disease unbearable to the clinician. The patient can offer the doctor nothing to satisfy his senses—he can only bring messages of pain to the doctor . . . The traditional remedy for this distress (I am of course talking about the distress of the doctor and not the distress of the patient) is to translate the illness language of diseases that do not require objects available to the doctor's eyes, ears or hands. I am talking about psychiatric language.

[Sickness is] the external and public mode of unhealth. Sickness is a social role, a status, a negotiated position in the world, a bargain struck between the person henceforward called "sick," and a society which is prepared to recognize and sustain him. The security of this role depends on a number of factors, not least the possession of that much treasured gift, the disease. Sickness based on illness alone is a most uncertain status. But even the possession of disease does not guarantee equity in sickness. Those with a chronic disease are much less secure than those with an acute one; those with a psychiatric disease than those with a surgical one. The diseases of the old are less highly regarded than those of the young; I do not dare to suggest that diseases of women are inferior to those of men. Best is an acute physical disease in a young man quickly determined by recovery or death—either will do, both are equally regarded.

Given these definitions of disorders, we can now consider the definition of "health." According to the World Health Organization (WHO): "Health is a state of complete physical, mental and social well-being and not merely the absence of disease or infirmity."[4] It is obvious that a policy focus on *this* definition will yield different priorities than a policy that relies on the ones above.

These definitions invite the question: What *are* the priorities of the U.S. healthcare system? In other words, what is its mission? After reading the examples in Exhibit 1.1, it should be obvious that one of the principle problems is that the United States does not have a mission statement that guides health policy.

EXHIBIT 1.1. Examples of Mission Features for Healthcare Systems

1. *Universal Declaration of Human Rights.* Adopted and proclaimed by U.N. General Assembly Resolution 217 A (III) of December 10, 1948 Article 25. (1): Everyone has the right to a standard of living adequate for the health and well-being of himself and of his family, including food, clothing, housing and medical care and necessary social services, and the right to security in the event of unemployment, sickness, disability, widowhood, old age or other lack of livelihood in circumstances beyond his control.

2. *National Health Service.* When former British Prime Minister Gordon Brown was Chancellor of the Exchequer, he said that taxation to fund healthcare is fair compared to:

   User Charges. "[I]t does not charge people for the misfortune of being sick."

   Private Insurance. It "does not impose higher costs on those who are predisposed to illness, or who fall sick."

   Social Insurance. "[I]t does not demand that employers bear the majority burden of health costs."[a]

---

[4]Constitution of WHO: principles. Retrieved March 28, 2018 from http://www.who.int/about/mission/en

3. Policy and administrative objectives for Canadian healthcare.

Public Administration. The provincial and territorial plans must be administered and operated on a nonprofit basis by a public authority accountable to the provincial or territorial government.

Comprehensiveness. The provincial and territorial plans must insure all medically necessary services provided by hospitals, medical practitioners and dentists working within a hospital setting.

Universality. The provincial and territorial plans must entitle all insured persons to health insurance coverage on uniform terms and conditions.

Accessibility. The provincial and territorial plans must provide all insured persons reasonable access to medically necessary hospital and physician services without financial or other barriers.

Portability. The provincial and territorial plans must cover all insured persons when they move to another province or territory within Canada and when they travel abroad. The provinces and territories have some limits on coverage for services provided outside Canada, and may require prior approval for non-emergency services delivered outside their jurisdiction.

Also: Efficiency, Value for Money, Accountability, and Transparency[b]

4. Principles of the Servizio Sanitario Nazionale (Italian National Health Service)

Human Dignity. Every individual has to be treated with equal dignity and have equal rights regardless of personal characteristics and role in society.

Protection. The individual health has to be protected with appropriate preventive measures and interventions.

Need. Everyone has access to healthcare and available resources to meet the primary healthcare needs.

Solidarity. Available resources have to be primarily allocated to support groups of people, individuals and certain diseases that are socially, clinically and epidemiologically important.

Effectiveness and Appropriateness. Resources must be addressed toward services whose effectiveness is grounded and individuals that might especially benefit from them. Priority should be given to interventions that offer greater efficacy in relation to costs.

Equity. Any individual must have access to the healthcare system with no differentiation or discrimination among citizens and no barrier at the point of use.[c]

[a] From speech given at the Social Market Foundation in London on March 20, 2002. At: http://www.ukpol.co.uk/2016/01/page/22/

[b] Canada Health Act and Commission on the Future of Healthcare in Canada, 2001, Romanow Report. https://www.canada.ca/en/health-canada/services/health-care-system/reports-publications/health-care-system/canada.html#a4

[c] http://www.salute.gov.it/portale/salute/p1_4.jsp?lingua=italiano&area=ll_Ssn

We can even go further in this analysis if we consider a definition for a healthcare *system* that will deliver those services and products for our desired goals.

When we turn to the definitions of "system" in Exhibit 1.2, the sense is of an orderly whole, working synchronously for a common purpose or, hopefully, positively influencing other parts.

EXHIBIT 1.2. Definition of System

According to the *Oxford English Dictionary*, a system is

- A set or assemblage of things connected, associated, or interdependent, so as to form a complex unity; a whole composed of parts in orderly arrangement according to some scheme or plan; rarely applied to a simple or small assemblage of things.

- An organized scheme or plan of action, especially one of a complex or comprehensive kind; an orderly or regular method of procedure.

According to the British Journal of Sociology,

- The idea of "system" has been used to imply that its parts (organizations or institutions) are interdependent with each other: that the performances of the parts have consequences or functions, consequences for the "performing" part, consequences for other "parts," consequences for the whole system.

Roemer[5] explained a further ideal:

The term *health system* or *system of health care* has been used with different meanings. Anthropologists use the terms systems of medicine to refer to various practices for healing the sick, according to diverse religious, philosophical, magical, and empirical doctrines. Many health observers analyzed the prevailing patterns of personal medical care in a country, defining these as the country's *health care system*. Government officials may describe the structure and functions of a country's ministry of health as its health system . . . we regard a health system as the *combination of resources, organization, financing, and management that culminate in the delivery of health services to the population.* (Emphases added.)

In contrast to this ideal, however, an accurate description of the U.S. healthcare system might be: an apparently ad hoc arrangement of small units, each with its own goals and incentives, whose purpose is treatment of acute diseases of insured populations. The deficiencies of focus, common purpose, and universality have significant implications for such tasks as structuring health insurance, building delivery organizations, designing continuity of care programs, aligning financial incentives, and choosing appropriate quality measures, among others.

The WHO provides a useful definition of a *healthcare system* as one that "encompasses all the activities whose primary purpose is to promote, restore, or maintain health . . . and include[s] patients and their families, health care workers and caregivers within organizations and in the community, and the health policy environment in which all health related activities occur."[6]

---

[5]Roemer, M. I. (1991). *National health systems of the world* (Vol. *1*, pp. 3, 4, 31). New York: Oxford University Press.
[6]WHO. (2002). *Innovative care for chronic conditions: Building blocks for action: Global report*, p. 29. Retrieved from http://www.who.int/chp/knowledge/publications/icccglobalreport.pdf

The word "system" will be used in future references to refer to healthcare schemes that have varying degrees of internal consistencies and coordination with one another.

One final consideration is not a definition per se but defining the elements that comprise a healthcare system. Simply stated by Sir Michael Marmot: "Every sector is a health sector."[7] This relationship is presented graphically in Exhibit 1.3. While the interrelationships among

EXHIBIT 1.3. Factors Influencing Healthcare Systems

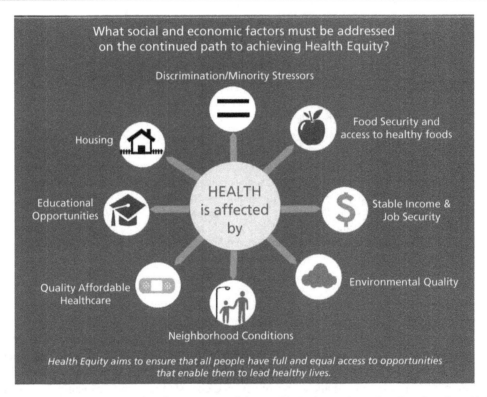

Source: Adapted and reprinted with permission of the Health Equity Institute, San Francisco State University. Retrieved March 30, 2018 from https://healthequity.sfsu.edu

---

[7]The original statement comes from M. Marmot (2005). Social determinants of health inequalities. *Lancet*. 365, 1099–1104. "A burgeoning volume of research identifies social factors at the root of much of...inequalities in health. Social determinants are relevant to communicable and non-communicable disease alike. Health status, therefore, should be of concern to policy makers in every sector, not solely those involved in health policy." Subsequently, Marmot shortened this assertion in a number of presentations, the earliest of which is perhaps: Taking forward action of the social determinants of health: WHO Commission on the Social Determinants of Health. Madrid, May 28, 2009. Retrieved from https://www.msssi.gob.es/profesionales/saludPublica/prevPromocion/promocion/desigualdadSalud/docs/presentacion Equidad.pdf

all these elements is extremely important, the scope of this book is limited to the healthcare inputs of such elements as provider and supplier organizations, professionals, and financing mechanisms.

HEALTH SYSTEM STRUCTURE AND FEATURES

First Lord.

> *The web of our life is of a mingled yarn, good and ill together...*
>
> —William Shakespeare, *All's Well That Ends Well*, Act 4, Scene 3

Deciphering the structure of any country's healthcare system can be a daunting and confusing task. Most approaches to understanding these complex systems use only the limited perspectives of economics and/or politics.[8] These approaches, however, often fail to include such important considerations as culture, politics, and underlying national demographics.

Exhibit 1.4 provides these additional dimensions in a systematic way to help you understand any nation's healthcare system. While this format may lead to some redundant questions and answers, it also ensures that you will not miss key aspects of a system. In order to better explain the use of this framework, some sample questions and comments

EXHIBIT 1.4. **Features of Healthcare Systems**

Domains for Analysis	Who Pays?	How Much Is Paid? (Costs/Budgets)	Who/What Is Covered?	Where Is Care Provided?	Who Provides Services and Products?
Political/regulatory/ judicial	1	6	11	16	21
Economic	2	7	12	17	22
Social/cultural	3	8	13	18	23
Technological	4	9	14	19	24
Population characteristics- demography and epidemiology	5	10	15	20	25

Source: Shalowitz, J. (2008). In P. Kotler, J. Shalowitz, & R. Stevens. *Strategic marketing for health care organizations: Building a customer-driven health system.* San Francisco: Jossey-Bass.

---

[8]Two classic views are those of Odin Anderson (Anderson, O. W. [1972]. *Health care: Can there be equity?* New York: Wiley) and Milton Roemer (Roemer, M. I. [1985]. *National strategies for health care organization.* Ann Arbor, MI: Health Administration Press).

for each numbered cell are presented. Users of this model are encouraged to ask additional questions and adapt its use to specific circumstances.

Who Pays?

Cell 1. Political/Regulatory/Judicial. The first question you can ask is: Where does the power reside to make decisions about payment for healthcare services and products? The answer depends on the degree of centralization or decentralization of the system. In the United States, except for strictly federal programs like Medicare, regulatory authority for health insurance resides at the state level. Even in countries with national health programs, there is often a regionalization of healthcare payment and delivery. For example, Canadian provinces and territories regulate their health insurance plans. (References to Canadian provinces below are also meant to include territories.) At the other extreme of local control, governmentally run healthcare systems in Sweden and Finland are managed at the level of municipalities.

Another question concerns the extent to which the public or private sectors pay for healthcare. In the United States, private insurance companies are largely responsible for healthcare payments. Most of this private insurance is purchased through employer and employee contributions at the workplace. At the opposite end of the spectrum is Cuba, where the entire healthcare system is publicly financed. Between these two limits there are a large number of variations. For example, in Canada, private insurance can provide coverage only for products and services that are not furnished by the provincial health insurance plans. In Chile, employees have the option to use the mandatory tax on wages to buy into either the state-sponsored health insurance plan (FONASA) or a private insurance company (ISAPRE). In yet another example, workers in Argentina (who purchase their health insurance with mandatory payroll deductions from their union) must use after-tax money if they want to enroll in a private insurance plan.

In all healthcare systems, private insurance can take on one of four roles vis-à-vis public insurance:

1. *Duplicate.* Public and private systems exist in parallel and cover same benefits (Chile)

2. *Substitute.* Private system replaces public system for certain population sectors (Germany)

3. *Complement.* Private system provides benefits the public sector does not cover (Canada)

4. *Supplement.* Private system extends benefits of the public sector in extent and/or payment (U.S., Medicare)

Cell 2. Economic. The state of a country's economy can also determine who pays for products and services, shifting the balance between government and private sources, such as employers and individuals. For example, in the 1990s, when the U.S. economy was rapidly expanding, many companies provided rich healthcare benefits for their employees. During the subsequent economic downturn, however, companies shifted more of the responsibility for payment to their workers. This pattern repeated itself after the market crash of 2008.

When the public sector is largely responsible for financing healthcare, during bad economic times it may withdraw considerable support, leaving individuals to shoulder substantial financial responsibility. Extreme examples of this latter situation are rural China and parts of the former Soviet Union. The opposite situation may also apply: When the economy is performing well and healthcare costs are rising, government often looks to increasing individual payments or enhancing the role of the private sector.

Cell 3. Social/Cultural. The social/cultural characteristics of a country can ultimately determine the mechanisms and sources of payment. In essence, these factors shape a country's healthcare "mission statement." (Please see Exhibit 1.1 and the Definitions section above.)

It is often difficult to determine which dimensions of culture are the most important in shaping a country's healthcare system. For purposes of comparing systems, however, analyzing measurable differences in culture can provide some guidance about which other countries may provide practical models for adoption. The most useful framework for such measurements is summarized in Exhibit 1.5. To demonstrate its utility, consider these two examples. Some American policy analysts advocate adoption of a Canadian model for the U.S. healthcare system; however, the two countries have substantial cultural differences. Specifically, the United States is distinguished from other countries as being the most individualistic nation. A pluralistic system with standard benefits is, therefore, not compatible with American culture.[9] Second, as Finland looks to other healthcare models for reform, it naturally studies Sweden. These countries share history (Finland was part of Sweden from the Middle Ages until 1809), language (Swedish is Finland's second official language), and structure of healthcare systems (Sweden and Finland base their systems at the municipal level). Also, in several cultural dimensions, Finland is similar to other Scandinavian countries. One important difference, however, is in the uncertainty avoidance index. Using this measure, Finland is very different from all other Scandinavian countries and is closer to Germany and Switzerland. If this dimension proves to be the most important cultural feature with respect to healthcare, the implication is that Finland needs to look to these latter two countries rather than (or in addition to) Sweden for healthcare system model reform. In fact, the recent Finnish reform proposal looks more like the Swiss system than that of Sweden.

Cell 4. Technological. In this context, technology incorporates drugs, devices, and procedures that are used in healthcare settings. The two key questions we must ask are: Who approves new technology? *and* How closely are safety and efficacy evaluations combined with cost considerations in determining whether a technology is approved and used? For example, in the United States, the Food and Drug Administration (FDA) will determine whether a pharmaceutical is safe and efficacious. This decision is totally independent of: (a) whether there are many similar pharmaceuticals in the same class already available in the marketplace or (b) if the newly approved drug is much more costly than similar ones, given

---

[9]For other views of cultural differences between the United States and Canada, see Adams, M. (2003). *Fire and ice: The United States, Canada and the myth of converging value*. Toronto: Penguin Canada.

EXHIBIT 1.5. Definition of Culture

According to Hofstede,[a] culture is defined "as the collective programming of the mind that distinguishes members of one group or category of people from another ... culture is the human collectivity what personality is to an individual."

Dimensions of Culture (from Hofstede)

Power distance. The extent to which the less powerful members of institutions and organizations within a country *expect* and *accept* that power is distributed unequally.

Uncertainty avoidance. The extent to which the members of a culture feel threatened by uncertain or unknown situations.

Individualism/collectivism. Individualism stands for a society in which the ties between individuals are loose: Everyone is expected to look after him-/herself and her/his immediate family only. Collectivism stands for a society in which people from birth onwards are integrated into strong, cohesive in groups, which throughout people's lifetime continue to protect them in exchange for unquestioning loyalty.

Masculinity/femininity. Masculinity stands for a society in which social gender roles are clearly distinct: Men are supposed to be assertive, tough, and focused on material success; women are supposed to be more modest, tender, and concerned with the quality of life. Femininity stands for a society in which social gender roles overlap: Both men and women are supposed to be modest, tender, and concerned with the quality of life.

Long-term orientation. The fostering of virtues oriented toward future rewards, in particular, perseverance and thrift. Its opposite pole, short-term orientation stands for the fostering of virtues related to the past and present, in particular, respect for tradition, preservation of "face," and fulfilling social obligations.

[a] Hofstede, G. (2001). *Culture's consequences: Comparing values, behaviors, institutions, and organizations across nations* (2nd ed.). Thousand Oaks, CA: Sage.

---

equivalent benefits. Contrast the FDA approval process with England's National Institute for Healthcare and Clinical Excellence (NICE). The NICE approves pharmaceuticals based not only on safety and efficacy but also on cost-effectiveness. This disparity exists principally because, in the former case, the U.S. federal government does not directly pay for most pharmaceuticals, whereas the British government does have such fiscal responsibility. Even for the United States' Medicare insurance scheme for pharmaceutical payment (Part D), the federal government has repeatedly decided not to bargain directly with pharmaceutical companies.

Once the technology is approved, who pays for it depends on site of use. For example, in the United States, patients with private health insurance usually share the cost of outpatient self-administered pharmaceuticals with the insurance company; for inpatient medications, however, the insurance company pays the hospital a negotiated rate that includes those items. By contrast, in Ontario, while hospital medications are fully covered through governmental payments, most individuals pay out of pocket for self-administered pharmaceuticals unless they have private insurance to cover that expense.

Cell 5. Population Characteristics. Demographic characteristics of the population will also determine who pays for products and services. For example, one of the key questions facing many countries is how they will care for their growing elderly populations. Who will pay for their care? How much will the elderly be expected to contribute themselves and how much will the public sector finance? While the United States is not among the world's most rapidly aging countries, due largely to past immigration policies, many other developed countries are facing changing demographics where covering elderly costs cannot be easily shifted to a young, working population.

How Much Is Paid?

Cell 6. Political/Regulatory/Judicial. In most countries, the political process is the origin of public healthcare budgets and fee schedules. Even in the United States, where most care is provided by the private sector, government-set global fees for hospitals (diagnosis-related groups [DRGs]) and per-service fees for physicians (resource-based relative value scale [RBRVS]) have been adopted by the private sector as benchmarks for paying those providers. (More will be said about those methods in later chapters.)

An example of judicial influence on costs comes from the debate on so-called gray markets for pharmaceuticals—the practice of importing drugs from lower-cost countries into higher-cost countries. While this issue has garnered much press and congressional attention in the United States (particularly with respect to importation of drugs from Canada), in Europe it has also been addressed by the European Union (EU) courts, where such practices were found to be legal.

Cell 7. Economic. Although politics will frame the debate about how much a country will spend on public programs, overall spending is most directly correlated with the state of a country's economy. Data from the Organisation for Economic Cooperation and Development (OECD) has consistently shown that globally, the highest correlative factor for per capita healthcare spending is gross domestic product (GDP) per capita.[10] (R^2 varies by year but averages about 0.9.) However, the United States is a conspicuous outlier, spending much more than the model predicts. The reason for this discrepancy is that prices have been higher than in other countries.[11] Another factor in this category is how much the government shifts payment responsibility to individuals. Not only do out-of-pocket amounts for each service vary widely by country, but so do the limits for how much an individual can be at financial risk. For example, in the United States, an individual covered by Medicare has unlimited financial responsibility for healthcare expenses beyond those covered by that program. In contrast, many countries put an upper limit on these amounts.

---

[10] OECD (2017), Health at a glance 2017: OECD indicators, OECD Publishing, Paris. doi: 10.1787/health_glance-2017-enRetrieved

[11] Papanicolas, I., Woskie, L. R., & Jha, A. K. (2018). Health care spending in the United States and other high-income countries. *JAMA 319*(10), 1024–1039.

Cell 8. Social/Cultural. Given the political and economic determinants for healthcare budgets, the social and cultural characteristics of a country lay the groundwork for what is possible regarding such factors as the government's role in providing healthcare benefits, extent of government support, types of services covered by insurance (both public and private), and relative amounts of payments. For example, in the United States, procedures are valued relatively more than cognitive services and hence are paid at higher rates. By contrast, in Sweden, the government raised caretaker salaries when it recognized the need for higher-quality workers in the long-term care sector.

Cell 9. Technological. As mentioned above, countries other than the United States consider the cost of technology along with its efficacy. Depending on the country, this cost analysis may occur simultaneously with the safety and efficacy evaluation or subsequent to it. Examples of some pharmaceutical pricing frameworks and cost-containment strategies are explained in Chapter 7, "Healthcare Technology."

Once the technology is approved and budgeted, its effect on healthcare costs can be determined by answering the question: How much does technology add to the cost of care as opposed to helping reduce overall expenses? One of the most significant factors contributing to rising healthcare costs across many countries is expenses related to new technology. This new technology is, by and large, layered on to the old technology rather than replacing it. A good example is balloon angioplasty and stenting of narrowed coronary arteries. These relatively less invasive techniques were supposed to replace many coronary artery bypass surgeries; in fact, the overall effect was to add a large number of patients who would not have been eligible for the latter procedure. In contrast, introduction of medication to treat peptic ulcer disease has all but eliminated surgery for that condition.

Cell 10. Population Characteristics. Demographic characteristics of the population will also determine who pays for products and services. For example, as mentioned above, one of the key questions facing many countries is how they will care for their growing elderly populations. Who will pay for their care? How much will the elderly be expected to contribute themselves and how much will the public sector finance?

Who and What Is Covered?

Cell 11. Political/Regulatory/Judicial. The political process plays a significant role in determining who will be covered and what healthcare benefits they will receive. For example, although all Canadian citizens are covered by government-sponsored insurance, the exact benefits vary by province. In the United States, examples in this category include state laws (called *mandates*) that require health insurance companies to offer certain benefits to their members. The Affordable Care Act (ACA) and Medicaid rules list categories of essential health services that must be covered by federally sanctioned plans, but the details are left to the states.

Cell 12. Economic. In addition to determining the amount of money allocated for the healthcare system, the economic climate will also determine what benefits are offered. In good economic times benefits may be added, but during downturns even government benefits may be withdrawn. For example, over several years of an economic pressure, Medicare limited the number of physical therapy visits; unlimited use was only reestablished in 2018.

Cell 13. Social/Cultural. These factors can have an important impact on whom and what is covered by public and private systems. For example, when economic conditions required benefit cutbacks in Germany, one of the most contentious programs that was eliminated was spa care—long a staple of that country's healthcare system. In the United States we would never consider eliminating pregnancy benefits; however, Japanese insurance usually does not cover such services.

Cell 14. Technological. The influence of technology in terms of coverage can be assessed by answering the following two questions: What technologies are lifesaving, life enhancing, or lifestyle enhancing *and* How are these technologies prioritized? An example is the U.S. government's decision to exclude drugs for erectile dysfunction as a covered benefit for Medicare's prescription drug plan (Part D).

Cell 15. Population Characteristics. Which populations require healthcare will also determine who or what is covered. The dilemma is: To what extent should the healthcare system focus on those with acute illnesses, those with chronic disease, and/or those who should receive preventive services? At this point, demographics intersect with epidemiology, and "what is covered" needs to reflect population disease patterns. For example, according to the Centers for Disease Control and Prevention (CDC), the leading causes of death in the United States are diseases of the heart, cancers, and chronic lower respiratory diseases.[12] Should we devote significant resources to treating these conditions or preventing them? Should we instead allocate these resources to other conditions that affect younger people, like accidents and mental illness?

Where Is Care Provided?

Cell 16. Political/Regulatory/Judicial. Governments may enact laws to ensure appropriate access to healthcare. These laws can promote establishment of healthcare facilities (e.g., by providing funding for community health centers) or restrict formation in areas of overabundance (e.g., by imposing certificate of need requirements for building or expanding hospital facilities). Other laws that affect access address portability of coverage across jurisdictions. For instance, the EU's courts have confirmed the rights of its citizens to obtain healthcare across the borders of member nations. In Canada, portability of coverage is guaranteed by the Canada Health Act. Another way access is guaranteed is through mandates for treatment. In the United States, the Federal Emergency Medical Treatment and Active Labor Act of 1986 (EMTALA) requires that a hospital with an emergency department provide "an appropriate medical screening examination" to any patient who "comes to the emergency department" for examination or treatment. Further, the emergency department (and hospital, in general) must provide ongoing care until the patient's condition is stabilized. It is important to note that the

---

[12]CDC. *Leading causes of death.* Retrieved March 31, 2018 from https://www.cdc.gov/nchs/fastats/leading-causes-of-death.htm

patient's insurance coverage status is not a factor that hospitals can take into consideration in accepting the patient for treatment.[13]

Cell 17. Economic. In countries with both public and private healthcare systems, during times of economic expansion, payers allow patients to receive care at and from nearly any licensed facility and provider. During more challenging economic times, however, payers tend to be more selective about where patients can receive their care. The example that epitomizes this concept is managed care, whereby a select group of primary care physicians will provide and coordinate services for members of such plans. This principle overlaps with the "who provides care" question below.

Cell 18. Social/Cultural. These considerations also have a strong influence on where care is provided. For example, many communities want a local hospital, even though regionalization would make more economic sense with respect to economies of scale. Also, in the United States, health insurers recognize that providing customers with freedom of choice of providers is an extremely important feature in marketing their plans.

Cell 19. Technological. In recent years, there have been two opposite major trends in technology with respect to location. The first has been consolidation to a single site for services to treat highly complex conditions. These sites have been commonly called *centers of excellence.* The simultaneous contrary trend has been a move away from centralized locations to points of care in the community. Technologies ranging from diagnostics to laser treatments have followed this latter pattern. In addressing the issue of where care is provided, one must also understand the extent to which technology *enables* care to be provided at "alternate" sites, such as in the home. A further trend is remote delivery of care, sometimes called *telemedicine.* (More will be said about this service in Chapter 8, "Information Technology.") Examples include consultations using audio and video conferencing over the Internet and robotic surgery performed by an off-site surgeon.

Cell 20. Population Characteristics. With respect to the demographic determinants of where care is provided, one must also address questions about physical access to care. For example, how do health-impaired elderly patients get to regular physician appointments? How are rural populations served when the closest healthcare facility or practitioner may be hours away? What is the role of telemedicine in providing care for the homebound and geographically remote populations?

Who Provides the Services and Products?

Cell 21. Political/Regulatory/Judicial. The first question one must ask in this category is: What are the regulations and laws defining who is allowed to care for patients and to handle and prescribe such products as pharmaceuticals and medical equipment? Related to this question is the matter of the scope of such practitioners; for example, what are nurse practitioners and physician assistants allowed to do vis-à-vis physicians? International

---

[13]CMS.gov Emergency Medical Treatment & Labor Act (EMTALA). Retrieved March 31, 2018 from https://www.cms.gov/Regulations-and-Guidance/Legislation/EMTALA/

examples demonstrate a great variance: The U.S. medical community makes extensive use of nurse practitioners and physician assistants, whereas these professionals are absent from the clinical scene in Japan (except for nurse midwives). Another related question is: Who licenses these professionals? In the United States and Canada, such licensure is conducted by states and provinces, respectively. With increased globalization, there is some pressure to make such licensure transnational. For instance, the European Economic Community Council Directive 93/16/EEC of April 5, 1993 states: "Each Member State shall recognize the diplomas, certificates and other evidence of formal qualifications awarded to nationals of Member States by the other Member States … by giving such qualifications, as far as the right to take up and pursue the activities of a doctor is concerned, the same effect in its territory as those which the Member State itself awards."[14]

Another major question in this category is: How is the supply of practitioners regulated, if at all? As an example, contrast the processes in the United States and Argentina for medical school admission. In the United States, admissions occur after a rigorous screening process; once students are admitted, however, few drop out. In Argentina, any student who can pass basic entrance requirements will be admitted to a public university, where tuition is free; however, the rigorous curriculum leads to a much higher dropout rate than in the United States. Further, the vast majority of medical school graduates in the United States go on to postgraduate residency training, whereas the numbers of such positions in Argentina are severely limited.

A related question is: Who accredits these training programs? In countries with public educational institutions, the government performs this function. In the United States, where most of these schools are in the private sector, a number of accrediting bodies review the quality of training. Ultimately, the U.S. Department of Education is responsible for oversight of these accrediting organizations.

Finally, what is the nature of the laws and regulations governing anticompetitive practices and fee sharing? For example, in some countries, it is perfectly legal and ethical for the referring physician to receive compensation from the specialist for sending patients. In the United States, this practice is considered both illegal and unethical. (This issue, of course, overlaps with the question of how much is paid.)

Cell 22. Economic. One could ask several questions to determine the extent economics influence who provides care. First, how are the fees for services and products determined (i.e., are they set by government regulation, subject to free market factors, or a combination of the two)? The payment structure is important, among other reasons, because it will determine equity between practitioners. For example, are procedural specialists (surgeons) and cognitive specialists (primary care doctors) paid at equal rates for similar services based on such factors as time, risk, and skill? Also, how are nonphysicians (such as nurse practitioners and physician assistants) paid compared to physicians for performing identical services? Finally,

---

[14]Council Directive 93/16/EEC of 5 April 1993 to facilitate the free movement of doctors and the mutual recognition of their diplomas, certificates and other evidence of formal qualifications. Retrieved April 2, 2018 from https://publications .europa.eu/en/publication-detail/-/publication/f211f687-d01e-42e3-b20a-2a224b2feb21/language-en

what is the role of the marketplace in determining the overall numbers of providers and their distribution both geographically and by specialty? In the United States, the marketplace largely determines the answers to these questions. In other countries, however, the government may have a more direct influence.

Cell 23. Social/Cultural. The two principal questions in this category are: How does a society determine and value who is accepted as a "legitimate" provider of care? *and* What are culturally valid treatments? For answers, one must look at who is allowed to provide nontraditional healthcare services in a country and how much of the overall care fits into the category of alternative and complementary medicine. One can also ask if these nontraditional providers and treatments are regulated or if there is any oversight by the government. For example, traditional Chinese medicine is regulated in Singapore, yet many nutritional supplements in the United States are not scrutinized in the same way. Also, how does the society view the integration of traditional and nontraditional practitioners and the services they provide?

Cell 24. Technological. The primary question here is: How do decisions about technology adoption and use affect who provides care? To answer this question, it is important to know who designs the educational content for training providers and who gets to use the technology based on training, licensure, or certification. For example, in some areas, interventional radiologists perform peripheral angioplasties (insertion of a balloon catheter into a blocked artery to restore flow), while in other locations, these procedures would be done by vascular surgeons. One must also know the process through which technologies are adopted, particularly when there is competition for resources. For instance, is the decision made based on population needs, return on investment, or political pressure from an individual or special interest groups?

Cell 25. Population Characteristics. The summary question one must pose here is: How do demographic and epidemiologic characteristics of the population determine who provides the care? Answering this question requires an assessment of where the providers are located, similar to the earlier question regarding *where* the care is provided. One also must look at the demographic characteristics of those who are delivering the care. Finally, the existing and projected population characteristics will determine the needed specialty mixes. For example, the aging population requires more practitioners who perform colonoscopies (gastroenterology), cataract removals (ophthalmology), and other geriatric services. Likewise, if diseases such as HIV/AIDS or other widespread infections occur, practitioners who focus on those conditions will be required.

While all of the above issues should be considered individually and expanded with follow-up questions, you should also consider how multiple categories interact simultaneously to uniquely define a healthcare system. As you read the remainder of this book, keep this defining framework in mind so you can apply principles to the healthcare system(s) you are studying, whether that of the United States or other countries.

Next we will assess how strategic planning can be applied to the above issues and consider how choices about multiple competing priorities simultaneously interact to uniquely define a healthcare system.

STRATEGIC PLANNING

Stakeholders

JAQUES.

> *All the world's a stage,*
> *And all the men and women merely players;*
> *They have their exits and their entrances;*
> *And one man in his time plays many parts.*

> —William Shakespeare, *As You Like It*, Act 2, Scene 7

One of the most important changes in strategic thinking about the healthcare sector is a shift from selling volumes of goods or services to understanding and delivering customer value. In order to understand this shift, we need to consider a few more definitions. With respect to healthcare, the term "customer" refers to those who purchase a product or service after determining that its characteristics meet a need or desire. By comparison, a "consumer" is the one who actually uses the product or service.

A customer may or may not be a consumer. For example, a parent would be the customer for snack food companies while the child might be the consumer. The healthcare setting is more complicated than that of consumer products, so we need to define more terms based on the roles individuals play in certain situations. Consider the following example.

A visiting aunt (aunt = *influencer*) tells the mother that the mother's child looks sick and should be taken to a doctor. The mother (mother = *decider*) takes the child (child = *patient*) to an emergency room where he is evaluated and treated by a physician. The physician decides the child needs medication and sends a prescription to the pharmacy (pharmacy = supplier). The physician and hospital (physician and hospital = providers) request payment from the health insurance company (insurance company = *payer*) to pay for the service that was rendered.

Aside from these direct participants in the scenario, other important participants are involved. For examples: Society as a whole might be interested if the child has a communicable infectious disease; the father may be involved if *his* health insurance is the one covering the child's care; whichever parent's insurance covers the cost, it is likely that insurance comes from an employer; and finally, all the products used to deliver the service (including the prescribed pharmaceutical) are manufactured by different companies. Further, the above designations depend on whose tale is being told. As presented, the story is one of the child receiving care. If, for example, the story were about pharmaceuticals, the decider would be the physician. Given these complex relationships, we need a term that encompasses all those persons and organizations having an interest in such matters as the funding, delivery, product development, and receipt of healthcare services and products. We call all interested parties *stakeholders*.

Following identification of its stakeholders, a healthcare business will inevitably confront conflicting needs and wants. For example, both payers and patients are important stakeholders for pharmaceutical companies and healthcare providers. Just as health plans may impose unreasonable constraints on the delivery of patient care, patients can express unrealistic demands for the provision of medical services and products. Balancing conflicting stakeholder requirements is a constant and difficult challenge.

From country to country, stakeholders vary in such important dimensions as power and scope. For example, in Cuba, physicians are employees of the state-owned and run system. By contrast, in Japan, the Japan Medical Association is a politically powerful organization that includes private practitioners. Given these broad disparities in health system designs, a descriptive model of stakeholders must be appropriately flexible. We can therefore divide stakeholders into three groups. (Please see Exhibit 1.6.)

The first set of stakeholders is individuals and their advocates in the private sector. Included in this group are not only the recipients of care (patients), but also other individuals who have an interest in these patients: family members, legal guardians, close friends, and community members. This category also includes private sector organizations that advocate on behalf of patients with similar characteristics, such as age, disease, or geographic location. For example, the Pediatric AIDS Foundation meets the first two criteria while the latter two criteria describe the American Lung Association of Metropolitan Chicago.

EXHIBIT 1.6. Stakeholders

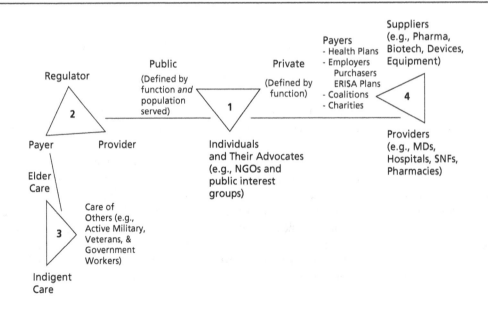

The second stakeholder is the public sector. The public sector acts as a regulator of healthcare products and services (e.g., handling licensure and approval of medical products) and also provides services through such institutions as veteran and county hospitals. The third public function, as payer, is noteworthy because it differentiates programs not only by what they do but for whom they cover healthcare benefits. Even in countries with universal coverage, separate systems of funding and care frequently exist for subcategories of the population, such as the elderly and the poor. Sometimes these categories are combined; for example, the Programa de Asistencia Medica Integral (PAMI) in Argentina covers the elderly and poor. These categories are exemplified in the United States by Medicare, Medicaid, and governmental programs for those who serve it in various capacities (i.e., active military, veterans, or government employees).

The third category of stakeholders is the private sector. *Constituents of the private sector define themselves by what they do.* The traditional division is among payers, providers, and suppliers. Payers include insurance companies, employers (who may self-fund all or part of employee health insurance), unions (the oldest form of health insurance and still the predominant method in Argentina), business associations, and charitable organizations. Pharmaceutical, biotechnology, device, medical supply, and diagnostic companies are significant producers of healthcare products. Providers comprise such categories as physicians, hospitals, nursing homes, pharmacies, and independent diagnostic facilities (e.g., laboratory and radiology).

Stakeholder categories were once fairly distinct. In the past couple of decades, however, there has been an acceleration of cross-category mergers, acquisitions, startups, joint ventures, and outsourcing, so that clear sector definition in many cases is no longer possible. Consider these few examples:

- A group of large hospitals systems decided to start its own generic pharmaceutical company to combat high and rising costs.[15]

- Large provider health systems have been entering the health insurance business so that they now own 52% of such products.[16] At the same time, health insurers are buying providers, including medical groups.[17]

- Health insurers and pharmaceutical companies are partnering to develop drugs for the insurers' customers.[18]

---

[15] Abelson, R., & Thomas, K. (2018, January 18). Fed up with drug companies, hospitals to start their own. A group of large hospital systems plans to create a nonprofit generic drug company to battle shortages and high prices. *New York Times*, B1.

[16] Morse, S. (2016). 25 biggest provider-sponsored health plans include some of the nation's biggest systems. Health system–owned plans now represent 52 percent of health insurance products, AIS said. *Healthcare Finance* (September 13). Retrieved from http://www.healthcarefinancenews.com/news/25-biggest-provider-sponsored-health-plans-includesome-nations-biggest-systems

[17] Abelson, R. (2017). In shift to care delivery, insurer buys doctors unit. *New York Times*, B3 (December 7).

[18] Humana. (2013). Humana and Astellas form research collaboration to improve health care delivery for seniors (February 19). Retrieved from http://press.humana.com/press-release/humana-and-astellas-form-research-collaborationimprove-health-care-delivery-seniors

- A pharmacy company decided to purchase a large health insurer.[19]

- Medicare contracts with private insurers to furnish insurance for one third of its membership.[20]

- In a study of 104 large patient-advocacy organizations, 83% were found to have received financial support from drug, device, and biotechnology companies.[21]

Health System Trade-offs and Value Propositions

Given these diverse and overlapping stakeholders, how can you formulate a strategy to address the needs of one or more of them? In other words, how can you develop a value proposition for your healthcare customers and other interested stakeholders? Before exploring the answer to this question, we must consider one more key term: *strategy*. We highlight three important characteristics of strategy. First, while businesses are often involved in many small, day-to-day decisions, strategy considers approaches to handling *major issues* with which the enterprise must deal now or in the future. Second, strategy involves setting the organizational direction for the medium to long term. These time frames are, of course, relative and vary by firm and industry. Third, useful strategies take into account that short-term decisions *do* need to be made. Strategy, therefore, provides a framework for making those decisions within the context of the organization's long-range goals.[22]

While a number of strategic approaches exist for organizational and industry analysis—for example, SWOT (strength/weakness/opportunity/threat) analysis and Five Forces Analysis[23]—the one used here (please see Exhibit 1.7) provides a useful framework for understanding the healthcare industry.

This model posits that in a Pareto optimal state (explained below), stakeholders' value positions are shaped by choices among Cost, Quality, and Access; any desired changes for one of these elements require changes (trade-offs) in one or both of the others.

Simply stated, for an individual stakeholder in a Pareto optimal state, any change in preferences results in a less desirable value position.[24] In other words, a healthcare stakeholder's overall value preference exists in an equilibrium state. As mentioned above, the implication

[19]de la Merced, M. J., & Abelson, R. (2017). CVS to buy Aetna for $69 billion in a deal that may reshape the health industry. *New York Times*, p. A1 (December 4).

[20]Henry, J. Kaiser Family Foundation. (2017). Medicare advantage enrollees as a percent of total Medicare population. Retrieved from https://www.kff.org/medicare/state-indicator/enrollees-as-a-of-total-medicare-population/?currentTimeframe=0&sortModel=%7B%22colId%22:%22Location%22,%22sort%22:%22asc%22%7D

[21]McCoy, M. S., Carniol, M., Chockley, K., Urwin, J. W., Emanuel, E. J., & Schmidt, H. (2017). Conflicts of interest for patient-advocacy organizations. *The New England Journal of Medicine*, 376, 880–885. Also see Kopp, E., Lupkin, S., & Lucas, E. (2018, April 6). Patient advocacy groups take in millions from drug makers. Is there a payback? *Kaiser Health News*. Retrieved from https://khn.org/news/patient-advocacy-groups-take-in-millions-from-drugmakersis-there-a-payback.

[22]For a good general strategy text, see: Besanko, D., Dranove, D., Shanley, M., & Schaefer, S. (2016). *Economics of strategy*, 7th ed. Hoboken, NJ: Wiley.

[23]Porter, M. (1980). *Competitive strategy*. New York: The Free Press.

[24]A more formal definition is: "... given the availability of information, neither agent's expected utility can be increased without decreasing the expected utility of the other agent." In Harris, M., & Raviv, A. (1978). Some results on incentive contracts with applications to education and employment, health insurance, and law enforcement, *The American Economic Review*, 68(1), 20–30.

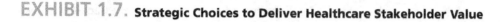

EXHIBIT 1.7. Strategic Choices to Deliver Healthcare Stakeholder Value

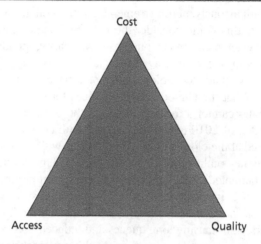

Source: Shalowitz, J. (2008). In P. Kotler, J. Shalowitz, & R. Stevens. *Strategic marketing for health care organizations: Building a customer-driven health system*. San Francisco: Jossey-Bass.

of this equilibrium is that if one wanted to lower cost, increase quality, and/or increase access, a trade-off in one or both other factors must occur. For example, if a stakeholder wants care at a lower cost, quality and/or access would need to be lowered.

The above explanation invites the question: Is it ever possible to improve one or more of these three elements *without* getting a worse overall value proposition? The answer is yes, but to do so requires health system restructuring or innovative technology. When either of these changes occur, a new Pareto optimal state results.

To illustrate this point, consider the portable glucose meter (glucometer) that helps diabetics measure their blood sugars with a finger stick. Blood sugars were originally only measured in hospitals or reference laboratories (freestanding centers where specimens were processed). If a physician saw a patient in the office and suspected diabetes, a blood sample would be drawn and sent to an off-site lab. The results would be available the next day. If the results were abnormal, the patient might be hospitalized for treatment to lower the sugars toward the normal range. During treatment in the hospital, blood could be drawn more frequently with results returning in about an hour rather than a day. Glucometer technology not only allowed faster in-hospital results but moved rapid testing into the physician's office. From there it quickly moved into the hands of patients. Overall, the cost was reduced (fewer hospital stays and lower test cost), the quality was improved (closer glucose monitoring led the potential for better diabetic control), and access was increased (the test can now be performed anywhere). The result of such technology implementation was a new Pareto optimal state. Further technological developments, such as glucose measurement without blood sampling,[25] have the potential to move the state again.

---

[25]Lipani, L., Dupont, B. G. R., Doungmene, F., Marken, F., Tyrrell, R. M., Guy, R. H., & Llie, A. (2018, April 9). Noninvasive, transdermal, path-selective and specific glucose monitoring via a graphene-based platform. *Nature Nanotechnology*. Published online. Retrieved from https://www.nature.com/articles/s41565-018-0112-4

For many years, academicians and policy makers have recognized these trade-offs. However, more often than not, stakeholders are not willing to make choices. They insist on having all three attributes simultaneously, putting tremendous stress on the system and causing periodic crises. To illustrate this point, consider the U.S. healthcare system, which is the most expensive in the world when measured by purchase price parity, spending per capita, and percentage of GDP. Technology is readily available and is not rationed. Further, as mentioned above, when the FDA evaluates technology (e.g., pharmaceuticals), cost is not a factor in the approval decision. What the United States sacrifices for access to this technology is its availability to those who cannot afford it. Although the passage of the Patient Protection and Affordable Care Act of 2010 (ACA) has helped with coverage, 12.2% of the population were still uninsured at the close of 2017.[26] Countries with national health systems, like England, spend less money on healthcare, not only because the service prices are lower but because healthcare is budgeted along with other governmental programs. Also, governmental agencies like the NICE incorporate cost into their analyses of technology approval. In such systems, all citizens are covered by public insurance, but the limited budget constrains the supply of providers, thus causing long queues and reduced access.

If these trade-offs were that easy to explain, healthcare marketing, strategy, and policy would be relatively simple; but each of these three characteristics must be further broken down into their components to fully appreciate them. These defining elements, in turn, can also require trade-offs, thus creating a cascade of interdependent attributes.

The remainder of this chapter will present a unified scheme after all system components have been explained. This scheme should be used as a heuristic device and not a rigid framework. For example, technology, which is presented in the cost section, could as easily be discussed under quality. Further, there is much overlap and many interrelationships among elements of different sections; a true representation would, therefore, appear as a complex web rather than elaborations of three discrete branches.

Cost. We will start by examining cost. (Please see Exhibit 1.8.) The word "cost" means different things to different people. Accountants often define the term as the *average* expenditure required to produce one unit of output (a good or service). Economists frequently refer to marginal costs, the resources required to produce *the next* unit of output. This latter concept leads to some unusual statements, such as: "The true costs of nonurgent care in the emergency department are relatively low."[27] There are other reasons for confusion over what we mean by the true cost of healthcare. For example, a provider lists an artificially high *charge* for a particular service; however, the *negotiated price* an insurance company pays is much lower. Further, the insurer will pay only a *portion* of the negotiated price determined by the contract with the purchaser of the insurance policy; the remainder of the bill is the patient's responsibility. To simplify the cost definition, in this book "cost" means *an actual payment* made by a specified stakeholder for a good or service.

---

[26] Auter, Z. (2018, January 16). U.S. uninsured rate steady at 12.2% in fourth quarter of 2017. *Gallup Well-Being.* Retrieved from http://news.gallup.com/poll/225383/uninsured-rate-steady-fourth-quarter-2017.aspx

[27] Williams, R. M. (1996). The costs of visits to emergency departments. *The New England Journal of Medicine, 334,* 642–646.

EXHIBIT 1.8. Components of Cost

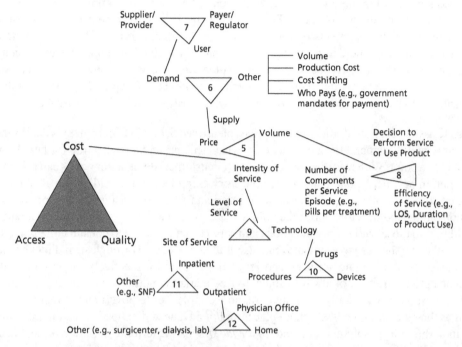

Source: Shalowitz, J. (2008). In P. Kotler, J. Shalowitz, & R. Stevens. *Strategic marketing for health care organizations: Building a customer-driven health system*. San Francisco: Jossey-Bass.

The total cost of products or services are governed by the following relationship:

$$Cost = f(P, V, I)$$

where P = price of the service or product; V = volume or number of units; and I = intensity of service or product.

Two brief examples will illustrate the use of this formula.

- Each year, national pharmaceutical expenditures are announced and increases are attributed to three categories: increase in prices of existing drugs (Price), increase in use of existing medications (Volume), and introduction of new products or technologies (Intensity).

- On a more micro level, the total cost of a hospitalization for a patient can be broken down into: level of care, e.g., intensive care unit versus a bed on a regular medical/surgical floor (Intensity); number of days (Volume); and price per day at different levels of care (Price).

Understanding these components can lead to important insights not only for making strategic decisions but also for public policy. Theoretically, one can attempt to check high costs by tackling any or all of these elements; however, addressing one without also confronting the other two is futile. For example, the U.S. government has been dealing with rising physician payments by lowering the fees for their services. Doctors respond by increasing volume or, more importantly, by increasing the technology applied to care, such as using newer, more expensive medications when older ones are as effective. More will be said about this issue when provider-induced demand is discussed in Chapter 2, "Determinants of Utilization of Healthcare Services." We will now deconstruct each of these three elements.

Price. Classical economics dictates that price (please see 5, 6, 7 in Exhibit 1.8) is determined by supply and/or demand for a product or service. This principle is also true for healthcare, but only to a point. With regard to *demand*, user (or customer) demand for goods can influence price but, in healthcare, that is not the whole story. Suppliers and providers can also manipulate customer demand by such measures as physician-requested visits. Recall from the discussion on stakeholders that one of the unique features of healthcare is the presence of parties in addition to those who supply the goods and services and those who consume them. Payers and regulators (such as governments) can also influence demand through such direct or indirect measures as rationing services and regulating pricing, respectively. *Supply* may also influence price, but it is not always subject to free market conditions. For instance, in many countries, supply is centrally regulated. As an example, some governments regulate such items as the number of medical school places and/or advanced diagnostic imaging machines.

In addition to supply and demand, *other factors* also determine the price of healthcare goods. At least four of these other factors are involved in determining prices.

1. *Volume.* As in other fields, volume discounts are often available. But lower costs with volume should also come with experience (so-called learning curve). In many cases, however, healthcare prices do not display this experience-related price deduction. For example, coronary artery bypass surgery prices have not decreased commensurate with the experience and standardization of the technology.

2. Prices are often linked to *production costs*. An example from the governmental domain (Medicare) illustrates this point. The federal government determines physician prices based on computation of practice costs and the work that goes into providing the service. This method is called a RBRVS, about which more will be said later.

3. Prices often have nothing to do with the good itself but with *other items* consumed in the same setting. For example, one hears about such hospital charges as the $5 aspirin. Obviously, the aspirin's cost is nowhere near that amount, but other hospital services are often paid below production cost. The hospital therefore cross-subsidizes its products and services in a practice called *cost shifting*. Some of these services are "loss leaders," like maternity care. Other services are truly underpaid, but the hospital must offer them in order to fulfill its mission of providing comprehensive care to the community. In addition to this "internal" cost shifting, "external" cost shifting also occurs in the form

of charging some payers more than others for the same products or services to make up for lower payments. For example, private insurance payments are almost always more than Medicare payments, which in turn are more than Medicaid payments.

4. *"Who pays"* can greatly influence the price, regardless of supply or demand for the good. This category reflects "buyer power" as well as "non-market" forces. For example, Medicare has set its reimbursement for injectable pharmaceuticals at 6% over "average sales price (ASP)" and in-patient hospital payments based on the patient's diagnosis (DRG). Providers cannot negotiate these rates, and Medicare is such an important payer that providers do not turn away these beneficiaries.

Volume. We now turn to the *volume* input of cost. (Please see 5 and 8 in Exhibit 1.8.) Determinants of volume can be divided into three components. The first portion of volume concerns the decision about whether to use a product or deliver/receive a service. While this notion seems simple, much debate has occurred over a variety of related issues in healthcare, prompting questions such as: Is the comprehensive "annual physical" really necessary for all adults? When is "watchful waiting" better than aggressive treatment?; and Are particular screening tests worthwhile?

An important related question is: Once experts agree that action is generally indicated (an exam must be performed, a test ordered, and/or treatment administered), which among the options is the best choice? Obviously, choosing *one* may mean the other actions do not occur. For example, assume a patient has blockages in the coronary (heart) arteries that require invasive intervention. Is the appropriate action stenting or coronary artery bypass graft surgery (CABG)? Although the answer depends on the extent of the blockages, where they occur, and how many arteries are involved, experts may not always agree on the best method for treating individual patients.

These issues only deal with professional decisions. Patients and other stakeholders also determine whether actions are taken or not. For example, patients often pressure physicians for antibiotics for viral infections, when none are needed. Public policies also may determine whether something is done or not. For instance, in the past, England's National Health Service did not pay for hemodialysis for persons over age 55.

Once the decision has been made to act, two further inputs will determine the overall volume. The first is the efficiency of its execution. For example, once the patient and physician agree that surgery is an appropriate option, how long is the patient to remain in the hospital and how many resources are used for that episode of care? The second issue is the necessary number of units of care once a specific action is chosen. For example, there are various antibiotic regimens for treatment of certain bacterial infections, ranging from 30 pills (1 pill three times a day of amoxicillin) to one dose of a liquid (ZMAX® form of the antibiotic azithromycin).

Intensity of Service. The third determinant of cost is the *intensity of service*. (Please see 5, 9, 10, 11, 12 in Exhibit 1.8.) The first part of intensity is *level of service*. For example, does a hospitalized patient require intensive care or is a regular medical/surgical bed sufficient?

Another illustration of this point is choice of antibiotics. Does a patient require a short course of oral medication or prolonged intravenous treatment?

Intensity of service also comprises use of medical *technology*, which consists of drugs, devices, and procedures. Sometimes these modalities are used in combination, while at other times they are substitutes for one another. For instance, different preferred treatments exist for diverse heartbeat irregularities. Some are best treated by medication; others should be cared for by devices (implantable defibrillators or pacemakers); still others require surgery (where the source of the rhythm disturbance is surgically ablated). Each of these different technologies carries its own cost.

Finally, the *site of service* is an important determinant of intensity and, hence, cost. Sites of care can be divided into institutional and noninstitutional settings. In the former category, hospitals come to mind first. We refer to the acute care hospital setting as "inpatient" care. Other institutional settings consist of skilled nursing facilities (sometimes just called SNFs) or long-term care settings, such as chronic ventilator facilities or long-term care centers. We refer to noninstitutional sites as "outpatient" care. Common sites are the physician's office, the patient's home (with varying degrees of skilled home healthcare), and various other locations for freestanding diagnostic and therapeutic services. In this latter category, we include same-day (ambulatory) surgery (whether at a hospital or freestanding surgicenter), dialysis facility, diagnostic laboratory, radiology facility, and physical therapy setting.

The different types of sites can be substitutes for one another or appropriate sequential choices. For example, an elderly patient should be hospitalized for repair of a hip fracture. After this treatment, she may recuperate and receive physical therapy in an SNF and then be sent home with appropriate services there. On the other hand, the majority of surgical procedures are now performed on a same-day basis, substituting for inpatient treatment. Further, as mentioned above, many diagnostic and therapeutic technologies are moving from centralized medical centers to outpatient points of care. For example, many tests that were formerly only done in a hospital laboratory can now be performed with the same quality in physicians' offices.

Quality. Since the subject of quality will be discussed in a separate chapter, just an outline will be presented here. (Please see Exhibit 1.9.) The dimensions of quality can be divided into the amenities, service aspects, and technical components. To illustrate and contrast these elements, consider a hospital stay.

- The *amenities* may consist of the items that form a first impression about the facility (e.g., building style, landscaping, and ease and cost of parking). While the marketing implications of these items are clear, these features bear no relation to the actual desired outcome (e.g., success of a surgical procedure).

- The *service* aspects come closer to affecting outcomes. To continue our example, inpatient service may consist of meals, how quickly personnel respond to patient requests, and housekeeping services. While these functions support the actual business of delivering care and can more strongly influence opinions about the institution than the amenities, they are not part of the core activities in delivering treatment.

EXHIBIT 1.9. Components of Quality

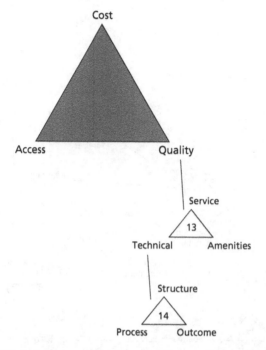

Source: Shalowitz, J. (2008). In P. Kotler, J. Shalowitz, & R. Stevens. *Strategic marketing for health care organizations: Building a customer-driven health system*. San Francisco: Jossey-Bass.

- The *technical* aspect is the work that is done that most directly affects outcomes. Examples of such activities are expertly performed surgery, choice of appropriate medication, and skillfully administered nursing care.

The technical component can be further divided into structure, process, and outcome. *Structure* refers to those items that are either present or absent and usually easy to measure. Examples include certification of specialists, presence of a piece of equipment, or adequate width of a doorway to accommodate a hospital bed. The meanings of process and outcome measures are self-explanatory.

Access and Equity. The third part of this strategic trade-off derives from a business model that can provide timely care of needed services and products. (Please see Exhibit 1.10.)

Availability. The first question regarding access/equity is whether certain resources are available. (Please see 15, 16, 17, 18 in Exhibit 1.10.) Availability can be assessed by answering the questions posed in 16 of Exhibit 1.10, starting with the question: *Who?* To expand on this

EXHIBIT 1.10. Components of Access/Equity

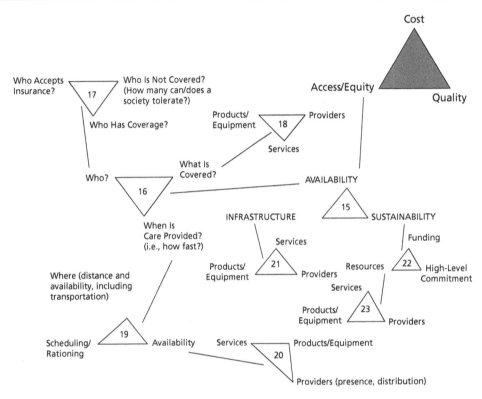

Source: Shalowitz, J. (2008). In P. Kotler, J. Shalowitz, & R. Stevens. *Strategic marketing for health care organizations: Building a customer-driven health system*. San Francisco: Jossey-Bass.

inquiry, we can ask: Who has health insurance coverage and who does not? These two issues, while apparently different sides of the same coin, address different strategic purposes. As an example of the former question, a pharmaceutical company will target the insured population for sales of a new product. The latter issue raises the question: How many uninsured people can a society accept? In virtually all countries except the United States, the answer to this question is *none*.

The third aspect of this dimension concerns who will accept the patient's insurance. For example, in the United States, the joint federal-state program for the poor and other select populations (Medicaid) ensures that eligible persons have at least a modicum of health insurance coverage. Unfortunately, this program often pays physicians so little and so late (9 months in accounts receivable aging is not unusual) that few may choose to see

Medicaid-insured patients. Also, not every commercial insurance plan will contract with every provider; patients must then seek those practitioners and institutions with whom their insurance companies contract in order to expect maximum payment for care.

"*What* is covered?" is the next question that defines availability. (Please see 18 in Exhibit 1.10.) Even though an individual has insurance, not all services, products/equipment, or providers are covered. As an example, most insurance plans in the United States do not pay for strictly cosmetic procedures.

The third aspect of availability is *when* care is able to be provided. (Please see 19 and 20 in Exhibit 1.10.) *When* care can be provided depends on whether services, providers, and products exist and/or are close enough to patients to be useful. In some developing countries, some technologies and practitioners skilled in their use may not exist. If the technologies do exist, where they are located is extremely important. The same conditions can also exist in urban centers. For example, making free prenatal care available to inner-city women is a pointless gesture unless they have an affordable and easy way to get to these services. Finally, even if healthcare is close and easy to reach, some services are in short supply so they are explicitly or implicitly rationed. Queues in the United Kingdom for certain services are examples of this problem.

Infrastructure. In addition to availability, the two other dimensions of access we must consider are *infrastructure* (please see 21 in Exhibit 1.10) and *sustainability*. These two topics are of particular concern for developing countries as well as rural and inner-city populations in developed nations. While thinking about infrastructure can raise similar questions as the "where" and "availability" themes, this topic refers more to the *supporting roles* played by services, providers, and products/equipment rather than the primary activity or product. For example, think about a program to deliver immunizations to children in rural locations in a developing country. Assume that a pharmaceutical company donates the supplies and healthcare practitioners volunteer time to administer injections. The infrastructure dimension of this program includes not only the traditional items, such as roads to get to needy populations, but also medical support services, such as an information system that logs and tracks who received the shots and when they are due for booster immunizations.

Another example concerns HIV/AIDS. Supplying medication is necessary but not sufficient to successful treatment programs. The infrastructure must also include healthcare personnel who make sure patients take the medication as prescribed and are available for support when side effects inevitably arise.

Wealthy nations also have infrastructure problems. Consider the following examples:

- A hospital advertises an innovative program, only to find it cannot accommodate the volume of phone calls or schedule the service in a timely fashion.
- Shortly after a pharmaceutical company gets approval to market a new "blockbuster" drug, its production plants cannot keep up with demand; in the meantime, a competitor releases a substitute and garners significant market share.

▩ A producer of unique diagnostic equipment experiences quality problems in its factory that cause a lengthy cessation of manufacturing, reduced revenue, and a plummeting stock price.

Sustainability. Contemplating the infrastructure problem naturally gives rise to consideration of *sustainability*. (Please see 22 and 23 in Exhibit 1.10.) Experts often use the metaphor that affecting lasting change in the healthcare arena is more like a marathon than a sprint. Sustainability starts with high-level commitment by appropriately empowered authorities. (While grassroots activities are worthwhile, their purpose is often to convince decision makers to act in the first place.) Funding is also critical. Institutions are often reluctant to accept large donations for buildings or equipment because of the anticipated (and unfunded) ongoing maintenance costs. Finally, decision makers and funders must commit appropriate resources for the long run. These resources must not only exist for episodic interventions but provide continuity.

Putting It All Together

In combining all these concepts, a few further considerations emerge. First, consider that each stakeholder has different preferences among the cost/quality/access dimensions *depending on a given issue*. When two or more stakeholders are involved in a strategic decision (as is almost always the case), conflicts often arise. The initial strategic choices you will need to make will, therefore, require answers to these questions:

Who are your stakeholders?

What is their relative importance to you given . . .

a) The specific issue/product under consideration (short-term view)?

b) The overall relationship (long-term view)?

What are your stakeholders' value propositions?

Who are your stakeholders' key stakeholders?

How can you help *your* key stakeholders deliver value to *their* key stakeholders?

How do your stakeholders prioritize your importance to *them*? (This question is asked last, since successfully acting on answers to the ones above will affect your importance.)

Another significant consideration is that when any one element in Exhibit 1.11 changes, it can have far-reaching effects on the entire system. For example, assume a state government lowers payment rates for physicians caring for Medicaid patients. How will that action affect the availability of physicians willing to care for those patients? As another example, consider a new diagnostic technology that can be used in the physician's office at the time of a patient's visit, providing quicker results. What are the implications of this test on volume, and hence cost, versus patient satisfaction?

EXHIBIT 1.11. Comprehensive View of Stakeholder Value Proposition Components

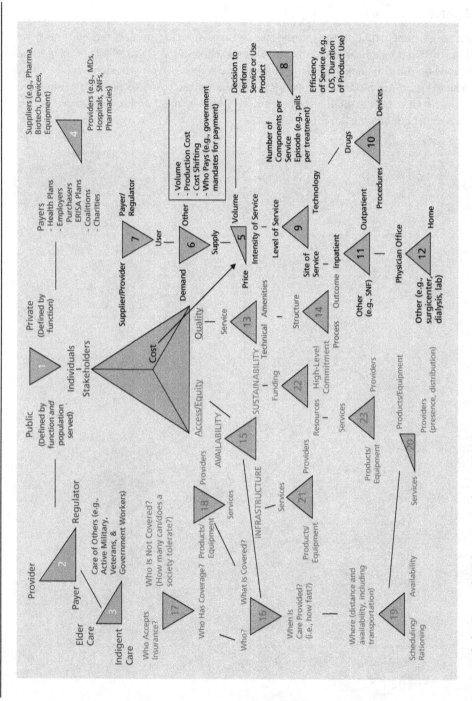

Source: Shalowitz, J. (2008). In P. Kotler, J. Shalowitz, & R. Stevens. *Strategic marketing for health care organizations: Building a customer-driven health system*. San Francisco: Jossey-Bass.

SUMMARY

This chapter presents some initial definitions and two working models that will help you understand different healthcare systems, relevant stakeholders, and the effects of their strategic decisions on other elements of the healthcare marketplace. You are encouraged to think about how to use these models in your sector of the industry and to practice using them, especially when it comes to challenging technology management and pricing decisions that are discussed in later chapters in this book.

CHAPTER

2

DETERMINANTS OF UTILIZATION OF HEALTHCARE SERVICES

Cassius.

> *The fault, dear Brutus, is not in our stars*
> *But in ourselves, that we are underlings.*

—William Shakespeare, *Julius Caesar*, Act 1, Scene 3

Given the frameworks of the previous chapter, it is now important for us to address the question: Why do people seek healthcare services and products? The answers to this question will help a firm to segment its market and allow development of better targeted services and products. The focus here will be on four types of segmentation, any or all of which can be used: all-stakeholder preferences for care, patients' personal characteristics, patient consumer behavior, and provider-induced demand.

REASONS STAKEHOLDERS SEEK HEALTHCARE

Consider the stakeholders mentioned in the previous chapter and the circumstances in which they might recommend or seek care. (Please see Exhibit 2.1.) Some examples in these categories are explained below.

The first obvious reasons to seek care are for known illnesses (either acute or chronic), accidents, or injuries. All of the stakeholders in Exhibit 2.1 have an interest in these motivations. While patients and those close to them obviously request services and products in this category, an employer also wants the patient (in this case, the employee) to return to work as soon as possible and reduce healthcare costs. The government's interest is represented by such federal agencies as the Food and Drug Administration (FDA), Centers for Disease

EXHIBIT 2.1. **Reasons Stakeholder Seek and Influence Care Decisions**

Stakeholder Reason	Patient	Family/ Partner	Friends	Employer	Public Health/ Safety	Insurance Company	Suppliers
Illness/Accident/Injury	X	X	X	X	X	X	X
Symptom	X	X	X	X	X		X
Prevention/"Checkup"	X	X	X	X	X	X	X
Second opinion	X	X	X	X		X	
Legal	X	X	X	X	X	X	X
Administrative	X			X	X	X	X
Discretionary	X	X	X				X

Control and Prevention (CDC), Occupational Safety and Health Administration (OSHA), and Environmental Protection Agency (EPA) as well as state and local public health departments. These agencies and departments are charged with the oversight and preservation of public health and safety and can request or require that an individual be treated. An example of this latter case is when an infection (such as tuberculosis or a sexually transmitted disease) may affect the public's health. Insurance companies have a significant financial stake in a patient seeking acute or chronic care, ranging from preventing unnecessary services to making sure timely and appropriate services are provided. Further, private and public insurers are now reminding patients to seek assistance to obtain preventive services, such as immunizations and screening for breast, colon, and cervical cancers. Finally, suppliers, particularly pharmaceutical companies, encourage patients to seek care for a variety of known diseases and symptoms. This encouragement may occur through such measures as public service announcements, sponsorship of health fairs, or direct-to-consumer (DTC) advertising.

The stakeholder concerns are the same for symptoms and preventive services, except insurance companies usually do not encourage individuals to seek care for specific *symptoms*. In this category, for example, the CDC may encourage patients with a high fever and cough to seek medical care during influenza season. Suppliers, such as those offering diagnostic tests, and pharmaceutical companies that manufacture vaccines are particularly interested in encouraging preventive services. The difference between suppliers and insurance companies with respect to symptoms is that the former may encourage use of their products (particularly by prescription) for self-limited conditions while the latter would prefer patients pay for over-the-counter remedies.

As far as second opinions are concerned, patients and those in their support network often want additional viewpoints about diagnoses and treatment recommendations. Insurance companies may request or require that a patient receive a confirmatory exam to avoid unnecessary care, such as surgery. Employers often require employees to obtain second opinions regarding the nature and treatment of work-related injuries and for return to work and functional expectations.

Legal reasons for seeking care can involve all stakeholders. Patients and those who are interested in them may believe they were physically or mentally harmed in some negligent fashion and initiate an encounter to verify or confirm this impression. Employers, governmental agencies, and insurance companies may initiate exams to determine disability payments. On the other side of the liability issue (i.e., the defendant side), stakeholders such as pharmaceutical companies may require exams to assess legal responsibility for damages.

Patients may be required to seek care for such administrative reasons as pre-employment physicals, documentation of immunization or treatment (this reason overlaps with some of those above), and for obtaining life and disability insurance. Of note is that since enactment of the Affordable Care Act (ACA), exams to determine eligibility for health insurance are no longer legal. Supplier interest is, for example, due to the requirement by pharmaceutical companies that certain patients must have specialist exams and/or certain tests to be eligible to receive medications (either FDA approved or experimental).

The discretionary category includes services that, strictly speaking, have little to do with health as we defined it in Chapter 1, "Understanding and Managing Complex Healthcare Systems." Services included in this category are procedures like cosmetic surgery. Products that may fall into this category comprise so-called lifestyle medications (such as those for erectile dysfunction and baldness). On an international perspective, a given country's culture will determine what is included in this category. For example, as mentioned in Chapter 1, until relatively recently, spa care was covered by the sickness funds in Germany. Such a benefit is unlikely to become standard in the United States. Individuals and concerned parties are obviously interested in these discretionary services, particularly when they have disposable income. Suppliers are eager to sell nonessential products or services by aggressively promoting their use via DTC advertising.

The strategic marketing lesson from this approach is: classify the type of service involved, understand the reason the patient is seeking care (e.g., self-motivated or required by a third party), and identify the relevant stakeholders.

PATIENT CHARACTERISTICS THAT INFLUENCE CARE-SEEKING

Given these reasons for requesting care and the role of relevant stakeholders, we must next ask about the *personal* characteristics that influence an individual's care-seeking behavior as well as his or her health status. A general overview of this topic is provided below. (Please see Exhibit 2.2 for some important personal characteristics that affect utilization of healthcare services.) Differences in health status due to these factors are called *health disparities*.[1]

EXHIBIT 2.2. **Personal Characteristics That Influence Care-Seeking Behavior and Health Status**

- Age
- Gender/sex
- Race
- Income
- Social status
- Education
- Culture/beliefs

[1] HealthyPeople.gov: "A health disparity is a health difference that is closely linked with social, economic, or environmental disadvantage." This website has much information comparing health disparities based on such factors as sex, age and race. Retrieved April 14, 2018, *from* www.healthypeople.gov

While general correlations exist between these attributes and utilization, you should be aware that correlation does not prove causation.

Age

With respect to age, across most countries, children (particularly those from birth to 2 years), women of child-bearing age, and the elderly use the most healthcare. Some of these relationships are displayed in Exhibit 2.3.

Age is also a factor for utilization of *specific* services. For example, "significant age-related disparities appear to exist for both evidence-based and non-evidence-based cancer-screening interventions."[2] Some differences in utilization of services and products are displayed in Exhibits 2.4 and 2.5.

Gender/Sex

A person's *sex* is a biological designation based on genetics at birth. *Gender* indicates a personally preferred societal role. The difference between men and women regarding utilization of healthcare is also displayed in Exhibit 2.3. Note that in every age category

EXHIBIT 2.3. **Total Personal Healthcare Spending (millions) by Gender and Age Group 2012**

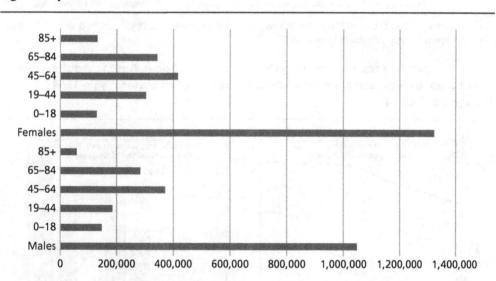

Source: CMS.gov, National Health Expenditure Data. Retrieved April 14, 2018 from https://www.cms .gov/Research-Statistics-Data-and-Systems/Statistics-Trends-and-Reports/NationalHealthExpendData/ Age-and-Gender.html

---

[2]Jerant, A. F., Erickson, J. E., & Doescher, M. P. (2004). Age-related disparities in cancer screening: Analysis of 2001 behavioral risk factor surveillance system Data. *Annals of Family Medicine*, 2, 481–487.

EXHIBIT 2.4. **Healthcare Visits in the Past 12 Months Among Children Aged 2–17 and Adults Aged 18 and Over, by Age and Provider Type: United States, 1997, 2006, and 2015**

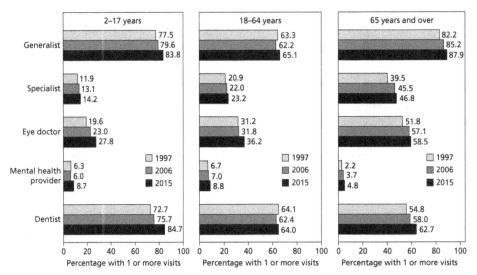

Source: Health, United States, 2016 NCHS, National Health Interview Survey. Retrieved April 14, 2018 from https://www.cdc.gov/nchs/data/hus/hus16.pdf

EXHIBIT 2.5. **Prescription Drug Use in the Past 30 days Among Adults Aged 18 and Over, by Age and Number of Drugs Taken: United States, 1988–1994 Through 2013–2014**

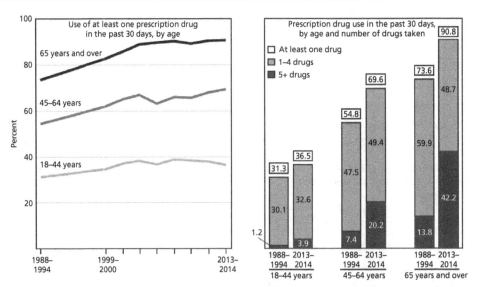

Source: Health, United States, 2016 NCHS, National Health Interview Survey. Retrieved April 14, 2018 from https://www.cdc.gov/nchs/data/hus/hus16.pdf

except childhood, women use healthcare more than men. Not only do men and women differ in their health-seeking behaviors, but providers order non–reproductive system–based services at different rates for the sexes. These differentials can be either beneficial or harmful, depending on the intervention studied. For example, women tend to be underdiagnosed concerning cardiovascular disease.[3] This category is only one of many where disparities for women lead to lower-quality care. With respect to cardiovascular disease, behavioral health, and access to care, "It is of concern that 83% of the measures showed a persistent disparity over time between men and women."[4]

One very important factor that cannot be inferred from these statistics is *the central role of women as the healthcare decision makers, not only for themselves but also their families.* This responsibility has critical marketing implications—from making sure mothers in developing countries know which products to use to treat childhood diarrhea (a leading cause of death) to persuading women in developed nations to direct their family's healthcare needs to a particular hospital or request a brand of medication. Recall the differences between customers and consumers explained in Chapter 1.

Race

When considering differences due to race, one must be aware of several caveats. First, race is a difficult category to define. Often people of mixed backgrounds identify with only one race, thus confounding studies that rely on self-reporting. Second, many findings associated with racial differences can be explained on the basis of socioeconomics or education (two other, independent, determinants of healthcare usage). For example, a study of adult preventive dental care showed that racial disparities among whites, African Americans, and Mexican Americans were "no longer significant when enabling resource variables are included in the model (income level, insurance, census region, and metropolitan statistical area)."[5] Third, the reason for racial disparities may be differences in *provider* care patterns. For example, a "study of a large, hospital-based sample suggests that modest racial differences in receipt of recommended breast cancer care persist even after adjustment for insurance and area-level SES [socioeconomic status]."[6]

Finally, as is probably obvious, one should not assume uniformity within any racial/ethnic group. An illustration of this principle in health-seeking behavior is the finding of

[3]Mehta, L. S., Beckie, T. M., DeVon, H. A., Grines, C. L., Krumholz, H. M., Johnson, M. N., … Wenger, N. K. (2016). Acute myocardial infarction in women. A scientific statement from the American Heart Association. *Circulation*, *133*, 916–947.

[4]Moore, J. E., Mompe, A., & Moy, E. (2018). Disparities by sex tracked in the 2015 National Healthcare Quality and Disparities Report: Trends across National Quality Strategy Priorities, Health Conditions, and Access Measures. *Women's Health Issues*, 28(1), 97–103. Retrieved from http://www.whijournal.com/article/S1049-3867(17)30043-9/pdf

[5]Doty, H. E., & Weech-Maldonado, R. (2003). Racial/ethnic disparities in adult preventive dental care use. *Journal of Health Care for the Poor and Underserved*, *14*, 516–534.

[6]Freedman, R. A., Virgo, K. S., He, Y., Pavluck, A. L., Winer, E. P., Ward, E. M., & Keating, N. L. (2011). The association of race/ethnicity, insurance status, and socioeconomic factors with breast cancer care. *Cancer*, *117*(1), 180–189.

variations among adolescents of different Latino origins with respect to frequency and reasons for obtaining routine physical examinations. For example, Cuban-origin adolescents in a single-parent household were *more* likely to get such an exam, while for those of Central/South American or Dominican background, the likelihood depended on higher income and having insurance.[7] These principles highlight the need to research the appropriate market segments for a product or service.

Despite these caveats, some overall differences can clearly be seen, one of which is life expectancies. (Please see Exhibit 2.6.)

EXHIBIT 2.6. **U.S. Life Expectancy, by Race, Hispanic Origin, and Sex: 2006–2015**

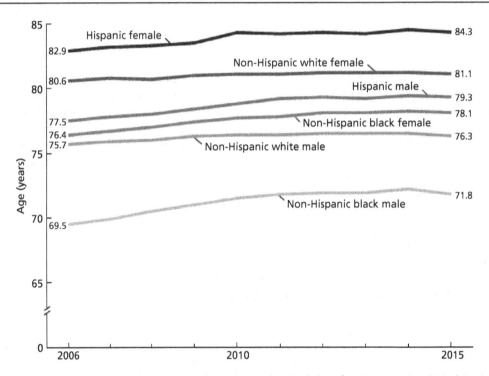

Source: Murphy, S. L., et al. (2017, November 27). Deaths: Final data for 2015. *National Vital Statistics Reports, 66*(6). Retrieved April 17, 2018 from https://www.cdc.gov/nchs/data/nvsr/nvsr66/nvsr66_06.pdf

---

[7] Sarmiento, O. L. (2004). Disparities in routine physical examinations among in-school adolescents of differing Latino origins. *Journal of Adolescent Health, 35*, 310–320.

Income

Income obviously affects use of healthcare products and services, a finding that exists across developed countries. For example: "In most countries, for the same health care needs, people with higher incomes are more likely to consult a doctor than those with lower incomes. Pro-rich inequalities in dental visits and cancer screening uptake are also found in nearly all countries, although the magnitude of these varies."[8]

Differences in use of professionals also vary by income strata. For example, specialist services "seem to be underused by lower socioeconomic groups."[9] Some international examples of income-related utilization are summarized in Exhibit 2.7. Note that this association has been recognized for a number of years.

EXHIBIT 2.7. Income and Healthcare Utilization—Some International Examples

- "Socioeconomic differences in utilization were present for all services [in the Netherlands] after we controlled for age, sex, and marital status."[a]

- "Although financial barriers may not directly impede access to healthcare services in Canada, differential use of physician services with respect to socio-economic status persists."[b]

- "Lower socio-economic groups [in Belgium] make more often use of the general practitioner and nursing care at home and are more often admitted to hospital than persons with a high socio-economic status. There is, however, no socio-economic gradient when the health status is taken into account. On the opposite, persons with higher socio-economic status report more often a visit to a specialist, a physiotherapist or a dentist."[c]

- "Women [in Britain] whose households were in the lowest income category were more likely to report back pain than those in the highest income group."[d]

[a] Van der Meer, J. B. W., van den Bos, J., &. Mackenbach, J. P. (1996). Socioeconomic differences in the utilization of health services in a Dutch population: The contribution of health status. *Health Policy, 37,* 1–18.
[b] Dunlop, S., Coyte, P. P., & McIsaac, W. (2000). Socio-economic status and the utilisation of physicians' services: Results from the Canadian National Population Health Survey. *Science & Medicine, 51,* 123–133.
[c] Van der Heyden, J. H. A., et al. (2003). Socio-economic differences in the utilisation of health services in Belgium. *Health Policy, 65,* 153–165.
[d] Croft, R., & Rigby, A. S. (1994). Socioeconomic influences on back problems in the community in Britain. *Journal of Epidemiology and Community Health, 48,* 166–170.

---

[8] Devaux, M. (2015). Income-related inequalities and inequities in health care services utilisation in 18 selected OECD countries. *European Journal of Health Economics, 16,* 21–33. Retrieved from https://link.springer.com/content/pdf/10.1007%2Fs10198-013-0546-4.pdf
[9] Veugelers, P. J., & Yip, A. M. (2003). Socioeconomic disparities in health care use: Does universal coverage reduce inequalities in health? *Journal of Epidemiology and Community Health, 57*(6). Retrieved from http://jech.bmj.com/content/57/6/424#ref-6

Social Status

While the term "socioeconomic status" is often used interchangeably with "income," it is also used as a synonym for "social status." Social status is defined as

> the relative rank that an individual holds ... in a social hierarchy based upon honor or prestige. Status may be ascribed—that is, assigned to individuals at birth without reference to any innate abilities—or achieved, requiring special qualities and gained through competition and individual effort. Ascribed status is typically based on sex, age, race, family relationships, or birth, while achieved status may be based on education, occupation, marital status, accomplishments, or other factors.
>
> The word *status* implies social stratification on a vertical scale. People may be said to occupy high positions when they are able to control, by order or by influence, other people's conduct; when they derive prestige from holding important offices; or when their conduct is esteemed by others. Relative status is a major factor in determining the way people behave toward each other.
>
> One's status tends to vary with social context.[10]

The most extensive analyses of the effects of status on health outcomes started in 1967, in what were subsequently called the Whitehall Studies (I and II). This research looked at health differences among members of different job grades of British civil servants. Starting in the 1980s, Sir Michael Marmot, the lead investigator, began publishing mortality difference results in this population. Among the most striking findings: "Compared with the highest grade (administrators), men in the lowest grade had three times the mortality rate from coronary heart disease, from a range of other causes, and from all causes combined."[11] This disparity persisted when adjusted for adverse health behaviors (such as smoking) that were more prevalent in the lower-grade employees. The follow-up (Whitehall II) study concluded that the reasons for these differences were higher job stress, lower degree of control, and higher pace of activities.[12] To summarize, Fitzpatrick noted that "accumulating evidence suggests that ... social status itself, regardless of associated material and economic advantages, may confer health benefits."[13]

Additionally, evidence has emerged that the *magnitude* of relative differences is also the source of stress that affects health status. One of these measures is *income inequality*,

[10]"Social Status," in Encyclopedia Britannica. Retrieved April 17, 2018, from https://www.britannica.com/topic/social-status

[11]Marmot, M., Shipley, M. J., & Rose, G. (1984). Inequalities in death—specific explanations of a general pattern? *The Lancet, 323*(8384), 1003–1006.

[12]See, for example, Bosma, H., Marmot, M. G., Hemingway, H., Nicholson A. C., Brunner E., & Stansfeld S. A. (1997). Low job control and risk of coronary heart disease in Whitehall II (prospective cohort) study. *British Medical Journal, 314*, 558; see also Kuper, H., & Marmot, M. (2003). Job strain, job demands, decision latitude, and risk of coronary heart disease within the Whitehall II study. *Journal of Epidemiology and Community Health, 57*(2) (February). Retrieved from http://jech.bmj.com/content/57/2/147

[13]Fitzpatrick, R. (2001). Social status and mortality. *Annals of Internal Medicine, 134*(10), 1001–1003.

defined as "the ratio of household income at the 80th percentile to that at the 20th percentile."[14] Higher levels of this inequality cause social stress that results in increased risk of mortality and poor health. As Sanger-Katz summarized, the literature on this subject suggests

> that it's stressful to live among people who are wealthier than you. That stress may translate into mental health problems or cardiac disease for lower-income residents of unequal places ... For every one-point increase in the ratio between high and low earners in a county, there were about five years lost for every 1,000 people. That's about the same difference they observed when a community's smoking rate increased by 4 percent or its obesity rate rose by 3 percent.[15]

Education

Apart from healthcare knowledge, education level attainment is also an independent determinant of use and health status.[16] (Please see Exhibit 2.8 for some international examples.)

In the United States as well: "People with fewer years of education have worse health than those with more education—even when they have the same access to health care ... And it's not true just for self-reports of problems—it's also true for verifiable health outcomes, like mortality."[17]

Lack of healthcare knowledge, which includes insurance terms, can also be harmful. Just after the start of the ACA in 2014, it became clear that people did not know how to make appropriate choices of insurance plans. As Garcia noted:

> An estimated 14 percent of English-speaking adults in the United States have below-basic literacy, or an inability to perform simple reading tasks. But 35 percent have only basic or below-basic health literacy. That means more than 77 million people have difficulty with common health-related reading tasks.
>
> Health literacy involves the ability to obtain, process, and understand the health information necessary to make appropriate decisions, and it's clearly essential to selecting health insurance ... This matters because those with low health literacy already tend to experience poorer health and to generate increased costs, estimated by some to amount to more than $100 billion annually.[18]

---

[14]CountyHealthRankings.org: Income Inequality. http://www.countyhealthrankings.org/explore-health-rankings/what-and-why-we-rank/health-factors/social-and-economic-factors/income/income-inequality Retrieved April 18, 2018.

[15]Sanger-Katz, M: How Income Inequality Can Be Bad for Your Health. *New York Times* March 31, 2015. P. A3.

[16]For a current academic study of the effects of education, race and sex on mortality, see: Case, A., & Deaton, A. (2017, Spring). Mortality and morbidity in the 21st century. *Brookings Papers on Economic Activity*, 397–476. Retrieved from https://www.brookings.edu/wp-content/uploads/2017/08/casetextsp17bpea.pdf

[17]VCU Center on Society and Health (2014, September). Health care: Necessary but not sufficient. Issue Brief. Retrieved from https://societyhealth.vcu.edu/work/the-projects/health-care-necessary-but-not-sufficient.html

[18]Garcia, S. (2014, January 22). Newly insured Americans don't understand basic healthcare terms: Why increasing health literacy should be a national priority. *The Atlantic*. Retrieved from http://www.theatlantic.com/health/archive/2014/01/newly-insured-americans-don-t-understand-basic-healthcare-terms/282914

EXHIBIT 2.8. Effect of Education on Healthcare Utilization—Some International Examples

- In a cross-sectional survey of 5556 patients from 15 European countries, "[p]atients with higher education had lower global coronary risk, than those with lower education."[a]

- In Israel, "those with high school educations were 1.18 times more likely to be hospitalized while those with elementary school educations experienced a risk of 1.32 ... Lower education was found to be a significant risk factor for hospitalization in most diagnostic categories."[b]

- In eastern Turkey, childhood "vaccination rates increased in parallel with maternal education level ... There was no difference in vaccination rates with respect to gender, paternal education level, number of siblings and socio-economic status."[c]

- In a survey of households in England, Wales, and Scotland, "women with no formal education qualification were more likely to report back pain than women who had a qualification. These associations were not explained by smoking, obesity, and co-existent depressive symptoms."[d]

- In Germany, education was "independently associated with severe current back pain."[e]

[a] Mayer, O., et al. (2004). Educational level and risk profile of cardiac patients in the EUROASPIRE II substudy. *Journal of Epidemiology and Community Health, 58,* 47–52.
[b] Huerta, D., Cohen-Feldman, C., & Huerta, M. (2005). Education level and origin as predictors of hospitalization among Jewish adults in Israel: A population-based study. *Harefuah, 144,* 407–412.
[c] Altinkaynak, S., Ertekin, V., Güraksin, A., & Kiliç, A. (2004). Effect of several sociodemographic factors on measles immunization in children of Eastern Turkey. *Public Health, 18,* 565–569.
[d] Croft, P. R., & Rigby, A. S. (1994). Socioeconomic influences on back problems in the community in Britain. *Journal of Epidemiology and Community Health, 48,* 166–170.
[e] Latza, U., Kohlmann T., Deck, R., & Raspe, H. (2004). Can health care utilization explain the association between socioeconomic status and back pain? *Spine, 29,* 1561–1566.

Culture and Beliefs

Finally, culture and patients' beliefs about the healthcare system have powerful effects on use of healthcare resources. (Please see Chapter 1 for a definition and some measurable characteristics of culture and Exhibit 2.9 for some international examples of how culture and beliefs affect health behavior.)

In the United States, perhaps the most infamous example of beliefs affecting healthcare behaviors is the Tuskegee Syphilis Study.[19] In 1932, the U.S. Public Health Service started to study African American men with syphilis and a control group without the disease in order to document the condition's progression. The study was curious in its design since the

---

[19]CDC. *U.S. Public Health Service Syphilis Study at Tuskegee.* Retrieved April 19, 2018, from https://www.cdc.gov/tuskegee/timeline.htm

EXHIBIT 2.9. Effects of Culture and Beliefs on Healthcare Behavior

- The perception that cancer treatment has advanced in Tunisia was positively associated with use of screening in that country.[a]

- The primary reason Swedes who need healthcare refrained from visiting a physician *was lack of* confidence in the healthcare system.[b]

- In a population of U.S. Chinese immigrants, one quarter of those surveyed believed cancer is contagious, and many believed it is caused by immoral behavior.[c]

- "Intercultural differences in perceiving or reporting back pain can be hypothesized is the most likely explanation of the markedly different prevalence rates of this disorder in the United Kingdom and East and West Germany [higher German prevalence]."[d]

- With regard to households from Tamil Nadu and Uttar Pradesh, "the status of women, and their exposures to and interaction with the outside world and control over decision-making at home explained the differences between the two groups," with the former being healthier than the latter.[e]

- "African-American women who had used religion/spirituality in the past year for health reasons ... were more likely to have seen a medical doctor during the year prior to the interview, compared to their counterparts."[f]

[a] Hsairi, M., Fakhfakh, R., Bellaaj, R., & Achour, N. (2003). Knowledge, attitudes and behaviours of women towards breast cancer screening. *East Mediterranean Health Journal, 9*, 87–98.
[b] Westin, M., Åhs, A., Bränd Persson, K., & Westerling, R. (2004). A large proportion of Swedish citizens refrain from seeking medical care—lack of confidence in the medical services a plausible explanation? *Health Policy, 68*, 333–344.
[c] Wong-Kim, M., Sun, A., &. DeMattos, M.C. (2003). Assessing cancer beliefs in a Chinese immigrant community. *Cancer Control, 10*(5 Suppl.), 22–28.
[d] Raspe, H., et al. (2004). Variation in back pain between countries: The example of Britain and Germany. *Spine, 29*, 1017–1021.
[e] Greenspan, A. (1994, March). Culture influences in demographic behavior: Evidence from India. *Asia Pacific Population Policy.* No. 28, np.
[f] Dessio, W., et al. (2004 Spring). Religion, spirituality, and healthcare choices of African-American Women: Results of a national survey. *Ethnicity & Disease, 14*, 189–197, 2004

course of untreated syphilis had been well documented in medical texts during the previous centuries. Informed consent was not obtained from any of the participants; this omission was standard practice at the time. Those in the infected group were told they were receiving treatment. The study continued until 1972, even though penicillin had been found to be an effective treatment for syphilis in 1945. This unethical practice, and others like it, has caused the African American community to distrust medical care. Lack of trust was at the heart of another infamous case. In 1951, Henrietta Lacks began treatment for advanced cervical cancer at The Johns Hopkins Hospital in Baltimore. The cells taken from her biopsy have been used for research purposes to the present day without permission from herself or her family. In her book, *The Immortal Life of Henrietta Lacks*,[20] Rebecca Skloot points out the ethical issues related to this lack of permission and highlights those who profited from discoveries using the cells in their research. Early in the book, however, Skloot mentions that Lacks had seen physicians at the hospital for vaginal bleeding before the cancer was found to be so advanced but did not return for follow-up. One reason for not returning was because the African American community feared it was being subjected to institutional experimentation.

Multifactorial Causes

Figuring out why people use healthcare services is not as simple as identifying *the single driver* for behavior. It is probably obvious by now that there are multiple factors that influence these activities. One of the key tasks of the effective healthcare strategist is to identify the relative importance of these reasons and realize that this analysis may not be generalized to other conditions or uses of products or services. Examples of multifactor influences are illustrated in Exhibit 2.10.

EXHIBIT 2.10. Some Multifactor Relationships in Healthcare Utilization

---

- With respect to asthma care, "age, gender, education level, and employment status all had a significant relationship to medical utilization."

- Delay in seeking care for cough in urban Lukasa, Zambia, "was associated with older age, severe underlying illness, poor perception of the health services, distance from the clinic and prior attendance at a private clinic. There was no relationship between delay and knowledge about tuberculosis, nor with education, socio-economic level or gender."

- Focusing on developing countries, Pakistan in particular, the authors concluded that "the utilization of a healthcare system, public or private, formal or non-formal, may depend on socio-demographic factors, social structures, level of education, cultural beliefs and practices, gender discrimination, status of women, economic and political systems, environmental conditions, and the disease pattern and healthcare system itself. Policy makers need to understand the drivers of health seeking behaviour of the population in an increasingly pluralistic health care system."

[a] Tinkelman, D. G., McClure, D. L., Lehr, T. L., & Schwartz, A. L. (2002). Relationships between self-reported asthma utilization and patient characteristics. *Journal of Asthma, 39*(8), 729–736. doi: 10.1081/JAS-120015796
[b] Godfrey-Faussett, P., et al. (2002). Why do patients with a cough delay seeking care at Lusaka urban health centres? A health systems research approach. *International Journal of Tuberculosis and Lung Disease, 6*(9), 796–805.
[c] Shaikh, B. T., & Hatcher, J. (2005, March 1). Health seeking behaviour and health service utilization in Pakistan: Challenging the policy makers, *Journal of Public Health, 27*(1), 49–54. doi: 10.1093/pubmed/fdh207

---

[20] Skloot, R. (2010). *The immortal life of Henrietta Lacks*. New York: Crown.

REDUCING PATIENT DEMAND FOR HEALTHCARE

Many companies in the healthcare field stop at this point and become expert at understanding all the reasons why people may tend to use more healthcare services or consume more products. Enhancing demand is, of course, the traditional role of healthcare marketing. However, many stakeholders may wish to *reduce* demand. Consider these stakeholders who may want to lessen utilization of healthcare products and services: public or private insurance payers that are at financial risk for paying for healthcare services and products; medical groups that assume financial risk for certain services by accepting advance payments (capitation or global payments—terms we will discuss more in detail later); and pharmaceutical benefit management companies (PBMs) or pharmacy companies that share some financial risk for overutilization of drugs with managed care companies. The profitability strategy in these instances changes from *revenue maximization* to one of *expense minimization*. (Please see Exhibit 2.11 for some strategies that stakeholders have used to mitigate customer demand.) Since there is an extensive literature on these topics, each category will be discussed only briefly. As with many other subjects in healthcare, the seminal literature is not new, though these techniques are currently being "rediscovered."

Increase Out-of-Pocket Expenses

The current approach to reducing healthcare costs is making customers more prudent about the types and amounts of healthcare they purchase, so-called consumer-driven healthcare. The proponents of this strategy recite the mantra that a more informed and price-sensitive customer will make "better" choices. The trend to shifting payment responsibility to individuals is illustrated in Exhibits 2.12 and 2.13. While these two exhibits provide information on deductibles, the same trends apply for other out-of-pocket expenses in the forms of copayments and coinsurance. (All these terms will be discussed in more detail in Chapter 6, "Payers.")

EXHIBIT 2.11. **Some Actions Used to Reduce Demand for Healthcare**

- Increase patient out-of-pocket payment responsibility (copays, deductibles, and coinsurance)
- Prevention
- Eliminate/reduce risky behaviors
- Self-management/education
- Managing end-of-life issues
- Healthy lifestyle promotion

EXHIBIT 2.12. **Average General Health Plan Deductibles for Single Coverage, 2006–2017**

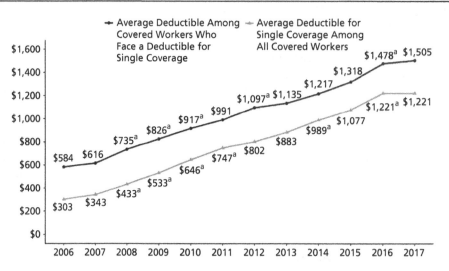

Source: Kaiser Family Foundation, Average General Health Plan Deductibles for Single Coverage, 2006–2017. Retrieved July 17, 2018 from https://www.kff.org/report-section/ehbs-2017-section-7-employee-cost-sharing/attachment/figure%207_10-11

[a] Estimate is statistically different from estimate for the previous year shown ($p < .05$).

EXHIBIT 2.13. **Percentage of Covered Workers Enrolled in a Plan with a High General Annual Deductible for Single Coverage, by Firm Size, 2017**

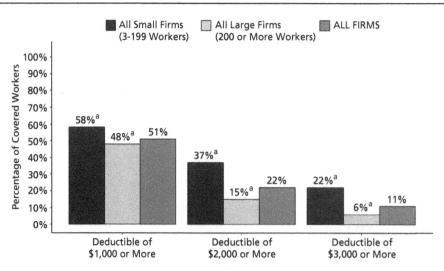

Source: Kaiser Family Foundation: Percentage of Covered Workers Enrolled in a Plan with a High General Annual Deductible for Single Coverage, by Firm Size, 2017. https://www.kff.org/health-costs/report/2017-employer-health-benefits-survey/view/print Retrieved July 17, 2018.

[a] Estimate is statistically different between All Small Firms and All Large Firms estimate ($p < .05$).

This strategy raises several questions: Does it work to reduce costs? If so, does price transparency (the ability of patients to see prices and "shop" before seeking care) offer the opportunity to lower costs? What are other consequences of shifting payment responsibilities to patients? Answers to these questions are addressed below.

■ *Does shifting payment responsibility to patients lower costs?*

The quick answer is yes, but the details are more multifaceted. This question has been asked for a number of years, but informed answers only started with the ground-breaking RAND Health Insurance Experiment (HIE). From 1971 to 1982, the RAND Corporation ran a still-unique health insurance experiment that remains a touchstone for health policy. The experiment was structured as follows:

- ■ 2,750 families were recruited from six states, each of which participated from 3 to 5 years.

- ■ RAND assumed the health insurer role so that it could get data from claims it processed.

- ■ Families were randomly assigned to one of five types of health insurance plans: three had coinsurance (a percentage of the charge for which the patient is responsible) of 25%, 50%, or 95%; one had free care; and one was a health maintenance organization (HMO) in which the care was more closely managed but was also free to the patients. The out-of-pocket maximum was $1,000. If these payments were more than the family's health plan before study participation, they would be paid the difference in the potential loss in advance, whether or not any services were used.

The study's results are summarized in Exhibit 2.14. As stated above, while out-of-pocket payments lower cost, the reasons and consequences are more nuanced.

■ *Does price transparency offer the opportunity to significantly lower costs?*

The current literature indicates that the answer is no. Consider the findings from three recent studies:

- ■ According to Mehrotra et al.,[21] "[o]nly 13 percent of respondents who had some out-of-pocket spending in their last health care encounter had sought information about their expected spending before receiving care, and just 3 percent had compared costs across providers before receiving care. The low rates of price shopping do not appear to be driven by opposition to the idea ... Common barriers to shopping included difficulty obtaining price information and a desire not to disrupt existing provider relationships."

---

[21] Mehrotra, A., Dean, K. M., Sinaiko, A. D., & Sood, N. (2017). Americans support price shopping for healthcare, but few actually seek out price information. *Health Affairs*, *36*(8), 1392–1400.

EXHIBIT 2.14. Summary of Some Key Findings of the RAND Health Insurance Experiment

---

- Averaged across all levels of coinsurance, participants (including both adults and children) with cost sharing made one to two fewer physician visits annually and had 20% fewer hospitalizations than those with free care. Declines were similar for other types of services as well, including dental visits, prescriptions, and mental health treatment.

- Consumers in the HMO-style cooperative had 39% fewer hospital admissions than consumers with free care in the fee-for-service system, but they had similar use of outpatient services. Spending reductions under the HMO plan were comparable to the effects of a higher rate of coinsurance in the fee-for-service system.

- Participants in cost sharing plans spent less on healthcare; this *savings came from using fewer services rather than finding lower prices.* Those with 25% coinsurance spent 20% less than participants with free care, and those with 95% coinsurance spent about 30% less. *Once care was accessed, there were no differences among the groups in treatment costs.*

- Reduced use of services resulted primarily from participants deciding not to initiate care. Once patients entered the healthcare system, cost sharing only modestly affected the intensity or cost of an episode of care.

- The analysis found that cost sharing reduced the use of effective and less-effective care across the board.

- Cost sharing did not significantly affect the quality of care received by participants.

- In general, the reduction in services induced by cost sharing had no adverse effect on participants' health. However, there were exceptions. The poorest and sickest 6% of the sample at the start of the experiment had better outcomes under the free plan for 4 of the 30 conditions measured. Specifically, for these patients, free care improved the control of *hypertension*, marginally improved *vision*, and increased the likelihood of receiving needed *dental care*.

- Cost sharing did not lead to better self-care. For example, rates of smoking and obesity were unchanged.

Source: Brook, R. H., et al. (2006). The health insurance experiment: A classic RAND study speaks to the current health care reform debate. Santa Monica, CA: RAND Corporation. Retrieved from https://www.rand.org/pubs/research_briefs/RB9174.html

- Desai[22] said: "We examined the experience of a large insured population that was offered a price transparency tool, focusing on a set of 'shoppable' services (lab tests, office visits, and advanced imaging services). Overall, offering the tool was not associated with lower shoppable services spending.... Simply offering a price transparency tool is not sufficient to meaningfully decrease health care prices or spending."

- According to the Health Care Cost Institute:[23]

  At most, 43% of the $524.2 billion spent on health care by individuals with ESI [employer-sponsored insurance] in 2011 was spent on shoppable services [those

---

[22]Desai, S. (2017). Offering a price transparency tool did not reduce overall spending among California public employees and retirees. *Health Affairs, 36*(8), 1401–1407.

[23]Health Care Cost Institute. (2016, March). *Spending on shoppable services in health care.* Issue Brief #11. Retrieved from http://www.healthcostinstitute.org/files/Shoppable%20Services%20IB%203.2.16_0.pdf

that are both the highest-spending and could be scheduled in advance of receiving the service] ...

About 15% of total spending in 2011 was spent by consumers out-of-pocket.

$37.7 billion (7% of total spending) of the out-of-pocket spending in 2011 was on shoppable services. ... Overall, the potential gains from the consumer price shopping aspect of price transparency efforts are modest.

■ *What are other consequences of shifting payment responsibilities to patients?*

This question is best answered by the Commonwealth Fund's Biennial Health Insurance Survey,[24] which asked respondents whether healthcare costs caused them to not visit a doctor or clinic if they had a medical problem; not fill a prescription; skip a recommended test, treatment, or follow-up; or not get needed specialist care. Overall, 63 million people in 2016 (34%) said yes to one of those questions. (By way of comparison, the numbers were 80 million and 43% in 2012, respectively, before the ACA was implemented in 2014.)

Putting the above answers together, we can say that out-of-pocket payments reduce costs but they also create barriers to care. The ideal amount for patient responsibility probably depends on individual disposable income. Making patients responsible for shopping for their care, even with accurate and accessible tools, may not have a significant impact on lowering costs.

Prevention

Because of public health concerns, governments are obviously interested in reducing illness by using preventive measures such as promoting or requiring immunizations. Pharmaceutical companies have responded to this need by developing new immunizations and combining existing ones in order to reduce the number of injections.

Some cost-saving examples are listed in Exhibit 2.15. Not all prevention-related savings are related directly to reductions, however. Sometimes lost wages and social factors must be considered. For example: A cost-effectiveness analysis was performed before initiation of the varicella vaccination program in the United States. The results of the study indicated a savings of $5.40 for each dollar spent on routine vaccination of preschool-aged children when direct and indirect costs were considered. When only direct medical costs were considered, the benefit-cost ratio was 0.9 : 1.0.[25]

Eliminate/Reduce Risky Behaviors

This category includes smoking cessation, wearing seatbelts, using car seats for young children, and reducing unprotected sex. Cigarette smoking alone adds more than $300 billion

[24]Commonwealth Fund (2016). *2016 Biennial Health Insurance Survey*. Retrieved from http://www.commonwealthfund .org/interactives-and-data/surveys/biennial-health-insurance-surveys/2017/2016-biennial-health-insurance-survey

[25]Marin, M., Güris, D., Chaves, S. S., Schmid, S., Seward, J. F., Advisory Committee on Immunization Practices, & Centers for Disease Control and Prevention. (2007, June 22). Prevention of varicella: Recommendations of the Advisory Committee on Immunization Practices (ACIP). *Morbidity and Mortality Weekly Report, 56* (RR04), 1–40. Retrieved from http://www.cdc.gov/mmwr/preview/mmwrhtml/rr5604a1.htm

EXHIBIT 2.15. **Examples of Cost-Saving Prevention**

- "Vaccination of the 23 million elderly people unvaccinated in 1993 would have gained about 78,000 years of healthy life and saved $194 million."[a]

- "A routine, universal rotavirus immunization program would prevent 1.08 million cases of diarrhea, avoiding 34,000 hospitalizations, 95,000 emergency department visits, and 227,000 physician visits in the first 5 years of life ... The program would provide a net savings of $296 million to society."[b]

- "The model was used to compare costs and benefits of a combined vaccination programme (CVP) including tetanus, diphtheria, and acellular pertussis (dTacp) administered at age 12, compared to current practice ... From the societal perspective, the CVP would be cost saving [Canadian]$858,106 at 10 years for the cohort."[c]

- If hepatitis A prevalence is 53% in patients with chronic liver disease, then immunizing this select group against this infection will save over $11,000 per 100 patients.[d]

[a] Sisk, J. E., et al. (1997). Cost-effectiveness of vaccination against pneumococcal bacteremia among elderly people. *JAMA, 278*(16), 1333–1339. doi: 10.1001/jama.278.16.1333.
[b] Tucker, A. W., et al. (1998). Cost-effectiveness analysis of a rotavirus immunization program for the United States. *JAMA, 279*(17), 1371–1376. DOI:10.1001/jama.279.17.1371
[c] Iskedjian, M., Walker, J. H., & Hemels, M. E. (2004). Economic evaluation of an extended acellular pertussis vaccine programme for adolescents in Ontario, Canada. *Vaccine, 22*, 4215–4227, 2004
[d] Duncan, M., Hirota, W. K., & Tsuchida, A. (2002). Prescreening versus empirical immunization for hepatitis A in patients with chronic liver disease: A prospective cost analysis. *American Journal of Gastroenterology, 97*, 1792–1795.

each year to U.S. healthcare costs.[26] The most effective measure to reduce risky behavior (like smoking) and other unhealthy practices (like consuming sugared drinks) is taxation.[27]

Unfortunately, sometimes attempts at legislating these behaviors runs into personal freedom issues. Examples of successes in this area have been seatbelt laws and smoking bans in public places. A typical example of failure is attempts in some states to pass laws requiring helmet use for motorcyclists.

End-of-Life Issues

One often hears the complaint that if we could reduce the cost of end-of-life care, there would be significant savings to the healthcare system. This issue has been a contentious one characterized by conflicting and sometimes confusing data.

Several measures have been taken over the years to address this issue: initiation of a hospice program for Medicare beneficiaries in 1983 (with a tripling of enrollees by the 1990s); changes in payment methods for skilled nursing homes and home care services; and increased

[26]CDC. *Economic trends in tobacco*. Retrieved April 21, 2018, from https://www.cdc.gov/tobacco/data_statistics/fact_sheets/economics/econ_facts/index.htm
[27]Summers, L. H. (2018). Taxes for health: Evidence clears the air. *The Lancet*. Retrieved from http://www.thelancet.com/pdfs/journals/lancet/PIIS0140-6736(18)30629-9.pdf?code=lancet-site

use of advanced directives (so-called do not resuscitate [DNR] orders). Although the rate of increase was not slowed by these measures, the *fraction* of Medicare costs this population comprised stabilized during the 1980s and 1990s.[28] By 2014, although Medicare spent nearly four times more on people who died that year than on those who lived the entire year, the share of *total Medicare spending* for people who die in a given year dropped from 18.6% of traditional Medicare spending in 2000 to 13.5% in 2014.[29]

With respect to reducing overall costs—that is, not just Medicare expenses—Aldridge and Kelley concluded that:

> Many proposals to reduce health care costs in the United States target the high cost of end-of-life care, yet at the population level the cost of caring for individuals in their last year of life accounts for only 13% of total annual health care spending. That is, although the majority of decedents are in the highest cost group, the majority of individuals in that group are not in their last year of life. Specifically, we estimate that only 11% of individuals in the highest cost group are in their last year of life.[30]

Even more recent studies showed reductions in end-of-life spending would not significantly help in lowering overall costs. For example, in an international study, French et al. found:

> The idea that reducing wasteful spending just before death can make the growth in health care costs sustainable is not supported by this study. Spending in the last twelve months of life accounted for 8.5–11.2 percent of overall spending in eight countries and Quebec, with the United States at the bottom of that ranking. Reducing this spending would thus have only a modest effect on total medical spending. In contrast, spending in the last three years of life accounted for as much as 24.5 percent of overall costs, which suggests that the focus should be on reducing the costs of caring for people with chronic conditions—many of whom are approaching death.[31]

Misunderstanding the potential savings in this category may be due to two factors. First, as French et al. mention, these costs are attributed to end of life when, in fact, they ought to be ascribed to chronic care. Second, as shown a number of years ago by Emanuel and Emanuel: "Even when patients refuse life-sustaining interventions, they do not necessarily require less medical care, just a different kind of care."[32] In other words, effective palliation

[28] Hogan, C., Lunney, J., Gabel, J., & Lynn, J. (2001). Medicare beneficiaries' costs of care in the last year of life. *Health Affairs, 20*, 188–195.

[29] Kaiser, H. J., Family Foundation (KFF). (2016, July 14). *Analysis finds end-of-life Medicare spending declines with age among seniors.* Retrieved from https://www.kff.org/medicare/press-release/analysis-finds-end-of-life-medicare-spending-declines-with-age-among-seniors

[30] Aldridge, M. D., & Kelley, A. S. (2015). The myth regarding the high cost of end-of-life care. *American Journal of Public Health, 105*(12), 2411–2415.

[31] French, E. B., McCauley, J., Aragon, M., Bakx, P., Chalkley, M., Chen, S. H., ... Kelly, E. (2017). End-of-life medical spending in last twelve months of life is lower than previously reported. *Health Affairs, 36*(7), 1211–1217.

[32] Emanuel, E. J., & Emanuel, L. L. (1994). The economics of dying: The illusion of cost savings at the end of life. *The New England Journal of Medicine, 330*, 540–544.

is not necessarily cheaper than curative attempts. Further, as the population ages, increased costs due to demographic effects are expected, balanced by "healthier aging." For example:

> Among beneficiaries who died in 2014, Medicare spent significantly more per person on medical services for seniors in their late sixties and early seventies than on older beneficiaries … The finding contradicts a popular assumption that Medicare … spends heavily on end-of-life medical care for the oldest beneficiaries.[33]

Two further distinctions on this topic must be made. We must first differentiate between rationing and the provision of futile care. "Rationing refers to the withholding of efficacious treatments which cannot be afforded. Futility refers to ineffective treatments."[34] Obviously, futile care needs to be examined along with other wasteful services. Next, the statistics mentioned above are *averages* across all patients and sites. Opportunities do exist for savings in this category by identifying best practices and reducing nonhelpful variations in care. For example, Wennberg et al. found that "[s]triking variation exists in the utilization of end of life care among US medical centres with strong national reputations for clinical care."[35]

Healthy Lifestyle Promotion

These measures complement the elimination of risky behaviors. They include such activities as eating a proper diet and exercising regularly. For example, the CDC estimates that "some 300,000 deaths each year in the U.S. likely are the results of physical inactivity and poor eating habits."[36]

CONSUMER BEHAVIOR—HEALTHCARE MARKET SEGMENTATION

Consumer behaviors, not unlike those in other sectors of the economy, also influence care-seeking. One of these models is presented in Exhibits 2.16 and 2.17 and is self-explanatory. With regard to introducing new products or services (or expanding current offerings), one should carefully consider which consumer segments would be most appropriate for initial and subsequent introductions.

Of further importance is that consumer behavior segments change over time. For example, from 2008 to 2015, the Sick and Savvy segment decreased to 11% and the Content and Compliant group decreased to 22%, while Casual and Cautious group increased to 34%.[37] Frequent reassessment of the market is therefore necessary, particularly with respect to these types of preferences.

---

[33] KFF. Analysis finds end-of-life Medicare spending declines with age among seniors.

[34] AMA Committee on Ethical and Judicial Affairs (1999). *JAMA, 281,* 937–941.

[35] Wennberg, J., Fisher, E. S., Stukel, T. A., Skinner, J. S., Sharp, S. M., & Bronner, K. K. (2004). Use of hospitals, physician visits, and hospice care during last six months of life among cohorts loyal to highly respected hospitals in the United States. *British Medical Journal, 328,* 607–611.

[36] CDC. (2017, September 15). *Physical inactivity: What's the problem?* Retrieved from https://www.cdc.gov/healthcommunication/toolstemplates/entertainmented/tips/PhysicalInactivity.html

[37] Deloitte, LLP. (2015). *Health care consumer engagement: No "one-size-fits-all" approach.* Retrieved from https://www2.deloitte.com/content/dam/Deloitte/us/Documents/life-sciences-health-care/us-dchs-consumer-engagement-healthcare.pdf

EXHIBIT 2.16. Profile of the Six Healthcare Consumer Segments

Factor	Content and Compliant	Sick and Savvy	Online Onboard	Shop and Save	Out and About	Casual and Cautious
Segment Size	29%	24%	8%	2%	9%	28%
System Use	Medium	Highest	High	Medium	Medium	Lowest
Preferences Regarding Care	Traditional	Traditional	Traditional but open to nonconventional settings	Traditional but open to alternative and nonconventional settings	Alternative approaches and nonconventional settings	Disengaged but currently leans toward traditional
Dependence on Providers	Accepts what doctor recommends	Takes charge of own care	Leans toward relying on self	Leans toward allowing doctor to make decisions	Makes own decisions/independent	Leans toward relying on self
Compliance with Treatment	Most compliant	Compliant	Compliant	Less compliant	Least compliant	Less compliant
Satisfaction with Providers and Plans	Most satisfied	Satisfied	Satisfied	Less satisfied	Least satisfied	Less satisfied
Other Important Distinctions	Less likely to seek information; less likely to use value-added services; least interested in shopping for and customizing insurance	Seeks information; sensitive to quality; uses some value-added services; wants to shop for and customize insurance	Seeks information; uses online tools the most; sensitive to quality; maximizes use of value-added services	Makes changes to insurance; price-sensitive; uses value-added services; most likely to travel for care	Seeks information; sensitive to quality; uses some value-added services; wants to shop for and customize insurance	Price-sensitive; unprepared financially for future needs; less likely to seek information; less likely to use value-added services

Source: Reproduced with permission of Deloitte, LLP. © 2008.

EXHIBIT 2.17. **Use of Healthcare Facilities and Services versus Willingness to Experience Innovation**

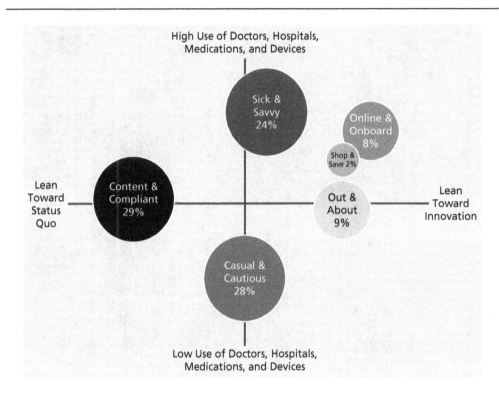

Source: Reproduced with permission of Deloitte, LLP. © 2008.

PROVIDER-INDUCED DEMAND FOR HEALTHCARE

While customers usually initiate contact with the healthcare system, understanding their behavior is only half the story. For decades, economists have been studying a phenomenon called *provider-induced demand* (PID)—providers stimulating use of their services or products, presumably for financial gain. Not surprisingly, physicians have been the subjects most studied. The foundational research on this topic was conducted in the 1980s and 1990s with policy makers only recently "rediscovering" their important implication on behavior and healthcare costs. The ongoing debate among academicians is whether this practice actually exists and, if so, to what extent. In interpreting the data, one must be aware of the following differences in studies: variation in analytical methods; environmental circumstances that would cause PID (e.g., increased density of physicians in a particular geographic area or changing payment amount or method); and cultural factors. With regard to problematic methodology, Dranove and Wehner, in an oft-cited paper, "proved" the thesis of their article, "Physician-Induced Demand for Childbirths."[38] The point of this research was to discredit a methodology (two-stage least squares regression) by confirming an obviously absurd notion.

Environmental events might include a change in the number of practicing physicians in a given specialty within a defined geographic area (physician density) or a shift from a fee-for-service payment system to capitation or salary. National cultural influences may account for differences highlighted by the following example: While an increase in physician density increases the number of services per visit in France,[39] under similar conditions this behavior did not occur in Norway.[40]

One must also realize that, while financial incentives have a powerful effect on physician behavior, they are only one of a number of influences on such conduct. As Eisenberg further noted:

> [T]he factors that influence physicians' use of medical services are complex. They include personal considerations of the physician, such as the aspiration for income, the enjoyment of a satisfying practice, and the desire for approval from peers. Characteristics of the patient and the clinical encounter are also influential, such as consideration of the patient's economic well-being, maintenance or improvement of the patient's health, and the understanding of the patient's perceived values and desires.[41]

Other factors that affect physician behavior include those that influence local area variations in practice patterns (which will be discussed further below), *organizational* cultural norms (which may be separate from peer approval issues), and professional uncertainty aversion, particularly in the context of malpractice fears. Although the focus here is on the behavioral implications of financial incentives, one must realize that these other issues are important for changing physician conduct and have their own situational advantages. As Eisenberg further notes: "Education, feedback, participation, administrative rules, incentives and penalties may each address different factors that govern medical decision making. Any one by itself is less likely to be successful than an orchestrated combination."[42] In interpreting the examples of PID in Exhibits 2.18 and 2.19, it is often difficult to separate the financial incentives from these other factors. Likewise, correlation does not prove causation. In this case, this caveat may mean that those physicians who respond to certain incentives may be most likely to practice in areas having compensation systems with which they feel most comfortable or seek locations having a growing demand for their services. Another

---

[38] Dranove, D., & Wehner, P. (1994). Physician-induced demand for childbirths. *Journal of Health Economics, 13*, 61–73.

[39] Delattre, E., & Dormont, B. (2003). Fixed fees and physician-induced demand: A panel data study on French physicians. *Health Economics, 12*(9), 741–754.

[40] Sorensen, R. J., & Grytten, J. (1999). Competition and supplier-induced demand in a health care system with fixed fees. *Health Economics, 8*(6), 497–508.

[41] Eisenberg, John M. (1986). *Doctors' decisions and the cost of medical care: The reasons for doctors' practice patterns and ways to change them.* Ann Arbor, MI: Health Administration Press Perspectives.

[42] Ibid.

EXHIBIT 2.18. Provider-Induced Demand: Some U.S. Examples

- "[L]arger fee differentials between caesarian and normal childbirth for the Medicaid program leads to higher caesarian delivery rates."[a]

- "Other things equal, a 10 percent increase in the surgeon/population ratio results in about a 3 percent increase in per capita utilization. Moreover, differences in supply seem to have a perverse effect on fees, raising them when the surgeon/population ratio increases."[b]

- "A 10 percent increase in surgeons per capita … results in a 0.9 percent increase in overall surgery per capita and 1.3 percent increase in elective surgery. The positive surgeon-availability elasticity, due primarily to elective surgery, supports the hypothesis that more discretionary surgical procedures are performed in areas of high surgeon concentration."[c]

- In an investor-owned ambulatory care center, changing compensation from an hourly salary to an hourly minimum plus bonus based on monthly gross charges resulted in increases in the following areas: laboratory tests per patient (+23%), number of X-ray films per visit (+16%), total charges per month (+20%), and average number of patient visits per month (+12%). The authors also noted that "all physicians in this study, including those who never received a bonus, increased the intensity of their practices after the bonus system was instituted."[d]

[a] Gruber, J., et al. (1999). Physician fees and procedure intensity: The case of cesarean delivery. *Journal of Health Economics, 18,* 473–490.
[b] Fuchs, V. R. (1978). The supply of surgeons and the demand for operations. *Journal of Human Resources, 13*(Suppl.), 35–56.
[c] Cromwell, J., & Mitchell, J. B. (1986). Physician-induced demand for surgery. *Journal of Health Economics, 5,* 293–313.
[d] Hemenway, D., et al. (1990). Physicians' responses to financial incentives—Evidence from a for-profit ambulatory care center. *New England Journal of Medicine, 322,* 1059–1063.

important factor to consider is quality of care effects. Although certain payment methods appear to increase PID, it is unclear whether services were underutilized before the change or overutilized after incentives were added. For all the above reasons, therefore, the conclusions in Exhibits 2.18 and 2.19, should be interpreted cautiously.

Payers, such as insurance companies and governments, that are aware of provider-induced demand have implemented one or more of the following five strategies to limit the costs that result from such behavior:

- *Decrease fees.* The first, and most common, approach is reduction of fees. For reasons explained in Chapter 1, this tactic will fail unless the number of patient visits and/or regulation of high-tech care are simultaneously implemented. (Recall that total costs are a function of price, volume, and intensity of service.)

- *Increase/decrease the number of providers.* In attempts to introduce market competition, payers encourage entry of more providers into each service area. In the public sector, that means training more professionals (e.g., physicians) or allowing construction of more facilities in otherwise regulated markets. States may control new construction by

EXHIBIT 2.19. Provider-Induced Demand: Some International Examples

- In France, where fees are fixed, when physician/population ratios increase, both general practitioners and specialists "counterbalance the fall of the number of encounters by an increase of the volume of care delivered in each encounter."[a]

- After the authors controlled for detailed characteristics of patients, they found that "increases in the relative numbers of [Japanese hospital and physician services were] significantly related to physician-initiated expenditures and the effect is higher for high-tech treatments."[b]

- After 1961, most Danish physicians were paid a mix of half capitation and half fee for service. Doctors in Copenhagen were paid primarily capitation until 1987, when they were able to bill patients for their services. Observing utilization patterns before and after the change and comparing those patterns to a comparable nearby group of practitioners, the authors found significant increases in many diagnostic and therapeutic services for the Copenhagen physicians after 1987.[c]

- "[W]e find evidence of induced demand since doctors that are paid fee-for-service tend to lengthen duration of the treatment."[d]

[a] Delattre, E., & Dormont, B. (2003). Fixed fees and physician-induced demand: A panel data study on French physicians. *Health Economics, 12*, 741–754.

[b] Noguchi, H., Shimizutani, S., & Masuda, Y. (2005, June). Physician-Induced demand for treatments for heart attack patients in Japan: Evidence from the Tokai Acute Myocardial Study (TAMIS). Economic and Social Research Institute, Cabinet Office, Tokyo, Japan. Discussion Paper Series No. 14.

[c] Flierman, H. A., & Groenewegen, P. P. (1992). Introducing fees for services with professional uncertainty. *Health Care Financing Review, 14*(1), 107–115.

[d] Jimenez-Martin, S., et al. (2004, January). An empirical analysis of the demand for physician services across the European Union. Fundacion Centro de Estudios Andaluces Documento de Trabajo Serie Economia. P. 455.

enacting laws that require review of projects costing more than a specified amount, so-called certificate-of-need (CON) legislation. However, increasing the number of physicians does not lower healthcare costs and frequently raises total expenditures. Likewise, measures such as CON laws have not had a significant effect on controlling healthcare costs, as evidenced by repeal of many of these measures in the 1970s.[43] In the private sector, attempts to control PID can take the form of contracting with more providers. Unfortunately, this strategy is not always successful either. For example, there is evidence that more hospitals in a concentrated geographic area will *increase* costs by duplicating technology to enhance their competitiveness. This paradox is sometimes called a "Medical Arms Race."[44]

---

[43]More will be discussed about CON in the section on hospitals. For now, the reader is referred to: Garrison, L. P. Jr. (1991). Assessment of the effectiveness of supply-side cost-containment measures. *Health Care Financing Review Annual Supplement, 1991*, 13–20.

[44]This topic is, in fact a bit more complex. A more detailed critique can be found in Dranove, D., Shanley, M., & Simon, C. (1992). Is hospital competition wasteful? *The RAND Journal of Economics, 23*, 247–262.

Reducing the number of providers can reduce spending, but the trade-off can be lowered quality due to treatment delays.

▪ *Change payment methods.* The third tactic to control PID is changing the payment method. Instead of paying providers on a per-item basis, methods such as capitation (a fixed amount per person, usually per month, for a specified set of services or products) or total payments per type of case have been successful in moderating overall cost. We will explain more about this topic when we discuss Medicare's Diagnosis Related Groups (DRGs) and managed care.

▪ *Employ utilization review/prior authorization methods.* Commercial insurance companies have often used utilization review to limit PID. These measures require providers to contact the payer for permission to perform a service (such as elective surgery), prescribe a drug, or order a medical device. Payers claim they have statistically valid criteria that will enable them to determine the appropriateness of a request. However, most of the methods these companies use are proprietary and have not been subject to valid study. One fact *is* commonly known: Well over 90% of requests are approved without further review. This piece of information should make us suspect that the "hassle factor" may be just as (or more) valuable a utilization technique as the actual criteria that companies use. In fact, in 1999, UnitedHealth Group, one of the largest healthcare companies in the United States, revealed that it was spending $100 million per year on preauthorization activities and was approving 99% of physician requests. As a result, the company announced it was eliminating this process for many types of services.

In subsequent years, utilization review has become more burdensome, especially for primary care physicians who do not benefit from what is being authorized but who still bear the cost of compliance. For example, in 2013, Morley et al. reported that the "mean annual projected cost per full-time equivalent physician for PA [prior authorization] activities ranged from $2,161 ... to $3,430."[45] On a more micro level, it is estimated that prior authorization costs providers $7.50 or $1.89 per transaction for, respectively, manual and electronic submissions.[46]

More recently, however, with rapidly rising healthcare costs, particularly for imaging studies and pharmaceuticals, this cost-containment strategy has resurfaced.

The physician community's current push-back against the cost and quality of care implications of this process started on January 25, 2015. On that date, the American Medical Association (AMA), on behalf of itself and 16 other provider organizations, called for insurer adherence to 21 principles in establishment and management of these reviews.[47] These principles are divided into five categories:

[45]Morley, C. P., Hickner, J., & Epling, J. W. (2013). The impact of prior authorization requirements on primary care physicians' offices: Report of two parallel network studies. *The Journal of the American Board of Family Medicine*, 26(1): 93–95.

[46]CAQH Index (2016). A report of healthcare industry adoption of electronic business. Retrieved from https://www .caqh.org/sites/default/files/explorations/index/report/2016-caqh-index-report.pdf

[47]AMA. *Prior authorization and utilization: Management reform principles—21 principles.* Retrieved April 22, 2018, from https://www.ama-assn.org/sites/default/files/media-browser/principles-with-signatory-page-for-slsc.pdf

1. Clinical validity

2. Continuity of care

3. Transparency and fairness

4. Timely access and administrative efficiency

5. Alternatives and exemptions

As an example, Principle 1 states: "Any utilization management program applied to a service, device or drug should be based on accurate and up-to-date clinical criteria and never cost alone. The referenced clinical information should be readily available to the prescribing/ordering provider and the public." To further protect individuals from unreasonable utilization review processes, states have enacted laws that outline allowed practices.[48]

■ *Implement practice guidelines.* Finally, practice guidelines have been tried with variable results in controlling cost. We will discuss this topic more in depth in Chapter 9, "Quality."

Local (Small Area) Variations

In view of all these consumer and provider factors, it should come as no surprise that patterns of care differ among nations and even different regions of a given country. (Please see Exhibit 2.20 for some international examples.) The variations are, in fact, much more extreme than one would imagine. For example, utilization of services can vary dramatically from town to town. The research that spurred interest in this topic dates to a landmark article in *Science* in 1973 by Wennberg and Gittelsohn,[49] who found marked differences in a wide variety of surgical procedures among different towns in Vermont, a state that, at that time, had a total population of 444,000. (Please see Exhibit 2.21.) This study, as well as numerous others that followed over the years, concluded that these differences were *not* due to variations in illness patterns. It is also important to realize that areas with higher utilization and/or cost do not necessarily have better outcomes. In fact, as Fisher and Wennberg pointed out: "Increased spending is associated neither with increased use of services known to be effective in reducing morbidity [sickness] or mortality [death], nor with increased use of surgical procedures where patients' preferences are important."[50] Numerous other studies have since come to the same conclusion.

In summarizing the reasons for these discrepancies, Detsky (and numerous subsequent authors) found that there "are three main reasons why there might be variation in the use of diagnostic and therapeutic procedures: differences in healthcare systems, physicians' practice styles, and patient characteristics."[51] We have already discussed factors related to the

---

[48] AMA (2018). Prior authorization state law chart. Retrieved from https://www.ama-assn.org/sites/default/files/media-browser/public/arc-public/pa-state-chart.pdf

[49] Wennberg, J., & Gittelsohn, A. (1973). Small area variations in health care delivery. *Science, 182* (4117), 1102–1108.

[50] Fisher, E., & Wennberg, J. E. (2003). Health care quality, geographic variations, and the challenge of supply-sensitive care. *Perspectives in Biology and Medicine, 46,* 69–79.

[51] Detsky, A. S. (1995). Regional variations in medical care. *The New England Journal of Medicine, 333,* 589–590.

EXHIBIT 2.20. **Local Area Variations: International Examples**

■ In Ontario, after "controlling for population characteristics and access to care (including the number of hospital beds, and the density of orthopaedic and referring physicians), orthopaedic surgeons' opinions or enthusiasm for the procedure was the dominant modifiable determinant of area variation."[a]

■ In Ontario, there was an "almost 10-fold difference between the areas with the highest and lowest rates [of tympanostomy tube placement. It] was the opinion of primary care physicians that predicted rates."[b]

■ "Following cardiac rehabilitation, there is a considerable regional variation in the prescription of cardiovascular medication in Germany. Beta-Blockers and lipid-lowering agents are prescribed more frequently in the West and ACE inhibitors in the East. Even after adjustment for differences in patient characteristics, region of residence remains an independent predictor for the prescription of lipid-lowering agents and ACE inhibitors."[c]

■ In the U.K., "[p]rescription rates for antiplatelet agents varied significantly between the RHAs [regional health authorities] for both TIA [transient ischemic attack] and stroke patients. Antiplatelets were prescribed for 15%–25% of stroke patients and for 30% to 45% of TIA patients over the 5 years, depending on region."[d]

[a] Wright, J. G. (1999). Physician enthusiasm as an explanation for area variation in the utilization of knee replacement surgery. *Medical Care, 37*, 946–995.

[b] Coyte, P. C., et al. (2001). Physician and population determinants of rates of middle-ear surgery in Ontario. *JAMA, 286*, 2128–2135.

[c] Muller-Nordhorn, J., et al. (2005). Regional variation in medication following coronary events in Germany. *International Journal of Cardiology, 102*, 47–53.

[d] Gibbs, R. G. J. (2001). Diagnosis and initial management of stroke and transient ischemic attack across UK health regions from 1992–1996. *Stroke, 32*, 1085–1090.

latter two reasons. To the explanation of physician practice styles we can add their own beliefs about effectiveness of care, their medical training, and beliefs in their own abilities. Examples of healthcare system characteristic differences include payment mechanisms and the organization of local provider groups and institutions. With respect to what might be different among systems, Fisher et al. indicate that the regional "differences in Medicare spending are largely explained by the more inpatient-based and specialist-oriented pattern of practice observed in high-spending regions. Neither quality of care nor access to care appear to be better for Medicare enrollees in higher-spending regions."[52] For more extensive data on local area variations, an excellent resource is *The Dartmouth Atlas* (http://www.dartmouthatlas.org).

---

[52] Fisher, E. S., Wennberg, D. E., Stukel, T. A., Gottlieb, D. J., Lucas, F. L., & Pinder, E. L. (2003). The implications of regional variations in Medicare spending. Part 1. *Annals of Internal Medicine, 138*, 273–287.

EXHIBIT 2.21. **Variation in Number of Surgical Procedures Performed per 10,000 Persons for the 13 Vermont Hospital Service Areas and Comparison Populations, 1969**

Surgical Procedure	Lowest Two Areas		Entire State	Highest Two Areas	
Tonsillectomy	13	32	43	85	151
Appendectomy	10	15	18	27	32
Hemorrhoidectomy	2	4	6	9	10
Males					
Hernioplasty	29	38	41	47	48
Prostatectomy	11	13	20	28	38
Females					
Cholecystectomy	17	19	27	46	57
Hysterectomy	20	22	30	34	60
Mastectomy	12	14	18	28	33
Dilation and curettage	30	42	55	108	141
Varicose veins	6	7	12	24	28

Note: Rates adjusted to Vermont age composition.

Source: Wennberg, J., & Gittelsohn, A. (1973). Small area variations in health care delivery. *Science, 182(4117)*: 1102–1108.

SUMMARY

In this chapter we have presented reasons why people seek care and how some stakeholders evaluate demand and act to reduce it. It is important for the healthcare marketer to understand that stakeholders may have different perspectives on these issues. While one is engaged enhancing demand for a product or service, another stakeholder may be just as active trying to counter those efforts.

CHAPTER

3

MANAGERIAL EPIDEMIOLOGY

MERCUTIO.

> I am hurt.

> A plague a' both your houses! ...

> > —William Shakespeare, *Romeo and Juliet*, Act 3, Scene 1

INTRODUCTION

Chapters 1 and 2 introduce the concepts of stakeholders and their interests in the healthcare system. This chapter provides some tools for assessing *patterns* of healthcare utilization.[1] Often this subject is considered only as a cornerstone of public health curricula; however, epidemiology also uses the management disciplines of statistics and marketing research. The aim of this chapter is to make this subject more understandable to general managers involved in healthcare management.

As with the other chapters in this book, we begin with a definition.

What Is Epidemiology?

Strictly speaking, epidemiology is the study of epidemics. The concepts and techniques used in epidemiology, however, reach far beyond public health into areas of clinical medicine, pharmaceuticals, medical products, and biotechnology. A broader definition of epidemiology is: "The study of the distribution and determinants of health-related states or events in specified populations, and the application of this study to control of health problems."[2]

Why Is It Important to Learn about Epidemiology?

The concepts and tools of epidemiology are important across the broad range of disciplines within the health industry. A brief listing of questions that an epidemiologic approach can help answer will illustrate its utility.

- Clinical Medicine

    Where did the outbreak of hospital-acquired infections originate?

    Can the source be found?

    What strains of influenza can we expect to infect this country next season, and when are the first infections likely to occur?

- Pharmaceutical Industry

    Given our finite, precious research budget, which diseases should we target for the development of treatments?

---

[1]For a good textbook on this subject, see: Fleming, S. T. (Ed.) (2015). *Managerial epidemiology: Cases and concepts.* Chicago: Health Administration Press.

[2]Stedman, T. L. (2006). *Stedman's medical dictionary.* Philadelphia: Lippincott Williams & Wilkins.

A recent case control study in a prominent medical journal raises important safety issues about one of our top-selling drugs; is there really a problem?

- Medical Products

    For what conditions will diagnostic devices most likely be used either in the patient's home or in the physician's office in the next several years?

    How good is your equipment at either diagnosing or ruling out a medical condition, particularly compared to other diagnostic options?

- Biotechnology

    What is the likelihood that a particular genetic mutation actually causes a disease and, hence, that genetic manipulation will lead to improvement or cure of that particular condition?

    To what extent are certain diseases caused by combinations of genetic and environmental factors?

DEFINITIONS AND USES OF PRINCIPLES

The core tools of epidemiology are acquired through study of probability and statistics. Since those topics are well covered by a number of texts, only terms specific to epidemiology will be explained here.

Morbidity and Mortality

"Morbidity" (from the Latin *morbidus*) refers to those who are sick. "Mortality" (from the Latin *mortalis*) refers to death. Both of these terms are used to convey such information as the illness and death rates in a particular population, respectively. These events can be caused by such factors as infections, complications from procedures, side effects from medications, or genetic mutations.

Incidence and Prevalence

Incidence is the number of *new* events (or cases) that occur *during a specified period of time*. Prevalence is the *total* number of events (or cases) in a population at a *point* in time.

Validity

"Validity" refers to the extent to which a test actually measures what it is supposed to measure. For example, while a thermometer is a valid testing instrument for temperature, it is not a valid tool for assessing blood pressure. One can also use the concept of validity to apply to surveys or questionnaires. For example, is a particular marketing survey a valid instrument to assess customer preferences about a particular product? Is the Spanish version of a valid survey written in English also valid?

Reliability

Used in the context of medical research, "reliability" means reproducibility. We can consider two types of reliability: intraobserver (or intrarater) and interobserver (or interrater). "Intraobserver reliability" means that the same person performing the test multiple times will get statistically similar results. Likewise, "interobserver reliability" means that when different people perform a test, all the results will be statistically similar.

Sensitivity, Specificity, Positive Predictive Value, and Negative Predictive Value

These concepts are best understood by use of an example. Suppose you are the marketing director of a biotech firm that develops and manufactures diagnostic equipment. The vice president of Research and Development (VP of R&D) comes to you with an interesting piece of equipment and insists that you get busy right away to develop a marketing plan. Before you develop this plan, you need to know something more about what the device does and how good it is in detecting or ruling out disease. The VP of R&D tells you that 10% of the U.S. population (the target market for this device) has a genetic mutation that puts them at very high risk for heart disease. If treated early and aggressively, morbidity and mortality for these people can be lowered significantly. When you ask how good this test is at detecting this genetic mutation, the answer you get is "90%." That means that if someone has the mutation, the test will pick it up 90% of the time. We refer to this percentage as the test's *sensitivity*. Translating this concept into a formula:

$$\text{True Positive} \div (\text{True Positives} + \text{False Negatives}) \times 100 = \% \text{ Sensitivity}$$

True positives are those people who really have the genetic mutation and the test finds the mutation. The false negatives are those people who also have the genetic mutation but, because of flaws in the test, the mutation is missed.

You also want to know how good the test is at picking up people who do not have the mutation. The VP of R&D says that if you do not have the mutation, then the test will be negative 80% of the time. We call this latter concept the *specificity* of a test, in this case 80%. The formula for the specificity of a test is:

$$\text{True Negatives} \div (\text{True Negatives} + \text{False Positives}) \times 100 = \% \text{ Specificity}$$

What this formula means is that if you do not have the genetic mutation, the test will be negative 80% of the time. However, because of flaws in the test, it *will* be positive 20% of the time (false positives).

You think about these properties of the test and then have a few more questions for the VP of R&D. It is nice to know that if you have a genetic mutation the test will pick it up 90% of the time. But what if you are part of a random screening process and your test comes back positive? Does that mean that you really have the mutation? This latter concept addresses the issue of *positive predictive value* (i.e., in the general population, if you use a screening test,

EXHIBIT 3.1. Scenarios for Measure Variations by Prevalence

Disease Prevalence	Scenario 1 10%		Scenario 2 5%		Scenario 3 1%	
	90,000 (TP)	180,000 (FP)	45,000 (TP)	190,000 (FP)	9,000 (TP)	198,000 (FP)
	10,000 (FN)	720,000 (TN)	5,000 (FN)	760,000 (TN)	1,000 (FN)	792,000 (TN)
	100,000	900,000	50,000	950,000	10,000	990,000
Sensitivity $\frac{(TP)}{(TP + FN)}$	90%		90%		90%	
Specificity $\frac{(TN)}{(TN + FP)}$	80%		80%		80%	
PPV $\frac{(TP)}{(TP + FP)}$	0.333		0.191		0.043	
NPV $\frac{(TN)}{(TN + FN)}$	0.986		0.986		0.999	

TP = true positive, FP = false positive, TN = true negative, FN = false negative, PPV = positive predictive value, NPV = negative predictive value

what are the chances that a positive result means that you really have a certain condition?). In order to answer that question in this particular case, please look at Exhibit 3.1, Scenario 1.

Assume you are screening 1 million people in your target population. You know that the disease prevalence (true positives plus false negatives) is 10%, or 100,000. You also know that the test's sensitivity is 90% and its specificity is 80%. Based on that information, you should be able to construct a 2 × 2 matrix as shown in Scenario 1. Now, back to the original question: If you do not know if you have the mutation and your test comes back positive, what is the likelihood that you really are affected? The answer can be calculated using the following formula:

True Positives ÷ (True Positives + False Positives) = Positive Predictive Value

In this case, a positive test tells you that you have a 1 in 3 chance (0.333) of having the mutation.

What if you would be just as satisfied knowing if you *didn't* have the mutation? If your test is negative, how confident are you that you are not affected? Answering this latter question involves calculating the *negative predictive value* of the test. It is calculated according to the following formula:

True Negatives ÷ (True Negatives + False Negatives) = Negative Predictive Value

Using the numbers provided in Scenario 1, you can see that the test is excellent at ruling out the mutation if you have a negative result (0.986; i.e., 98.6% likelihood that one is not affected).

Now that you have an idea about the test's capability, you really want to know more about its potential market. You ask the VP of R&D if she is *really* certain that 10% of the population is affected. She hedges a bit and says that what she really meant was that *up to* 10% of the population might have mutation. She says the company's epidemiologists estimate that anywhere from 1% to 10% of the population may have the mutation. The next question that you want to ask is: If the mutation prevalence is less than 10%, does it affect the test characteristics and, hence, the ability to market the device? The VP of R&D first assures you that the sensitivity and specificity are unchanged by the prevalence of the mutation in the population, since sensitivity and specificity are innate characteristics of the test. This statement is correct. The positive predictive value and negative predictive value, however, can change *substantially* with a different prevalence. In order to understand what those differences are, you calculate two more scenarios, using 5% and 1% prevalences. Again, you can use a survey size of the same 1 million people. (Please see Exhibit 3.1, Scenarios 2 and 3 for the results of those calculations.) When comparing positive and negative predictive values across the three prevalences, two results should be obvious. First, the *higher* the prevalence of a condition in a population, the higher will be a test's positive predictive value. Second, the *lower* the prevalence of a condition in a population, the higher will be a test's negative predictive value.

Knowing what you now know about these testing concepts, you can more effectively design a marketing campaign. For example, if the marketing strategy involves direct-to-consumer advertising, you may want to focus on the fact that if the results of a person's test are negative, the person can be nearly certain that he or she does not have the particular genetic mutation. This strategy is very different from one where you tell people to have the test performed so the mutation could be detected.

Other examples for the use of these methods are mammography, stress tests for coronary artery disease screening, and prostate specific antigen (PSA) for prostate cancer screening.

CLINICAL STUDY DESIGNS

Using the terms and concepts mentioned above, as well as the tools from studies of probability and statistics, three major study designs used in epidemiology are now presented. It is important to note that these methods are the same ones that are used extensively in the pharmaceutical and biotech sectors.

Case Control Studies

Case control studies are sometimes called *retrospective observational studies* because they look at affected persons in the present and then search the past to find out if those people had an *exposure* different from those who are unaffected. We refer to those who are affected as *cases* and those who are unaffected as *controls*. You should be aware that there is no value judgment assigned to cases versus controls. For example, with regard to tobacco use, cases may represent those who have lung cancer and, therefore, are worse off than controls who do not have cancer. On the other hand, cases can be healthier than controls; for example, cases could be those who do not have heart disease, and controls could be those who have had heart attacks.

Now that you understand the concept of a case, consider the control population. In all types of study designs, one wants to eliminate as many variables as possible and focus on the exposure being studied. Therefore, the control population should be as similar as possible to the cases with respect to such factors as age, gender, geographic location, race, socioeconomic status, income, and educational level, to name a few. One also needs enough cases and controls to be able to infer a statistical difference between those populations. (More will be discussed later about the importance of large numbers in this type of study.)

In considering the word "exposure," one usually thinks of some environmental toxin, such as radiation, toxic waste, or tobacco smoke. Remember, however, that cases need not be worse off than controls. Exposure can also mean that one population exercised more, ate a better diet, used a drug, or had a particular genetic mutation.

Please see Exhibit 3.2 for a schematic representation of the case control method. From this study design, it should be obvious that anyone involved in this type of research will fall into one of the four categories in the matrix presented in Exhibit 3.3.

Given this background material, the question we really want to answer is this: Is there any difference between cases and controls due to the exposure being studied? The numerical answer to this question is called the *relative risk*: Incidence of cases ÷ Incidence of controls. A relative risk >1 implies the exposure causes more cases to occur than controls; likewise, if the relative risk is <1, the exposure may lower the rate of cases compared to the control population. A relative risk = 1 obviously means there is no difference between the groups. In order to accurately determine the relative risk, one needs to factor out the

EXHIBIT 3.2. **Case Control Study Design**

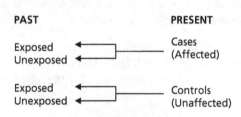

PAST	PRESENT
Exposed	Cases
Unexposed	(Affected)
Exposed	Controls
Unexposed	(Unaffected)

EXHIBIT 3.3. **Case Control Study Matrix**

	CASES	CONTROLS
Exposed	a	c
Unexposed	b	d

natural occurrence of the condition being studied (i.e., the occurrence without the exposure); therefore, one needs to know such factors as the incidence of the condition in the general population *as well as* the incidences in both cases and controls. Remember that incidence is the number of *new* events occurring over a specified time period (such as the length of the study). With this design, however, we do not always know the exact duration, magnitude, or timing of the exposure or when the condition being observed occurred (e.g., when did the cancer start or when did high blood pressure develop: viz. when did the "case became a case."). All we know is that an exposure occurred in the past and at present we have a certain number of cases. We also need to know the general incidence to make sure the sample size is adequate to detect differences between cases and controls.

Because of these problems, we can only *estimate* the relative risk using this type of study. This estimate of relative risk in a case control study is called the *odds ratio*. Referring to Exhibit 3.3, the odds ratio is calculated according to the following formula: ad ÷ bc. This formula should make some intuitive sense. The ideal result of a case control study is that all cases should have been exposed and none of the controls will have been exposed ("a" and "d," respectively). Likewise, in the ideal situation, almost none of the cases ("b") will have been unexposed and very few of the controls ("c") will have been exposed.[3]

Now that you understand some of the mechanics of a case control study, we can summarize some of the drawbacks and benefits of conducting this and other types of observational research.

Problems with Observational Research

Measurement Bias. For the reasons stated above, one cannot precisely calculate the relative risk in this type of study but can only estimate it through calculation of the odds ratio.

Selection Bias. It is important that both cases and controls have an equal probability of being selected for the study. Often, however, the method or place of selection will favor one or the other group. For example, studying a hospitalized population with respect to response rates to blood pressure medication may yield a very different sample profile than conducting the same survey from a group drawn from physician offices.

Classification of Exposure. As mentioned above, it is often very difficult for the researcher to ascertain, or the individual to recall, such factors as the timing, nature, duration, or magnitude of exposure. Within this category, *recall bias* is often cited as a major problem with observational research.

Determination of Endpoints. In conducting observational research, we have to ask: Is the endpoint we are measuring a valid indicator? Also, is it truly an *end*point or merely a transitional stage? More will be mentioned about this issue in the discussion of the randomized control trial below.

---

[3]The odds ratio is a good approximation of the relative risk *only* when the incidence of the outcome you are studying in a particular population is low (i.e., < 10%). When the outcome is more frequent, the odds ratio will overestimate the relative risk when it is more than one or underestimate the risk when it is less than one. See: Zhang, J., & Yu, K. F. (1998). What's the relative risk? A method of correcting the odds ratio in cohort studies of common outcomes. *JAMA*, 280, 1690–1691.

Confounding Factors. When considering this problem, we need to ask: Are there factors other than the exposure we are studying that could contribute to our results? For example, if we found in a particular population that cases with heart disease had a poorer diet, we may have missed that the incidence of cigarette smoking in the population was also higher than that of controls.

Chance. As in any other type of study with observational research, we would like to know: What is the chance that differences between cases and controls could be attributable to chance alone? Answering this question involves the calculation of *p* values.

Causality. While research studies can very strongly imply that there is a *correlation* between exposure and the appearance of a case, proving *causality* is often difficult or impossible and often must be inferred. Causality becomes more likely when one or more criteria in Exhibit 3.4 are satisfied.

Benefits to Employing Observational Research

Given all these problems, why do we bother at all with doing case control studies? The several benefits are listed below.

Hypothesis Generation. Sometimes we would like to know whether there is an association between an exposure and a given condition. Given the possibility of this association, we may be able to design a more rigorous experimental protocol to prove causality.

Removal of Multiple Confounding Factors. Sometimes there are so many confounding factors, both known and unknown, that removing them from the study design becomes nearly impossible. Many epidemiologists believe that if you use large enough populations and appropriately assign cases and controls, the effect of these confounding factors becomes relatively negligible. If the resultant relative risk estimate (odds ratio) is moderate to large

EXHIBIT 3.4. **Evidence That an Association Is More Likely Causal**

Criterion	Comments
Temporality	Cause precedes effect
Strength	Large relative risk
Dose-response	Higher exposure associated with higher rate of effect
Reversibility	Reducing exposure lowers risk of disease
Consistency	Similar results in different studies in different places, time, etc.
Plausibility	Makes sense

Source: Philip Greenland, M.D. Director, Institute for Public Health and Medicine, Center for Population Health Sciences, Harry W. Dingman Professor of Cardiology, Northwestern University. Personal communication. Used with permission.

(e.g., greater than 1.5), then there is a fairly good likelihood that the exposure is causal and not caused by confounding factors.

Ethical Considerations. Because of ethical considerations, some problems cannot be rigorously researched using an experimental design. For example, we cannot expose one population to potentially harmful toxins and then compare that group to those who have not been exposed. It is noteworthy that tobacco industry executives always argued that no controlled experimental research existed to prove that tobacco use causes lung cancer and other diseases. Their contention was that all of the "evidence" was based on case control studies and were therefore subject to the problems mentioned above. The executives obviously knew that it is ethically impossible to conduct clinical trials to prove that tobacco use substantially adds to the population's morbidity and mortality.

Study of Rare Diseases or Results. If an outcome is rare, in order to obtain statistical significance compared to a controlled population, one must include very large numbers in a study. It may be very difficult to find enough cases in a general population to do a controlled trial so that useful inferences can be obtained. Instead, starting with cases of a known, rare condition, a case control trial can be conducted so that one may at least be able to draw appropriate hypotheses.

Cost. For some of the reasons listed above, large numbers of enrollees are often necessary to obtain valid results. Rigorously conducted, randomized controlled trials (explained below) can therefore often cost billions of dollars. Case control studies can frequently be conducted for substantially less.

Cohort Study

As mentioned above, the case control method focuses on the occurrence of cases in the general population at present and then looks for exposures in the past. The cohort study, by contrast, begins with an investigation of the *exposure* and then determines its consequence. The classic type of cohort study is done prospectively. Two populations, one exposed and the other unexposed, are followed over time and, at certain endpoints, one or more outcomes are assessed. The scheme for this type of investigation is displayed in Exhibit 3.5.

EXHIBIT 3.5. **Prospective Cohort Study**

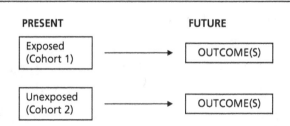

The most famous of these investigations is the Framingham Heart Study, which started in 1948 and is still ongoing with third-generation participants. These participants did not have cardiovascular disease (CVD) at the start; the purpose of the study is to follow them and discover the major factors that lead to its development. The study

> led to the identification of major CVD risk factors, as well as valuable information on the effects of these factors such as blood pressure, blood triglyceride and cholesterol levels, age, gender, and psychosocial issues. Risk factors for other physiological conditions such as dementia have been and continue to be investigated. In addition, the relationships between physical traits and genetic patterns are being studied.[4]

Another type of cohort study uses the retrospective method depicted in Exhibit 3.6. Using this research design, exposed and unexposed cohorts are identified in the past and one or more outcomes are assessed in the present. Note that with the cohort study, the terms "exposed" and "unexposed" have the same meaning as they did in the case control method.

Since the cohort study method focuses on measuring exposures, we can more precisely compute the incidence of the outcomes in the exposed and unexposed populations. Therefore, instead of indirectly estimating the relative risk using an odds ratio, we can calculate it. (Please see Exhibit 3.7.)

As we saw with the case control method, there are four possible outcomes in a cohort study. Exposed individuals may or may not develop an outcome; likewise, unexposed individuals may or may not be affected. The incidence, therefore, of those who are exposed and develop the outcome is: $a \div (a + c)$. The incidence of those who did not have the exposure but did show the outcome is: $b \div (b + d)$. The relative risk of the occurrence of the outcome for those exposed compared to those who are unexposed is therefore: (incidence of the outcome in the exposed cohort) ÷ (incidence of the outcome in the unexposed cohort).

Interpretation of the possible numerical results is the same as explained in the case control study method: relative risks >1 tend to indicate the exposure causes the outcome, values <1 imply the exposure prevents the outcome, and values = 1 imply the exposure has no effect on the outcome.

EXHIBIT 3.6. **Retrospective Cohort Study**

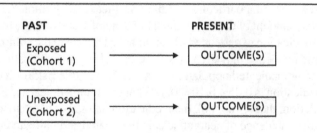

---

[4] About the Framingham Heart Study. Retrieved May 1, 2018 from https://www.framinghamheartstudy.org/fhs-about

EXHIBIT 3.7. **Relative Risk Calculation**

OUTCOME

	YES	NO
Exposed	a	c
Unexposed	b	d

Incidence of outcome in exposed cohort = a ÷ (a + c)
Incidence of outcome in unexposed cohort = b ÷ (b + d)
Relative risk = incidence in exposed cohort ÷ incidence in unexposed cohort

Since the cohort study allows us to measure the incidence of outcomes in the exposed and unexposed populations and enables us to directly calculate the relative risk, we can get even more information from this type of study. For example, we can answer the question: What *percentage* of people in the population have an outcome that is due to the exposure? The answer to this question involves calculation of the *attributable fraction*. It is calculated according to the following formula:

$$[f (RR - 1)] \div [f (RR - 1) + 1] \times 100 = \% \text{ attributable to the exposure}$$

where f = fraction of the entire population who are exposed and RR = relative risk.

Using incidence data, we can also determine how *many* cases in the population are due to the exposure. This number, called the *attributable risk*, is calculated by subtracting the incidence of the disease in the unexposed group from the incidence in the exposed population. The formula is:

$$[a \div (a + c)] - [b \div (b + d)] = \text{Attributable Risk}$$

An example will illustrate how a cohort study can be used. Assume that you are working for a pharmaceutical company that is conducting a trial on a medication to see whether it prevented heart attacks in a particular population. (Please see Exhibit 3.8.)

After a certain amount of time, you find that 50 out of 1,000 of these high-risk people who have taken the medication experienced a heart attack. The rate in the control population is 200 out of 2,000. The incidence of heart attack for those taking the medication is, therefore, 0.05 while that of the unmedicated population is 0.10. The relative risk for having a heart attack while on the medication is 0.05 ÷ 0.10 = 0.5. What this number means is that compared to the untreated population, those who took the medication had fewer heart attacks (RR < 1). If we look at the relative incidence of heart attacks in the treated and untreated population, we find

EXHIBIT 3.8. **Example of Results of a Heart Attack Outcome Study**

	YES	NO
Medication (Exposed)	50	950
No Medication (Unexposed)	200	1800

Incidence on medication = 50 ÷ (50 + 950) = .05
Incidence without medication = 200 ÷ (200 + 1800) = .10
Relative Risk = .05 ÷ .10 = 0.5
Attributable risk = .05 − .10 = −.05
Attributable fraction = $\dfrac{.50\,(.50-1)}{.50\,(.50-1)+1} \times 100 = 33\%$
(where $f = .50$)

that the attributable risk is: $0.05 - 0.10 = -0.05$. What this number means is that 5 out of every 100 heart attacks in this population could be prevented if everyone took this medication. Let's assume, however, that only half of the people who would benefit from this medication will actually take it (reasons range from tolerability to affordability). In this case, the fraction of the exposed population (i.e., the fraction who can or does take the medication) is 0.5. Using this number, we can calculate the attributable fraction using the formula in Exhibit 3.8. We find, therefore, that if only 50% of the people in this population can take the medication, a 33% reduction in heart attacks will occur.

Because of the design method, the cohort study design has the following advantages:

- Unlike the case control method, you can directly measure the relative and attributable risks.

- Because the exposure is the focus of the investigation, you know its exact nature, timing, strength, and duration.

- Because you know the exposure came before the outcome, it is easier to hypothesize causality than with a case control study.

- Because a cohort study is designed to gather information regarding an exposure, recall bias is minimized.

- This type of study design can measure multiple outcomes.

The cohort study method, however, also has some drawbacks. These drawbacks are mainly related to the long amount of time that is necessary to determine outcomes, particularly in a well-designed prospective study. This length of time not only delays knowledge about outcomes but causes the study to be much more costly than the case control method. Also, because of the length of the study, a sample bias may be induced that is due to those who drop out before it is completed. A self-selection bias can also occur since those who choose an exposure may vary in one or more characteristics from those who do not; those characteristics can influence the outcome. For example, people who consume more beta-carotene may be more likely to take better care of themselves, smoke less, get regular preventive exams, and so on, and thus will be less likely to develop or die from certain malignancies. If one is not aware of these factors, it may appear that beta-carotene lowers the risk of certain cancers. Finally, because of the limitation in number of enrollees and a design that targets exposures and not outcomes, this type of study is not well suited to investigation of rare diseases.

Randomized Controlled Trial

The hallmark of the randomized controlled trial (RCT) is randomization of the intervention. What this statement means is that each participant in the study has an equal chance of being assigned to either the intervention group or the control group. (Please see Exhibit 3.9 for a representation of this study design.)

Unlike the other types of studies that were discussed above, in the RCT, subjects do not have a choice of the groups into which they are assigned, and the investigator takes a much more active role in determining the study design (protocol) of the trial. What makes this type of design the gold standard among research projects is that it enables the investigator to control for more of the confounding variables than is possible with the other types of research studies. For example, properly done randomization will eliminate selection bias by both subjects and investigators.

It is important to note from Exhibit 3.9 that the outcomes of an RCT are often called endpoints. The reason for making this distinction is that these endpoints are not always the same as outcomes in the other types of studies. For example, the endpoint of a pharmaceutical study might be normalization of blood cholesterol levels or blood pressure measurements. However, these studies may not measure the ultimate desired outcome, which is the reduction of stroke or heart attack rates in the intervention group compared to the control population. It should also be noted that since one can calculate the incidences of these endpoints with the same precision as in a cohort study, the calculation of relative risk can be performed as was previously explained.

In the classic type of RCT, the intervention is compared to a no-treatment group. The purpose of this design is to provide information about whether or not treatment is safer and

EXHIBIT 3.9. **Randomized Control Trial Study Design**

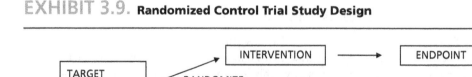

better than no treatment. In the case of pharmaceuticals, it is often easy to formulate a pill that closely resembles the appearance and taste of the experimental medication. This type of pill, called a placebo, however, is inert. It is not always possible, though, to compare an intervention with a placebo. The obvious example would be a surgical intervention, though sham operations had been used in the past to determine the efficacy of certain surgical procedures. Another reason that using a placebo might not be possible is for ethical reasons. For example, we cannot withhold appropriate antibiotic treatments for patients who are gravely ill from bacterial infections. In this latter case, investigators may use historical controls, or the control population can be comprised of a group using standard therapies.

In a further refinement of the RCT, the intervention and control groups are switched after a certain period, called the *washout time*, where neither receives the intervention; the intervention group then becomes the control group and the control group receives the intervention. This type of trial is called a *cross-over study*. An example might be where the intervention group initially receives a medication for treatment of mild, chronic pain with the desired endpoint being pain control. The control group would receive a placebo. After a certain amount of time where neither receive an intervention, the intervention group would receive the placebo and the control group would receive the test medication. In a study where the test subjects do not know what type of medicine they are receiving, but the evaluators do, the trial is called *single blinded*; where neither the test subjects nor the evaluators know which medication a given individual is receiving, the trial is called *double blinded*. Blinded studies are obviously easy with pharmaceutical agents; for methodological as well as ethical reasons, it is virtually impossible to blind a surgical procedure.

Results of RCTs can be complicated by the *placebo effect*. It has long been known that using placebos can achieve the results desired by the intervention. For example, in a study of headaches in children, "[p]lacebo was effective in reducing headaches. Other commonly used drugs have no evidence supporting their use in children and adolescents."[5] Further, this beneficial effect can occur even if the patient is aware that the treatment is a placebo.[6]

Since RCTs can require a large number of enrollees to achieve statistical significance, which is expensive, researchers have frequently combined many small randomized studies to get meaningful information. Special statistical techniques are required to ensure the validity of the results from these combined studies. To address this issue, in 1976 Glass coined the term "meta-analysis" to mean "the statistical analysis of a large collection of analysis results from individual studies for the purpose of integrating the findings."[7] In some cases, this analysis of many studies can give useful information where the individual reports lacked sufficient statistical power. However, it should be noted that this type of analysis may combine RCTs that have different protocols and are thus not directly comparable.

---

[5]El-Chammas, K., Keyes, J., Thompson, N., Vijayakumar, J., Becher, D., & Jackson, J. L. (2013). Pharmacologic treatment of pediatric headaches: A meta-analysis. *JAMA Pediatrics*, 67(3), 250–258.
[6]See, for example: Kaptchuk T. J., Friedlander, E., Kelley, J. M., Sanchez, M. N., Kokkotou, E., Singer, J. P., ... Lembo, A. J. (2010). Placebos without deception: A randomized controlled trial in irritable bowel syndrome. *PLoS One*, 5(12), e15591. Retrieved from http://journals.plos.org/plosone/article?id=10.1371/journal.pone.0015591
[7]Glass, G. V. (1976). Primary, secondary and meta-analysis of research. *Educational Researcher*, 10, 3–8.

SUMMARY

The tools and concepts of epidemiology can provide valuable benefits to those in healthcare management beyond the public health sector. Many of these concepts are not at first obvious and must be used and reviewed often to derive their full benefits. The rewards can be not only successful products and services but avoidance of costly and dangerous ventures.

CHAPTER

4

HOSPITALS AND
HEALTHCARE SYSTEMS

BIRON.

　　And what to me, my love? and what to me?

ROSALINE.

　　You must be purged too, your sins are rack'd,

　　You are attaint with faults and perjury:

　　Therefore if you my favour mean to get,

　　A twelvemonth shall you spend, and never rest,

　　But seek the weary beds of people sick . . .

BIRON.

　　A twelvemonth! well; befall what will befall,

　　I'll jest a twelvemonth in an hospital.

　　　　　　　—William Shakespeare, *Love's Labour's Lost*, Act 5, Scene 2

A BRIEF HISTORY OF WESTERN HOSPITALS

For a great part of recorded history, care of the ill and injured has been provided in either the patient's home or where the "healer" practiced his/her art. The word "hospital" comes from the Latin *hospes* (host); its usage referring to a place to care for sick and injured is rather modern. In fact, the *Oxford English Dictionary* (*OED*) gives the first definition to the oldest meaning of the word and current usage to its third reference:

1.　A house or hostel for the reception and entertainment of pilgrims, travelers, and strangers; a hospice. Hence, one of the establishments of the Knights Hospitallers . . .

3a.　An institution or establishment for the care of the sick or wounded, or of those who require medical treatment. (The current sense.) Such institutions are either public or private, free or paying, —or combined, —general or special with respect to the diseases treated.

　　The ancestor of Western[1] hospitals is generally considered to be the temples of Asclepius (Aesculapius in Latin),[2] the Greek god of medicine and healing. While a temple at Titanus

---

[1]Considerable evidence exists for ancient institutions in the Middle East and India; however, their relationship to the foundations of healthcare institutions in the United States is not as direct. Therefore, the focus here will be on Western institutions.

[2]The Staff of Aesculapius (a single snake wound around a staff) often signifies the profession of medicine. For example, this symbol is on the logo of the American Medical Association. Medicine is often erroneously represented by the caduceus, which is two snakes wound around each other and separated by a staff; this symbol belongs to Hermes (Mercury), the messenger and god of commerce. The U.S. military uses the caduceus as a designation for its healthcare personnel.

is said to have existed since 1134 BCE,[3] the cult of Aesculapius was founded in the fifth century BCE in Epidaurus (Greece) before spreading to other sites around the Greek and Roman empires.[4] Patients went to a temple and slept there overnight, often with the aid of a soporific, such as opium.[5] In the morning, the temple priests would interpret dreams and recommend cures. Evidence also exists that actual procedures were performed there: "Three large marble boards dated to 350 BC preserve the names, case histories, complaints, and cures of about 70 patients who came to the temple with a problem and shed it there . . . such as the opening of an abdominal abscess or the removal of traumatic foreign material."[6]

These temple practices were adopted by the Romans as that empire grew. The first permanently constructed *secular* hospitals (*valetudinaria*) were built as parts of Roman forts in strategic locations in order to treat sick and injured soldiers. The first *valetudinarium* was built about 100 BCE at Carnuntum (near Vienna).[7] In addition to these permanent structures, field hospitals were also established closer to combat lines. What is noteworthy about these places of care is that they were administered by junior military officers (*optio valetudinarii*) rather than physicians or priests; thus, these officers were the first lay hospital administrators.

The establishment of hospitals for general public use originated with the spread of Christianity, particularly after Roman Emperor Galerius' Edict of Serdica (Edict of Toleration) in 311 CE ordered religious tolerance for Christians. As the religion became more prevalent, shelters (*xenodochia*) for travelers and for messengers between bishops were established. These shelters were primarily housed in monasteries, where care for the poor and sick was also provided. The word "xenodochia" became synonymous with what we now would call a hospital.[8] Further, these monasteries grew herbs and medicinal plants, becoming the foundation of the first hospital-based pharmacies.

The First Council of Nicaea in 325 CE encouraged further diffusion of these institutions when it ordered the construction of a hospital in every cathedral town. In order to abolish pagan competition from the still-extant Aesculapian temples, in 331 CE Constantine ordered their closure.

Until this time, hospitals had been set up with religious or governmental sponsorship. The first privately funded hospital is generally recognized to have been established in 390 CE

---

[3]Dates will be referenced here in the format of archaeological scholarship. BCE refers to before the common era and CE refers to the common era: BC and AD, respectively. When no suffix appears, the date is CE.

[4]MacEachern, M. T. (1949). *Hospital organization and management* (2nd ed.). Berwyn, IL: Physicians Record.

[5]Askitopoulou, H., Konsolaki, E., Ramoutsaki, I. A., & Anastassaki, M. (2002). Surgical cures by sleep induction as the Asclepieion of Epidaurus. In J. C. Diz, A. Franco, D. R. Bacon, J. Rupreht, & J. Alvarez (Eds.), *The history of anesthesia: Proceedings of the fifth international symposium.* Elsevier Science B.V., International Congress Series, 1242, 11–17.

[6]MacEachern, M. T. (1949). *Hospital organization and management* (2nd ed.). op. cit.

[7]Retief, F. P., & Cilliers, L. (2005). The evolution of hospitals from antiquity to the renaissance. *Acta Theologica Supplementum*, 7, 213–232.

[8]The place in the monastery where the monks cared for the sick may have been the same rooms set aside for their own brothers. The place was called the *infirmarium*, from whence we get the word "infirmary," another term that has been used for "hospital."

by a penitent, wealthy Roman woman named Fabiola (later, St. Fabiola) who became a disciple of St. Jerome. (This type of facility is now sometimes called a voluntary hospital, after the voluntary nature of contributions to establish it.) According to St. Jerome's eulogy for Fabiola: "Et primo omnium νοσοκομεῖν instituit, in quo aegrotantes colligeret de plateis et consumpta languoribus atque inedia miserorum membra refoveret." [And first of everyone, established a nosocomiun in which she brought together the sick from the streets, to restore the wretched whose limbs were consumed by disease of weakness and destroyed by starvation.][9] Fabiola thus also founded a tradition of religious women caring for the sick in hospitals.

After the fall of Rome in 476 and the beginning of the so-called Dark Ages, monastic stewardship of hospitals continued for the next six to seven centuries.

Religion continued to be the dominant influence in the proliferation of hospitals during the Middle Ages, and their establishment accelerated during the Crusades. Starting at the end of the 11th century, hospitals and orders of knights were established throughout Europe to care for the sick and injured on the path to and from Jerusalem. One of the most famous is the Hospitallers of the Order of St. John, which founded a hospital in the Holy Land for 2,000 patients in 1099. The order has come down to us today as the St. John Ambulance Corps in Britain and some of its former colonies.

These institutions received further stimulus in 1198 when Pope Innocent III encouraged establishment of Hospitals of the Holy Spirit (Santo Spirito) in major towns. Some of their cost was covered by church-levied commercial taxes.[10]

Hospitals as places of learning and patient care by *nonreligious* medical practitioners started in the 12th and 13th centuries with several events. First, a church edict of 1163 forbade clergy from performing operations where blood was shed. This action eliminated many centuries of clerical practice, though administration of medications was still allowed. Into this void stepped a few skilled surgeons with university training; but it was mostly less well educated barber surgeons who bled patients, lanced abscesses, and removed teeth.[11] Second, schools of medicine were established and affiliated with hospitals. Finally, this age was the dawn of medical licensure, when a physician was required to show competence by examination before local medical school professors or appointees of the towns. Training to obtain this competence was partially achieved in hospitals.

The Western system most relevant to American hospitals is that of the United Kingdom (particularly England and Scotland). Like most of Europe, until the 16th century, British hospitals were primarily religious institutions run by monks. When Henry VIII established

---

[9]St. Jerome: *Ad Oceanum De Morte Fabiolae. Epistula lxxvii*. Retrieved November 15, 2011 from http://www.perseus.tufts.edu/hopper/text?doc=Perseus%3Atext%3A2008.01.0566%3Aletter%3D77 The Greek word translates as "nosocomiun," a term for a small Roman-type hospital. From this word we derive "nosocomial," which refers to conditions or events that occur in a hospital (e.g., nosocomial infections). Source of the Latin translation is Professor Heather Vincent, Eckerd College.

[10]MacEachern, M. T., *Hospital organization and management*. op. cit.

[11]The red-striped barber pole, simulating blood running down an arm, is a reminder of their trade.

the Church of England, he also eliminated the monasteries. MacEachern[12] describes what happened next:

> The previous years of association with the Catholic Church caused hospitals to be objects of spoliation by the crown, and Henry VIII ordered them to be given over to secular uses or destroyed. The sick were turned into the streets. Conditions became so intolerable that the Londoners petitioned the king to return to them one or two of the buildings for the care of patients, pledging financial support. Henry acceded and restored St. Bartholomew's in 1544... but in other parts of England, hospitals were forced to close their doors... In fact, twenty-three of the principle counties had no general hospitals until 1710.

After that time, privately funded, charity hospitals started to be built, most notably, the Westminster Hospital in 1719, Guy's Hospital in 1724, and the London Hospital in 1740. Admission to such hospitals often required the patient to obtain a ticket from a trustee testifying to the bearer's good character.

Following the European pattern, religious sponsorship was responsible for the first hospitals in the Western Hemisphere;[13] however, the British secular hospital system is the one that early settlers brought with them to what would become the United States.

In 1663, a hospital for soldiers was established on Manhattan Island, apparently the first such institution on American soil. The first nonmilitary American hospital is considered to be the Philadelphia General Hospital (1732), descended from an almshouse founded in 1713 by William Penn for the benefit of Quakers. New York's Bellevue Hospital (now affiliated with New York University) was founded in 1736 and holds the claim to be America's oldest public hospital. The legal and structural prototype for subsequent institutions, however, is the Pennsylvania Hospital in Philadelphia, the first incorporated hospital in the United States. This hospital, which still operates as part of the University of Pennsylvania, was established with the help of Benjamin Franklin (who also contributed to its design). It received its charter from the English king in 1751 and opened to the public in 1755. As was the case with the London Hospital, moral worthiness and political connections often determined who could be admitted. According to Rosenberg:[14]

> One of the fundamental motivations in founding America's first hospitals was an unquestioned distinction between the worthy and unworthy poor... Thus, it was only natural that the Pennsylvania Hospital should, in the late 18th century, have demanded a written testimonial from a "respectable" person attesting to the moral worth of an applicant before he or she could be admitted to a bed.

---

[12]MacEachern, M. T., *Hospital organization and management*. op. cit.

[13]The first hospital in the Americas was the Hospital San Nicolás de Bari in Santo Domingo. It was authorized on December 29, 1503, by Fray Nicolás de Ovando, Spanish governor and colonial administrator (1502–1509). Like its European counterparts, it was also affiliated with a church (the first built of stone in the Americas). Due to earthquakes in the 19th century, it is now in ruins. The earliest, still-extant hospital in the Americas was founded in 1524 by Conquistador Hernán Cortés: the Immaculate Conception Hospital, now the Hospital de Jesús Nazareno in Mexico City.

[14]Rosenberg, C. R. (1987). *The care of strangers, the rise of America's hospital system*. New York: Basic Books, p. 19.

Establishment of other hospitals in major cities followed. They included public, secular institutions (e.g., Massachusetts General Hospital, established in 1811); nonreligious organizations for the benefit of certain nationalities (e.g., New York's French Hospital, established in 1809); and specialty hospitals (e.g., the Boston Lying-In, established in 1832 [now part of Brigham & Women's Hospital in Boston]). Religious hospitals began to proliferate in the 19th century. Particularly noteworthy are Catholic systems that are still prominent, such as those founded by the Sisters of Mercy and Daughters of Charity. Because of religious discrimination, Jewish hospitals started to appear in the mid-19th century, often with names like Jewish Hospital, Mount Sinai, and Beth Israel.[15] Among other functions, these institutions provided a place for Jewish physicians, who were barred from medical staffs elsewhere, to practice medicine.[16] Racial issues also contributed to hospital development in the United States. Care of African Americans was established around three organizational models: general hospitals with a segregated ward (The Georgia Infirmary, 1832); demographically determined, black-controlled hospitals (Freedmen's Hospital, in Washington, DC, 1863); and black-founded hospitals (Provident Hospital and Training School in Chicago, 1891). In addition to providing a site for care, these hospitals were also the place black physicians could practice medicine, as they were excluded from segregated hospital staffs elsewhere.

Despite the long history of these institutions, until the 20th century, not much could be done for patients in hospitals that could not also be accomplished at home. The simple reason was that medical science was not yet sufficiently advanced. In fact, hospitals were still places mostly poor people went for care; the "best" care was delivered at home. Exhibit 4.1 summarizes some of the scientific developments that enabled hospitals to become the preferred and higher quality centers for medical attention.

EXHIBIT 4.1. **Some Technologies That Consolidated Care in Hospitals**

- *Anesthesia.* Crawford Long, MD, used diethyl-ether anesthesia for the first time on 30 March 1842 to remove a neck tumor of a patient in Jefferson, Georgia. Anesthesia allowed longer and safer surgeries.

- *Radiology.* W. C. Roentgen, MD, published *Über eine neue Art von Strahlen* (On a New Kind of Rays) in the *Sitzungsberichte der Physikalisch-Medizinischen Gesellschaft* in Germany in January 1896. His work heralded the practice of radiology.

- *Blood banking.* In 1901, Karl Landsteiner identified three blood groups, A, B, and O (which he called C), and found that transfusions between persons with the same type did not cause agglutination of red blood cells (a transfusion reaction that can be fatal).[a] Based on this finding, the first successful blood transfusion was performed by Reuben Ottenberg at Mount Sinai Hospital in New York in 1907. While the problem of incompatibility had been clarified, transfusions were not helpful unless a person was on hand who could

---

[15]The first Jewish hospitals in the United States were the Jewish Hospital in Cincinnati (1850) and the Jews' Hospital in New York City (1855), later renamed Mt. Sinai.

[16]Katz, R. (2008). Continuing their mission, Jewish hospitals continue to invest in philanthropy. *The Forward* (June 18). Retrieved May 2, 2018 from http://www.forward.com/articles/13591

donate enough blood of the same type as that of the patient. In 1915, Richard Lewisohn, also at Mount Sinai Hospital, used sodium citrate to keep blood from coagulating, and Richard Weil demonstrated the feasibility of refrigerated storage of anticoagulated blood. Two years later, during World War I, Oswald Hope Robertson used these storage techniques to found what is recognized as the first blood bank.

- *Laboratory*. Diagnostic laboratory tests (particularly examination of urine) were performed in ancient Egypt. Physicians conducted simple tests at the patient's bedside while more complex ones were carried out in a chemistry lab. It was only after the mid-20th century, with advent of sophisticated and expensive automated analyzers, that hospital laboratories were the main focus of such studies.

  Examination of tissue removed from a patient for diagnostic purposes took on clinical significance only after the latter half of the 19th century, when special stains were developed to identify different normal and abnormal cellular structures. The tissue processing was carried out in a hospital laboratory. Subsequent introduction of immunochemical and electron microscopic studies consolidated the role of the hospital laboratory in high-technology diagnostics.

- *Professional nursing*. While Dr. Valentine Seaman at New York Hospital is credited with establishing the first nursing school in the United States (1798), it was in 1872 that the first permanent school was founded at the New England Hospital for Women in Boston.[b] The nursing schools that were created after that time were hospital based and had varying amounts of lecture and scientific content; however, they were all founded on the professional teachings of Florence Nightingale. The Yale School of Nursing, established in 1923, claims to be "the first school within a university to prepare nurses under an educational rather than an apprenticeship program."[c] Professional nursing enables high-quality and technologically enabled attention for critically ill patients, promoting the hospital as a preferred, and often essential, site for provision of care.

- *Aseptic technique*. The importance of cleanliness while performing surgery (particularly hand washing) was known since Ignaz Semmelweis introduced the concept in Vienna in 1847. The scientific basis for this practice was not known until the 1860s, when Louis Pasteur formulated the germ theory of disease. British surgeon Joseph Lister pioneered antiseptic surgery and dressing treatments using carbolic acid in the mid-1860s.[d] Despite the demonstrated benefits of these theories and practices, physicians were very slow to adopt antiseptic methods, making hospitals very dangerous places to have surgery or deliver a baby. In fact, even after Lister presented his scientific findings in Philadelphia at the U.S. Centennial in 1876, many prominent American surgeons were still skeptical of the benefits of his practices. It was only after the 1880s that antiseptic surgery became widespread.[e]

- *Teaching hospitals*. While not all hospitals serve as teaching facilities for medical students and those studying specialties after graduation (residents), the emergence of institutions serving that purpose enhanced the reputation of all hospitals as a safe, high-quality place to obtain care. Although a few such establishments existed in the late 19th century (such as the Hospital of the University of Pennsylvania), it was the newly built Johns Hopkins Hospital (1889), modeled on European teaching institutions, that set the standard. The proliferation of teaching hospitals dates from 1910, when Abraham Flexner published his highly influential report that reformed medical school teaching.[f] Prominent examples built at that time include Peter Bent Brigham Hospital (Harvard) and Barnes Hospital (Washington University).

[a] In 1939, Landsteiner and colleagues discovered another category of blood types (the Rh factor) that was causing unexplained reactions in patients receiving blood from a donor with a compatible ABO match.

[b] Goodnow, M. (1916). *Outlines of nursing history*. Philadelphia: W.B. Saunders.

[c] Yale School of Nursing (2018). About YSN. Retrieved May 2, 2018 from http://nursing.yale.edu/about-ysn

d Lister, J. (1867). Illustrations of the antiseptic system of treatment in surgery. *The Lancet* 90, 668–669.

e Millard, C. (2011). *Destiny of the republic: A tale of madness, medicine and the murder of a president*. NY: Doubleday. The author claims that President Garfield would have survived his assassination attempt were it not for his physician's unsterile probing of his wound, which led to the massive infection that eventually killed him. Aseptic techniques were widely adopted thereafter in the United States.

f Ludmerer, KM. (1983). The rise of the teaching hospital in America. *Journal of the History of Medicine and Allied Sciences* 38, 389–414. Flexner, A. (2002). Medical education in the United States and Canada. From the Carnegie Foundation for the Advancement of Teaching, Bulletin 4, 1910 Bulletin of the World Health Organization, 80, 594–602.

AMERICAN HOSPITAL EXPANSION IN THE 20TH CENTURY

By the early 1900s, hospitals were well established as a desired place for care; their payment sources, however, started to change over the next 50 years.[17] Early in the 20th century, these institutions were still largely philanthropic organizations whose trustees were more than a governing board; they were the financial backers and administrators. With the emergence of commercial insurance in the 1930s and beyond, hospitals started to make more of their money from that source, and the organizational culture shifted from charity care to more of a for-profit model. This trend accelerated after World War II with a substantial increase in coverage by private insurance. In addition to changes in financing, a need arose for construction of more hospital beds,[18] particularly in rural areas. Subsequent government policy to correct this problem was directed at both encouraging construction of more hospitals and adding more beds to existing institutions, thus promoting community hospitals as the centers of the healthcare system. The hope was also that with more rural community hospitals, physician supply in these areas would increase. Hospitals, however, were concerned about how they were going to pay for this construction, especially given the looming possibilities of national health insurance.[19] They also faced the threat of expansion of *government hospital* capacity, thus increasing competition with the private sector. In order to ensure a funding source and continued strength of the private sector, hospitals lobbied the federal government for subsidies. According to Rosemary Stevens, "the instigating force for the hospital construction bill was George Bugbee, the AHA's [American Hospital Association's] executive director."[20] Bugbee successfully garnered bipartisan support for

---

[17] For more details about these events, see the section in Chapter 6, "Origins and Current Status of Private Health Insurance in the United States."

[18] Rufus Rorem highlighted this maldistribution as early as 1930 in *The Public's Investment in Hospitals* (Chicago: University of Chicago Press). Action to address the problem only came after July 1944, when the U.S. Surgeon General, Dr. Thomas Parran, told the Senate Subcommittee on Wartime Health and Education that 1,200 U.S. counties with a population over 15,000 persons had no recognized hospital facilities. He estimated that 419,400 new and replacement beds were needed. The testimony was covered in *JAMA* 125 (12): 856–857, 1944.

[19] President Roosevelt included such a possibility in his "Second Bill of Rights Message," as part of his January 11, 1944, State of the Union Speech when he stated that every family has "the right to adequate medical care and the opportunity to achieve and enjoy good health." He reinforced this message in his January 1945 budget message to Congress. Also in 1945, the Wagner-Murray-Dingell bill included a proposal for a national insurance plan.

[20] Stevens, R. (1989). *In sickness and in wealth, American hospitals in the twentieth century*. New York: Basic Books.

passage in August 1946 of the Hospital Survey and Construction Act (Public Law [P.L.] 79–95), called the Hill-Burton Act, after its sponsors, Senators Lister Hill (D-Alabama) and Harold H. Burton (R-Ohio).[21] It is important to note that the act (passed in the Truman administration) originally had a universal insurance coverage provision, which was eliminated because of anticipated costs.[22] The Hill-Burton program required states to conduct hospital need assessments, formulate construction plans, and build the facilities by contributing $2 for every $1 of federal money.[23] Preference was given to rural facilities and university hospitals that served as referral centers; only governmental and nonprofit facilities were eligible. Funds were also available under this program for other types of healthcare organizations, including skilled-nursing facilities, rehabilitation facilities, nursing schools, and public health centers.

In exchange for funding, recipients had two obligations. First, all facilities were required by the Community Service Assurance of Title VI of the Public Health Service Act "to make services provided by the facility available to persons residing in the facility's service area without discrimination on the basis of race, color, national origin, creed, or any other ground unrelated to the individual's need for the service or the availability of the needed service in the facility."[24] Application of this requirement means that the facility must make emergency services available to *all* patients regardless of their ability to pay. Prior to the enactment of civil rights legislation, the "separate but equal" doctrine was acceptable in fulfillment of this condition.

In addition to the community service requirement, many facilities were also subjected to the "uncompensated care provision." In return for governmental financing, they were "required to develop an uncompensated care allocation plan, indicating the type of services available to persons unable to pay . . . [and] publish a notice of their obligation to provide free medical care in a local newspaper, post notices within their facility, and provide individual notices of the availability of free care to all patients."[25]

The Public Health Service (PHS) determined the total amount of uncompensated care a hospital was required to pay back and prorated it over 20 years, starting with the date of completion of construction of the facility. At least once in 3 years, these institutions are required to report to the Department of Health and Human Services (DHHS) the amount of free care they provide. The PHS could also determine whether the facility can accelerate or extend its payback obligation. Each year, DHHS determines the poverty guidelines that

---

[21] Senator Burton was appointed to the Supreme Court before the bill was introduced. Much of the credit for its passage belongs to the other Ohio senator, Robert Taft.

[22] Mantone, J. (2005, August 15). The big bang: The Hill-Burton Act put hospitals in thousands of communities and launched today's continuing healthcare building boom. *Modern Healthcare, 15*, 35, 6–7, 16

[23] The federal contribution portion increased in subsequent years.

[24] U.S. Office of Civil Rights. (2018). *Medical treatment in Hill-Burton funded healthcare facilities*. See this site for a full list of obligations. Retrieved May 2, 2018 from www.hhs.gov/ocr/civilrights/understanding/Hill-Burton

[25] Department of Health and Human Services Office of Inspector General. (1992, August). *Public health service's oversight of the Hill-Burton program*, 1.

apply to pay-back of Hill-Burton obligations.[26] Of note is that these requirements are very similar to the current community service requirements described below.

> After the enactment of Hill-Burton, more than $4.6 billion in grants and $1.5 billion in loans were allocated to projects that led to the construction of or equipment for roughly 6800 health-care facilities in more than 4000 communities ... The bulk of the funding was provided from 1960 to 1979, with $3.5 billion being issued. From 1980 to 1997, the last time money was issued, $200 million was allocated.[27]

As of December 2011, there were still 181 facilities in 40 states that had Hill-Burton obligations.[28] Virtually all of these facilities are expected to pay back their obligations by 2020.

The results of this program have been somewhat mixed. The program did not achieve the goal of bringing more physicians to underserved areas; but, at best, "the program might have prevented the more deprived areas from falling even farther behind in the availability of doctors."[29] The program was more successful in stimulating hospital construction, particularly in poorer areas. "A nearly complete equalization of bed supplies had occurred by 1970 across states ranked in the lowest, middle and highest thirds for bed supplies in 1950."[30] This benefit was statistically significant even accounting for the country's increase in affluence and the rapid emergence of private health insurance.

After the Hill-Burton Act, the second major financial impetus for hospital construction occurred in 1963 with the issuance of Internal Revenue Service (IRS) Revenue Ruling 63-20, 1963-1 C.B. 24. This ruling allowed private, nonprofit hospitals to issue tax-free bonds. (The implications for this benefit are explained below.) The conditions allowing issuance of such debt are explained in Exhibit 4.2.

EXHIBIT 4.2. IRS Conditions Allowing Issuance of Tax-Exempt Hospital Debt

According to the IRS, 63-20 corporations are formed under state nonprofit law for purposes of issuing obligations on behalf of a political subdivision and must meet five criteria:

1. The corporation must engage in activities which are essentially public in nature.

2. The corporation must be one which is created under the state's general nonprofit corporation law (and is not organized for profit except to the extent of retiring indebtedness).

---

[26] For example, see: U.S. DHHS Program Policy Notice No. 11-02 (revision), March 1, 2011.

[27] Mantone, J. (2005, August 15). The big bang: The Hill-Burton Act put hospitals in thousands of communities and launched today's continuing healthcare building boom. *Modern Healthcare*, 6–7, 16

[28] Health Resources and Services Administration. (2018). *Hill-Burton facilities waiver and recovery*. Retrieved from www.hrsa.gov./gethealthcare/affordable/hillburton/waiver.html

[29] Hochban, J., Ellenbogen, B., Benson, J., & Olson, R. M. (1981). The Hill-Burton program and changes in health services delivery. *Inquiry, 18*, 61–69.

[30] Clark, L. J., Field, M. J., Koontz, T. L., & Koontz, V. L. (1980). The impact of Hill-Burton: An analysis of hospital bed and physician distribution in the United States, 1950–1970. *Medical Care, 18*, 532–550.

3. The corporate income must not inure to any private person.

4. The state or political subdivision thereof must have a "beneficial interest" in the corporation while the indebtedness remains outstanding and it must obtain legal title to the property of the corporation with respect to which the indebtedness was incurred upon the retirement of such indebtedness.

5. The corporation must have been approved by the state or political subdivision thereof, either of which must also have approved the specific obligations issued by the corporation.

The rules for determining whether the governmental unit has the requisite "beneficial interest" in the nonprofit corporation are:

1. The governmental unit must have exclusive beneficial possession and use of at least 95% of the fair market value of the facilities; *or*

2. If the *nonprofit corporation* has exclusive beneficial use and possession of 95% of the fair market value of the facilities, the governmental unit appoints 80% of the members of the board of the corporation and has the power to remove and replace members of the board; *or*

3. The governmental unit has the right at any time to get unencumbered title and exclusive possession of the financed facility by defeasing (paying off or providing for payment of) the bonds.[31]

The third financial spur to hospital growth came when the Medicare program became operational in 1966. Reimbursement for Medicare beneficiaries was based on the costs the hospitals incurred for taking care of them, including allocated capital expenditures and interest payment on debt.[32] These payments made the tax-free financing of facility expansion even cheaper. As explained below, these payments lasted until 1985, when they were fully replaced by payments based on Diagnosis Related Groups (DRGs).

By the mid-1960s, three types of concerns arose from these sponsored expansion activities. The first problem was the uncontrolled proliferation of facilities and lack of coordination of clinical programs. This coordination problem created a barrier to efficient delivery of services and posed an obstacle to tackling issues of national healthcare importance. (Note that this problem persists and is one of the reasons for Accountable Care Organizations [ACOs], described below.) To address this situation, Congress passed P.L. 89-749 on November 3, 1966: "An Act to amend the Public Health Service Act to assist in combating heart disease, cancer, stroke and related diseases."[33] Among the purposes of this law was "[t]hrough grants, to encourage and assist in the establishment of regional cooperative arrangements among medical schools, research institutions, and hospitals for research and training (including continuing education) and for related demonstrations of patient care in the field of heart disease,

---

[31] IRS. *Introduction to Federal Taxation of Municipal Bonds,* B16. Retrieved May 2, 2018 from https://www.irs.gov/pub/irs-tege/teb_phase_1_course_11204_-3module_b.pdf

[32] For an amusing, but clear, explanation of how this financing worked, see: Fisher, G. R. (1979). The hospital that ate Chicago. *New England Journal of Medicine, 301,* 56–57.

[33] Public Laws Enacted During the Second Session of the Eighty-Ninth Congress of the United States. PL 89-749. Government Printing Office, pp. 1180–1190. November 3, 1966. Retrieved May 2, 2018 from http://uscode.house.gov/statutes/pl/89/749.pdf

cancer, stroke, and related diseases." The grants established 56 Regional Medical Programs (RMPs), which were cooperative arrangements "among a group of public or nonprofit private institutions or agencies engaged in research, training, diagnosis, and treatment relating to heart disease, cancer, or stroke." This law was refunded and renewed in 1970 with

> new provisions [that] reflected an emphasis on primary care and regionalization of health care resources; added prevention and rehabilitation services; added kidney disease treatment programs; *added authority for new construction*; *required review of RMP applications by Area-wide Comprehensive Planning agencies* [emphasis added]; and emphasized health services delivery and human resource utilization.[34]

The National Health Planning and Resource Development Act of 1974, P.L. 93-641, consolidated RMPs with the Hill-Burton and Comprehensive Health Planning federal programs. The main purpose of the new law was to mandate a nationwide program of state-based Certificate of Need (CON) reviews to evaluate the necessity for new facility expansion, particularly projects that used federal funds. The object of CON regulations is to set criteria for expansion of health facilities in order to prevent their unregulated growth. The fear regulators had was that this type of growth caused healthcare costs to rise rapidly and prevented coordination and cooperation among existing organizations. By the late 1970s, all states had CON initiatives in place.

The second concern came from the hospital industry: fear about increased competition coming from new facilities. Because of this worry, states adopted hospital association-initiated CON reviews at the same time the federal government drafted its legislation. New York became the first state to enact a CON law in 1964, followed 5 years later by California, Connecticut, Maryland, and Rhode Island. Other states followed, linking their efforts with federally initiated health planning agencies.[35]

The results of reviews of these activities have been quite mixed, particularly because of the state-by-state differences in the types of institutions that are reviewed as well as the specific methodologies.

> Several older studies concluded that CON regulations have either had minimal or no direct effect on healthcare expenditures. Recent studies have found that CON regulations appear to raise the volume of procedures and average cost for specific services like cardiac and cancer care, while other research indicates that states with CON laws have lower hospital prices and flat or reduced procedure volume for certain elective surgical procedures and cardiac care. Given these disparate findings, it is no surprise that the need for CON laws remains in dispute.[36]

---

[34]U.S. National Library of Medicine. *The regional medical programs collection*. Retrieved May 2, 2018 from http://profiles.nlm.nih.gov/ps/retrieve/Narrative/RM/p-nid/94

[35]Congressional Budget Office. (1997, August). *Expenditures for health care: Federal programs and their effects*. Retrieved May 2, 2018 from https://www.cbo.gov/sites/default/files/95th-congress-1977-1978/reports/77doc566.pdf

[36]Yee, T., Stark, L. B., Bond, A. M., & Carrier, E. (2001, May). Health care certificate-of-need laws: Policy or politics? *National Institute for Health Care Reform Research Brief* 4.

As a result of the questionable benefit of this process, the federal government withdrew its requirement for CON programs in 1986. Subsequently, 14 states dropped their requirements, leaving the remaining 36 states and the District of Columbia with some type of review process.[37]

The third problem was the rapidly rising hospital costs associated with filling all those newly constructed beds. The concern was stated most famously by Shain and Roemer and came to be known as Roemer's Law: "[H]ospital beds that are built tend to be used."[38] As these authors go on to explain: "Before hospital insurance became common, family income largely determined which cases would go to hospitals. With widespread insurance, however, the kinds of cases that are hospitalized in any community reflect the number of beds provided." Both admission rates and lengths of stay accounted for the increased occupancies. The expanding utilization could not be explained just by the *availability* of beds in the community; for example, the occupancy rate was not highest where bed supply (measured in beds per 1,000) was lowest, or vice versa. Nor could the increase be attributed to an increased incidence of disease or patients from more remote sites coming to these newly built or expanded facilities.[39] While attention to this problem and proposed solutions came with the growing prominence of utilization review in the 1980s, more recent evidence indicates this problem persists.[40]

In the first decade of the 21st century, after a long lull in hospital construction, a flurry of activity occurred due to new programmatic opportunities, changing patterns in care, and the need to replace aging facilities. The differences between this more recent building surge and those of the past are twofold. First, the source of building funds has changed: more equity, less debt, and no major government sponsorship. According to the 2012 Health Facilities Management/American Society for Healthcare Engineering (HFM/ASHE) annual survey:

> Organizations are relying less on bank loans and other debt to finance construction projects than at any time since the HFM/ASHE survey began in 2005. Just 17 percent are using debt, down from 20 percent a year ago, compared with 42 percent drawing on cash reserves . . . Use of tax-exempt bonds also is at its lowest in at least six years, accounting for just 21 percent of construction financing among survey respondents.[41]

The second difference is the types of construction have changed:

1. Newer hospitals have fewer beds than their predecessors and a higher ratio of intensive care beds to general medical/surgical beds.

---

[37] See the American Health Planning Association website for a current list of which states have CON programs and what they cover. Retrieved May 2, 2018 from http://www.ahpanet.org/matrix_copn.html

[38] Shain, M., & Roemer, M. I. (1959). Hospital costs relate to the supply of beds. *Modern Hospitals, 92*, 71–73, 168.

[39] Roemer, M. I. (1961). Bed supply and hospital utilization: A natural experiment. *Hospitals, 35*, 36–42.

[40] Delamater, P. L., Messina, J. P., Grady, S. C., WinklerPrins, V., & Shortridge, A. M. (2013, February 13). Do more hospital beds lead to higher hospitalization rates? A spatial examination of Roemer's law. *PLoS One*. doi:10.1371/journal.pone.0054900

[41] Carpenter, D., & Hoppszallern, S. (2012). Time to build? Reform uncertainties drive financial scrutiny for new projects. *Health Facilities Management, 25*(2), 12–18, 20.

2. More outpatient than inpatient facilities are being built. Recently, this construction has been in the form of urgent care centers (freestanding emergency departments) and physician offices.
3. More renovation than new construction.

The reason for these structural changes is the trend toward delivery of more care outside the hospital (outpatient care). More recent trends also include a surge in behavioral health facility construction and "resilient design" projects to help buildings withstand natural disasters.[42]

Regardless of the form these construction projects take, they all share one common theme: redesign of facilities around patient perceptions and needs. One of the earliest institutions in this redesign trend was Northwestern Memorial Hospital, which completed a new facility in 1999. In describing the new focus for hospital design, then-CEO Gary Mecklenburg said:

> Health care today is a consumer service, no different from a whole host of others ... consumers don't want to go to a cold, sterile, unfriendly environment. Part of what drove the design of our building was the recognition that people wanted something different in the environment. We asked people what they thought about hospitals and they told us they didn't like hospitals. People expected a different environment, different décor, a different delivery system.[43]

This consumer-driven approach has persisted. According to a 2016 report:

> More than 86 percent of survey respondents said that patient satisfaction is "very important" in driving design changes to health facilities and/or services. Another 12 percent said patient satisfaction is "somewhat important" in driving changes. No respondents said patient satisfaction was "not at all important" in design.[44]

HOSPITAL DEFINITION AND CLASSIFICATIONS

Definition

In addition to the OED description, the legal definition of a hospital varies from state to state. Exhibit 4.3 provides some examples. The common features are capabilities to provide overnight (or longer) care to two or more unrelated persons for a variety of

---

[42]Burmahl, B., & Morgan, J. (2018, March 7). Hospital Construction Survey: Resilient design takes center stage as a top project consideration for health care facilities. *Health Facilities Management.* Retrieved May 2, 2018 from https://www.hfmmagazine.com/articles/3291-hospital-construction-survey

[43]Weinstock, M. (2006). Taking stock. Interviews with Gary Mecklenburg and Anthony Barbato. *Hospital and Health Networks, 80*(9), 42–45.

[44]Hoppszallern, S., Vesely, R., & Morgan, J. (2016, February 3). Hospital Construction Survey: Patient experience drives design and construction. *Health Facilities Management.* Retrieved May 2, 2018 from https://www.hfmmagazine.com/articles/1878-2016-hospital-construction-survey

EXHIBIT 4.3. Examples of Legal Definitions of Hospitals

California

"General acute care hospital" means a hospital, licensed by the Department, having a duly constituted governing body with overall administrative and professional responsibility and an organized medical staff which provides 24-hour inpatient care, including the following basic services: medical, nursing, surgical, anesthesia, laboratory, radiology, pharmacy, and dietary services. A general acute care hospital shall not include separate buildings which are used exclusively to house personnel or provide activities not related to hospital patients.

Illinois

"Hospital" means any institution, place, building, buildings on a campus, or agency, public or private, whether organized for profit or not, devoted primarily to the maintenance and operation of facilities for the diagnosis and treatment or care of two or more unrelated persons admitted for overnight stay or longer in order to obtain medical, including obstetric, psychiatric and nursing, care of illness, disease, injury, infirmity, or deformity . . .

The term "hospital" does not include:

1. Any person or institution required to be licensed pursuant to the Nursing Home Care Act, the Specialized Mental Health Rehabilitation Act, or the ID/DD Community Care Act;

2. Hospitalization or care facilities maintained by the State or any department or agency thereof, where such department or agency has authority under law to establish and enforce standards for the hospitalization or care facilities under its management and control;

3. Hospitalization or care facilities maintained by the federal government or agencies thereof;

4. Hospitalization or care facilities maintained by any university or college established under the laws of this State and supported principally by public funds raised by taxation;

5. Any person or facility required to be licensed pursuant to the Alcoholism and Other Drug Abuse and Dependency Act;

6. Any facility operated solely by and for persons who rely exclusively upon treatment by spiritual means through prayer, in accordance with the creed or tenets of any well-recognized church or religious denomination;

7. An Alzheimer's disease management center alternative healthcare model licensed under the Alternative Health Care Delivery Act; or

8. Any veterinary hospital or clinic operated by a veterinarian or veterinarians licensed under the Veterinary Medicine and Surgery Practice Act of 2004 or maintained by a State-supported or publicly funded university or college.

Massachusetts

"Hospital" means any institution in the Commonwealth of Massachusetts, however named, whether conducted for charity or for profit, which is advertised, announced, established, or maintained for the purpose of caring for persons admitted thereto for diagnosis or medical, surgical, or restorative treatment which is rendered within said institution. This definition shall not include any hospital operated by the Commonwealth of Massachusetts or by the United States.

conditions. Because these features also describe such organizations as skilled nursing facilities, the laws say, in effect: It is a hospital unless it is not; that is, unless it is covered by another licensing law.[45] The American Hospital Association will list a facility in its hospital guide if it is accredited by one of several organizations (see Chapter 9, "Quality") or meets a long list of features about size (at least six beds) and operational requirements (e.g., presence of a responsible governing authority, pharmacy, continuous nursing services, etc.).[46]

Ways Hospitals May Be Classified and Special Related Issues

Although all licensed hospitals have a single legal definition in each state, they are obviously quite different from one another. It is, therefore, important to understand some of the different ways hospitals can be categorized for such purposes as peer group comparisons, quality evaluations, and market segmentation activities.

It should be noted, however, that despite these differences, all hospitals are facing the same environmental forces, particularly shrinking number of beds due to expanded outpatient treatment capabilities and increasing costs. Two major reasons for the cost increases are increases in acuity of care and the nature of the hospital business: very personal and personnel-intensive care. Contrary to popular opinion that hospital expenses are driven by costs of technology, a significant portion of costs is due to wages and benefits. When hospital cost containment is considered, one must account for the effect on quality of reducing people. Exhibit 4.4 displays categories of typical hospital costs.

Some of the common ways hospitals are classified, with brief descriptions of each, are presented next.

Size. The usual metric for hospital size is total number of beds. This number can be confusing, however, since bed size can be expressed as number of licensed beds (what the state allows the hospital to operate) or the number of beds actually available for use. For example, the hospital may be licensed for 100 beds, but because of cost overruns or staff shortages, it operates 80 beds. The wide distribution of hospitals by bed size is displayed in Exhibit 4.5.

Levels of Care. Levels of care have been traditionally divided into primary, secondary, tertiary, and quaternary. The definition of primary care usually mentions that it is the first point of contact patients have with the healthcare system. (Please see Chapter 6, "Payers," for a full definition and explanation of this term.) For purposes of hospital classification, "a primary care hospital offers basic services, such as an emergency department and limited intensive care facilities. A secondary care hospital generally offers primary care, general

---

[45] See, for example, the exceptions listed in the Illinois statute in Exhibit 4.3. Some facilities are excluded not because they are not hospitals, but they are not subject to the state licensing statute, for example, "facilities maintained by the federal government or agencies thereof."

[46] AHA Guide 2012 edition. P. A2 Health Forum LLC. An American Hospital Association Company. 155 N. Wacker Drive, Chicago, IL 60606-1725.

EXHIBIT 4.4. **Percentage of U.S. Hospital Costs in 2016, by Type of Expense[a]**

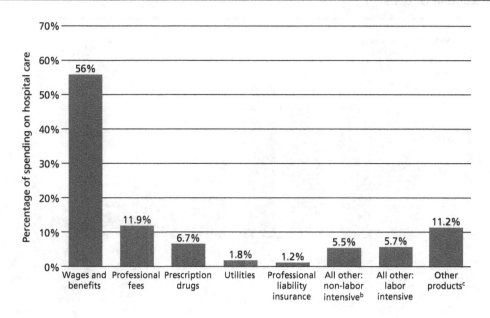

[a] Does not include capital.

[b] Includes postage and telephone expenses.

[c] For example food, medical instruments, etc.

Source: CMS and American Hospitals Association Data. © 2018 by Statistica Used with permission.

internal medicine, and limited surgical and diagnostic capabilities. A tertiary care hospital provides a full range of basic and sophisticated diagnostic and treatment services, including many specialized services."[47]

The term "secondary care" is not much used in the United States but is particularly common in European countries. It generally refers to the type of care provided at a community hospital. The "specialized services" of the tertiary care hospital often include such procedures as cardiovascular surgery and transplantation. An additional term used by some people is "quaternary care," which refers to a tertiary care center that is extensively involved in research and experimental treatments.

Many tertiary and quaternary care centers are also teaching hospitals (some of which are also called academic medical centers). A useful definition for these organizations comes

---

[47] Federal Trade Commission, Department of Justice. (2004, July). *Improving health care: A dose of competition. A report by the Federal Trade Commission and the Department of Justice*. Retrieved May 2, 2018 from http://www.justice.gov/atr/public/health_care/204694/chapter3.htm#3

EXHIBIT 4.5. **Number of Registered Hospitals in the United States in 2016, by Number of Beds**

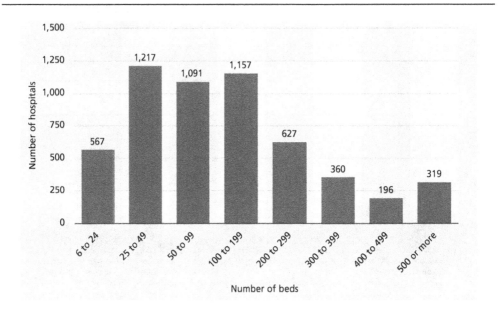

Source: American Hospital Association 2018 Hospital Data. © 2018 by Statistica. Used with permission.

from the membership requirements for the Council on Teaching Hospitals (COTHs) section of the American Hospital Association:

> Membership in COTH is limited to organizations having a documented affiliation agreement with a medical school accredited by the Liaison Committee on Medical Education (LCME) [the organization that accredits medical schools in the United States and Canada]. Typically, these organizations must sponsor, or participate significantly in, at least four approved, active residency programs. At least two of the approved residency programs should be in medicine, surgery, obstetrics/gynecology, pediatrics, family practice, or psychiatry.[48]

Ownership of these facilities varies widely. They can be independent corporations (frequently but not exclusively nonprofit) or owned by the affiliated university. According to the American Association of Medical Colleges,[49] while the nearly 400 teaching hospitals represent only 6% of all U.S. hospitals, they provide:

- 40% of neonatal intensive care units,
- 61% of pediatric intensive care units,

---

[48] AAMC. Council of Teaching Hospitals and Health Systems. Retrieved May 2, 2018 from https://www.aamc.org/download/333616/data/cothmemberservices.pdf
[49] Ibid.

- 79% of all burn care units,
- 48% of the surgical transplant services,
- 44% of Alzheimer centers,
- 22% of all cardiac surgery services,
- 41% of all hospital charity care, and
- Are the sites for approximately 28% of all Medicaid hospitalizations.

In addition to the usual insurance payments described below, teaching hospitals receive supplemental funds from Medicare Part A that are called Medicare Direct Graduate Medical Education (DGME) Payments. These payments started with the beginning of Medicare[50] and were initiated for two reasons: recognition of the importance of training medical specialists and an inducement for teaching hospitals to participate in the Medicare program. The amount of Graduate Medical Education (GME) support was capped by the Balanced Budget Act of 1997. According to Iglehart:[51]

> Medicare remains the largest supporter of GME, providing both direct payments to hospitals that cover medical education expenses related to the care of Medicare patients (about $3 billion per year) and an indirect medical education (IME) adjustment to teaching hospitals for the added patient-care costs associated with training (about $6.5 billion).

Annual amounts are modified by an update factor (with slightly more support going to primary care residency programs)[52] and cover about 100,000 physician trainees. Federal agencies and state Medicaid agencies spent over $16.3 billion in 2015 to fund GME training for physicians—commonly known as residency training. According to a 2018 study, the Government Accountability Office (GAO) found that in 2015 the "federal government spent $14.5 billion through five programs, and 45 state Medicaid agencies spent $1.8 billion. About half of teaching sites that received funding—such as teaching hospitals—received funds from more than one of the five programs."[53] (Please see Exhibit 4.6.)

Increasing economic pressures have caused many states to cut back on their GME funding.[54] In addition, the federal government is considering reduction of the IME portion of its subsidies. Of note is that the Departments of Veterans Affairs and Defense also support GME at their own teaching hospitals.

---

[50] House Report, Number 213, 89th Congress 1 Session 32 (1965), and Senate Report, Number 404, Pt. 1 89th Congress 1 Session 36 (1965).

[51] Iglehart, J. K. (2012). Financing graduate medical education-mounting pressure for reform. *New England Journal of Medicine, 366*, 1562–1563.

[52] For more details about DGME payments see: Medicare Direct Graduate Medical Education (DGME) Payments. Retrieved May 2, 2018 from https://www.aamc.org/advocacy/gme/71152/gme_gme0001.html

[53] GAO. (2018, March 29). *Physician workforce. HHS needs better information to comprehensively evaluate graduate medical education funding*. Retrieved May 2, 2018 from https://www.gao.gov/assets/700/690580.pdf

[54] Association of American Medical Colleges. (2016). *Medicaid graduate medical education payments—A 50-state survey*. Retrieved May 2, 2018 from https://www.documentcloud.org/documents/4392445-Medicaid-Graduate-Medical-Education-Payments-a.html

EXHIBIT 4.6. **Federal Spending on Graduate Medical Education Training, 2015**

Program	Total GME Spending ($in millions)	Percentage of Total Spending (%)
HHS programs		
Medicare	10,335	71
Medicaid (federal share)	2,351	16
Children's Hospital GME Payment Program	249	2
Teaching Health Center GME Program	76	1
VA program	1,499	10
Total	**14,509**	**100**

Source: GAO: Physician workforce. HHS needs better information to comprehensively evaluate graduate medical education funding. March 2018. Retrieved from https://www.gao.gov/assets/700/690581.pdf

In addition to the common hospital definition, teaching hospitals also share three essential features in their mission statements: patient care, education of healthcare professionals (such as physicians and nurses), and research. (Please see Exhibit 4.7 for examples of these statements.) Despite the clarity of these three elements, members of the organization will prioritize them differently. For example, in a teaching hospital without a nursing school, nurses will put patient care far ahead of teaching and research. On the other hand, a junior faculty member will give top priority to research, since productivity in that area alone will determine promotion, tenure, and salary. The other activities merely take time away from research. Leaders in this setting often have conflicting priorities depending on which role they play in a given situation. For example, the dean of a medical school must prioritize research because it affects rankings in the popular press. However, in order to attract medical students, teaching must get high marks. Further, if the dean is head of the faculty medical group, patient care takes priority because it is the largest source of the group's income. All these different priorities result in mission conflicts. While they cannot always be resolved, they must be appreciated when these organizations formulate their strategies and allocate resources.

Corporate Status/Sponsorship. One of the most common distinctions among hospitals is whether they are operated as for-profit or nonprofit enterprises. (Please see Exhibit 4.8 for trends and relative numbers of these institutions.)

For-profits can be held either privately or by shareholders who trade ownership on stock exchanges. Many of the largest for-profit systems are headquartered in the Nashville area because of their connections with the largest such system located there, Hospital Corporation of America (HCA). Consider these examples: In 2007, Community Health Systems cemented

EXHIBIT 4.7. Sample Mission Statements of Teaching Hospitals

Mission Statement of St. Michael's Hospital, Toronto, Ontario[a]

At St. Michael's Hospital, we recognize the value of every person and are guided by our commitment to excellence and leadership. We demonstrate this by:

- Providing exemplary physical, emotional, and spiritual care for each of our patients and their families
- Balancing the continued commitment to the care of the poor and those most in need with the provision of highly specialized services to a broader community
- Building a work environment where each person is valued, respected, and has an opportunity for personal and professional growth
- Advancing excellence in health services education
- Fostering a culture of discovery in all of our activities and supporting exemplary health sciences research
- Strengthening our relationships with universities, colleges, other hospitals, agencies, and our community
- Demonstrating social responsibility through the just use of our resources

The commitment of our staff, physicians, volunteers, students, community partners, and friends to our mission permits us to maintain a quality of presence and tradition of caring, which are the hallmarks of St. Michael's.

Mission Statement of Northwestern Medicine (Academic System) Chicago, IL[b]

Northwestern Medicine is a premier integrated academic health system where the patient comes first.

- We are all caregivers or someone who supports a caregiver.
- We are here to improve the health of our community.
- We have an essential relationship with Northwestern University's Feinberg School of Medicine.
- We integrate education and research to continually improve excellence in clinical practice.
- We serve a broad community and bring the best in medicine closer to where patients live and work.

[a] stmichaelshospital.com/about/mission.php.
[b] https://www.nm.org/about-us.

its corporate location by its purchase of Triad, an HCA spin-off; Lifepoint was founded in 1999 as a spin-off of 23 HCA hospitals; and Vanguard Health Systems was formed in July 1997 by group of healthcare executives led by Charles Martin, Jr., a former HCA executive.

One of the hallmarks of a nonprofit hospital is its tax-exempt status. According to Castro:[55]

The policies that initially conferred tax-exempt status on hospitals can trace their roots to the Elizabethan Statute of Charitable Uses of 1601. This British statute commonly bestowed

---

[55] Castro, A. I. (1995). Overview of the tax treatment of nonprofit hospitals and their for-profit subsidiaries: A short-sighted view could be very bad medicine comment. *Pace Law Review, 15,* 501–505.

EXHIBIT 4.8. Number of Hospitals in the United States from 2009 to 2016, by Ownership Type

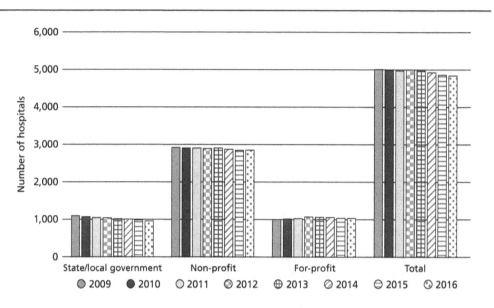

Source: American Hospital Association © Statistica 2018. Used with permission.

exemptions upon hospitals and other "charitable" organizations which promoted the common general welfare. The United States initially adopted this interpretation through its early common law. The federal government subsequently recognized income tax exemption with the enactment of the Revenue Act of 1894, and afterward with the ratification of the Sixteenth Amendment.

By 1959, the statutes dealing with the tax-exempt status of charitable organizations were consolidated into IRS code 501(c)(3). Nonprofit hospitals are currently incorporated under this code. (Please see Exhibit 4.9 for a full explanation of this category.) The portions that apply directly to hospitals are the charitable, religious, educational, or scientific missions and the requirement that they not be organized or operated for the benefit of private interests. (Hospitals are also evaluated for nonprofit status by state/local governments. Since the criteria for these evaluations can be very different, they will be considered separately.)

Because the U.S. Tax Code does not contain a definition for the word "charitable," the IRS has used two standards over the years to evaluate whether a hospital meets the criteria of 501 (c) (3): the "charity care standard" and the "community benefit standard." From 1956 to 1969, IRS Revenue Ruling 56–185 was the statute that spelled out the requirements a hospital needed to meet in order to qualify for 501(c)(3) status. Under this Ruling, a hospital had to provide, within its financial ability, free or reduced-cost care to patients unable to pay for it. It did not specify a minimum requirement for dollars spent or number treated.

EXHIBIT 4.9. Exemption Requirements—Section 501(c)(3) Organizations

To be tax-exempt under section 501(c)(3) of the Internal Revenue Code, an organization must be organized and operated exclusively for exempt purposes set forth in section 501(c)(3), and none of its earnings may inure to any private shareholder or individual. In addition, it may not be an action organization, i.e., it may not attempt to influence legislation as a substantial part of its activities and it may not participate in any campaign activity for or against political candidates.

Organizations described in section 501(c)(3) are commonly referred to as charitable organizations. Organizations described in section 501(c)(3), other than testing for public safety organizations, are eligible to receive tax-deductible contributions in accordance with Code section 170.

The organization must not be organized or operated for the benefit of private interests, and no part of a section 501(c)(3) organization's net earnings may inure to the benefit of any private shareholder or individual.

The exempt purposes set forth in section 501(c)(3) are charitable, religious, educational, scientific, literary, testing for public safety, fostering national or international amateur sports competition, and preventing cruelty to children or animals. The term *charitable* is used in its generally accepted legal sense and includes relief of the poor, the distressed, or the underprivileged; advancement of religion; advancement of education or science; erecting or maintaining public buildings, monuments, or works; lessening the burdens of government; lessening neighborhood tensions; eliminating prejudice and discrimination; defending human and civil rights secured by law; and combating community deterioration and juvenile delinquency.

Source: Internal Revenue Service Exemption Requirements, Section 501(c)(3) Organizations. Retrieved May 2, 2018 from https://www.irs.gov/charities-nonprofits/charitable-organizations/exemption-requirements-section-501c3-organizations

With the advent of Medicare and Medicaid in 1966, and the further availability of private health insurance, charity care and philanthropy were becoming even less of a factor in hospital finances. So, in 1969, the IRS issued Revenue Ruling 69-545, replacing the "charity standard" with a new "community benefit standard." Under the newer rule:

> A nonprofit organization whose purpose and activity are providing hospital care is promoting health and may, therefore, qualify as organized and operated in furtherance of a charitable purpose ... The promotion of health, like the relief of poverty and the advancement of education and religion, is one of the purposes in the general law of charity that is deemed beneficial to the community as a whole even though the class of beneficiaries eligible to receive a direct benefit from its activities does not include all members of the community, such as indigent members of the community, provided that the class is not so small that its relief is not of benefit to the community.[56]

The specific criteria mentioned in the ruling require that the hospital uses "its surplus funds to improve the quality of patient care, expand its facilities, and advance its medical training, education, and research programs."[57] It must also operate an accessible emergency

---

[56]Rev. Rul. 69-545, 1969-2 C.B. 117.
[57]Rev. Rul. 83-157, 1983-2 C.B. 94 set conditions for hospitals to maintain their 501(c)(3) status without having an emergency room, for example, if it would duplicate existing services or the hospital was very specialized (like a rehabilitation facility) and provided its community benefits in other ways.

room, maintain a medical staff open to all qualified physicians, and vest control of the hospital in its board of trustees, composed of independent civic leaders.

In subsequent years, Congress and the public have become more skeptical about the tax-exempt status of these institutions. Particular areas of suspicion include:

> the prices charged to low-income uninsured patients for medical care in comparison to those charged patients paying through insurance; the methods used by hospitals to collect payment from patients and the classification of bad debt as a community benefit; an increasing number of partnerships between tax-exempt hospitals and for-profit entities; and the amount of compensation paid to high-level employees.[58]

Research has shown some justification for these worries. "In 2009, tax-exempt hospitals varied markedly in the level of community benefits provided, with most of their benefit-related expenditures allocated to patient care services. Little was spent on community health improvements."[59]

Of further concern, particularly in bad economic times, are lost direct tax revenues from these institutions. Calculating the exact amount of this loss is difficult because of lack of current data, differences in what studies include in the community benefits hospitals provide, and differences in assigning an actual dollar value for those benefits. Given these caveats, what is currently claimed about the trade-off between tax benefits and community benefits can be summarized as follows:

- "The Congressional Joint Committee on Taxation estimated the value of the nonprofit hospital tax exemption at $12.6 billion in 2002—a number that included forgone taxes, public contributions, and the value of tax-exempt bond financing ... [W]e estimate that the size of the exemption reached $24.6 billion in 2011."[60]

- Tax exempt giving to nonprofit hospitals and healthcare systems in 2016 was $10.143 billion.[61]

- "In 2013, the estimated tax revenue forgone due to the tax-exempt status of nonprofit hospitals is $6.0 billion. In comparison, the benefit tax-exempt hospitals provided to their communities ... is estimated to be $67.4 billion, 11 times greater than the value of tax revenue forgone."[62]

---

[58]Lunder, E. K., & Liu, E. C. (2010, May 12). *501(c)(3) Hospitals and the community benefit standard.* Congressional Research Service. Retrieved May 2, 2018 from https://www.everycrsreport.com/files/20100512_RL34605_461b539b090d997945e30d4e85afd42cc90294ff.pdf

[59]Young, G. J. (2013). Provision of community benefits by tax-exempt U.S. hospitals. *The New England Journal of Medicine, 386,* 1519–1527.

[60]Rosenbaum, S., Kinday, D. A., Bao, J., Byrnes, M. K., & O'Laughlin, C. (2015). The value of the nonprofit hospital tax exemption was $24.6 billion in 2011. *Health Affairs, 34*(7): 1225–1233.

[61]Association for Healthcare Philanthropy. (2017, October 5). Healthcare organizations raised over $11 billion in FY 2016. [The $11 billion was for U.S. and Canadian institutions combined]. Retrieved May 2, 2018 from https://www.prnewswire.com/news-releases/healthcare-organizations-raised-over-11-billion-in-fy-2016-300531776.html

[62]American Hospital Association: Estimates of the federal revenue forgone due to the tax exemption of nonprofit hospitals compared to the community benefit they provide, 2013. Prepared for the American Hospital Association October 2017 by

- "The incremental community benefit exceeds the tax exemption for only 62% of non-profits. Policymakers should be aware that the tax exemption is a rather blunt instrument, with many nonprofits benefiting greatly from it while providing relatively few community benefits."[63]

In order to address these concerns, the IRS began studying the nonprofit activities of these hospitals in 2006. Further, passage of the Patient Protection and Affordable Care Act (ACA) in 2010 offered the possibility that a much larger number of people would be insured through Medicaid expansion and government-sponsored Health Insurance Exchanges; thus, as was the case after Medicare and Medicaid became operational, the definitions of charitable care and its potential reduced impact needed reexamination and redefinition. Anticipating these changes, the ACA included the recommendations for the IRS to formalize community health needs assessment (CHNA) requirements described in Sections 501(r) and 4959 of the IRC. In brief, hospitals[64] must now perform the activities detailed in Exhibit 4.10 in order to preserve their 501(c)(3) status and provide documentation on IRS Form 990 Schedule H.[65]

EXHIBIT 4.10. Hospital Activities to Preserve 501(c)(3) Status

- A hospital organization must conduct a CHNA at least once every three taxable years, starting with its first taxable year beginning after March 23, 2012.

- The CHNA must include:

  (1) A description of the community served by the hospital facility and how it was determined.

  (2) A description of the process and methods used to conduct the assessment, including a description of the sources and dates of the data and other information used in the assessment and the analytical methods applied to identify community health needs. The report should also describe information gaps that impact the hospital organization's ability to assess the health needs of the community served by the hospital facility.

  (3) A description of how the hospital organization took into account input from persons who represent the broad interests of the community served by the hospital facility. It must, at a minimum, take into account input from—

      (a) Persons with special knowledge of or expertise in public health;

Ernst and Young. Retrieved May 2, 2018 from https://www.aha.org/system/files/2018-02/tax-exempt-hospitals-benefits.pdf The reader should look at the study in more detail because it makes certain assumptions, such as that charitable contributions would be made to other organizations if not donated to nonprofit hospitals—so this item is not included in lost governmental benefit.

[63] Herring, B, Gaskin, D., Zare, H., & Anderson, G. (2018). Comparing the value of nonprofit hospitals' tax exemption to their community benefits. *Inquiry, 55*, 1–11. Retrieved May 2, 2018 from https://www.ncbi.nlm.nih.gov/pmc/articles/PMC5813653

[64] If a hospital organization operates more than one hospital facility, each facility must meet these requirements (IRS Section 501(r)(2)(B)(i)).

[65] IRS. 2017 Instructions for Schedule H (Form 990). Hospitals. Retrieved May 2, 2018 from https://www.irs.gov/pub/irs-pdf/i990sh.pdf

    (b)   Federal, tribal, regional, State, or local health or other departments or agencies with current data or other information relevant to the health needs of the community served by the hospital facility; and

    (c)   Leaders, representatives, or members of medically underserved, low income, and minority populations, and populations with chronic disease needs in the community served by the hospital facility.

(4)   A prioritized description of all of the community health needs identified through the CHNA, as well as a description of the process and criteria used in prioritizing such health needs.

(5)   A description of the existing healthcare facilities and other resources within the community available to meet the community health needs identified through the CHNA.

- A CHNA must be made widely available to the public, for example by posting the written report on the hospital facility's website.

- A hospital must adopt a written "implementation strategy" to meet the community health needs identified through the CHNA. An implementation strategy will:

(1)   describe how the hospital facility plans to meet the health need; or

(2)   identify the health need as one the hospital facility does not intend to meet and explain why the hospital facility does not intend to meet the health need.

        The implementation strategy must tailor the description to the particular hospital facility, taking into account its specific programs, resources, and priorities. The date the implementation strategy is considered approved by the IRS is when it is accepted by an authorized governing body of the hospital organization.

- Hospitals that fail to satisfy the CHNA requirements in any consecutive 3-year period will incur a $50,000 excise tax.[a]

- A hospital organization must establish a written financial assistance policy (FAP) and a written policy relating to emergency medical care.[b] The FAP must include:

(1)   eligibility criteria for financial assistance, and whether such assistance includes free or discounted care;

(2)   the basis for calculating amounts charged to patients (It is important to note that for those patients who qualify for its FAP, the hospital cannot use gross charges. Instead, it must limit the amounts to not more than the amounts generally billed to individuals who have insurance covering such care.);

(3)   the method for applying for financial assistance;

(4)   the actions the hospital organization may take in the event of nonpayment, including the reasonable efforts to determine whether an individual is FAP-eligible before engaging in extraordinary collection actions (ECAs); and

(5)   measures to widely publicize the FAP within the community to be served by the hospital organization.

[a] IRS: Part III—Administrative, Procedural, and Miscellaneous Notice and Request for Comments Regarding the Community Health Needs Assessment Requirements for Tax-Exempt Hospitals Notice 2011-52. Retrieved May 2, 2018 from www.irs.gov/pub/irs-drop/n-11-52.pdf

[b] Internal Revenue Service 26 CFR Part 1 RIN 1545-BK57, Additional Requirements for Charitable Hospitals. Notice of proposed rulemaking. June 22, 2012. Retrieved May 2, 2018 from https://www.irs.gov/pub/irs-drop/reg-130266-11.pdf

Given these extensive and often vague criteria, why would a hospital organization want to maintain its 501(c)(3) status? The benefits of federal nonprofit status are fourfold. The first two were mentioned above: These hospitals do not have to pay federal taxes on their earnings, and donors can deduct their contributions from taxable income (perhaps encouraging donations). The third reason is that borrowing costs are reduced because lenders (e.g., bondholders) to these institutions do not have to pay federal taxes on the interest payments they receive from borrowers; therefore, they can charge a lower rate for the loans.[66] Finally, these institutions are exempt from paying federal unemployment tax.

Since nonprofit hospitals often engage in for-profit activities, the organizational structure of these institutions must separate those latter businesses to preserve the tax exempt status of the nonprofit activities. For example, if the hospital owns and manages non-healthcare properties, that activity should be isolated from the hospital itself in a distinct corporation (with a separate tax number) that pays taxes.

As mentioned above, since states and localities have their own levies (such as state income taxes and local property taxes), they can set their own criteria for nonprofit status without regard to federal guidelines. The wide variance of criteria is exemplified by two decisions in the 1980s. In the first, the Supreme Court of Utah[67] found that just because a hospital takes charitable donations and provides free care to some of its patients, it is not entitled to full property tax exemption. Instead, the *extent* of free care must be determined annually; if it exceeds the value of the property tax, the hospital does not owe any state taxes. This decision emphasized that a hospital can lose its tax-exempt status not only by engaging in for-profit activities but also by not providing sufficient charitable services (both solely defined by the state). In Vermont, by contrast, its Supreme Court[68] decided that the property tax exemption could stand if the hospital is "open to all who need it regardless of ability to pay." Exhibit 4.11 compares the two states' criteria.

More recently, financially stressed states and localities have been reevaluating their tax-exempt policies. For example, on June 14, 2012, then–Illinois Governor Pat Quinn signed Senate Bill 2194 that changed the tax exemption status of hospitals, requiring them to furnish charity care in amounts at least equal to the value of their property taxes. As the economy and the roles of insurance subsidies change, further state reevaluations of their policies will undoubtedly occur.

Public/Private Status. Most hospitals in the United States are both private and nonprofit. Public hospitals are, by definition, owned by governmental agencies. For example, the federal government owns hospitals for military veterans; many states own psychiatric hospitals; and

---

[66] For example, a lender with a tax rate of 33% is indifferent to charging a borrower 6% interest for fully taxable payments and 4% if the interest income is tax exempt.

[67] Utah County v. Intermountain Health Care Inc., 709 P.2d 265 (Utah 1985).

[68] Medical Center Hospital of Vermont v. City of Burlington. No. 87–501; October 13, 1989.

EXHIBIT 4.11. **Comparison of Criteria between Utah and Vermont Whether an Institution Is Using a Property "Exclusively ... for Charitable Purposes"***

Comparison of Utah Decision and *Vermont Decision*

1. whether the stated purpose of the entity is to provide a significant service to others without immediate expectation of material reward;

    Healthcare institution need not dispense any free care in order to be considered charitable for purposes of tax exemption; relevant inquiry is whether healthcare was made available to all who needed it, regardless of ability to pay.

2. whether the entity is supported, and to what extent, by donations and gifts;

    Healthcare institution need not show that the majority of its income is derived from charitable sources in order to claim charitable use tax exemption.

3. whether the recipients of the "charity" are required to pay for the assistance received, in whole or in part; *see (1) above.*

4. whether the income received from all sources (gifts, donations, and payment from recipients) produces a "profit" to the entity in the sense that the income exceeds operating and long-term maintenance expenses;

    Not-for-profit institutions may generate revenues in excess of their expenses in order to maintain the organization and still retain charitable use tax exemption, the criteria being only that such revenues not be passed through to shareholders as profits but put back into operating expenses.

5. whether the beneficiaries of the "charity" are restricted or unrestricted and, if restricted, whether the restriction bears a reasonable relationship to the entity's charitable objectives; and

6. whether dividends or some other form of financial benefit, or assets upon dissolution, are available to private interest, and whether the entity is organized and operated so that any commercial activities are subordinate or incidental to charitable ones.

*Note: Text in regular font is from the Utah decision. Text in italic type is from the Vermont decision. Both states agree on criteria 5 and 6.

many highly populated counties own their own hospitals, such as Kings County (Brooklyn), Cook County (Chicago), and Los Angeles County (in California).

General/Specialty Hospitals. This distinction separates institutions with many different services from those that tend to specialize according to some market segment, such as age (children's hospitals), sex (women's hospitals), or clinical specialty (psychiatry or rehabilitation). Identifying a specialty hospital is not often obvious, however. For example, some places designated as children's hospitals are in freestanding facilities while others are in a section of a larger institution.

In addition to those obvious distinctions, specialty hospitals can be segmented by lengths of stay, particularly those of longer duration. Many of these specialty hospitals have their origins as disease-specific facilities, such as tuberculosis sanitaria. The modern movement to long-term acute care hospitals (LTCHs; pronounced "el tax") started in the 1980s. At that time, technology began to allow many patients to survive for long times on ventilators, thus crowding hospital intensive care units. Further, after 1982, Medicare started to pay hospitals by diagnosis rather than on a fee-for-service (FFS), cost-based system. (See the section in Chapter 6 devoted to Medicare for a full discussion of DRGs.) Therefore, patients with serious and long-term health needs were putting space *and* financial stresses on hospitals. In order to address these problems, the federal government created the category of LTCHs to qualify for Medicare payment.[69] This payment source accounts for about two thirds of the income of these facilities. Currently, three types of organizations can have an LTCH designation: freestanding facilities usually owned by for-profit corporations (such as Kindred[70] or Select Medical Holdings,[71] which, as the largest two for-profit chains, own more than half of this market's facilities); satellite facilities usually owned by nonprofit hospitals; and "hospitals within hospitals" (HwHs), facilities that are physically part of a hospital (like a floor or wing) but designated for this purpose.

Like acute care hospitals, these facilities are licensed as hospitals according to different state laws; however, to

> qualify as an LTCH for Medicare payment, a facility must meet Medicare's conditions of participation for acute care hospitals and have an average length of stay greater than 25 days for its Medicare patients. (By comparison, the average Medicare length of stay in acute care hospitals is about five days.) There are no other criteria defining LTCHs, the level of care they furnish, or the patients they treat.[72]

In 2014, 391 LTCHs treated about 134,000 Medicare beneficiaries. Most of these stays are for a few conditions; in 2014, the top 25 LTCH diagnoses made up 65% of all LTCH discharges. (Please see Exhibit 4.12 for the top 10 diagnoses.) CMS estimates that total Medicare spending for LTCH services was $5.4 billion in fiscal year 2014. Compared with all Medicare beneficiaries, those admitted to LTCHs are disproportionately under age 65, over age 85, disabled, and diagnosed with end-stage renal disease. They are also more likely to be African American.

Because of rising costs for these facilities, since 2002[73] Medicare has paid LTCHs by a prospective payment system[74] that is adjusted by relative weights. These weights reflect the

[69]CMS. *Long-term care hospital prospective payment system.* Retrieved May 3, 2018 from https://www.cms.gov/Outreach-and-Education/Medicare-Learning-Network-MLN/MLNProducts/Downloads/Long-Term-Care-Hospital-PPS-Fact-Sheet-ICN006956.pdf

[70]Retrieved May 3, 2018 from https://www.kindredhealthcare.com

[71]Retrieved May 3, 2018 from https://www.selectmedical.com

[72]MedPAC. (2016, October). *Long-term care hospitals payment system.* Retrieved May 3, 2018 from http://www.medpac.gov/docs/default-source/payment-basics/medpac_payment_basics_16_ltch_final.pdf

[73]The Medicare, Medicaid, and SCHIP [State Children's Health Insurance Program] Balanced Budget Refinement Act of 1999 (BBRA) (Pub. L. 106-113) and the Medicare, Medicaid, and SCHIP Benefits Improvement and Protection Act of 2000 (BIPA) (Pub. L. 106-554).

[74]The payments are, by law, budget neutral (i.e., total expenditures are the same as if the previous method of payment were used). Also, some facilities, such as veterans' hospitals and others having existing prospective payment, are exempt.

EXHIBIT 4.12. **Top 10 Diagnoses for LTCHs (2014)**

MS–LTC–DRG	Description	Discharges	Percentage
189	Pulmonary edema and respiratory failure	16,017	12.0
207	Respiratory system diagnosis with ventilator support 96+ hours	15,224	11.4
871	Septicemia without ventilator support 96+ hours with MCC	8,809	6.6
177	Respiratory infections and inflammations with MCC	3,733	2.8
592	Skin ulcers with MCC	3,663	2.7
208	Respiratory system diagnosis with ventilator support <96 hours	3,105	2.3
949	Aftercare with CC/MCC	2,864	2.1
539	Osteomyelitis with MCC	2,785	2.1
662	Renal failure with MCC	2,437	1.8
919	Complications of treatment with MCC	2,321	1.7

MS–LTC–DRG: Medicare severity, long-term care, diagnosis-related group; LTCH: long-term care hospital; MCC: major complication or comorbidity; CC: complication or comorbidity; OR: operating room.
MS–LTC–DRGs are the case-mix system for LTCH facilities.

Source: MedPAC: Chapter 10: Long-term care hospital services. Report to the Congress: Medicare payment policy 2016, p. 284. Retrieved May 3, 2018 from http://www.medpac.gov/docs/default-source/reports/chapter-10-long-term-care-hospital-services-march-2016-report-.pdf?sfvrsn=0.AU

different costs in the LTCH setting as well as outlier payments for especially expensive cases. Unlike other prospective payment schemes, payments to LTCHs are adjusted downwards for cases whose length of stay are shorter than average for a given diagnosis.

After establishment of LTACHs, hospital costs continued to rise, and CMS was concerned that hospitals were referring many of their acute cases to their satellites or HwHs in order to be able to bill for the long term as well as acute care parts of the hospital stay. In fiscal year 2005, CMS modified the payment to these affiliated facilities so that if more than 25% of their referrals came from their owner, payments would be the lower of the LTCH prospective payment or the inpatient prospective payment. In 2007, the rule was changed to apply to referrals from any source.[75] Further, from 2007 to 2017 (when the law expired), federal legislation mandated (with certain exceptions) a moratorium on the establishment of new LTCHs, LTCH satellites, and increase in the number of LTCH beds. This latter policy change caused consolidation in the sector due to for-profit acquisitions.

---

[75]"In special situations (i.e., admissions from rural and urban single or Metropolitan Statistical Area [MSA] dominant hospitals), the payment threshold was raised to 50 percent." Long Term Care Hospital Prospective Payment System: Payment Adjustment Policy (Revised, 4/16/2013). Retrieved May 3, 2018 from http://www.cms.gov/LongTermCareHospitalPPS/01_Overview.asp

Despite all these changes, research commissioned by CMS found that "patients transferred to LTCHs had longer stays, higher total payments, and higher provider costs than clinically similar patients who did not use LTCHs, with the smallest proportional differences seen for patients in the ventilator condition group."[76] The payment differences were much less if the LTCH care evaluation focused on the most severely ill patients.

Going forward, the key policy issues regarding these institutions are:

- *Clear and uniform admission criteria need to be set for patients and facilities.* Research has not been able to distinguish many complex LTCH patients from those receiving services in acute care hospitals and some skilled nursing facilities.

- *Uniform payment schedules need to be established for like services.* Since the patient populations in LTCHs and other facilities are similar, this uniformity is needed to avoid "selective gaming." Both major chains, and other owners, have been diversifying into other post-acute care sectors (i.e., intensive rehab facilities, outpatient rehabilitation centers, skilled nursing facilities [SNFs], and home health agencies). These strategies are intended to improve the ability of chains to control costs and limit the impact of payment policy changes.

- *Quality measures need to be implemented on the scale of acute care hospitals.* The ACA requires CMS to collect data on quality in LTCHs. The Improving Medicare Post-Acute Care Transformation Act of 2014 (the IMPACT Act)[77] mandates that LTCHs submit standardized patient assessment data with regard to quality measures, resource use, and other measures. However, the requirements are just for reporting purposes and are not as rigorous or extensive as those for acute care hospitals.[78]

Location. This category can have at least four groups. The first group is a region—for example, New England, Upper Midwest, Northwest, and so on. No consistency exists among companies or government agencies with respect to this definition. The second classification is by state. The third location dimension is by Metropolitan Statistical Areas (MSAs) (i.e., aggregations of populations around high-population density centers). These designations are standardized by the U.S. Census Bureau.[79]

Fourth is the distinction among urban, suburban, and rural hospitals. Because rural areas have fewer beds than do their urban counterparts, federal policies give them special exemption from certain laws or extra compensations. (More about these institutions is included in the section of this chapter titled "Safety Net Providers.") One special consideration will be

---

[76]Kandilov, A., & Dalton, K. (2011). *Utilization and payment effects of Medicare referrals to long-term care hospitals (LTCHs)*. Prepared under contract to the Centers for Medicare & Medicaid Services. Research Triangle Park, NC: RTI International.

[77]Public Law 113-185. (2014, October 6): *Improving Medicare Post-Acute Care Transformation Act of 2014*. Retrieved May 3, 2018 from https://www.gpo.gov/fdsys/pkg/PLAW-113publ185/pdf/PLAW-113publ185.pdf

[78]CMS.gov. (2018, April 10). *Long-Term Care Hospital (LTCH) Quality Reporting (QRP)*. Retrieved May 3, 2018 from https://www.cms.gov/Medicare/Quality-Initiatives-Patient-Assessment-Instruments/LTCH-Quality-Reporting/index.html

[79]Wilson, S. G. (2012, September). United States Census Bureau: Patterns of metropolitan and micropolitan population change: 2000 to 2010: *2010 Census Special Reports*. Retrieved May 3, 2018 from https://www.census.gov/content/dam/Census/library/publications/2012/dec/c2010sr-01.pdf

mentioned here: the swing bed exemption. "Swing beds" are those beds in a hospital that are used for acute care patients but can also be used for post-acute care, like skilled nursing facility services. As mentioned in the LTCH section, hospitals can game their reimbursement by quickly discharging Medicare patients to a long-term care facility they own. Many rural hospitals, however, are not filled to capacity, and the local area often lacks post-acute care institutions. Recognizing that these hospitals are in a special, vulnerable position, Congress included a provision in the Omnibus Budget Reconciliation Act of 1980 allowing Medicare and Medicaid to pay for swing-bed care in rural hospitals that had fewer than 50 beds.

Hospital Systems. According to the American Hospital Association,[80] a health [hospital] system is defined as "[h]ospitals belonging to a corporate body that owns and/or manages health provider facilities or health-related subsidiaries. The system may also own non-health-related facilities." "Sixty percent of AHA member hospitals are part of health systems, the majority consisting of three to 10 hospitals...Three-quarters are not-for-profit, with another 10% identifying as Catholic church-related and 10% as for-profit investor-owned. The remaining are non-federal government of varying types."[81]

The three types of systems that will be discussed here are wholly owned systems, alliances, and group purchasing organizations (GPOs). It is important to note that hospitals can belong to one or more of these arrangements. Since the large majority of hospitals belong to some type of system (please see Exhibit 4.13), the nature of the affiliation will drive institutional strategy and product/service purchasing. It is therefore critical for healthcare managers to understand these organizational arrangements and where the decision-making authority rests.

Wholly owned/singly managed systems. The most obvious type of system exists when a single entity owns or manages two or more hospitals. (Please see Exhibit 4.14 for a list of the 10 largest systems in this category.)

Six reasons exist for formation of these systems:

1. Economies of scale
2. Economies of scope
3. Vertical integration
4. Capture populations
5. Market power over payers
6. Bureaucratization

These reasons are discussed next.

Economies of scale. The benefits of economies of scale result from major savings derived by sharing support functions like payroll, accounting, logistics management, and volume

---

[80]American Hospital Association. (2016). *Trendwatch chartbook: Glossary*. Retrieved May 3, 2018 from https://www.aha.org/system/files/research/reports/tw/chartbook/2016/glossary.pdf

[81]American Hospital Association. *Healthcare systems*. Retrieved May 3, 2018 from https://www.aha.org/advocacy/health-care-systems

EXHIBIT 4.13. **Number of Nonprofit Hospital Systems in the United States from 1995 to 2016**
Total Number of Hospitals in Systems: At least 3,200

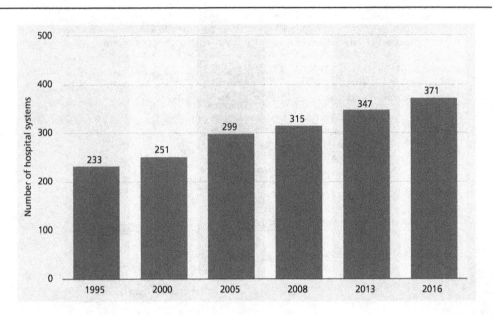

Source: The Governance Institute © Statistica 2018. Used by permission.

purchasing (although this latter benefit can also be gained from GPO membership, described below). Some shared equipment, such as centralized computers and vehicles, can also achieve this goal. This benefit often accrues with horizontal integration: mergers of like organizations, in this case, hospitals merging with other hospitals. Despite these potential cost savings, research findings are clear and consistent about the results of these mergers: They raise costs without providing other societal benefits. Gaynor recently summarized these findings:

> Extensive research evidence shows that consolidation between close competitors leads to substantial price increases for hospitals, insurers, and physicians, without offsetting gains in improved quality or enhanced efficiency. Further, recent evidence shows that mergers between hospitals not in the same geographic area can also lead to increases in price. Just as seriously, if not more, evidence shows that patient quality of care suffers from lack of competition.[82]

---

[82]Gaynor, M. (2018, February 14). *Examining the impact of health care consolidation.* Statement before the Committee on Energy and Commerce Oversight and Investigations Subcommittee, U.S. House of Representatives. Retrieved May 5, 2018 from https://docs.house.gov/meetings/IF/IF02/20180214/106855/HHRG-115-IF02-Wstate-GaynorM-20180214.pdf

EXHIBIT 4.14. **Ten Largest U.S. Health Systems Based on Number of Hospitals (as of December 2017)**

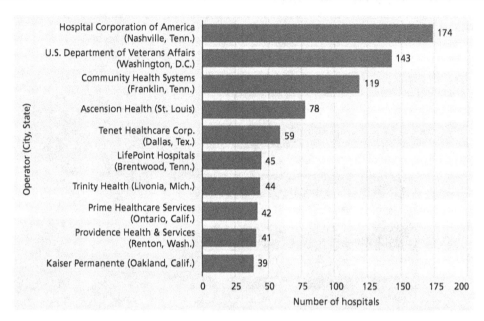

Source: *Becker's Hospital Review*: Top U.S. health systems based on number of hospitals as of 2017 © 2018 Statistica. Retrieved May 2, 2018 from https://www.statista.com/statistics/245010/top-us-for-profit-hospital-operators-based-on-number-of-hospitals Used with permission of Statistica.

Economies of scope. When two or more different services can be produced using common resources at a lower cost than if created individually, then economies of scope exist. For example, a radiology department can produce a variety of diagnostic and therapeutic services using the same staff and equipment. Another way to look at scope is when system members are geographically close (a relative term that will vary case by case), they can diversify the types of services each offers without the expense of duplication. For example, one facility may provide high-level neonatal care, while another might offer invasive cardiac treatments. This advantage is not always possible, however, since expensive diagnostics (such as CT and MRI scanners) often need to be available on-site in the event of an emergency. In addition, many system hospitals are located across a large geographic area so that each serves a different community; each facility must, therefore, be relatively self-sufficient with a diverse portfolio of services. Because systems can draw from and service a larger area than a single hospital, certain types of system-owned, non-acute care facilities/programs can better demonstrate economies of scope. (Please see Exhibits 4.15 and 4.16 for examples.)

EXHIBIT 4.15. **Types of Facilities Owned by Systems**

Acute care hospitals

Assisted living facilities

Continuing-care retirement communities

Freestanding psychiatric hospitals

Home care facilities

Long-term acute care facilities

Physician organizations

Rehabilitation

Skilled nursing facilities

EXHIBIT 4.16. **Types of Programs Run by Systems**

Adult day care

Behavioral clinics

Cancer treatment

Chest pain clinics

Diagnostic imaging

Dialysis

Emergency service facility

Hospice

Laboratories

Mobile imaging

Occupational health

Pain management

Pediatrics

Pharmacy

Physical therapy/sports medicine

Physician offices/clinics

Rehabilitation centers

Sleep centers

EXHIBIT 4.16. *(Continued)*

Surgery centers

Urgent care

Wellness centers

Women's health centers

Wound care

Vertical integration. Because vertical integration is a bit more complex than the other reasons for system formation, it will be explained in more detail. Vertical integration occurs when one organization acquires (or creates) another that is elsewhere along the value chain from production of the product (or service) to its delivery to (or consumption by) the end user. Vertical integration primarily occurs when it is not economically advantageous or feasible to create bilateral agreements, such as purchasing/sales contracts or alliances/joint ventures. Backward integration arises when the other entity supplies inputs to the organization, while forward integration occurs when the other entity receives the outputs from the organization. The simplest general examples of vertical integration are when an auto manufacturer buys a parts supplier (backward integration) or a dealership (forward integration). Hospitals have vertically integrated by such activities as buying physician practices (backward integration) and creating home health agencies (forward integration). In addition to these patient care services, vertical integration is also occurring when hospital systems set up their own health insurance capability. Exhibits 4.14 and 4.15. also provide examples of vertical integration.

Given the theme of this chapter, the relevant questions are: Should hospitals vertically integrate and, if so, when? Stuckey and White[83] posit that there are four reasons for vertical integration. These reasons are discussed below in the context of hospital systems.

1. A vertical market "fails" when transactions within it are too risky and the contracts designed to overcome these risks are too costly (or impossible) to write and administer.

2. Companies in adjacent stages of the industry chain have more market power than companies in your stage.

    The transactions necessary for a hospital to assume financial and clinical risk are characterized by high frequency and the potential of certain participants to slow care or make it costlier to deliver. The best-studied vertical integration strategy is hospital purchase of physician practices. Consider the following two examples of reasons for vertical integration: If a hospital is taking global financial risk for a population but its physicians demand high fees, the system will not be viable. If a hospital wishes to contract with a payer for global fees for cardiovascular services but the surgeons do not want to participate, the enterprise will fail. In these cases, the power of suppliers (or more correctly, business partners) is disproportionately large.

---

[83] Stuckey, J., & White, D. (1993, April 15). When and when not to vertically integrate. *MIT Sloan Management Review, 341*(3) (Spring), reprint #3435. Retrieved May 3, 2018 from http://sloanreview.MIT.edu/article/when-and-when-not-to-vertically-integrate

3. Integration would create or exploit market power by raising barriers to entry or allowing price discrimination across customer segments.

4. The market is young and the company must forward integrate to develop a market, or the market is declining and independents are pulling out of adjacent stages.

Organized delivery systems (ODSs) can successfully differentiate themselves and access risk contracts only if they are clinically integrated. (See the Organized (Integrated) Delivery Systems/Accountable Care Organizations section later in this chapter.) If the delivery systems can achieve this clinical integration, they can raise barriers to entry for others who cannot accomplish it. The price discrimination occurs when the system develops market power over payers and can command higher fees.

Of note is that, with respect to hospitals, vertical integration has historically not been challenged on antitrust grounds as much as has horizontal integration, though that laissez-faire attitude is changing.[84] The reason was succinctly stated by Spengler in a classic and oft-quoted article: "Horizontal integration may, and frequently does, make for higher prices and a less satisfactory allocation of resources than does pure or workable competition. Vertical integration, on the contrary, does not, as such, serve to reduce competition and may, if the economy is already ridden by deviations from competition, operate to intensify competition."[85] Given this statement, one must ask what the research shows about benefits or harms of vertical integration. Three relationships have been studied: hospital–physician, hospital–post-acute care, and hospital–insurance.

Studies on the effects of hospital–physician integration come mainly from the 1990s. Using data from Arizona, Florida, and Wisconsin for 1994 to 1998, Cuellar and Gertler[86] found that "integration has little effect on efficiency, but is associated with an increase in prices, especially when the integrated organization is exclusive and occurs in less competitive markets." On the other hand, using data from California for 1994 to 2001, Ciliberto and Dranove[87] found "no evidence of higher prices. If anything, integration is associated with lower prices, though the estimated price reductions are neither precise nor statistically significant."

Hospitals bought many physician practices in the 1990s, but the strategy mostly failed and systems lost a great deal of money. More recently, attempts to replicate this integration have not fared much better. "Hospitals lose $150,000 to $250,000 per year over the first 3 years of employing a physician—owing in part to a slow ramp-up period as physicians establish themselves or transition their practices and adapt to management changes. The losses decrease by approximately 50% after 3 years but do persist thereafter."[88]

---

[84] One of the earliest challenges in antitrust litigation for vertical integration was reported in: FTC and Idaho Attorney General Challenge St. Luke's Health System's Acquisition of Saltzer Medical Group as Anticompetitive. Retrieved May 3, 2018 from http://www.ftc.gov/opa/2013/03/stluke.shtm

[85] Spengler, J. J. (1950). Vertical integration and antitrust. *Journal of Political Economy, 58*(4), 347–352.

[86] Cuellar, A. & Gertler, P. J. (2006). Strategic integration of hospitals and physicians. *Journal of Health Economics, 25*, 1–28.

[87] Ciliberto, F., & Dranove, D. (2006). The effect of physician–hospital affiliations on hospital prices in California. *Journal of Health Economics, 25*, 29–38.

[88] Kocher, R. & Sahni, N. R. (2011). Hospitals' race to employ physicians—The logic behind a money-losing proposition. *New England Journal of Medicine, 364*, 1790–1793.

Research studies have also consistently shown that after hospitals purchase physician practices, insurance and patient costs increase. For example: "For certain cardiology, ortho-pedic, and gastroenterology services, hospital employment of physicians results in up to 27% higher costs for Medicare and 21% higher costs for patients."[89]

With respect to post-acute care, David et al.[90] found that:

> hospitals that are vertically integrated tend to discharge patients to their own HHA [home health agency] and skilled nursing facilities sooner and in poorer health compared with non-integrated hospitals; yet, health outcomes are actually better for patients who transi-tion to hospitals' own skilled nursing facilities and no worse for patients who transition to hospital's own HHA.

In other words, the shift to the lower-cost settings does not result in reduced quality of care.

The last type of vertical integration discussed here is a payer (insurance)–hospital combi-nation, called provider-sponsored health plans.[91] Payer-provider combinations, such as group or staff model HMOs (discussed in the Managed Care section of Chapter 6), are well known and have been shown to lower costs compared to indemnity coverage. Kaiser-Permanente is a prominent example. However, these older organizations were designed from their start to integrate functions and harmonize incentives. In the past, when hospitals purchased insur-ers or set up their own companies, the efforts largely failed. (Please see Exhibit 4.17 for an example.) More recent efforts have not been much more successful. In an oft-quoted study, Baumgarten concluded:

> Dozens of provider systems have established their own health plans since 2010...Based on the analysis reported here, it is hard to identify any of the new cohort of provider-sponsored health plans that show strong promise...A few new plans have enjoyed some success, reaching enrollments of 100,000 in just a few years. However, almost all these plans continue to operate at a loss, in some cases reporting very large losses...The key to success for provider-sponsored health plans is the ability to enunciate and then deliver on a value proposition: a provider system and its affiliated physicians and hospitals providing high-quality medical care at a lower cost...But, so far, the plans reviewed in this research are only able to price competitively by paying their own providers below market rates. That is not a strategy that can be sustained for long.[92]

---

[89] Avalere Health, LLC. (2017, November). Implications of hospital employment of physicians on Medicare beneficiaries. Retrieved May 6, 2018 from http://www.physiciansadvocacyinstitute.org/Portals/0/assets/docs/PAI_Medicare%20Cost %20Analysis%20--%20FINAL%2011_9_17.pdf

[90] David, G., Rawley, E., & Polsky, D. (2011). Integration and task allocation: Evidence from patient care. *Journal of Economics & Management Strategy, 22*(3), 617–639.

[91] For a list of some of the largest plans, see: Morse, S. (2016, September 16). 25 biggest provider-sponsored health plans include some of the nation's biggest systems. *Healthcare Finance*. Retrieved May 5, 2018 from http://www .healthcarefinancenews.com/news/25-biggest-provider-sponsored-health-plans-include-some-nations-biggest-systems

[92] Baumgarten, A. (2017, June). Analysis of Integrated Delivery Systems and New Provider Sponsored Health Plans. Study for the Robert Wood Johnson Foundation. Retrieved May 5, 2018 from https://www.rwjf.org/content/dam/farm/ reports/reports/2017/rwjf437615

EXHIBIT 4.17. **Example of Early Failure of Provider-Sponsored Health Insurance Plan**

HealthChicago was a commercial HMO incorporated on January 2, 1984, by four suburban Chicago-area hospitals: Central Du Page Hospital in Winfield, Elmhurst Memorial Hospital in Elmhurst, Ingalls Memorial Hospital in Harvey, and Northwest Community Hospital in Arlington Heights. The plan grew rapidly, so that at its peak in 1988 it had 85,000 members. Despite success in enrollment, the hospital-owned plan ran into early financial troubles. Financial statements ending December 31, 1986, showed a negative net worth of $2.21 million because of $6.3 million in losses. The following year was worse, when the plan had a $23 million loss. In order to maintain state-mandated reserve requirements, owners needed to come up with $14 million in early 1988, bringing their total investment to $41 million. By the end of September 1988, Northwest Community Hospital announced it was pulling out of the venture. According to one news report[a]: "The hospital said its directors concluded that ownership of an HMO isn't consistent with its role as a care provider." In 1992, membership declined to 65,000 and losses persisted. On January 22, 1992, Humana announced its acquisition of the plan for an undisclosed amount. The lack of insurance expertise as the principal cause of the failure is demonstrated by a postscript to this story. In August 1993, an Illinois Appellate Court dismissed a lawsuit HealthChicago had originally brought against its former auditors Touche, Ross and Company (a predecessor organization to Deloitte). "In its original complaint, plaintiff alleged that defendant failed to inform it of the need for changes in its pricing structure and levels of claims reserves and that such failure cost plaintiff approximately $25 million."[b] These activities are routine practices for any insurance company.

[a] Moore, P. (September 28 1988). One of Health Chicago's part owners calls it quits. *Chicago Sun Times.*
[b] *HealthChicago, Inc. v. Touche, Ross and Co.*, 625 N.E.2d 706 (1993) 252 Ill. App.3d 608, 192 Ill. Dec. 551.

In summary, what can now be said is that the outcome of vertical integration may depend on highly specific market characteristics, including method of physician compensation. Stuckey and White caution: "*Do not vertically integrate unless absolutely necessary. This strategy is too expensive, risky, and difficult to reverse.*"[93] Other models with aligned financial incentives, such as joint ventures or strategic alliances, could be employed instead of vertical integration, but the power among participants would be more equal, a situation not always to the liking of hospital administrators.

Capture populations. It is important for individual hospitals to develop patient loyalty so that no matter what services are needed, the institution stays top of mind. One way systems can accomplish this goal is by developing strong brand recognition. Another way is by providing geographic coverage. For example, patients often wonder if they should choose a physician or hospital close to work or home. Systems with a strong brand identity and geographic coverage can offer themselves to patients across a variety of settings.

Market power over payers. This advantage is a separate outgrowth of the previous one but can be an independent motivator for system formation. With geographic coverage and a large, loyal patient base, insurance companies will need to include these systems in their networks. The one caveat systems face in this strategy is the possibility of antitrust.

---

[93] Stuckey, J., & White, D. (1993, April 15). When and when not to vertically integrate. *MIT Sloan Management Review, 341*(3) (Spring), reprint #3435. Retrieved from http://sloanreview.MIT.edu/article/when-and-when-not-to-vertically-integrate

Bureaucratization. The advantage of bureaucratization is mainly seen in public institutions and in countries that have regionalized their hospitals into de facto systems. Examples include the Veterans Administration, hospital clusters of the Hong Kong Hospital Authority, Local Health Integrated Networks in Ontario, and the Agences Régionales de Santé in France.

Alliances. Alliances form for the same reasons as do single-owned/operated systems (except for bureaucratization). In *pooling alliances*, entities bring together similar resources to achieve economies of scale. *Trading alliances* are formed when participants bring different resources to the enterprise to achieve economies of scope. Proponents of alliances see these arrangements as a way to address the increasingly complex healthcare environments while maintaining individual participant autonomy. However, this autonomy is also the source of the greatest weakness of this type of arrangement, and it has been estimated that 50% to 80% of all alliances fail.[94]

Three major reasons exist for failure. First, participants may enter the alliance with divergent goals that can cause conflict over strategic direction of the overall organization. These disagreements can be over such matters as different types of capital investments, location of deployed resources, or incorporation of additional partners (e.g., those with additional expertise or in a different location). Second, the governing structure may be unstable. Governing boards are usually comprised of member organizations with equal or near-equal votes. This problem has caused the failure of systems that need to make decisions but are paralyzed by democracy. A third potential problem is clash of organizational cultures. In this case, culture can dictate which issues are major problems, how problems are addressed, and how conflicts are handled.

An example of an alliance that failed for these reasons was the teaching hospitals of Northwestern University, called Northwestern Healthcare Network, which operated in the 1990s before dissolving. One of the reasons it failed was predicted in an interview with Gary Mecklenburg, then CEO of Northwestern Memorial Hospital: "Voluntary organizations continue to have a very important place in health care. But they don't have the ability to make the hard decisions when health care is changing, and we must make hard decisions in terms of organization, structure, cost, etc. I start off with a premise that says regional networks or systems must have some degree of substantial authority to make them work."[95]

Successful, large national alliances include Premier[96] and Vizient-owned hospitals.[97] Reasons for their success include large national presences, provision of services highly

[94]Zajac, E. J., D'Aunno, T. A., & Burns, L. R. (2011). Managing strategic alliances. In L. R. Burns, E. H. Bradley, & B. J. Wiener (Eds.), *Shortell and Kaluzny's healthcare management: Organization design and behavior* (pp. 321–346). Clifton Park, NY: Delmar. This reference provides an excellent discussion of healthcare alliances.

[95]Johnson, D. E. (1992). CEO interview: Gary A. Mecklenburg—Networks help assure survival. *Health Care Strategic Management, 10,* 12–17.

[96]Retrieved May 6, 2018, from www.premierinc.com

[97]"Vizient was founded in 2015 as the combination of VHA Inc., a national health care network of not-for-profit hospitals; University HealthSystem Consortium, an alliance of the nation's leading academic medical centers; and Novation, the health care contracting company they jointly owned." Retrieved May 6, 2018, from https://www.vizientinc.com/About-us

valued by their stakeholders (such as supply chain management, revenue cycle management, and quality benchmarking information), and health policy involvement. From empirical observation, it appears that alliances succeed when they focus on cost savings (such as economies of scale) and quality improvement. Failure occurs more often when conflicts arise over ways to increase revenues (such as resource allocations among member institutions).

Group purchasing organizations. According to the group purchasing organization (GPO) trade group, the Healthcare Supply Chain Association (HSCA), "GPOs date back to 1909, when the Hospital Superintendents of New York first considered establishing a purchasing agent for laundry services. In 1910, the first GPO was created, the Hospital Bureau of New York."[98] These organizations provide members not only with buying power but also such services as supply chain management (i.e., assistance with acquisition, inventory management, clinical evaluation, standardization of products, and evaluations of new technology). A GAO study of the services provided by the six largest GPOs is displayed in Exhibit 4.18. Many firms are owned by members; others are patronized by those who only pay membership fees. Some specialize in certain merchandise types while others offer a broad range of products. Most of these arrangements are voluntary; members are able but not required to make purchases from the GPO to which they belong. Hospitals and systems typically belong to two to four organizations and make 96% to 98% of their purchases through them.[99] On average, GPO contracts account for about 73% of nonlabor purchases that hospitals make.[100] The business model for these companies derives principally from "administrative fees" vendors pay based on the purchase price that the healthcare provider pays; Exhibit 4.19 provides a typical scheme for payment flows. Membership charges also contribute to revenue.

The largest organizations by annual spending volume are:[101]

1. Vizient (Irving, TX)—$100 billion
2. Premier (Charlotte, NC)—>$50 billion
3. HealthTrust (Nashville, TN.)—$30 billion
4. Intalere (St. Louis, MO)—$9 billion

The benefit of these organizations to their members has been highlighted in a number of studies. For example, Burns and Lee[102] found that GPOs lower product prices, particularly

---

[98]Retrieved May 6, 2018, from http://www.supplychainassociation.org/?page=FAQ

[99]Healthcare Supply Chain Association (HSCA). *A primer on group purchasing organizations: Questions and answers.* Retrieved May 6, 2018, from http://c.ymcdn.com/sites/www.supplychainassociation.org/resource/resmgr/research/gpo_primer.pdf

[100]Schneller, E. S. (2009, April). *The value of group purchasing—2009: Meeting the need for strategic savings.* Scottsdale, AZ: Health Care Sector Advances.

[101]Gooch, K. (2017, February 6). *Four of the largest GPOs, 2017. Becker's hospital CFO report.* Retrieved May 6, 2018, from https://www.beckershospitalreview.com/finance/4-of-the-largest-gpos-2017.html

[102]Burns, L. R., & Lee, J. A. (2008). Hospital purchasing alliances: Utilization, services, and performance. *Health Care Management Review, 33,* 201–215.

EXHIBIT 4.18. **Services the Six Largest Group Purchasing Organizations (GPO) Reported Providing in 2008**

Service[a]	GPO					
	A	B	C	D	E	F
Custom contracting	✓	✓	✓	✓	✓	✓
Clinical evaluation and standardization	✓	✓	✓	✓	✓	✓
Technology assessments	✓	✓	✓	✓	✓	✓
Supply-chain analysis	✓	✓	✓	✓	✓	
Electronic commerce	✓	✓	✓	✓	✓	
Materials management consulting	✓	✓	✓	✓	✓	
Benchmarking data	✓	✓	✓	✓	✓	
Continuing medical education	✓	✓		✓	✓	✓
Market research	✓	✓	✓	✓		
Materials management outsourcing	✓	✓			✓	
Patient safety services	✓	✓	✓			
Marketing products or services	✓	✓		✓		
Insurance services	✓	✓				
Revenue management	✓	✓				
Warehousing	✓					
Equipment repair	✓					
Other[b]			✓		✓	✓

Note: The six largest GPOs were selected based on their reported 2007 purchasing volume in Health Industry Distributors Association, *Group Purchasing Organization & Integrated Delivery Network: Market Brief*, Alexandria, Va., July 2009.

[a] This list includes services that may be offered through affiliates of the GPO.
[b] Other reported services included, for example, contracting for environmentally friendly products, energy-related services and education, and public policy services.

Source: GAO structured data collection protocol. GAO (2010, August). *Group purchasing organizations. Services provided to customers and initiatives regarding their business practices.* Retrieved May 6, 2018 from www.gao.gov/new.items/d10738.pdf.

for commodity and pharmaceutical products, and reduce transaction costs. GPOs are less successful in lowering prices of other valued services, do not reduce costs for expensive physician preference items, and do not impede contracting with innovative firms or restrict desired products. These benefits as well as ownership in GPOs and payment of rebates to purchasers make entry into this sector very difficult. For example, in 2017, Amazon announced

EXHIBIT 4.19. **Hypothetical Flow of Contract Administrative Fees**

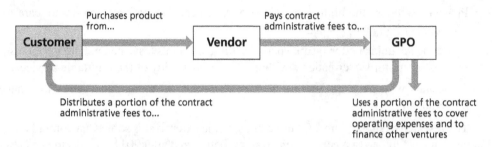

Source: GAO (2010, August). Group purchasing organizations. Services provided to customers and initiatives regarding their business practices. August 2010. Retrieved May 6, 2018 from www.gao.gov/new .items/d10738.pdf

it would enter the hospital supply business; by April 2018, the company pulled back this initiative.[103]

The message here for healthcare product and service firms is that in addition to direct customer sales, they must also develop a marketing strategy that involves multiple GPOs in their channels.

Physician-Owned Hospitals. Although this category could be included in either the ownership or specialty sections, some distinct issues warrant its separation. Like many healthcare issues, physician-owned hospitals are not new. Many prominent organizations that own or control hospitals are named for their physician-founders, including the Mayo, Menninger, and Ochsner clinics.[104] After decades of stagnation, starting in the 1990s there was rapid growth in these organizations. In 2017, there were about 250 such hospitals, with a heavy concentration in Texas. According to the Physician Hospitals of America[105] (the trade organization for these institutions), the top five categories of these hospitals (in declining frequency) are: Surgical, General Care, Orthopedic, Cardiac, and Long-Term Acute Care.

Proponents of these hospitals cite the following benefits compared to non-physician-owned establishments:

- Better clinical outcomes due to specialization
- Lower costs
- Higher patient satisfaction
- More procedural efficiency

---

[103] See, for example: Aungst, T. (2018). Amazon withdraws plans for medication distribution. *Pharmacy Times* (April 19). Retrieved May 7, 2018, from http://www.pharmacytimes.com/contributor/timothy-aungst-pharmd/2018/04/amazon-withdrawals-plans-for-medication-distribution

[104] These institutions are nonprofit, as distinguished from current for-profit physician-owned hospitals.

[105] Retrieved May 7, 2018, from http://www.physicianhospitals.org

Critics (especially the American Hospital Association and Federation of American Hospitals) claim:

- Physicians choose the highest-margin services to care for patients and do not care for Medicaid or indigent patients.

- By taking healthier, better-insured patients, these hospitals leave general, nonprofit institutions to care for sicker patients without the cross-subsidy of the profitable services.

- Physicians who have an interest in these facilities do more unnecessary/low-value procedures.

The research to support any of these claims, while extensive, is somewhat contradictory. Further, studies fall into two general time frames: before and after 2011 (i.e., during and after a period of rapid expansion and competitive pressures, respectively). The reason to divide the research into these time periods is that, starting in 2011, the ACA restricted new construction or expansion of existing physician-owned hospitals:

- The number of operating rooms, procedure rooms, and beds is frozen except for certain counties with high population growth and/or low bed capacity. Medicare and Medicaid stopped payment for services at such facilities if they were built or expanded after December 31, 2010.

- Referring and treating physicians must disclose to patients their ownership interests (if any) in the hospital, giving patients enough time to make a "meaningful decision" about the place of care.

- "Ownership or investment returns [cannot be] . . . distributed to each owner or investor in the hospital in an amount that is directly proportional to the ownership or investment interest of such owner or investor in the hospital." In other words, profits cannot be distributed based on the number or profitability of the patients referred or treated by physician-owners.[106]

Currently, the federal government is considering lifting this freeze; however, some of the important recommendations still rely on older studies.[107] Before policy makers enact changes, a thorough statistical and methodologic review of more current studies should be conducted. However, since the debate continues using studies over the past two decades, it is worthwhile to selectively analyze some of them.

---

[106]PPACA (Consolidated) (2010, June 9). Title VI—Transparency and Program Integrity. Subtitle A—Physician Ownership and Other Transparency. Sec. 6001. Limitation on Medicare Exception to the Prohibition on Certain Physician Referrals for Hospitals, pp. 619–624. Retrieved May 7, 2018, from https://www.cms.gov/Medicare/Fraud-and-Abuse/PhysicianSelfReferral/Downloads/Section_6001_of_the_ACA.pdf

[107]See, for example: Letter from MedPAC to Seema Verma [CMS Director], May 23, 2017, which largely relies on its 2005 report. Retrieved May 8, 2018, from http://medpac.gov/docs/default-source/comment-letters/05232017_medpac2018ippscommentletterfinal.pdf?sfvrsn=0 This memo's recommendation with respect to these hospitals largely relies on a 2005 MedPAC study: MedPAC: Physician-owned Specialty Hospitals. March 2005. Retrieved from http://www.medpac.gov/documents/Mar05_SpecHospitals.pdf

In a widely cited paper, Mitchell[108] found: "The consistent finding of higher use rates by physician owners across time clearly suggests that financial incentives linked to ownership of either specialty hospitals or ambulatory surgery centers influence physicians' practice patterns." Although the results make some intuitive sense, the study was done in one state (Idaho), with data from one insurer, and analyzed one specialty. Further, causality cannot be determined: Did the physicians use their facilities solely to make money, or did these facilities provide a more efficient way to treat patients in an area where shortages prevented timely service provisions? Three additional criticisms of these types of studies exist. First, they focus on ownership but not whether referring physicians (as distinguished from those performing the procedures) have an interest in the facilities. Second, in most studies, utilization and other measured parameters are not correlated with degree of ownership interest. This question is especially important since the vast majority of physicians have ownership shares in these facilities of less than 5%.[109] Further, according to Greenwald et al.:

> [A]lthough we found that physician-owners do tend to favor their own specialty hospitals, they also refer patients to competitor hospitals; the size of the ownership share appears to be an important factor, not the fact of ownership per se. We also found that most physician-owners have very small shares in their specialty hospital and, possibly as a consequence, make few referrals to the facility.[110]

Third, almost all the studies contributing to this debate were conducted prior to implementation of the Medicare Severity-Diagnosis Related Groups (MS-DRGs) in 2007. (Please see Chapter 6 for an explanation of this method.) Briefly, prior to this time, facilities could profit by doing the same procedures on healthier patients. After this time, payments have been adjusted depending on the severity of each case, thus limiting (though not eliminating) the ability to "cream skim" the patients with the lowest resource use.

The research in this area has focused not just on the term "physician-owned hospitals" but also on "single-specialty hospitals" (SSHs). Specific definitions have varied, but Medicare has used the term "SSH" to designate facilities that are largely physician-owned and that primarily treat patients with cardiac, orthopedic, or general surgical services; physician ownership varies by type of hospital and ranges from about 33% to 100%.

---

[108]Mitchell, J. (2010). Effect of physician ownership of specialty hospitals and ambulatory surgery centers on frequency of use of outpatient orthopedic surgery. *Archives of Surgery*, 145, 732–738. In another article (Mitchell, J. [2008]. Do financial incentives linked to ownership of specialty hospitals affect physicians' practice patterns? *Medical Care*, 46, 732–737), the author comes to the same conclusions based on a sample of Oklahoma workers' compensation cases for back/spine disorders.

[109]Schneider, J. E., Ohsfeldt, R. L., & Li, P. (2010). The effects of endogenous market entry of physician-owned hospitals on medicare expenditures: An instrumental variables approach. *Contemporary Economic Policy*, 29, 151–162.

[110]Greenwald, L., Cromwell, J., Adamache, W., Bernard, S., Drozd, E., Root, E., & Devers, K. (2006). Specialty versus community hospitals: Referrals, quality, and community benefits. *Health Affairs*, 25(1), 106–118.

An example of a study using this terminology provides further insights. Carey et al.[111] found that:

> SSHs are entering less regulated markets; virtually all SSH growth nationally since 1990 has been in states without certificate of need (CON) laws.
>
> [R]esults did not show an overall statistical effect of either growing or declining safety-net services among general hospitals. [In other words, if SSHs take the most profitable patients, the provision of necessary community services were not reduced due to loss of profitable cross subsidies.]
>
> SSH entry is associated not only with more cardiac services being performed, but with *more* hospitals performing cardiac services since some that did not offer these services prior to the SSH entry added them. Competition from orthopedic and surgical SSHs also is associated with the growth of freestanding outpatient centers that are affiliated with general hospitals.
>
> [H]igh-technology diagnostic services showed a very strong pattern of growth in markets with increasing SSH competition compared to markets without SSH competition.

Further, numerous studies have concluded that after adjustments for lower severity and higher procedure volume, "specialty hospitals appear to offer levels of [technical] quality at least comparable and in some cases better than their general hospital counterparts."[112] Proponents of these hospitals claim the results are from the specialization in a particular service and process, so-called focused factories.[113] Critics point out that even after clinical risk adjustment, differences in such factors as race and insurance status skew these results in favor of the SSH. Some even criticize the comparability of populations after risk adjustment.[114]

Using another type of measure, patient satisfaction, SSHs have enjoyed high scores compared to general hospitals in the same market.[115]

---

[111]Carey, K., Burgess, J. F., & Young, G. J. (2009, Summer). Single specialty hospitals and service competition. *Inquiry*, *46*, 162–171.

[112]Several of these studies are summarized in: Schneider, J. E., Miller, T. R., Ohsfeldt, R. L., Morrisey, M. A., Zeiner, B. A., & Li, P. (2008). The economics of specialty hospitals. *Medical Care Research and Review*, *65*, 531–553.

[113]Herzlinger, R. (1997). *Market-driven healthcare: Who wins, who loses in the transformation of America's largest service industry*. Reading, MA: Addison-Wesley.

[114]O'Neill, L., & Hartz, A. J. (2012). Lower mortality rates at cardiac specialty hospitals traceable to healthier patients and to doctors' performing more procedures. *Health Affairs*, *31*(4), 806–815.

[115]See, for example: Dunn, L. (2012, January 27). Press Ganey honors 20 physician-owned hospitals with summit award. *Becker's Hospital Review*. Retrieved from http://www.beckershospitalreview.com/news-analysis/press-ganey-honors-20-physician-owned-hospitals-with-summit-award.html; and, more recently, Dyrda, L. (2017, February 13). 38 physician-owned hospitals receive top patient ratings. *Beckers Hospital Review*. Retrieved from https://www.beckershospitalreview.com/rankings-and-ratings/38-physician-owned-hospitals-receive-top-patient-ratings.html

As far as cost, while higher profitability of SSHs has been linked to choice of higher reimbursed services, there is evidence that they are more efficient than general hospitals.[116] Further, Schneider et al.[117] concluded:

> Much of the policy concerns over physician ownership, particularly those arguing that the "demand inducement" aspects of physician ownership drive up costs, are likely overstated. Conversely, taking the quality and expenditure savings estimates together, POHs [physician-owned hospitals] would generate about $10 billion in savings over a 10-year period.

Other, more recent, studies reached these conclusions:

- "Although POHs may treat slightly healthier patients, they do not seem to systematically select more profitable or less disadvantaged patients or to provide lower value care."[118]

- "Certain models consistently outperformed others based on the VBPP [Medicare Value Based Purchasing Program] methodology. In general, smaller physician-owned hospitals outscored larger tertiary centers, teaching hospitals, and safety-net providers."[119]

- "[P]hysician-owned hospitals are associated with lower mean Medicare costs, fewer complications, and higher patient satisfaction following THA [total hip arthroplasty] and TKA [total knee arthroplasty] than non-physician-owned hospitals."[120]

In summary, the two objections to physician-owned hospitals that have led to government regulation, namely that taking the most profitable patients causes a decrement in the ability of general hospitals to care for poorer patients and increases overall expenses, have not been conclusively proved.[121] More current analyses need to be performed to enlighten healthcare policy. However, in the absence of such data, the future of such facilities will depend as much on which political party controls Congress and the lobbying power of their critics as it does on their cost and quality performances.

---

[116] Kumar, K. (2010). Specialty hospitals emulating focused factories. *International Journal of Health Quality Assurance*, *23*, 94–109.

[117] *The effects of physician-owned hospitals on medical care quality and expenditures: A review and update* ("Avalon Health Economics Study") (July 2015). Retrieved May 8, 2018, from http://waysandmeans.house.gov/wp-content/uploads/2016/08/20150519HL-SFR-Johnson-PHA-Summary-Value-Manuscript-.pdf N.B.: "This research received partial support from an unrestricted research grant from Physician Hospitals of America."

[118] Blumenthal, D., Orav, E. J., Jena, A. B., Dudzinski, D. M., Le, S. T., & Jha, A. K. (2015). Access, quality, and costs of care at physician-owned hospitals in the United States: Observational study. *BMJ, 351*, h4466. doi:10.1136/bmj.h4466.

[119] Ramirez, A., Tracci, M. C., Stukenborg, G. J., Turrentine, F. E., Kozower, B. D., & Jones, R. S. (2016). Physician-owned surgical hospitals outperform other hospitals in the medicare value-based purchasing program. *Journal of the American College of Surgeons*, *223*(4), 559–567.

[120] Courtney, P. M., Darrith, B., Bohl, D. D., Frisch, N. B., Della Valle, C. J. (2017). Reconsidering the affordable care act's restrictions on physician-owned hospitals: Analysis of CMS data on total hip and knee arthroplasty. *Journal of Bone and Joint Surgery*, *99*(22), 1888–1894.

[121] For a detailed economic analysis of this issue, see: Schneider, J. E., Miller, T. R., Ohsfeldt, R. L., Morrisey, M. A., Zeiner, B. A., & Li, P. (2008). The economics of specialty hospitals. *Medical Care Research and Review, 65*, 531–553.

Safety Net Providers. Many public and private facilities are included in a group called *safety net providers*. The Institute of Medicine[122] described these institutions as those that:

> deliver a significant level of health care to uninsured, Medicaid, and other vulnerable patients . . . These providers have two distinguishing characteristics:
>
> 1. Either by legal mandate or explicitly adopted mission, they offer care to patients regardless of their ability to pay for those services; and
> 2. A substantial share of their patient mix are uninsured, Medicaid, and other vulnerable patients. Core safety net providers typically include public hospitals, community health centers, and local health departments, as well as special service providers such as AIDS and school-based clinics.[123]

Additionally, the hospital's financial condition and the provision of selected services (e.g., trauma, burn, and neonatal intensive care) may be considered.[124]

Within this group are a number of classifications distinguished by payer mix, geography, and the method of federal payment for their services. These types of institutions are subject to their own Medicare Conditions of Participation in addition to the eligibility requirements that distinguish each one.

Disproportionate share hospitals. Medicare and Medicaid have separate programs to help hospitals who care for a disproportionate number of poorer Medicare patients (those on Supplemental Security Income [SSI]) and Medicaid (non-dual eligible) patients, respectively. Prior to 1981, the payment method for Medicaid services was a vaguely worded "reasonable costs" standard, and the federal government gave states leeway to set eligibility and payments standards. To establish a more solid footing for payments and address increasing costs, the Disproportionate Share Hospital (DSH) program was started by the Omnibus Budget Reconciliation Act of 1981. It was strengthened by the Omnibus Budget Reconciliation Act of 1987 (P.L. 100-203), which required state Medicaid agencies to make additional payments to hospitals that serve disproportionate numbers of low-income patients with special needs. (Its permanence was codified in Section 1923 of the Social Security Act.) However, because the payments were not capped, program costs began to rise rapidly, causing the federal government to gradually institute three measures to control spending. First, national and state-specific ceilings were placed on special payments to DSH hospitals.[125]

---

[122] Institute of Medicine. (2000). *America's health care safety net: Intact but endangered*. Washington, DC: The National Academies Press. doi:10.17226/9612

[123] Two important organizations that represent these facilities are the National Association of Community Health Centers (http://www.nachc.org) and the National Association of Public Hospitals and Health Systems (http://www.naph.org). Both retrieved May 8, 2018.

[124] Bachrach, B., Braslow, L., & Karl, A. (2012). Toward a high performance health care system for vulnerable populations: Funding for safety-net hospitals. *The Commonwealth Fund* (March 8). Retrieved April 29, 2018, from http://www.commonwealthfund.org/Publications/Fund-Reports/2012/Mar/Vulnerable-Populations.aspx?view=print&page=all

[125] Medicaid Voluntary Contribution and Provider-Specific Tax Amendments of 1991 (P.L. 102–234).

Second, hospital-specific ceilings were set on payments.[126] Finally, limits to DSH allotments were set at 12 % of states' total annual Medicaid expenditures.[127] Except for some adjustments in 2003, the structure remained the same until passage of the Affordable Care Act (ACA) in 2010. Since the government anticipated that many more people would be insured under the ACA, the law contains provisions to scale back DSH payments through 2020. In addition to the change in amounts, Section 3133 of the ACA also revises the *method* for computing the Medicare DSH adjustment for discharges occurring on or after October 1, 2013:

1. Instead of the amount that would otherwise be paid as the DSH adjustment, hospitals receive 25 percent of the amount determined under the current Medicare DSH payment method beginning in fiscal year (FY) 2014 (for discharges occurring on or after October 1, 2013).

2. The remainder, equal to 75 percent of what otherwise would have been paid as Medicare DSH, becomes available for an uncompensated care payment after the amount is reduced for changes in the percentage of individuals who are uninsured. The Centers for Medicare & Medicaid Services (CMS) is currently using uncompensated care costs reported on Worksheet S-10 in combination with insured low-income days (the sum of Medicaid days and Medicare SSI days) to develop hospital uncompensated care payments. Each hospital eligible for Medicare DSH payments receives an uncompensated care payment based on its relative share of total uncompensated care costs and low-income days reported by Medicare DSHs.[128]

Subsequent laws provide examples of legislative delay, indecision, and bowing to political pressures. First, the payment reductions were extended to 2021[129] and 2022.[130] In 2013, the lowered payments were put on hold until 2016, but the reductions were extended to 2023.[131] The following year, the reductions were delayed until 2017 and extended to 2024.[132] In 2015, the reductions were revised further to cover 2018 to 2025, with increasing reductions in payments reaching $8 billion for the final 2 years. Finally, in 2018, the 2018–2019 reductions were eliminated and the cutbacks for 2020 to 2025 were adjusted.[133] Under current law, federal DSH allotments are scheduled to be reduced in fiscal year (FY) 2020 by $4 billion, which is 31% of states' unreduced DSH allotment amounts. DSH allotment reductions are scheduled to increase to $8 billion a year in FYs 2021 to 2025.

---

[126] The Omnibus Budget Reconciliation Act of 1993 (P.L. 103–66).

[127] Balanced Budget Act of 1997 (BBA 97, P.L. 105–33).

[128] Medicare Learning Network Fact Sheet. (2018, May) *Medicare disproportionate share hospital*. Updated May 2018. Retrieved from https://www.cms.gov/Outreach-and-Education/Medicare-Learning-Network-MLN/MLNProducts/Downloads/Disproportionate_Share_Hospital.pdf

[129] Middle Class Tax Relief and Job Creation Act of 2012 (P.L. 112–96).

[130] American Taxpayer Relief Act of 2012 (P.L. 112–240).

[131] Bipartisan Budget Act of 2013 (P.L. 113–67).

[132] Protecting Access to Medicare Act of 2014 (P.L. 113–93).

[133] Bipartisan Budget Act of 2018 (P.L. 115–123).

Future payments will take into account the Medicaid and Children's Health Insurance Program (CHIP) Payment and Access Commission (MACPAC) assessments of the program. Most recently, MACPAC reported that it:

> continues to find little meaningful relationship between DSH allotments and the number of uninsured individuals; the amounts and sources of hospitals' uncompensated care costs; and the number of hospitals with high levels of uncompensated care that also provide essential community services for low-income, uninsured, and vulnerable populations. Total hospital charity care and bad debt continue to fall, especially in states that expanded Medicaid coverage.[134]

Specifically, the study found that in the years since implementation of the ACA, total hospital charity care and bad debt fell by $8.6 billion (23%) between 2013 and 2015, with the largest declines occurring in states that expanded Medicaid.

Currently, eligibility is determined according to the formula below. "If a hospital's DPP [Disproportionate Patient Percentage] equals or exceeds a specified threshold amount, the hospital qualifies for the Medicare DSH adjustment. The Medicare DSH adjustment is determined by using a complex formula (the applicable formula is also based on a hospital's particular DPP)."[135]

Alternatively, a hospital can qualify if it is located in an urban area, has 100 or more beds, and can demonstrate that more than 30% of total net inpatient care revenues come from state and local government sources for indigent care (other than Medicare or Medicaid).

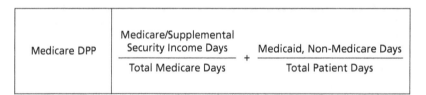

According to MACPAC, in fiscal year 2017, "a total of $12 billion in federal funds was allotted for DSH payments. Similar to other types of Medicaid payments, federal DSH funds must be matched by state funds; in total, $21 billion in state and federal DSH funds were allotted in FY 2017."[136]

Despite these delays and particularly in the face of subsequent adjustments, six issues must still be considered with regard to reduced DSH's financial impact. First, in order to keep their volumes up and provide a source of funding that currently comes from DSH payments, these facilities will need to obtain contracts with the companies participating in

[134]MACPAC (Medicaid and CHIP Payment and Access Commission). (2018, March). *Report to Congress on Medicaid and CHIP*. Retrieved May 9, 2018, from https://www.macpac.gov/wp-content/uploads/2018/03/Report-to-Congress-on-Medicaid-and-CHIP-March-2018.pdf

[135]Medicare Learning Network Fact Sheet, op. cit.

[136]MACPAC. (2017, June). Issue Brief https://www.macpac.gov/wp-content/uploads/2017/06/Medicaid-DSH-Allotments-How-Could-Funding-for-Safety-Net-Hospitals-Change-in-2018.pdf

the Health Insurance Exchanges that the ACA created. Second, when DSH payments are reduced or eliminated, the Medicaid payments may remain inadequate, since each state has wide discretion in its own program's design, including scope of benefits and payment amounts. Third, about 15.5% of adults aged 19 to 64 remain uninsured, higher than in 2016.[137] Current DSH payments may no longer be available to subsidize their care. Fourth, many of these hospitals provide specialty care to currently insured patients. For example, Cook County Hospital has one of the area's few burn care units. With subsidy removals for services that are undercompensated (like burns), hospitals may be hard-pressed to continue offering them. Fifth, reduction in DSH payments was based on anticipated full enrollment in Medicaid expansion. However, with states being able to opt out, these uninsured persons will still seek uncompensated care, but now without DSH payments. The uninsured rate in states that did not expand their Medicaid programs is 21.9%.[138] Finally, a significant number of these hospitals' patients are Medicare beneficiaries. Medicare's payment structure is increasingly incorporating a "value-based" purchasing scheme that reduces payment if patient evaluations of the process of care fall below target values.[139] Because safety-net hospitals (SNHs) have lower scores than non-SNHs on measures of patient-reported experience,[140] their Medicare payments will suffer, thus reducing yet another source of funds.

Medicare-dependent hospitals. Medicare-dependent hospitals (MDHs) have 100 or fewer beds, are not also classified as a sole community hospital (SCH) (see below), and at least 60% of their inpatient days or discharges are attributable to individuals receiving Medicare Part A benefits.[141] Because hospitals have claimed that Medicare payments do not adequately compensate them for their expenses, MDHs can receive inpatient payments based on the greater of the Medicare Prospective Payment Rate (PPR) or a blend of the PPR (25%) and their historical costs (75%).[142]

Although most of these facilities are rural, a subset are designated Urban Medicare Dependent Hospitals (UMDHs). Section 3142 of the ACA defines an UMDH as a hospital that

> does not receive any additional Medicare payments or adjustments under section 1886(d)
> of the Social Security Act, such as indirect graduate medical education payments

[137]Collins, S. R., Gunja, M. Z., Doty, M. M., & Bhupal, H. (2018, May 1). First look at health insurance coverage in 2018 finds ACA gains beginning to reverse. Retrieved May 9, 2018, from http://www.commonwealthfund.org/publications/blog/2018/apr/health-coverage-erosion

[138]Ibid.

[139]HCAHPS (Hospital Consumer Assessment of Healthcare Providers and Systems). Retrieved May 9, 2018, from https://www.cms.gov/Medicare/Quality-Initiatives-Patient-Assessment-Instruments/HospitalQualityInits/HospitalHCAHPS.html

[140]Chatterjee, P., Joynt, K. E., Orav, E. J., & Jha, A. K. (2012). Patient experience in safety-net hospitals: Implications for improving care and value-based purchasing. *Archives of Internal Medicine, 172*(16), 1204–1210.

[141]42 C.F.R. § 412.108 Special treatment: Medicare-dependent, small rural hospitals. Title 42—Public Health.

[142]MedPAC. (2017, October). *Critical access hospitals' payment system.* Retrieved May 10, 2018, from http://www.medpac.gov/docs/default-source/payment-basics/medpac_payment_basics_17_cah_final09a311adfa9c665e80adfff00009edf9c.pdf?sfvrsn=

under subsection (d)(5)(B), disproportionate share payments, payments to a rural referral center (RRC), payments to a sole community hospital (SCH), or payments to a Medicare-dependent small rural hospital. In addition, the hospital must not be a critical access hospital (CAH).[143]

This program was extended by the Bipartisan Budget Act of 2018 through September 30, 2022, and the terms are discussed in the 2019 Medicare Inpatient Prospective Payment System (IPPS) rule.[144] CMS projected that the MDH program extension should have paid hospitals about $119 million in 2018.

Sole community hospitals. Congress created the Sole Community Hospital (SCH) program in 1983 to support small rural hospitals that, "by reason of factors such as isolated location, weather conditions, travel conditions, or absence of other hospitals, [are] the sole source of inpatient hospital services reasonably available in a geographic area to Medicare beneficiaries."[145] CMS defines an SCH as a hospital paid under the Medicare IPPS that meets *one* of the following criteria:

1. The hospital is located at least 35 miles from other like hospitals, i.e., those that furnish short-term, acute care; are paid under the Medicare Acute Care Hospital PPS; and are not Critical Access Hospitals *or*

2. The hospital is rural, located between 25 and 35 miles from other like hospitals, and meets one of these criteria:

   a) No more than 25 percent of residents who become hospital inpatients or no more than 25 percent of the Medicare beneficiaries who become hospital inpatients in the hospital's service area are admitted to other like hospitals located within a 35-mile radius of the hospital or, if larger, within its service area *or*

   b) The hospital has fewer than 50 beds and would meet the 25 percent criterion above if not for the fact that some beneficiaries or residents were forced to seek specialized care outside of the service area due to the unavailability of necessary specialty services at the hospital *or*

   c) The hospital is rural and located between 15 and 25 miles from other like hospitals but because of local topography or periods of prolonged severe weather conditions, the other like hospitals are inaccessible for at least 30 days in each of 2 out of 3 years *or*

   d) The hospital is rural and because of distance, posted speed limits, and predictable weather conditions, the travel time between the hospital and the nearest like hospital is at least 45 minutes.[146]

---

[143] Sibelius, K. (2010). Report to Congress. Department of Health and Human Services Study of Urban Medicare-Dependent Hospitals. Retrieved May 10, 2018, from http://www.cms.gov/Research-Statistics-Data-and-Systems/Statistics-Trends-and-Reports/Reports/downloads/Riley_UMDH_RTC_2010.pdf

[144] Department of Health and Human Services (2018, May 7). Centers for Medicare & Medicaid Services 42 CFR Parts 412, 413, 424, and 495. *Federal Register,83*, 88. Proposed Rules, pp. 20172–20175. Retrieved from https://www.gpo.gov/fdsys/pkg/FR-2018-05-07/pdf/2018-08705.pdf.

[145] Section 405.476, Title 42 of the 1983 Code of Federal Regulations.

[146] Medicare Learning Network: Acute Care Hospital Inpatient Prospective Payment System. March 2018. https://www.cms.gov/Outreach-and-Education/Medicare-Learning-Network-MLN/MLNProducts/Downloads/AcutePaymtSysfctsht.pdf Retrieved May 10, 2018.

3. The hospital is rural and located between 15 and 25 miles from other like hospitals but because of local topography or periods of prolonged severe weather conditions, the other like hospitals are inaccessible for at least 30 days in each of 2 out of 3 years or

4. The hospital is rural and because of distance, posted speed limits, and predictable weather conditions, the travel time between the hospital and the nearest like hospital is at least 45 minutes . . .

A hospital's service area is the area from which it draws at least 75% of its inpatients during the most recent 12-month cost reporting period ending before it applies for classification as an SCH.

Rural SCHs are paid for inpatient care on a cost basis rather than by DRG and are allowed to choose from several years on which to base these payments.[147] Starting in 2016, rural SCHs received an additional 7.1% above standard payment rates for outpatient prospective payment services excluding drugs, biologics, brachytherapy sources, and devices paid under the pass-through payment policy (devices that receive temporary extra payment because of their newness and uniqueness).

Critical access hospital. The Balanced Budget Act of 1997 (P.L. 105-33) created the category of critical access hospitals (CAHs), expanding and replacing the Essential Access Community Hospital/Rural Primary Care Hospital Program and the Medical Assistance Facilities demonstration in Montana.[148]

A Medicare-participating hospital must meet the following criteria for CMS to designate it a CAH:[149]

- Be located in a state that has established a State Medicare Rural Hospital Flexibility Program.

- Be designated by the state as a CAH.

- Be located in a rural area or an area that is treated as rural.

- Be located either more than 35 miles from the nearest hospital or CAH or more than 15 miles in areas with mountainous terrain or only secondary roads; OR prior to January 1, 2006, was certified as a CAH based on state designation as a "necessary provider" of healthcare services to residents in the area.

- Maintain no more than 25 inpatient beds that can be used for either inpatient or swing-bed services. In addition to the 25 inpatient CAH beds, a CAH may also operate a psychiatric and/or a rehabilitation distinct part unit of up to 10 beds each. These units must comply with the Hospital Conditions of Participation.

---

[147]Code of Federal Regulations. Title 42—Public Health. Vol. 2, Date: 2017-10-01 Title: Section §412.92—Special treatment: Sole community hospitals. Retrieved May 10, 2018, from https://www.gpo.gov/fdsys/pkg/CFR-2017-title42-vol2/xml/CFR-2017-title42-vol2-sec412-92.xml

[148]Since a number of legislative changes shaped this program over the years since its establishment, see CAH Legislative History. Retrieved May 10, 2018, from http://www.aha.org/advocacy-issues/cah/history.shtml

[149]Critical Access Hospitals. Retrieved May 3, 2018, from http://www.cms.gov/Medicare/Provider-Enrollment-and-Certification/CertificationandComplianc/CAHs.html

- Maintain an annual average length of stay of 96 hours or less per patient for acute inpatient care (excluding swing-bed services and beds that are within distinct part units).

- Demonstrate compliance with the critical access hospitals conditions of participation found at 42 Code of Federal Regulations (CFR), Part 485 subpart F.

- Furnish 24-hour emergency care services 7 days a week.

These facilities may also be health clinics or centers (as defined by the state) that previously operated as a hospital before being downsized to a health clinic or center.

Like MDHs and SCHs, the CAHs are not subject to the fixed Inpatient Prospective Payment System (IPPS) or Outpatient Prospective Payment System. Instead, a CAH may bill Medicare under one of two methods. The Standard Payment Method allows the hospital to bill for facility services (inpatient and outpatient) based on 101% of reasonable costs.[150] Under the Optional Payment Method, the hospital can bill for both facility and physician services, the latter at 115% of local Medicare rates. In order to be eligible for the optional method, a physician must assign Part B billing rights to the CAH. Additionally, since 2007, physicians and other practitioners electing the optional method can bill Medicare for telehealth services.[151]

These higher payment levels (compared to Medicare inpatient and outpatient prospective payment methods) are supposed to enable these facilities to furnish services in scarcity areas while maintaining quality care. Research on this topic shows that for most services, CAHs furnish comparable care; however, this finding does not necessarily hold as complexity increases. For example:

- With respect to Medicare beneficiaries, prior to 2002, CAHs and non-CAHs had similar mortality rates. However, for "beneficiaries with acute myocardial infarction, congestive heart failure, or pneumonia, 30-day mortality rates for those admitted to CAHs, compared with those admitted to other acute care hospitals, increased from 2002 to 2010."[152]

- "Among Medicare beneficiaries undergoing common surgical procedures, patients admitted to critical access hospitals compared with non–critical access hospitals had no significant difference in 30-day mortality rates, decreased risk-adjusted serious complication rates, and lower-adjusted Medicare expenditures, but were less medically complex."[153]

---

[150]The Medicare Prescription Drug, Improvement, and Modernization Act (MMA) of 2003 (P.L. 108–173, Section 405). This Act increased payment to 101% of costs and created the Optional Payments method.

[151]Medicare Learning Network. (2017, August). Critical Access Hospital. Retrieved May 10, 2018, from https://www.cms.gov/Outreach-and-Education/Medicare-Learning-Network-MLN/MLNProducts/downloads/CritAccessHospfctsht.pdf

[152]Joynt, K. E., Orav, E. J., & Jha, K. A. (2013). Mortality rates for Medicare beneficiaries admitted to critical access and non–critical access hospitals, 2002–2010. *JAMA, 309,* 1379–1387.

[153]Ibrahim, A. M., Hughes, T. G., Thumma, J. R., Dimick, J. B. (2016). Association of hospital critical access status with surgical outcomes and expenditures among Medicare beneficiaries. *JAMA, 315*(19), 2095–2103.

■ "Compared with PPS hospitals, CAHs are significantly less likely to have any observed (unadjusted) adverse event on 4 of the 6 indicators. After adjusting for patient mix and hospital characteristics, CAHs perform better on 3 of the 6 indicators. Accounting for the number of discharges eliminated the differences between CAHs and PPS hospitals in the likelihood of adverse events across all indicators except one . . . The study suggests there are no differences in surgical patient safety outcomes between CAHs and PPS hospitals of comparable size."[154]

■ "For emergency colectomy procedures, Medicare beneficiaries in critical access hospitals experienced lower mortality rates but more frequent re-operation and readmission. These findings suggest that critical access hospitals provide safe, essential emergency surgical care, but may need more resources for postoperative care coordination in these high-risk operations."[155]

The relative numbers of the three types of hospitals described above are displayed in Exhibit 4.20.

EXHIBIT 4.20. Share of Hospitals and Medicare Payments by Rural Hospital Type, 2015

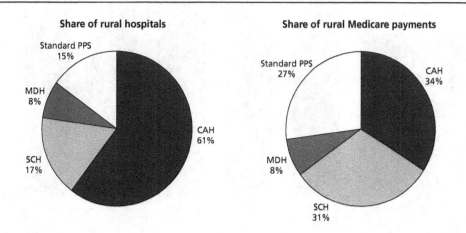

Share of rural hospitals

Standard PPS
15%

MDH
8%

SCH
17%

CAH
61%

Share of rural Medicare payments

Standard PPS
27%

CAH
34%

MDH
8%

SCH
31%

Religious-sponsored (faith-based) hospitals. The origins of these hospitals are discussed in the history section above, and they share many of the same issues as other hospitals. What

---

[154]Natafgi, N., Baloh, J., Weigel, P., Ullrich, F., & Ward, M. M. (2017). Surgical patient safety outcomes in critical access hospitals: How do they compare? *The Journal of Rural Health, 33*(2), 117–126.

[155]Ibrahim, A. M., Regenbogen, S. E., Thumma, J. R., Dimick, J. B. (2018). Emergency surgery for medicare beneficiaries admitted to critical access hospitals. *Annals of Surgery, 267*(3), 473–477, 2018.

distinguishes them from the other types of hospitals is that religious beliefs guide not only what care they provide but *how* they provide the care (e.g., with compassion and attention to the individual's spiritual, as well as physical, needs). The number of these organizations has continued to grow, as shown in Exhibit 4.21.

The predominant affiliation of these hospitals is Catholic. The more than 600 Catholic hospitals make up over 14% of the all acute care hospitals and 1 in 6 acute care beds. CMS has identified 46 of them as being "sole community" providers. Further, Catholic systems own more than 1,400 long-term care facilities across 50 states.[156]

These hospitals control what is provided to patients in such areas as reproductive services and end-of-life care. The principles that guide their actions are dictated by the United States Conference of Catholic Bishops.[157]

EXHIBIT 4.21. Number of Faith-Based Hospitals in the United States from 1995 to 2016

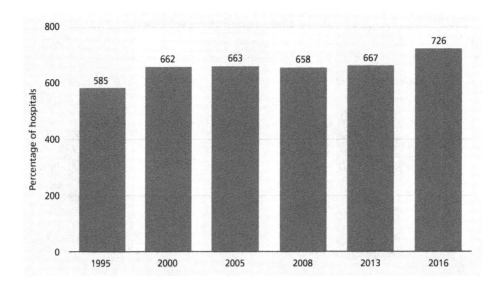

Note: In 2016, 17% of all U.S. hospitals were faith-based.

Source: The Governance Institute. © Statistica. Used with permission.

[156] Johnson, S. R. (2017, September 14). As Catholic systems grow by acquiring other hospitals, abortions plummet. *Modern Healthcare*. Retrieved May 10, 2018, from http://www.modernhealthcare.com/article/20170914/NEWS/170919931
[157] United States Conference of Catholic Bishops. (2009). Ethical and Religious Directives for Catholic Health Care Services (5th ed.). Retrieved May 10, 2018, from http://www.modernhealthcare.com/article/20170914/NEWS/170919931

HOSPITAL INPATIENT PAYMENT METHODS

Hospitals include in their descriptions of financial conditions and projections a metric called *payer mix*, or what percentage of their services are paid by private payers, Medicare, Medicaid, self-pay (direct patient payments), and charity (free) care. Of equal importance, though often lacking, is a description of the mix of the *methods* of payment. The frequency of these methods on a geographic or hospital-specific level can vary dramatically, depending on such population factors as economics (Medicaid eligibility) and age (Medicare) and on such insurance market factors as penetration of types of managed care and degree of competition among payers and providers.

The following eight methods (which are not mutually exclusive for a given institution) are used to pay hospitals for inpatient services; they may also be used in other countries as well as in the United States.

1. *Fee for service*. This arrangement is the traditional retail model where the payer pays charges. This method is best for hospitals since markups are significant and can cover uncompensated/undercompensated care. It is obviously the worst method for payers.

2. *Discount fee for service*. This scheme is not quite a "wholesale" model since the charges on which the discounts are based can be raised significantly to make payments substantial. It is very favorable for hospitals and only slightly better for payers.

3. *DRGs*. Please see the Medicare section in Chapter 6 for a discussion of DRGs. Briefly, this method is a single payment for inpatient services based on the reason (diagnosis) the patient was in the hospital. DRGs cover only the hospital portion while bundled/global payments (see below) cover physician services and possibly some post-discharge care as well. This method is better for payers since it can help predict hospital costs given the mix of expected illnesses in a population. It also limits payment for particularly costly patients.[158]

4. *Per diems*. Before discussing this topic, it should be noted that hospital expense for providing inpatient care is typically greatest in the first day or two of the stay, when costly procedures and/or tests are usually performed. As patients recuperate or receive ongoing treatment (such as intravenous medication), costs are lower than at the beginning of the stay. When payment is by DRG or global rate, shorter times are more profitable for the hospital, since revenue does not increase with longer stays but expenses do accumulate. With FFS-like payments, however, longer stays are much more lucrative for hospitals since (barring complications) their margins are higher nearest the time of discharge.

   When managed care plans such as health maintenance organizations (discussed in more detail in the Managed Care section in Chapter 6) started to become more prevalent in the 1980s, they were looking for clearer, easier, and presumably cheaper alternatives to FFS hospital payments. While some companies negotiated payments based

---

[158]If patients are very ill and require prolonged services, Medicare will pay extra amounts called "outlier payments."

on discount charges or DRG-like schemes, others crafted a method based on a flat, all-inclusive, daily (per diem) fee. Each level of service (such as intensive care, regular medical/surgical care, maternity care, and psychiatric care) has its own daily charge. Total payment is, therefore, the sum of all the daily charges. The method for calculating these fees was simple: With adjustments for days spent at different levels of care, the per diem was the quotient of total costs divided by total days.

While this method is simple, for three reasons it led to inadequate compensation for hospitals. First, the patients who were being admitted were sicker than the average case used to calculate the average payments. This situation was due to an increased capability to treat many illnesses in the outpatient setting and increased scrutiny of the appropriateness of hospitalization (utilization review). Second, the lengths of stay were shortened and patients were being transferred to less expensive sites of care, such as skilled nursing facilities. The "profitable" part of the hospital stay was, therefore being truncated. Finally, when most of the payers compensated hospitals on an FFS basis, no shortfall existed (or it was insignificant); all fixed costs were essentially being covered by these traditional plans, and these per diem contracts were more than covering marginal costs. However, when many private payers switched to per diem payments after the late 1980s, hospitals began to feel the economic strains.

5. *Budgets.* Many government hospitals, such as those of the Veterans Administration (VA) and counties, are given annual budgets with which they must deliver all their services. These hospitals are not prohibited from collecting from private payers when such coverage is available; however, frequently they are not equipped or are unwilling to do so because of the relatively low volume of these patients. For example, a 2009 GAO study found that for patient services at 18 VA medical centers: "Although some medical services are not billable, such as service-connected treatment, management had not validated reasons for related unbilled amounts of about $1.4 billion to assure that all billable costs are charged to third-party insurers."[159]

The advantage to the payer of this method is the ability to budget expenses. The disadvantage is that the hospitals have a disincentive to be more efficient; if they do not spend their budgeted money in the designated year, their next allocation is reduced at least by the amount of the savings.

6. *Risk.* This arrangement is more fully explained in the next section on organized delivery systems/accountable care organizations. Briefly, this scheme requires hospitals to accept financial risk for caring for patients (akin to insurance risk) as well as clinical risk (i.e., responsibility for the quality of care). In the latter case, the payer financially rewards the organization with additional payments if certain targets are met. Monies may also be deducted from payments if hospitals do not achieve certain thresholds.

---

[159]Government Accountability Office Document GAO-10-152T: VA Health Care: Ineffective Medical Center Controls Resulted in Inappropriate Billing and Collection Practices. October 15, 2009. Retrieved May 8, 2018, from https://www.gao.gov/assets/130/123540.pdf

7. *Bundled/global/packaged payments.*[160] Instead of receiving a bill for multiple services from multiple providers, the payer negotiates one fee for an *episode of care*. As mentioned above, while DRGs refer only to in-patient services, bundled payments can refer to outpatient care as well as combined inpatient and outpatient care for the same episode of illness. Bundled payments often include professional charges (such as physician fees) and ancillaries (laboratory and radiology). While private payers have been paying in this fashion for a number of years (e.g., for such services as transplantation and coronary artery bypass surgery), as a result of provisions in the ACA, Medicare has been at the forefront of initiating a bundled payments program based on the success of previous pilot studies. For example, in the Medicare Acute Care Episode (ACE) Demonstration project, which bundled certain in-hospital cardiac and orthopedic procedures in selected states, Medicare achieved a per- episode savings of $319 and total net savings of approximately $4 million.[161] The Medicare bundled payment programs have undergone many politically motivated changes in the past several years. Most recently, CMS announced voluntary Bundled Payments for Care Improvement Advanced (BPCI Advanced) for 32 clinical episodes in order "to align incentives among participating health care providers for reducing expenditures and improving quality of care for Medicare beneficiaries."[162] The program began October 1, 2018, and will run through December 31, 2023. Exhibit 4.22 provides a list of these episodes. Note the diversity of conditions, which provides the opportunity for businesses to partner with provider organizations to deliver cost-effective care.

8. *Quality payments.* In addition to the above methods, hospitals are also paid or penalized for their performance of clinical care. Please see Chapter 9 for details of this process.

ORGANIZED (INTEGRATED) DELIVERY SYSTEMS/ACCOUNTABLE CARE ORGANIZATIONS

Origins and Definition

In the 1990s, a number of researchers conducted studies on what were then called integrated or organized delivery systems (IDSs or ODSs). These systems were formed for the same reasons listed above for hospital systems. An ODS was defined as "[a] network of organizations which provides or arranges to provide a coordinated continuum of services to a

---

[160]These three terms are often used interchangeably or idiosyncratically. Since Medicare has a program that it calls Bundled Payment, this term will be used for this concept.

[161]Centers for Medicare & Medicaid Services Final Evaluation Report Evaluation of the Medicare Acute Care Episode (ACE) Demonstration. May 31, 2013. Retrieved May 10, 2018, from https://downloads.cms.gov/files/cmmi/ACE-EvaluationReport-Final-5-2-14.pdf Of note is that the savings from the acute care episode (physician and hospital charges) were more substantial; post-acute care costs *reduced* savings by 45%.

[162]CMS.gov. (2018, April 30). BPCI Advanced. Retrieved May 10, 2018, from https://innovation.cms.gov/initiatives/bpci-advanced

EXHIBIT 4.22. **Clinical Episodes for the Bundled Payments for Care Improvement Advanced Program—29 Inpatient Clinical Episodes**

1. Disorders of the liver excluding malignancy, cirrhosis, alcoholic hepatitis
2. Acute myocardial infarction
3. Back and neck except spinal fusion
4. Cardiac arrhythmia
5. Cardiac defibrillator
6. Cardiac valve
7. Cellulitis
8. Cervical spinal fusion
9. COPD, bronchitis, asthma
10. Combined anterior posterior spinal fusion
11. Congestive heart failure
12. Coronary artery bypass graft
13. Double joint replacement of the lower extremity
14. Fractures of the femur and hip or pelvis
15. Gastrointestinal hemorrhage
16. Gastrointestinal obstruction
17. Hip and femur procedures except major joint
18. Lower-extremity/humerus procedure except hip, foot, femur
19. Major bowel procedure
20. Major joint replacement of the lower extremity
21. Major joint replacement of the upper extremity
22. Pacemaker
23. Percutaneous coronary intervention
24. Renal failure
25. Sepsis
26. Simple pneumonia and respiratory infections
27. Spinal fusion (noncervical)
28. Stroke
29. Urinary tract infection

Three outpatient clinical episodes:

1. Percutaneous coronary intervention (PCI)
2. Cardiac defibrillator
3. Back and neck except spinal fusion

defined population and is willing to be held clinically and fiscally accountable for the outcomes and health status of the population served. An ODS will own or be closely aligned with an insurance product."[163]

The ideal structure of these systems is outlined in Exhibit 4.23.

Noteworthy about this scheme are the following observations:

1. The stakeholders are the same ones discussed in Chapter 1, "Understanding and Managing Complex Healthcare Systems."

2. The end states are cost, quality, and access.

EXHIBIT 4.23. The Value Chain of Healthcare Delivery

Stakeholders	Communities Patients Employees Employers Purchasers Government Investors
	↑
End States	Ease of Interpersonal Accurate Competent Positive Affordable More access satisfaction diagnosis treatment outcomes cost knowledgeable consumer
	↑
Competencies	Disease Health Primary Acute Rehabilitative Chronic Supportive Prevention promotion care care care care care management management management management
	↑
Underlying Capabilities	Functional Physician-system Clinical Integration Integration Integration

Source: Shortell, S., Gillies, R. R., Anderson, D. A., Erickson, K. M., & Mitchell, J. B. (2000). *Remaking healthcare in America: The evolution of organized delivery systems* (2nd ed.). San Francisco: Jossey-Bass.

Functional Integration. The extent to which the supported functions and activities (e.g., financial management, human resources management, information technology management, strategic planning, quality improvement) are coordinated across operating units so as to add greatest overall value to the system.

Physician Integration. The extent to which physicians and the ODSs with which they are associated agree on the aims in purposes of the system and work together to achieve mutually shared objectives.

Clinical Integration. The extent to which patient care services are coordinated across people, functions, activities, and sites over time so as to maximize the value of services delivered to patients.

---

[163] Shortell, S., Gillies, R. R., Anderson, D. A., Erickson, K. M., & Mitchell, J. B. (2000). *Remaking healthcare in America: The evolution of organized delivery systems* (2nd ed.). San Francisco: Jossey-Bass.

3. The competencies represent care across the spectrum of services (from prevention to end-of-life support).

4. Functional integration is the low-hanging fruit of integration—easy to achieve and recognize its financial benefits. It mainly derives from economies of scale.

5. Physician integration requires not just shared culture and goals between those professionals and the system but also a compensation scheme that aligns them.

6. Clinical integration is the hardest alignment to achieve. It requires that the organizations not only have a process in place to learn and develop best practices, but also has a mechanism to spread those best practices and make them part of how the firm works.

7. In order to ensure that these systems accept not only clinical risk for care but also financial risk, they must assume an insurance-like function, either directly by owning an insurance plan or by contracting on some type of risk basis with one.

Despite the success of long-standing, mostly private systems (such as Geisinger, Intermountain Healthcare, Cleveland Clinic, Mayo Clinic, and others), for reasons explained below, this concept did not fulfill the promise of transforming the way care was delivered. More recently, Section 3022 of the ACA[164] added Section 1899 to the Social Security Act that requires the Secretary to establish a Medicare Shared Savings Program, which is the origin of federal ACO initiatives. This change spurred a more recent attempt at using these ODSs (now often called ACOs) to address large regional variations in costs and quality of care. While Medicare funding is the underpinning of this program, the topic is discussed here since it has created a large, renewed impetus for systems to form and integrate. The structures of these newer arrangements are also shaped by the different payment mechanisms described below.

The goal of the ACO initiative is to reward quality performance and operational efficiency rather than sheer volume of services. Also, federal budget deficits made shifting financial risk for the provision of care to providers more attractive to CMS.

According to CMS: "ACOs are groups of doctors, hospitals, and other health care providers, who come together voluntarily to give coordinated high-quality care to the Medicare patients they serve."[165]

In addition to addressing Medicare issues, other provisions in the ACA create a number of constraints on the profitability of *private* payers (e.g., regulated premiums, reduced ability to charge different rates to older and higher risk members, mandated benefits, limits on members' out-of-pocket payments and bounds on profit margins). Consequently, these commercial plans are also very interested in shifting more risk to providers. The result is

---

[164] Section 3022 of the Affordable Care Act added a new section 1899 to the Social Security Act that requires the Secretary to establish a Medicare Shared Savings Program, which is the origin of federal ACO initiatives.

[165] Like many other facts in this book, these provisions are subject to change. The provisions were taken from the CMS publication of the Shared Savings Program: Accountable Care Organizations, October 11, 2011. Retrieved May 13, 2018, from http://www.cms.gov/sharedsavingsprogram

private ACO arrangements whereby the health delivery system takes substantial clinical and financial risk for patient care. Since private payer contracts can vary considerably, the next section focuses on operational requirements of Medicare ACOs.[166]

Eligibility

ACO participants or combinations of ACO participants must qualify as one, or more, of the following providers or suppliers or participate through an ACO formed by one or more of these groups:[167]

- Professionals in group practice arrangements
- Networks of individual professional practices
- Partnerships or joint venture arrangements between hospitals and ACO professionals
- Hospitals employing ACO professionals
- CAHs that bill for both Medicare Part A and B (such as inpatient and physician components)
- Rural health clinics (RHCs)
- Federally Qualified Health Centers (FQHCs)

In 2018, there were 561 ACOs that enrolled 10.5 million beneficiaries; the distribution of types of these organizations in the Shared Savings Program (see below) were:[168]

- Physicians only: 171 (30%)
- Physicians, hospitals, and other facilities: 324 (58%)
- FQHCs/RHCs: 66 (12%)

CMS identifies providers using their National Provider Identifier (NPI) and Taxpayer Identification Number (TIN)—either an Employer Identification Number or a Social Security number. While specialists can contract with multiple organizations, primary care doctors can join only one ACO. Members of a group with one TIN must join the same ACO regardless of their office locations. The only way to avoid this situation is if each group member has a different TIN.

Financial Arrangements

In order to achieve its goals, Medicare withholds parts of its usual payments to ACOs and pays them back as bonuses if those organizations meet certain financial and quality

---

[166] See, also, the website for the National Association of ACOs, the trade group of these organizations. Retrieved May 15, 2018, from https://www.naacos.com

[167] For more details on eligibility, see: CMS Eligibility Requirements Checklist for MSSP ACO Participation. Retrieved May 13, 2018, from https://www.hcca-info.org/Portals/0/PDFs/Resources/Conference_Handouts/Compliance_Institute/2014/mon/101handout1.pdf

[168] CMS. (2018, January). *Medicare Shared Savings Program Fast Facts*. Retrieved May 13, 2018, from https://www.cms.gov/Medicare/Medicare-Fee-for-Service-Payment/sharedsavingsprogram/Downloads/SSP-2018-Fast-Facts.pdf

benchmarks. Patients are assigned to an ACO based on whom they recently saw for primary care services (as determined by certain procedure codes). Except for the Pioneer and Next Generation ACOs (see below), these organizations often do not know which patients are assigned to them until the end of the assessment period, when CMS calculates the bonuses (or deficits). The benchmarks are adjusted using a severity-of-illness measure for the local county population (as opposed to individual patients). One important characteristic of these plans is that, like traditional Medicare, patients are free to seek care from any provider; if they do so, the financial and quality performance of the non-ACO providers are attributed to the ACO to which the patient is assigned.

Eligible providers are able to enroll in one of three types of ACOs, described next.

The first, and most common, type of ACO is the *Medicare Shared Savings Program (MSSP)*, which offers participants several options that allow for varied amounts of downside risk. These options are explained in Exhibit 4.24.

EXHIBIT 4.24. **Shared Savings Program ACO Participation Options**

Track (% of ACOs)	Financial Risk Arrangement	Description
1 (82%)	One-sided	Track 1 ACOs do not assume downside risk (shared losses) if they do not lower growth in Medicare expenditures.
Medicare ACO Track 1+ Model[a] (10%)[a]	Two-sided	Medicare ACO Track 1+ Model (Track 1+ Model) ACOs assume limited downside risk (less than Track 2 or Track 3).
2 (1%)	Two-sided	Track 2 ACOs may share in savings or repay Medicare losses depending on performance. Track 2 ACOs may share in a greater portion of savings than Track 1 ACOs.
3 (7%)	Two-sided	Track 3 ACOs may share in savings or repay Medicare losses depending on performance. Track 3 ACOs take on the greatest amount of risk but may share in the greatest portion of savings if successful.

[a] The Track 1+ Model is a time-limited CMS Innovation Center model. An ACO must concurrently participate in Track 1 of the Shared Savings Program in order to be eligible to participate in the Track 1+ Model. See: CMS: FACT SHEET: New Accountable Care Organization Model Opportunity: Medicare ACO Track 1+ Model. July 2017. Retrieved May 14, 2018 from https://www.cms.gov/Medicare/Medicare-Fee-for-Service-Payment/sharedsavingsprogram/Downloads/New-Accountable-Care-Organization-Model-Opportunity-Fact-Sheet.pdf See also CMS: Medicare Program; Revisions to Payment Policies Under the Physician Fee Schedule and Other Revisions to Part B for CY 2018; Medicare Shared Savings Program Requirements; and Medicare Diabetes Prevention Program November 15, 2017 *Section H. Medicare Shared Savings Program*. Regulations effective January 1, 2018. Retrieved May 14, 2018 from https://www.federalregister.gov/documents/2017/11/15/2017-23953/medicare-program-revisions-to-payment-policies-under-the-physician-fee-schedule-and-other-revisions

Source: CMS.gov (2018, March 27). *Shared savings program: About the program*. Retrieved May 14, 2018 from https://www.cms.gov/Medicare/Medicare-Fee-for-Service-Payment/sharedsavingsprogram/about.html

The second type of plan is the Advanced Payment ACO. Recognizing that smaller and/or rural hospitals may have financial constraints in developing the systems and infrastructure needed for an ACO, starting in 2012, CMS offered the Advanced Payment ACO model option. This subset of the MSSP provided advanced payments to these organizations as well as monthly, population-based payments. Hospitals were to repay these advances out of future savings. This program was terminated in 2015 and replaced with the *ACO Investment Model* with the same aims and general financial structure.[169] CMS is accepting applications for the latter model in 2019, with future operations dependent on further evaluations.

The third model is the Pioneer ACO. This program was designed for experienced, integrated systems that wanted to accept more risk and share more in the upside of savings. It was launched in 2012 with 32 organizations and closed at the end of 2016 with 8 (by some accounts, 9). It is useful to understand how Pioneer ACOs differed from MSSPs for two reasons: CMS is now moving to have MSSPs accept more risk, and some of the new features may reprise the terms of Pioneer participation; and the Next Generation ACO model described below is the successor to these plans.

> The Pioneer ACO Model differed from the Medicare Shared Savings Program in some of the following ways:
>
> The first 2 years of the Pioneer ACO Model were a shared savings payment arrangement with higher levels of savings and risk than in the Shared Savings Program.
>
> In year three of the program, those Pioneer ACOs that elected to and showed savings over the first 2 years were eligible to move to a population-based payment model. Population-based payment is a per-beneficiary per month payment amount intended to replace some or all of the ACO's fee-for-service (FFS) payments with a prospective monthly payment.
>
> Pioneer ACOs were encouraged to negotiate similar outcomes-based payment arrangements with other payers by the end of the second year, and fully commit their business and care models to offering seamless, high quality care.
>
> Pioneer ACOs were generally responsible for the care of at least 15,000 aligned beneficiaries (5,000 for rural ACOs)...
>
> Population-based payments were per-beneficiary per-month payments intended to replace a portion of the ACO's fee-for-service (FFS) payments with prospective payments.[170]

---

[169]CMC.gov. (2017, March 27). *ACO investment model*. Retrieved May 15, 2018, from https://innovation.cms.gov/initiatives/ACO-Investment-Model

[170]CMS.gov. (2017, February 17). *What was the Pioneer ACO Model?*). Retrieved May 15, 2018, from https://innovation.cms.gov/initiatives/Pioneer-ACO-Model/Pioneer-ACO-FAQs.html

At the end of the program, eight Pioneer ACOs produced gross savings of $68 million and six earned enough to participate in shared savings. CMS published a final report in December 2016 with cumulative evaluation and performance data.[171]

The *Next Generation ACO*[172] was introduced in 2016 as a replacement for Pioneer ACOs; these plans are authorized to run until 2020. In 2018, 51 organizations covering about 1.4 million beneficiaries were participating under multiple risk arrangements (up to 100%) for achieving spending and quality[173] performance benchmarks.[174] In 2016 (the only data currently available), the original 18 Next Generation ACOs generated net savings of $63 million.[175] All participants scored 100% across 33 quality measures, and 11 of the original 18 ACOs in this program received $58 million in shared savings bonuses. However, the other 7 sites had to pay back $20 million.[176] By participating in this model, organizations gain four advantages[177] over the MSSP offerings:

1. *Telehealth expansion waiver.* The enhanced ability to bill for these services normally reserved for rural and underserved areas.

2. *Post discharge home visit waiver.* Relaxes supervision requirements for billing for home visits by ancillary personnel.

3. *Three-day skilled nursing facility waiver.* Normally Medicare only pays for skilled nursing home visits after a 3-day inpatient stay. This provision waives the requirement to receive this benefit.

4. *Voluntary alignment assistance.* In the MSSP, patients are most often unaware they are part of an ACO (see below for problem discussion). Under the voluntary alignment assistance, Next Generation ACOs are able to offer their assigned patients the option to confirm (or deny) their relationships with specific providers.

Beginning in 2017, under an arrangement called the All-Inclusive Population-Based Payments (AIPBPs), the Next Generation ACOs were offered the option of receiving capitation for Medicare beneficiaries enrolled with those plans. In other words, the ACO receives a

---

[171]L&M Policy Research, LLC. (2016). Evaluation of CMMI Accountable Care Organization Initiatives Pioneer ACO, Final Report (December 2). Retrieved May 15, 2018, from https://innovation.cms.gov/Files/reports/pioneeraco-finalevalrpt.pdf

[172]For more details, see: CMS. *Next Generation Accountable Care Organization (ACO) Model: Frequently Asked Questions.* Retrieved May 16, 2018, from https://innovation.cms.gov/Files/x/nextgenacofaq.pdf

[173]CMS. (2018). *33 ACO quality measures.* Retrieved May 16, 2018, from https://www.cms.gov/Medicare/Medicare-Fee-for-Service-Payment/sharedsavingsprogram/Downloads/ACO-Shared-Savings-Program-Quality-Measures.pdf

[174]Participation in this option counts as an Advanced Payment Mechanism (APM) under the Medicare and CHIP Reauthorization Act (MACRA) and is thus eligible for additional payments not based on the ACO formula. More details on this program are explained in the Quality Chapter.

[175]Kaiser Family Foundation. *8 FAQs: Medicare accountable care organizations (ACOs).* Retrieved May 16, 2018, from http://files.kff.org/attachment/Evidence-Link-FAQs-Accountable-Care-Organizations

[176]Leventhal, R. (2017, October 16). CMS releases 2016 next generation ACO data with positive financial, quality results. *Healthcare Informatics.* Retrieved May 18, 2018, from https://www.healthcare-informatics.com/article/value-based-care/cms-releases-2016-next-generation-aco-data-positive-financial-quality

[177]For more details about these benefits, see: CMS.gov. *Next generation ACO model.* Retrieved May 18, 2018, from https://innovation.cms.gov/initiatives/Next-Generation-ACO-Model

per-person, per-month payment for those assigned to that organization. Under this scheme, the ACO is responsible for paying all bills for its assigned patient members.

Future Issues. A number of problems exist for this program now and in the future:

1. *Readiness for a risk-based model.* Eighty-two percent of ACOs are in the MSSP Track 1, which does not have any downside payment risk. These plans are allowed to remain in this track for two periods of 3 years each before they are required to convert to a risk-based model. The 82 ACO that started operations in 2012 or 2013 are, therefore, confronting this transition. The problem is that all the losses in this program occurred in this track. *In other words, only ACOs that assumed financial risk saved money for Medicare.* (Please see Exhibit 4.25.) The Association of ACOs has appealed to CMS, saying that 71% of respondents to a poll said they are slightly to very likely to drop out of the program if forced to go at risk.[178] Many will not be able to demonstrate they

EXHIBIT 4.25. **Savings and Losses of Risk-Based and No-Risk ACOs**

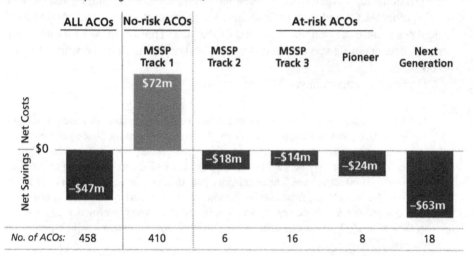

Net Medicare spending on ACO models, in millions:

| | ALL ACOs | No-risk ACOs | At-risk ACOs | | | |
		MSSP Track 1	MSSP Track 2	MSSP Track 3	Pioneer	Next Generation
Net Savings — Net Costs	−$47m	$72m	−$18m	−$14m	−$24m	−$63m
No. of ACOs:	458	410	6	16	8	18

Analysis excludes Comprehensive ESRD (End-Stage Renal Disease) Care Model. Advance Payment (AP) and Accountable Care Organization Investment Model (AIM) ACOs are included in their respective MSSP tracks.

Source: The Henry J. Kaiser Family Foundation. (2018, January). *8 FAQs: Medicare accountable care organizations (ACOs)*. Retrieved May 18, 2018 from http://files.kff.org/attachment/Evidence-Link-FAQs-Accountable-Care-Organizations

---

[178] National Association of ACOs. (2018, May 2). Press Release. Retrieved May 20, 2018, from https://www.naacos.com/assets/docs/pdf/PressReleaseonT1ExtensionSurvey050218.pdf

have the financial resources to pay back CMS if required to do so. CMS administrator Seema Varma responded with the government's position on these organizations: "The presence of these upside-only tracks may be encouraging consolidation in the marketplace, reducing competition and choice for our beneficiaries. While we understand that systems need time to adjust, our system cannot afford to continue with models that are not producing results."[179]

2. *Unclear responsibility.* Medicare beneficiaries do not choose to belong to an ACO. CMS identifies primary care providers (general practitioner, family practitioner, internist, or geriatrician as well as a nurse practitioner or physician assistant) who belong to an ACO and then assigns their patients to that ACO. This assignment is based on claims that use primary care billing codes[180] linked to the provider's NPI. If beneficiaries do not see a primary care provider, then they are assigned to an ACO based on whomever is providing primary care services, such as a cardiologist, pulmonologist, rheumatologist, oncologist, and so on. However, it is not always clear which patients fall under ACO responsibility. For example, a healthy patient who sees her personal physician every few years may have visited an urgent care center for a minor problem. She may, therefore, be enrolled with the ACO that employs the urgent care physician rather than with her personal physician. Except for the Next Generation model, other ACOs and their patients may know the affiliation status only when CMS calculates bonuses or deficits at the end of the year. Thus, if an ACO wants to inform its members about its services in order to try to keep them in its network, it is unable to do so.

Despite this uncertainty, CMS requires that:

> Providers participating in an ACO must notify beneficiaries that they are participating in an ACO, and that the provider is eligible for additional Medicare payments for improving the quality and coordination of care the beneficiary receives while reducing overall costs or may be financially responsible to Medicare for failing to provide efficient, cost-effective care. The beneficiary may then choose to receive services from the provider or seek care from another provider that is not part of the ACO. A provider may not require a beneficiary to obtain services from another provider or supplier in the same ACO, as beneficiaries maintain the freedom to choose which providers they see.[181]

---

[179]Dickson, V. (2018, May 12). Heading for the exit: Rather than face risk, many ACOs could leave. *Modern Healthcare.* Retrieved May 20, 2018, from http://www.modernhealthcare.com/article/20180512/NEWS/180519966

[180]The primary care codes are 99201 to 99215 (new visit and follow-up office visits), 99304 to 99340 (new, follow-up or discharge services for skilled nursing facility or domiciliary care), 99341 to 99350 (home visits) and G0402 (Welcome to Medicare Visit).

[181]CMS. (2012, December 11). *Accountable care organization 2012 program analysis: Quality performance standards narrative measure specifications, final report.* Retrieved May 20, 2018, from http://www.cms.gov/Medicare/Medicare-Fee-for-Service-Payment/sharedsavingsprogram/Quality_Measures_Standards.html

3. *Lack of control.* The Medicare program is based on complete freedom for beneficiaries to seek care from any Medicare-affiliated physician. This freedom is preserved with all ACO models. It means that ACOs are responsible for care over which they have no control. The potential magnitude of this problem was highlighted by McWilliams et al.:[182] "Among ACO-assigned beneficiaries, 8.7% of office visits with primary care physicians were provided outside of the assigned ACO, and 66.7% of office visits with specialists were provided outside of the assigned ACO. Leakage of outpatient specialty care was greater for higher-cost beneficiaries."

4. *Inadequate risk adjustment.* Many of potentially at-risk organizations believe they take care of sicker populations. Since the financial risk is calculated on a county-wide basis (as opposed to a per-individual basis), these ACOs are worried that their costs of care have a high probability to register losses without a concomitant upside potential.

5. *Need to coordinate care across the continuum of services.* Proponents of integration believe ACOs are well positioned to improve quality and lower costs for populations with specific chronic conditions and expensive, acute diseases. While this notion is attractive, there is little systematic evidence to support the effectiveness of disease management programs. For example, in a large study of such efforts, RAND Corporation researchers found that "although disease management seems to improve quality of care, its effect on cost is uncertain."[183] Further, since ACO formation often involves hospital mergers, such consolidation must also be assessed. One study of cardiac patients that considered 40 mergers in California from 1990 to 2006 found that "merger completion is associated with a 3.7 per cent increase in utilization of bypass surgery and angioplasty and a 1.7 per cent increase in inpatient mortality."[184] Further, programs such as those geared to lower readmissions have not consistently proven successful.[185] In short, these benefits are not self-evident.

6. *Shortage of primary care physicians.* In order to succeed, ACOs need a core of primary care physicians who will coordinate care. In the case of Medicare patients, internists or family physicians with a geriatric specialty are necessary; they are already in short supply, and the situation is getting worse. This problem is discussed further in the Physicians section of Chapter 5, "Healthcare Professions."

---

[182]McWilliams, J. M., Chernew, M. E., Dalton, J. B., & Landon, B. E. (2014). Outpatient care patterns and organizational accountability in Medicare. *JAMA Internal Medicine, 174*(6), 938–945.

[183]Mattke, S., Seid, M., & Ma, S. (2007). Evidence for the effect of disease management: Is $1 billion a year a good investment? *American Journal of Managed Care, 13*, 670–676. See also Weintraub, A., & Terhune, C. (2010). Take your meds, exercise—and spend billions. *Businessweek* (February 4). Retrieved May 20, 2018, from http://www.businessweek .com/magazine/content/10_07/b4166046292556.htm

[184]Hayford, T. (2012). The impact of hospital mergers on treatment intensity and health outcomes. *Health Services Research, 47*(1): 1008–1027.

[185]Center for Health Research and Transformation. (2013, May). Acute care readmission reduction initiatives: Major program highlights. Retrieved May 20, 2018, from https://www.chrt.org/publication/acute-care-readmission-reduction-initiatives-major-program-highlights

7. *Alignment of incentives.* Successful ACOs must reward physicians for practicing cost-effective, high-quality medicine—a shift from so-called volume to value. However, according to physician placement firm Merritt Hawkins (which recruits mainly for hospitals): "Despite the rise in value/quality-based incentives, volume-based incentives . . . continue to be the most frequently utilized physician productivity metric . . . value-based incentives only account for about four percent of overall physician compensation."[186] Further, hospital administrators are also still largely paid for volume performance.[187] Clearly, hospitals have not made the appropriate shift in incentive payments necessary for ACO success.

8. *Startup costs.* According to CMS, startup costs for ACO formation average $1.7 million per organization. While many established systems can start a shared savings ACOs with minimum additional costs, smaller organizations that want to enter the program may find it too costly to participate; recall that startup funding is limited to the ACO Investment Model. A further problem is that ACOs wishing to move to a risk basis may need to incur further significant expenses, such as information systems and additional administrative personnel.

9. *Dealing with different insurance models.* While MSSP ACO models are now largely paid on a cost-saving basis using fee-for-service (FFS) data, the government's intention is that eventually all will move toward global payments based on capitation (AIPBPs). ODSs employed these payment models without much success; ACOs have generally not yet adapted to make them work. One of the important questions ACOs must address is how they will distribute capitated or bundled payments among both independent and institutionally-based providers. Another unresolved problem is the system's ability to collect and analyze the data needed to handle these payment models.

In transitioning to a new payment model, ACOs must recognize that in addition to inpatient care, they bear risk for other potentially costly services, such as home health and skilled nursing facility care.

Past experience has shown that four elements can challenge these systems' ability to profit by taking insurance risk: low enrollment, inadequate funding, adverse selection (enrollment of sicker patients), and lack of expertise managing insurance products. With respect to low enrollment, Medicare has put a lower membership limit on ACOs; the 5,000 members that Medicare requires should be sufficient to mitigate size-related risk. The initial shared-savings mode of payment provides FFS compensation at Medicare rates, diminishing the payment adequacy problem (at least until capitation is phased-in). However, the latter two risks remain as significant barriers to ACO success.

---

[186] Merritt, H. (2017). *2017 review of physician and advanced practitioner recruiting incentives.* Retrieved May 20, 2018, from https://www.merritthawkins.com/uploadedFiles/MerrittHawkins/Pdf/2017_Physician_Incentive_Review_Merritt_Hawkins.pdf

[187] Hancock, J. (2013, June 13). Hospital CEO bonuses reward volume and growth. *Kaiser Health News.* Retrieved May 20, 2018, from http://www.kaiserhealthnews.org/Stories/2013/June/06/hospital-ceo-compensation-mainbar.aspx?utm_source=khn&utm_medium=internal&utm_campaign=skybox2

The issue of adverse selection was discussed above. What could go wrong is highlighted by the experience of The Greater Marshfield Community Healthplan, a Medicare HMO prototype in the early 1980s.[188] The plan was based around the tertiary care center, Marshfield Clinic, in rural central Wisconsin. Because patients were sicker than at other demonstration sites in that state and around the country, and because capitation was based on rural Wisconsin rates, the plan folded after experiencing significant losses.

The last problem is that insurance risk and management are not core competencies of these hospital-based organizations. (See the HealthChicago example in Exhibit 4.16 above.) Outsourcing will not completely help since the ACO needs to understand and oversee companies that perform these services on their behalf.

10. *Information system needs.* While current information systems are a vast improvement over those of the past two decades, at least two major problems remain. First, for ACOs to operate efficiently and effectively, systems across the enterprise must be able to talk to one another, an issue called *interoperability.* Despite the promises of health information exchanges, this requirement has not yet been realized to the extent necessary. Second, before information systems can enhance efficiency, the underlying processes which they automate must be evaluated and often reengineered. Too often, this latter process has not been accomplished.[189] More will be said about this topic in Chapter 8, "Information Technology."

11. *Culture.* Hofstede defined culture "as the collective programming of the mind that distinguishes members of one group or category of people from another.... Culture is to a human collectivity what personality is to an individual."[190] While mergers are considered and then executed after financial issues are extensively vetted, few merging institutions assess cultural compatibility. This oversight is puzzling because it can lead to failure of the merged organization. Perhaps the most famous example was the merger of University of California at San Francisco (UCSF) and Stanford University Medical Centers in 1997. The reason for its dissolution in 2000 was succinctly stated by Nathan Nayman of the Hospital Council, a trade organization representing Northern California hospitals: "Comparing Stanford and UCSF is like comparing apples and oranges. The two hospitals had radically different institutional cultures, which made the merger impossible in the end."[191]

---

[188]Iglehart, J. K. (1982). The greater Marshfield community health plan: The future of HMOs. *The New England Journal of Medicine, 307,* 451–456.

[189]Carayon P., Karesh, B.-T., & Cartmill, R. S. (2010, October). *Incorporating health information technology into workflow redesign—summary report.* (Prepared by the Center for Quality and Productivity Improvement, University of Wisconsin–Madison, under Contract No. HHSA 290-2008-10036C). AHRQ Publication No. 10-0098-EF. Rockville, MD: Agency for Healthcare Research and Quality.

[190]Hofstede, G. (2001). *Culture's consequences: Comparing values, behaviors, institutions, and organizations across nations* (2nd ed.). Thousand Oaks, CA: Sage Publications.

[191]Pyati, A. (2000). UCSF/Stanford: Marriage was rough; divorce is expensive. *San Francisco Business Times* (April 23). Retrieved May 20, 2018, from http://www.bizjournals.com/sanfrancisco/stories/2000/04/24/focus4.html?page=all

12. *Antitrust.* Antitrust concerns have always threatened integration efforts; however, from 1994 to 2007, the Department of Justice (DOJ) failed to prevent any nonprofit hospital mergers. Richman[192] noted that "confidence that nonprofit hospitals' market concentration does not lead to higher prices largely drives judicial sympathy for nonprofits in merger cases, and in turn a tolerance of nonprofits' market power." Governmental successes in challenging these combinations began on August 7, 2007 when the Federal Trade Commission (FTC) commissioners unanimously ruled that the 2000 acquisition by Evanston Northwestern Healthcare (ENH) of Highland Park Hospital violated Section 7 of the Clayton Act by creating a highly concentrated market, thereby increasing hospital prices and harming consumers. (The system is now known as NorthShore University HealthSystem.) The philosophical change in attitude about nonprofits is summarized by the FTC's conclusion: "ENH's nonprofit status did not affect its efforts to raise prices after the merger, and . . . does not suffice to rebut complaint counsel's evidence of anticompetitive effects."[193] Even though ENH claimed it spent more than $120 million on integration improvements with the extra charges, the FTC said quality improvements must result from cost-saving efficiencies, not higher prices. Since then, the FTC has been successful in a number of challenges to horizontal and vertical integration of hospitals and medical groups.[194] As Carlson[195] pointed out: "The collision of old-world antitrust enforcement and new ideas like accountable care, bundled payments, value-based purchasing and patient-centered medical homes has ratcheted up the uncertainty over healthcare needs." Although the DOJ and FTC have developed joint antitrust guidelines for the ACO shared savings program, the interpretation and application of these rules is still unclear. A further wrinkle on this issue came in 2013 when the U.S. Supreme Court ruled that even a government-owned hospital is not exempt from antitrust when it seeks to purchase a local for-profit hospital.[196]

13. *Achieving physician alignment.* This issue is discussed above but is worth another mention because it is critical to organizational success. Of particular relevance here is realizing that when the ACO assumes full risk and is receiving only global payments, the problem of dividing the money will emerge as an important issue. Further, since

---

[192] Richman, B. D. (2007). Antitrust and nonprofit hospital mergers: A return to basics. *University of Pennsylvania Law Review, 156,* 121–150. Retrieved May 20, 2018, from https://pdfs.semanticscholar.org/804b/26c7ece7119ec5bc10c8ec99b96d284efaaa.pdf

[193] Federal Trade Commission. Commission Rules that Evanston Northwestern Healthcare Corp.'s Acquisition of Highland Park Hospital Was Anticompetitive. Retrieved May 20, 2018, from http://www.ftc.gov/opa/2007/08/evanston.shtm

[194] Meier, M. H., Albert, B. S., & Monahan, K. (2018, September). *Overview of FTC actions in health care services and products.* Health Care Division, Bureau of Competition, Federal Trade Commission. Washington DC. Retrieved May 20, 2018, from https://www.ftc.gov/system/files/attachments/competition-policy-guidance/overview_health_care_september_2017.pdf

[195] Carlson, J. (2012) Pulled in two directions. Providers pursuing coordinated care confused by antitrust actions. *Modern Healthcare, 42,* 6–7, 16.

[196] Federal Trade Commission v. Phoebe Putney Health System, Inc., et al. Supreme Court Docket No. 11-1160 [Internet]. Retrieved from http://www.supremecourt.gov/opinions/12pdf/11-1160_1824.pdf

the enterprise is at increased risk for losses, it must deal with the problem of which part of the system will bear the burden if those shortfalls occur. Like many of these issues, achieving physician alignment is not new. This latter issue was one of the core difficulties in the above-mentioned UCSF-Stanford breakup. According to Stanford University president Gerhard Casper, "one of the largest problems was administrators' failure to achieve physician buy-in. Faculty members at both institutions resisted the merger from the beginning, refusing to combine their practices and share financial risk."[197]

Because of some of these problems (particularly items 2, 3, and 4), many well-respected, mature organizations decided from the program's beginning not to participate.[198] How many more will drop out or be reluctant to participate will be seen in the near future as they must decide whether to continue with the program on a risk basis.

HOSPITAL GOVERNANCE

This section will address hospital governance by focusing on its board of trustees or directors. Since the literature on corporate governance is extensive, the focus here is primarily on the essentials as they relate to nonprofit hospitals.

Definition and Purpose

The relevant origin of the word "board" is the table where a communal meal is served. Hence, according to the *Oxford English Dictionary*, a board is "[t]he company of persons who meet at a council-table; the recognized word for a body of persons officially constituted for the transaction or superintendence of some particular business." The importance of the definition is that the board decides and acts *communally*, in distinction from management members whose day-to-day function is frequently as individuals, though as part of a larger team. Early hospital boards were made up of philanthropist trustees who raised and donated money for the institution. As the first board of Massachusetts General Hospital stated in 1814 when trying to raise $100,000: "We shall instance, in both classes of objects, to which this Institution relates, *the sick poor and the insane* [emphasis in the original] . . . It purposes to afford the best medical aid; the best nurses; the most suitable apartments; all the assistance which sickness requires; and all the comforts, which are subsidiary to convalescence."[199]

Once the money was secured, trustees were responsible for proper stewardship of the charitable funds according to the institutional mission. More recently, as nonprofits have become more complex organizations, their success has depended on performance of a larger

---

[197]"We Took on Too Much": Stanford-UCSF System Breaks Up. *California Healthline*. Friday, October 29, 1999. Retrieved February 10, 2018, from http://www.californiahealthline.org/articles/1999/10/29/we-took-on-too-much--stanforducsf-system-breaks-up.aspx

[198]Alonso-Zaldivar, R. (2011, May 11). Obama plan for health care quality dealt a setback: Mayo Clinic, other top health providers say "accountable care" is too complex. Retrieved May 20, 2018, from http://www.nbcnews.com/id/42997540/ns/health-health_care/t/obama-plan-health-care-quality-dealt-setback

[199]Quincy, J., Perkins, T. H., Sargent, D., May, J., Barnard, T., Higginson, S., . . . Sullivan, R. (1814, January 8). *Address of the board of trustees of the Massachusetts General Hospital to the public* Boston: J. Belcher.

and more complex portfolio of tasks. Green and Griesinger[200] succinctly stated that the practitioner literature:

> reveals significant consensus that the activities of effective nonprofit boards should at least include (1) determining or setting the organization's mission, purpose, and policies; (2) strategic planning; (3) determining or evaluating the organization's programs and services; (4) board development; (5) selecting, evaluating, and terminating the CEO; (6) ensuring adequate resources, including fund development; (7) financial management (operating budget); (8) interaction with the community; and (9) serving as a court of appeal for the resolution of disputes involving staff, clients, or both.

Legal Requirements

Most of the legal requirements covering boards derive from state hospital licensure laws that mandate a governing board for each institution. Further, corporate laws describe standards for stewardship, setting three interrelated fiduciary requirements for board members:[201]

1. *Duty of Care*

   Requires action in good faith (primarily without self-interest) that any ordinarily prudent person would take in the best interests of the organization. In taking this action, the board member must make sure that sufficient information is available. It is reasonable to rely on management and other experts' reports for this information except when there is reason to believe problems exist with its truthfulness. Although the courts require that a corporate information and reporting system is in place, they do not specify the exact content and methods. Each institution must, therefore, develop its own compliance plan that satisfies its unique needs.

2. *Duty of Loyalty*

   Prohibits action in self-interest, particularly that which would result in economic gain to a board member doing business with the institution.

3. *Duty of Obedience to Purpose*

   Requires action to further the purposes of the institution in accordance with its mission statement, articles of incorporation, and bylaws.

   Legal adherence to these duties is not always straightforward.

> The difficulty in articulating a standard for nonprofit board business accountability is that the legal concept of duty is ambiguous and the judicial tests are muddled, forging a rather odd hybrid standard mixing charitable and nonprofit law. Such ambiguity in

---

[200]Green, J. C., & Griesinger, D. W. (1996). Board performance and organizational effectiveness in nonprofit social services organizations. *Nonprofit Management and Leadership, 6*(4), 381–402.

[201]American Health Lawyers Association (2011, August 29). *The health care director's compliance duties: A continued focus of attention and enforcement.* A joint publication from the Office of the Inspector General, U.S. Department of Health and Human Services, and the American Health Lawyers Association. © 2010. Updated.

nonprofit board decision making hampers good faith business judgment, particularly for multi-state hospital systems.[202]

Further, sometimes these duties clash. One of the major sources of such conflict arises when board members seek to fulfill the institution's charitable mission while maintaining its financial sustainability. On this theme, the late Sister Irene Kraus (who was president of the Daughters of Charity National Health System and AHA board chair) is said to have exhorted her staff: "No margin, no mission."[203] The seriousness of this dilemma was highlighted when the Minnesota attorney general sued Accretive Health for "compromising patient privacy and using strong-arm tactics to collect payments from patients at a health system [Fairview Health Services] in Minneapolis."[204]

In response to prominent violations of these corporate duties, Congress passed the American Competitiveness and Corporate Accountability Act of 2002, commonly known as the Sarbanes-Oxley Act. Except for provisions prohibiting retaliation against whistleblowers and the destruction, alteration, or concealment of certain documents or the impediment of investigations, Sarbanes-Oxley does not generally apply to nonprofit organizations. Its influence, however, has caused many nonprofit hospital boards to reconsider the level and mechanism of oversight. In this respect, the American Bar Association suggestions are listed in Exhibit 4.26.

EXHIBIT 4.26. Nonprofits and Sarbanes-Oxley

Ten general principles of corporate governance emerging from the Sarbanes-Oxley reforms may be worthy of consideration for the governance of nonprofit organizations:

Principle 1. Role of Board. The organization's governing board should oversee the operations of the organization in such manner as will assure effective and ethical management.

Principle 2. Importance of Independent Directors. The independent and non-management board members are an organizational resource that should be used to assure the exercise of independent judgment in key committees and general board decision-making.

Principle 3. Audit Committee. An organization with significant financial resources should have an audit committee composed solely of independent directors, which should assure the independence of the organization's financial auditors, review the organization's critical accounting policies and decisions and the adequacy of its internal control systems, and oversee the accuracy of its financial statements and reports.

---

[202]Blum, J. (2010). The quagmire of hospital governance, finding mission in a revised licensure model. *Journal of Legal Medicine, 31,* 35–57.

[203]Bryant-Friedland, B. (1998, August 25). Sister Irene Kraus remembered for vision, leadership. *The Florida Times-Union.*

[204]Schorsch, C. (2018, April 4). Investors cool to Accretive's management shakeup. *Crain's Chicago Business.* Retrieved May 20, 2018, from http://www.chicagobusiness.com/article/20130404/NEWS03/130409891/investors-cool-to-accretives-management-shakeup

Principle 4. Governance and Nominating Committees. An organization should have one or more committees, composed solely of independent directors, that focus on core governance and board composition issues, including: the governing documents of the organization and the board; the criteria, evaluation, and nomination of directors; the appropriateness of board size, leadership, composition, and committee structure; and codes of ethical conduct.

Principle 5. Compensation Committee. An organization should have a committee composed solely of independent directors that determines the compensation of the chief executive officer and determines or reviews the compensation of other executive officers, and assures that compensation decisions are tied to the executives' actual performance in meeting predetermined goals and objectives.

Principle 6. Disclosure and Integrity of Institutional Information. Disclosures made by an organization regarding its assets, activities, liabilities, and results of operations should be accurate and complete, and include all material information. Financial and other information should fairly reflect the condition of the organization, and be presented in a manner that promotes rather than obscures understanding. CEOs and CFOs should be able to certify the accuracy of financial and other disclosures, and the adequacy of their organizations' internal controls.

Principle 7. Ethics and Business Conduct Codes. An organization should adopt and implement ethics and business conduct codes applicable to directors, senior management, agents, and employees that reflect a commitment to operating in the best interests of the organization and in compliance with applicable law, ethical business standards, and the organization's governing documents.

Principle 8. Executive and Director Compensation. Executives (and directors if appropriate) should be compensated fairly and in a manner that reflects their contribution to the organization. Such compensation should not include loans, but may include incentives that correspond to success or failure in meeting performance goals.

Principle 9. Monitoring Compliance and Investigating Complaints. An organization should have procedures for receiving, investigating, and taking appropriate action regarding fraud or noncompliance with law or organization policy, and should protect "whistleblowers" against retaliation.

Principle 10. Document Destruction and Retention. An organization should have document retention policies that comply with applicable laws and be implemented in a manner that does not result in the destruction of documents that may be relevant to an actual or anticipated legal proceeding or governmental investigation.

Source: American Bar Association Coordinating Committee on Nonprofit Governance (2005), *Guide to Nonprofit Corporate Governance in the Wake of Sarbanes-Oxley.* Chicago: American Bar Association, pp. 17–18.

Responsibilities

In addition to legal requirements, boards are responsible for ensuring institutional payment and accreditation, the latter being closely linked to evaluations of quality. Perhaps the most important obligation of the board with respect to payment is its responsibilities delineated by the Medicare Conditions of Participation and Conditions for Coverage.[205]

---

[205]CMS.gov. *Conditions for coverage (CfCs) & conditions of participations (CoPs).* Retrieved May 21, 2018, from http://www.cms.gov/Regulations-and-Guidance/Legislation/CFCsAndCoPs/index.html?redirect=/cfcsandcops

Medicare standards require six areas in which boards must act: (1) overseeing the medical staff, including credentialing and approval of bylaws; (2) appointing the hospital chief executive officer; (3) ensuring appropriate patient care; (4) developing an institutional budget; (5) providing oversight of contracted services; and, (6) if emergency services are offered, conducting them in a high-quality fashion. The relevant parts of these requirements for the governing body are excerpted in Exhibit 4.27.

EXHIBIT 4.27. Medicare Conditions of Participation and Conditions for Coverage

§ 482.12 Condition of Participation: Governing Body

The hospital must have an effective governing body legally responsible for the conduct of the hospital as an institution . . .

(a) *Standard: Medical staff.* The governing body must:

  (1) Determine, in accordance with State law, which categories of practitioners are eligible candidates for appointment to the medical staff;

  (2) Appoint members of the medical staff after considering the recommendations of the existing members of the medical staff;

  (3) Assure that the medical staff has bylaws;

  (4) Approve medical staff bylaws and other medical staff rules and regulations;

  (5) Ensure that the medical staff is accountable to the governing body for the quality of care provided to patients;

  (6) Ensure the criteria for selection are individual character, competence, training, experience, and judgment . . .

(b) *Standard: Chief executive officer.* The governing body must appoint a chief executive officer who is responsible for managing the hospital.

(c) *Standard: Care of patients.* In accordance with hospital policy, the governing body must ensure that the following requirements are met:

  (1) Every Medicare patient is under the care of [a licensed practitioner in accordance with state laws]:

  (2) Patients are admitted to the hospital only on the recommendation of a licensed practitioner permitted by the State to admit patients to a hospital . . .

  (3) A doctor of medicine or osteopathy is on duty or on call at all times.

  (4) A doctor of medicine or osteopathy is responsible for the care of each Medicare patient with respect to any medical or psychiatric problem . . .

(d) *Standard: Institutional plan and budget.* The institution must have an overall institutional plan that meets the following conditions:

  (1) The plan must include an annual operating budget that is prepared according to generally accepted accounting principles.

(2) The budget must include all anticipated income and expenses. This provision does not require that the budget identify item by item the components of each anticipated income or expense.

(3) The plan must provide for capital expenditures for at least a 3-year period . . .

(6) The plan must be reviewed and updated annually.

(7) The plan must be prepared—

   (i) Under the direction of the governing body; and

   (ii) By a committee consisting of representatives of the governing body, the administrative staff, and the medical staff of the institution.

(e) *Standard: Contracted services.* The governing body must be responsible for services furnished in the hospital whether or not they are furnished under contracts . . .

(f) *Standard: Emergency services.* (1) If emergency services are provided at the hospital, the hospital must . . . meet the emergency needs of patients in accordance with acceptable standards of practice . . . organized under the direction of a qualified member of the medical staff [and] . . . integrated with other departments of the hospital.

Source: 42 C.F.R. Part 482—Conditions of Participation for Hospitals. Retrieved May 21, 2018 from https://law.justia.com/cfr/title42/42-3.0.1.5.21.html#42:3.0.1.5.21.2.199.2.

In most hospitals (for-profit as well as nonprofit), the board's oversight of quality originated from the governance criteria of the Joint Commission, a principal organization responsible for accrediting hospitals. (See Chapter 9, "Quality," for more information about accreditation and the Joint Commission.) More recently, however, the board has needed to take a more active interest in quality performance due to Medicare-imposed financial penalties for certain clinical events, such as catheter-related sepsis, pressure sores, and hospital readmissions within 30 days of discharge, to name a few. Further, with increased transparency of hospital quality data,[206] the board is more engaged with the issue of quality as a competitive strategy. Unfortunately, hospital boards are not always as involved as they should be in this latter regard. For example, Jha and Epstein[207] found that:

> Among our nationally representative sample of chairs of boards from [1,000] nonprofit U.S. hospitals, a little over half identified clinical quality as one of the two top priorities for board oversight. Although 69 percent of board chairs thought that the CEO had great influence on quality of care, just 44 percent identified quality performance as one of the two most important criteria for evaluating the CEO's performance. Programmatic emphasis on quality was not uniformly high. Also, although only a few board chairs had work experience in the health care sector, fewer than one-third of nonprofit boards sampled had formal training programs that include clinical quality.

---

[206] See, for example, http://www.medicare.gov/hospitalcompare (accessed May 21, 2018).

[207] Jha, A., & Epstein, A. (2010). Hospital governance and the quality of care. *Health Affairs, 29*(1), 182–187.

Since that study was published in 2010, little progress has been made in this area. As Pronovost et al.[208] note: "In most organizations outside health care, the Board of Trustees (or Directors) assumes ultimate accountability for performance. This is rarely the case in health care, where boards have traditionally fixated on financial performance and delegated quality of patient care to the medical staff, often with limited board oversight."

Board Structure and Activities

Given the importance of the board in institutional oversight, and the many possibilities for its structure and operational features, one might ask what model(s) works best. Board practices found to be associated with better performance in both process of care and mortality include (1) having a board quality committee; (2) establishing strategic goals for quality improvement; (3) being involved in setting the quality agenda for the hospital; (4) including a specific item on quality in board meetings; (5) using a dashboard with national benchmarks that includes indicators for clinical quality, patient safety, and patient satisfaction; and (6) linking senior executives' performance evaluation to quality and patient safety indicators. Involvement of physician leadership in the board quality committee also enhances the hospital's quality performance.[209]

Further insight into this question involves examination of the corporate mission and structures of hospitals. For example, as hospitals moved way from strictly philanthropic organizations, the purpose and expertise of their boards needed to change. Alexander et al.[210] draw a distinction between philanthropic and corporate models for hospital boards. "The philanthropic model stresses community participation, due process, and stewardship, whereas the corporate model stresses strategy development, risk taking, and competitive positioning."[211] While their research showed that corporate model institutions were associated with enhanced operational efficiency, higher volume of adjusted admissions, larger market share, better strategic adaptivity, and quicker responses to changing environmental conditions, hospital occupancy and cash flow were generally unrelated to the governing board's configuration. Despite these advantages, institutions should not necessarily move to the corporate model. One reason for this caution is the relationship of the institution to its stakeholders. Hospitals (even nonprofits) that are part of a system will be subject to a corporate model board at the parent's organizational level; thus, local institutions that have their own boards may want to

---

[208] Pronovost, P., Armstrong, M., Demski, R., Peterson, M. H. A., & Rothman, M. D. (2018). Taking health care governance to the next level. *NEJM Catalyst*. Retrieved May 21, 2018, from https://catalyst.nejm.org/healthcare-governance-next-level-quality-committee

[209] Jiang, H. G., Lockee, C., Bass, K., & Fraser, I. (1988). Board oversight of quality: Any differences in process of care and mortality? *Journal of Healthcare Management, 54*(1), 15–29; discussion 29–30.

[210] Alexander, J., Morlock, L. L., & Gifford, B. D. (1988). The effects of corporate restructuring on hospital policymaking. *Health Services Research, 23*(2), 311–337.

[211] Alexander, J., & Lee, S. D. (2006). Does governance matter? Board configuration and performance in not-for-profit hospitals. *The Milbank Quarterly*, 84(4), 733–758. The authors add this cautionary note to their findings and recommendations: "... the hospital governance data for this study were based on surveys conducted in the mid to late 1980s, and the dependent variables reflected hospital performance in the period between 1986 and 1994. Accordingly, our findings should be generalized with caution to NFP hospitals in recent years."

retain a philanthropic focus that is more community oriented. A similar reason applies to public hospitals, which have other layers of governmental oversight.

In addition to the nature of stakeholders and corporate status, the overall environment (including location and resources) also plays an important part in the board's structure and direction. In a comprehensive description of hospital boards, Shoou-Yih et al.[212] identified three overarching board responsibilities: mission and strategy setting, performance evaluation and oversight, and external relations.

> Mission and strategy setting includes definition and maintenance of hospital mission, and the board's role in the approval of strategic plans for fulfilling mission. Performance evaluation and oversight role comprises the assessment of hospital and CEO performance in areas such as financials, care quality, patient safety, community health outcomes, and physician and staff relationships. External relations role includes such activities as community and government relations, public accountability, and fundraising.

While all three activities would seem important, the authors give the following caveat: "[H]igh levels of activity in multiple governance roles may not be synonymous with effectiveness...the effectiveness of the board and its impact on hospital performance may...be determined by the match between governing board roles and the organizational and environmental conditions of the hospitals." In implementing any governance model, it is important to note the interdependency of its characteristics (viz., the components are complex and symbiotic). Changing features piecemeal may therefore destroy the effectiveness of the whole. Even so, other studies have identified independent features and practices of higher performing boards; for example, they tend to have more physician members. [213]

Research[214] into a number of other characteristics of higher performing boards yields some useful, and occasionally counterintuitive, findings:

- *Size.* Size of the boards and marginal profit were unrelated.

- *Terms of service.* Limiting term *length* for board members but not board officers was associated with higher profit margin. Limiting the *number* of terms had no effect for either officers or board members.

- *Compensation.* Compensating board members of a nonprofit has been controversial. Study results do not indicate that payment (even travel or conference reimbursement) has any effect on profitability.

---

[212]Shoou-Yih, D. L., Alexander, J. A., Wang, V., Margolin, F. S., & Combes, J. R. (2008). An empirical taxonomy of hospital governing board roles. *Health Services Research, 43*(4), 1223–1243. The authors also provide a taxonomy of five types of boards and their characteristics.

[213]Prybil, L. D. (2006). Size, composition, and culture of high-performing hospital boards. *American Journal of Medical Quality, 21*, 224–229.

[214]Culica, D., & Prezio, E. (2009). Hospital board infrastructure and functions: The role of governance in financial performance. *International Journal of Environmental Research and Public Health, 6*, 862–873. Note: Performance was measured using the average profit margins over the three years of the study.

- *Standing committees.* Paradoxically, the presence of audit and finance/budget committees is highly *negatively* correlated with higher profit margins, as is the regular review of financial statements. Likewise, the presence of the CFO as a board member is slightly negatively correlated with higher profit margins. The presence of a governance committee is also slightly negatively correlated with profitability. Routine review of capital planning, however, was associated with greater profitability.

- *Benchmarks.* Consistent with the above findings, market share is a more useful benchmark than strict financial performance.

- *Individual board member expertise.* Knowledge of finance, insurance, or managed care was not correlated with higher profit margins.

- *Frequency of meetings.* Greater frequency of meetings is negatively correlated with profitability, with fewer than six meetings a year being optimal.

"One limitation of the study was the potential issue of reverse causality (i.e., the governance variables may themselves be affected by the hospital performance)."[215] For example, hospitals in better financial shape may require only a few meetings per year, while poorer organizations may need to meet more often to correct problems.

In summary, while the general legal and regulatory requirements of a hospital board are similar across institutions, the most effective ways to meet obligations are not straightforward. Hospitals must consider the issues mentioned above and create a board that meets its current, unique needs but is flexible enough to change as the organization's internal and external environments evolve.

SUMMARY

Prior to the 20th century, hospitals played a peripheral part in the provision of most healthcare. In the last 100 years, a confluence of advances in technology, new organizational models, and emergence of insurance payments placed these institutions at the centers of care. These same forces, however, are refocusing where care is and should be delivered. Technology is increasingly enabling outpatient services; organizational models are incorporating nonhospital sites of care; and payers are promoting noninstitutional care to drive down costs. The questions that remain are: How far can these trends proceed? Can hospitals adapt and still be able to provide high-quality care?

---

[215]Ibid.

CHAPTER

5

HEALTHCARE PROFESSIONALS

The delivery of high-quality healthcare requires many different types of professionals and ancillary personnel working together. To allow for an in-depth discussion of this topic, only a few of these occupations will be discussed. The Bureau of Labor Statistics of the U.S. Department of Labor provides a comprehensive list and description of health professions.[1]

PHYSICIANS

MACBETH.

> *... How does your patient, doctor?*

DOCTOR.

> *Not so sick, my lord, as she is troubled with thick-coming fancies that keep her from rest.*

MACBETH.

> *Cure her of that! Canst thou not minister to a mind diseased, pluck from the memory a rooted sorrow, raze out the written troubles of the brain, and with some sweet oblivious antidote cleanse the stuffed bosom of that perilous stuff which weighs upon her heart.*

DOCTOR.

> *Therein the patient must minister to himself.*

MACBETH.

> *Throw physic to the dogs; I'll none of it ...*

—William Shakespeare, *Macbeth*, Act 5, Scene 3

History of Western Medical Care

The extensive history of medicine is often inseparable from the persons who practiced their craft during the past several millennia. Many practitioners in Europe, the Middle East, India, China, and elsewhere made significant contributions to the field. Because the focus here is on the American healthcare system, only its origins in "Western" medicine will be presented.

The *Oxford English Dictionary* defines a physician[2] as "[a] person who is trained and qualified to practise medicine." But the term carries many additional meanings, shaped by such factors as culture, religion, and law.

---

[1] Bureau of Labor Statistics. *Healthcare occupations*. Retrieved May 22, 2018, from http://www.bls.gov/ooh/healthcare/home.htm

[2] The origin of the word is the Greek φύσις. The sense of its meaning is related to nature or natural characteristics, in this case, of the body. It is closely related, therefore, to the *OED* obsolete definition of "[a] person who studies natural science or physics." The term is also very closely linked to the measures physicians use for treatment, viz. the Latin *physicum* became the English *physic*, or medicinal treatment. One commonly used word for this practitioner is "doctor." Since the Latin origin of this word is "teacher," it is not a precise term. Even Chaucer used the term "Doctour of Physic" when describing a physician. The word "physician" is also used to distinguish practitioners who use medication from those who cut to achieve a cure (surgeons). As an aside, the Greeks used the word ἰατρός (iatros)—one who heals—for a physician.

It is first important to understand how societies understood illness. Belief in the supernatural was accompanied by the idea that illness was due to something put into or taken out of the body by a deity. In order to remedy these problems, the role of the physician was at first vested in the religious leader, often called shaman.[3] The shaman's role was to remove the evil or restore whatever was lacking. For example, ancient skulls with trephined openings have been found in cultures as wide-ranging as South America and the Middle East; lore explains the holes were made to let out evil spirits. The healing role of the religious leader transferred to European monarchs in the 11th century, particularly in England and France. The "royal touch" of the French or English monarchs was said to cure diseases, particularly scrofula.[4] The laying-on of royal hands long retained a religious aspect, as evidenced by inclusion of the service for the ceremony in the English Book of Common Prayer until the early 18th century.[5] The practice lasted until 1714 in England with Queen Anne and 1825 in France on the coronation of Charles X. Today, the faith healer has taken the place of monarchs in curing by touch.

The role of the secular practitioner begins with Imhotep, the polymath Egyptian vizier to Pharaoh Zoser (ca. 2600 BCE), who is often identified as the first architect, engineer, and physician. Imhotep separated diseases for which treatments existed from those of unknown origin, thus distinguishing the roles of physician and priest, respectively. He also separated the origins of some diseases from magic. Although he was a scribe, Imhotep did not leave any clearly identified writings; however, the Edwin Smith Surgical Papyrus (written around 1700 BCE) is thought to be a partial compendium of his surgical teachings.[6] In a strange twist on the stories of gods taking human form, Imhotep was subsequently deified as an Egyptian god after the Persian conquest in 525 BCE. "Imhotep's cult reached its zenith during Greco-Roman times, when his temples in Memphis and on the island of Philae (Jazīrat Fīlah in Arabic) in the Nile River were often crowded with sufferers who prayed and slept there with the conviction that the god would reveal remedies to them in their dreams."[7]

In addition to medicinal (and very few surgical) remedies, the Egyptians contributed several medical practices that have survived to modern times. The first practice is specialization. Herodotus[8] noted: "The art of medicine among them is distributed thus: each physician is a physician of one disease and of no more; and the whole country is full of physicians, for

---

[3] The word "shaman" has been historically gender-neutral, reflecting the healer role women have played from ancient times. By the time Greek medical influence prevailed, however, women were not allowed to assume the role of physician.

[4] Scrofula is chronic enlargement of the lymph glands of the neck due to tuberculosis; called the king's evil.

[5] Cummings, B. (Ed.) (2011). *The book of common prayer, the texts of 1549, 1559, and 1662.* New York: Oxford University Press.

[6] Not all treatments were surgical. For example, the Ebers Papyrus (ca. 1550 BCE) describes a treatment for (possibly) asthma as follows: "[Y]ou should then bring 7 stones and heat them on fire. Take one of them, place parts of these drugs [honey, cream, milk, carob, colocynth and date kernels] over it, cover with a new jar with a pierced bottom. Introduce a tube of reed through this hole and put your mouth on this tube so that you swallow its fumes."

[7] Rogers, Kara (Ed.) (2011). *Medicine and healers through history.* New York: Britannica Educational Publishing. Please see Chapter 4, "Hospitals," for similarity to temples of Aesculapius.

[8] Herodotus (1890). *History of herodotus*, Vol. 1. Translated by G.C. Macaulay (p. 152, para. 84). London: MacMillan and Company.

some profess themselves to be physicians of the eyes, others of the head, others of the teeth, others of the affections of the stomach, and others of the more obscure ailments."

Second is the practice of triage. The Ebers Papyrus (ca. 1550 BCE)[9] divides injuries into three categories: "An ailment which I will treat; an ailment with which I will contend; an ailment not to be treated." Diodorus Siculus[10] (ca. 90–ca. 30 BCE) reports the third and fourth Egyptian innovations: a system of free care (financed by taxes) and protection against medical discipline if the physician follows established expert guidelines:

> On a military campaign or a journey inside the country everybody must be healed without special remuneration, as the physicians receive their wages from the state. They have to follow a written law when healing which was composed by many of the most famous physicians. When following the laws which are read out from the holy book they are beyond guilt and safe from any accusation, even when they cannot save the patient. But if they act counter to the regulations they are liable to mortal accusation.

The Greeks adopted the cult of Imhotep, changing his name to Imhoutes, who some believe was the prototype for the Greek Asclepius. Like Imhotep, Asclepius was first believed to be human; in fact, Homer mentions his physician-sons Machaon and Podalirius, though with contradictory descriptions of professional status. In *The Iliad*, Homer recounts Nestor praising these practitioners as "the worth of many other men,"[11] while in *The Odyssey*, the swineherd Eumaeus groups them with "masters of some public craft, builders and minstrels."[12] Between 500 BCE and 100 CE, both Asclepius and these sons became divine, with different myths about them laying the foundations for popular expectations of physician behavior.[13] Apollodorus describes Asclepius becoming so skilled a surgeon "that he not only saved lives but even revived the dead … "; however, "Zeus was afraid that men might learn the art of medicine from Aesculapius … so he hit him with a thunderbolt."[14] The legend says the physician treated all without regard to status or potential divine punishment for himself.

A warning to physicians comes from a tale by Pindar,[15] who said that Zeus killed Asclepius for bringing Hippolytus back to life. The reason was not as described above but because Asclepius acted for "a lordly bribe, gold flashing in the hand … "; hence, a punishment for physicians driven by greed.

Although Imhotep's temples predated those of Asclepius, as mentioned in Chapter 4, "Hospitals," the latter's are generally recognized as the first hospitals and their priests the

---

[9]Nunn, J. F. (2002). *Ancient Egyptian medicine*. London: British Museum Press; Tulsa: University of Oklahoma, p. 28.

[10]Diodorus Siculus (2009). *Brief history of vision and ocular medicine*. In W. H. Vogel & A. Berke, *Historical Library*, Vol. 1 (46). Amsterdam: Kugler Publications.

[11]Homer. *The Iliad*. Book XI. Verse 514. Retrieved May 22, 2018, from http://www.perseus.tufts.edu/hopper/text?doc=Perseus%3Atext%3A1999.01.0134%3Abook%3D11%3Acard%3D489

[12]Homer. *The Odyssey*. Book XVII. Verse 384. Retrieved May 22, 2018, from http://www.perseus.tufts.edu/hopper/text?doc=Perseus%3Atext%3A1999.01.0136%3Abook%3D17%3Acard%3D380

[13]Bailey, J. E. (1996). Asklepios: Ancient hero of medical caring. *Annals of Internal Medicine, 124*, 257–263.

[14]Pseudo-Apollodorus, Bibliotheca 3. 118–122. Retrieved May 22, 2018, from http://www.theoi.com/Ouranios/Asklepios.html

[15]Pindar, Pythian, Ode 3. 54 ff 4. Ibid.

first healing practitioners. In addition to the aforementioned sons of Aesculapius, the Greeks extended deification and roles to his other family members: his wife Epione eased pain; daughters Hygeia[16] and Panacea were responsible for, respectively, health/disease prevention and cure; and another son, Telesphoros, symbolized convalescence.

While not remembered as a physician, the Greek philosopher Empedocles (ca. 492–432 BCE) had a profound and lasting influence on medical practice. Writing more than a century before Aristotle, he posited that the universe (and hence all humans) was made of four "roots" (which Plato later called elements): earth, air, fire, and water. The structure of humans relied not only on the amount of each but also on their relative proportions. Each of the elements was subsequently associated with a bodily "humor": fire—yellow bile, earth—black bile, water—phlegm, and air—blood. Predominance of a specific humor was responsible for personality characteristics and an overabundance caused disease, requiring measures specifically linked to rebalancing the four elements. (Please see Exhibit 5.1 for the linkage of these features and treatments of excesses.) Herbals and foods also aided this rebalancing; for example, citrus fruits were thought to counter too much phlegm. This rebalancing became the basis of medical therapeutics (especially bleeding) that lasted at least into the 19th century.

The physician considered the father of Western medicine is Hippocrates (ca. 460–ca. 375 BCE), who taught and practiced on the Greek island of Cos. Although Hippocrates was

EXHIBIT 5.1. The Four Humors (Elements)

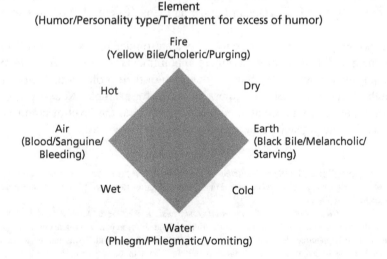

Element
(Humor/Personality type/Treatment for excess of humor)

Fire
(Yellow Bile/Choleric/Purging)

Hot   Dry

Air
(Blood/Sanguine/
Bleeding)

Earth
(Black Bile/Melancholic/
Starving)

Wet   Cold

Water
(Phlegm/Phlegmatic/Vomiting)

---

[16]In later mythology, Hygeia was sometimes identified as his wife. One of the Orphic hymns (67) refers to: "[Asklepios] husband of blameless Hygeia (Health)."

mentioned by both Plato and Aristotle, most of what we know him about is from stories and attributed writings. His status comes from several noteworthy accomplishments:

- *Writings.* A compendium of treatments and diagnostic insights (*Corpus Hippocratum*) attributed to Hippocrates was compiled at the Great Library in Alexandria in the fourth century BCE. (This collection most certainly also contained works by other practitioners from around the Mediterranean.)[17]

- A philosophy of natural (nondivine) causes of illnesses. For example, with regard to epilepsy, he said: "It is thus with regard to the disease called Sacred: it appears to me to be nowise more divine nor more sacred than other diseases, but has a natural cause .... Men regard its nature and cause as divine from ignorance and wonder."[18]

- *A professional code of conduct (the so-called Hippocratic Oath).* This code prohibits, among other things: euthanasia ("I will neither give any deadly drug, having been asked for it, nor will I guide the same advice."); abortion ("I will not give an abortifacient pessary to a woman."); practicing beyond one's skills ("I will not use the knife ... but I will give way to those who are practitioners of this work."); and breach of confidentiality ("That which I may see or hear during treatment, or even outside of treatment concerning the life of men, which must not in any way be divulged outside, I will not speak, regarding such things to be unutterable.").[19]

Among other contributions of Greek medicine to its Western descendants are medical schools and government-sponsored healthcare. The four most important centers of medical learning in the Greek sphere were Cnidus (in the southwest coast of Anatolia, modern Turkey, founded about 700 BCE), Croton (in the southeastern coast of Italy), Cyrene (on the eastern part of current Libya's Mediterranean coast), and Cos (where Hippocrates was born and taught).

The Greeks adopted the Egyptian concept of state-funded physician care but used a more democratic method.[20] Instead of government appointments, Greek citizens directly elected their public physicians, who were generally the best of their profession. A city's population determined the number of these elected practitioners; for example, Athens was said to have six. They were paid from a special annual tax (*iatrikon*) at the level of compensation of a skilled artisan. Private physicians were also available on a fee basis.

[17]Lyons, A. S., & Petrucelli II, R. J. (1987). *Medicine, an illustrated history*. New York: Abrams.

[18]Hippocrates (ca. 400 BCE). *On the sacred disease*. Trans. Francis Adams. Retrieved May 22, 2018, from http://classics.mit.edu/Hippocrates/sacred.html

[19]Herrell, H. (2000). *The Hippocratic Oath: A commentary and translation*. Retrieved May 22, 2018 from http://utilis.net/hippo.htm. See further commentary in this article about euthanasia and abortion in its historical context. One saying often incorrectly attributed to Hippocrates is "primum non nocere," or "first, do no harm." Although he writes in Epidemics (Book I, Chapter XI): "As to diseases, make a habit of two things—to help, or at least to do no harm," the phrase was certainly not in Latin. Smith dates its common use to the mid-1800s in the United States and England. (Smith, C. M. [2015]. Origin and uses of *Primum Non Nocere—Above All, Do No Harm!*. *Journal of Clinical Pharmacology, 45,* 371–377).

[20]Woodhead, A. G. (1952). The state health service in Ancient Greece. *Cambridge Historical Journal, 10*(3), 235–253.

When the Roman Empire rose to prominence, its physicians tended to come from Greece. Because these foreigners were not always trusted to treat illness, the Romans relied to a great extent on herbal and medicinal home remedies as well as prayer to household gods.[21] In summarizing this situation, Pliny the Elder (23–79 CE) stated that "the Roman people for more than six hundred years were not, indeed, without medicine, but they were without physicians."[22] Rome's contributions to the practice of medicine shifted the focus from individual patient care to significant public health initiatives, including:[23]

1. *Official oversight of physicians.* Even though no licensure existed, the Romans reviewed the qualifications of physicians. This practice originated not to ensure the quality of care, but for financial reasons. Because Augustus (63 BCE–19 CE) granted physicians exemption from public taxes, there were many fraudulent claims and thus a diminution in treasury funds. Antoninus Pius (86–161 CE) subsequently restricted this tax relief to a fixed number of qualified physicians (*archiatri*) in each community. While medical quackery persisted among private practitioners, penalties for negligent damages were severe, as was the custom in the ancient world from the time of Babylonia.

2. *Clean water.* By the end of the first century CE, at least nine aqueducts brought clean water to Rome. Subsequently, many more were built there and across the empire. The water supplied public fountains and baths; for an extra fee, private citizens could have a home connection.

3. *Drainage.* The best-known system is the Cloaca Maxima, which the Etruscans built in the sixth century BCE to drain swamps. It subsequently became the sewage system for Rome, though not all homes were connected. Public toilets also helped keep the waste from food and drinking water.

4. *Public baths.* The Romans stressed cleanliness not only for the nobility but also for commoners and slaves.

5. *Public hospitals.* Please see Chapter 4.

6. *Government organization of public health.* Augustus established numerous boards and commissions to supervise public health initiatives, including the Water Board, Health Commission, and various commissions of public supervisors (*aediles*) responsible for supervising the public baths, cleaning the streets, and overseeing the food supply.

7. *Support of medical education.* Vespasian (9–79 CE) provided salaries to physicians who taught others the profession; before that time, students paid their instructors directly. Severus Alexander (208–235 CE) supplied space in which to teach and subsidies for poorer students.

---

[21] Cato (234–149 BCE), who rejected Greek ideology and, as a result, Greek medical care, recommended cabbage and wine to prevent and treat ills.

[22] Elliott, J. S. (1971). *Outlines of Greek and Roman medicine.* Boston: Milford House (Full republication of text originally published in 1917), 14.

[23] Ciliers, L. (2006). Where were the doctors when the Roman Empire died? *Acta Theologica, 26*(2), 62–78.

While the Egyptian and Greek systems of national health schemes were not adopted by the Romans, some services were provided. For example, in 368, Valentinian I decreed that public doctors must provide free treatment for the poor.

One practitioner of note from this period is the Greek physician Galen (131–201 CE). His influential medical texts included 9 books on anatomy, 17 on physiology, 6 on pathology, 16 essays on the pulse, 14 books on therapeutics, and 30 books on pharmacy. In therapeutics, his focus was his own successful treatments, particularly polypharmacy (use of multiple drugs simultaneously), which included plant extracts. His anatomic observations, however, were less than accurate since he based his writings largely on dissections of apes and swine. His real contribution was in experimental physiology; as Garrison notes: "His contributions to the physiology of the nervous, respiratory, and circulatory systems, however faulty, were the only real knowledge for seventeen centuries."[24]

For the next 1,000 years, the practice of medicine was dominated by the church and its doctrines. "This dogma ... overthrew the science of medicine, and reduced its economy to the most abject dependence on divine manifestations.... Development, or even preservation, of medical science was therefore impossible."[25] Medical practice and training became the province of the monasteries, but the individual abbots decided whether such education would be provided. In 805, Charlemagne decreed that medicine must be taught in monastic schools; however, the content was limited to the teachings of such figures as Galen and Hippocrates. In 816, Abbot Gozpert founded what became a model school and hospital at St. Gall monastery (in present-day Switzerland). This monastery was a pioneer in hospital architecture (e.g., separating infectious patients from others) as well as in establishment of a pharmacy stocked from an on-site botanical garden.

As long as medical attention was provided at these religious sites, the church was content with this professional model of care. What happened, however, was anything but ecclesiastical. Monks who received medical training often left the monasteries and became wandering physicians who kept the payments for their services. To change this practice, in 1139, Pope Innocent II's Second Lateran Council declared:

> [T]he evil and detestable practice has grown ... whereby monks and canons regular, after receiving the habit and making their profession, are learning civil law and medicine with a view to temporal gain, in scornful disregard of the rules of their blessed teachers Benedict and Augustine ... There are also those who, neglecting the care of souls, completely ignore their state in life, promise health in return for hateful money and make themselves healers of human bodies ... Therefore, we forbid by apostolic authority this practice to continue, so that the monastic order and the order of canons may be preserved without stain in a state of life pleasing to God, in accord with their holy purpose.[26]

---

[24] Garrison, F. H. (1921). *An introduction to the history of medicine.* Philadelphia: WB Saunders.

[25] Fort, G. F. (1883). *Medical economy during the Middle Ages: A contribution to the history of European morals from the time of the Roman Empire to the close of the fourteenth century.* New York: J. W. Bouton

[26] *Second Lateran Council—1139 A.D.* Para. 9. Retrieved May 22, 2018, from http://www.papalencyclicals.net/councils/ecum10.htm This ruling confirmed a previous prohibition at the Council of Rheims in 1131.

Similar subsequent prohibitions reinforced this doctrine.[27] Of particular note was the interdiction on regular clergy from *teaching* law or medicine.[28] As a result of this change in church policy, the need for more lay medical practitioners became necessary; hence, there was a shift from monastic medical teaching and practice to the university setting.

The first medical school of "modern" times and the one subsequently emulated by others across Europe was at Salerno. The school was founded in the 9th century, formally organized in the 10th, and reached its pinnacle at the end of the 12th. A confluence of four factors led to its formation:

1. Because of its climate, Salerno was a health destination for invalids from all over Europe. As a result, it had a high concentration of physicians.

2. Benedictine monks ran a well-known school there.

3. The location was at the nexus of trade among many cultures (including Greek and Arab culture), which brought diverse ideas about medical practice to the university.

4. The ruling Norman kings provided enlightened leadership.

In addition to the quality of its physicians, the school was renowned for its liberality and rigor. Some of the more innovative features of the school and city included:

- *Acceptance of women and Jews, who were otherwise excluded from other schools.* They were not only accepted as students but also welcomed as teachers. As Walsh[29] points out: "Women were given opportunities for the higher education at practically all of the Italian universities … No century from the twelfth down to the nineteenth was without some distinguished women professors at Italian universities." This situation was not replicated for many centuries in other European institutions.[30]

- *Prescribed courses of study.* Starting with King Roger II (1095–1154) and subsequently codified by his grandson, Frederick II, Holy Roman Emperor (1194–1250), premedical studies of 3 years[31] and medical studies of 4 years were required for a doctor of medicine degree. This degree allowed the recipient to teach medicine. In order to be able to practice, the law required an additional year of supervised practice with an

---

[27] For example, the Fourth Lateran Council (1215) stated: "nor may a subdeacon, deacon or priest practise the art of surgery, which involves cauterizing and making incisions …" Para. 18. Retrieved May 22, 2018, from http://www.papalencyclicals.net/Councils/ecum12-2.htm

[28] Synod of Tours, 1179 under Pope Alexander III.

[29] Walsh, J. J. (1920). *Medieval medicine*. London: A. & C. Black.

[30] Ibid. Walsh explains this exclusion in this way: "[T]here seems, however, to have been not nearly so much freedom or so much encouragement for women in medicine in France as in Italy … One reason for this was doubtless the Héloïse-Abélard incident early in the history of the University of Paris. This seems to have discouraged efforts in the direction of the securing of the higher education for women in most of the Western Universities. Oxford was the daughter University of Paris, and Cambridge of Oxford, and they and all the other universities of the West were more deeply influenced in their customs and organization by Paris than by Italy, and as a consequence we hear little of feminine education in the West generally."

[31] Topics included logic, grammar, rhetoric, mathematics, astronomy, theology, and music.

established physician. Further, surgeons were obliged to prove they had 1 year of anatomy study.[32]

▪ *Enactment of licensure rules*. According to Friedenwald:[33]

> In 1140 Roger II, King of the two Sicilies, issued the first known legal enactment for the regulation of medical practice in Europe:

> "Whosoever will henceforth practise medicine, let him present himself to our officials and judges to be examined by them; but if he presume of his own temerity, let him be imprisoned and all his goods be sold by auction. The object of this is to prevent the subjects of our kingdom incurring peril through the ignorance of physicians."

▪ *Issuance of conflict of interest standards*. In 1241, Emperor Frederick II issued the Edict of Salerno, in which he stated that a physician "must not enter into any business relations with the apothecary [pharmacist] nor must he take any of them under his protection nor incur any money obligations in their regard. Nor must any licensed physician keep an apothecary's shop himself." Despite this prohibition, it is noteworthy that as early as the 14th century, physicians in many European cities regularly saw patients in apothecary shops,[34] predating medical care in American pharmacies by over 600 years.

▪ *Fee schedules*. The Edict of Salerno also fixed prices for medications and medical services.

From Salerno, the medical school model spread to Bologna (early 13th century) and then to other Italian cities. French universities followed the Italian model, and Salerno[35] was eclipsed in prominence by Montpellier starting in the 13th century. This school rose to prominence for reasons similar to Salerno: it was at the crossroads of trade (and hence medical knowledge) and the salubrious climate made it the destination of those in need of recovery. Further, academics fled there (and elsewhere) from Paris after a police attack on rioting students in 1229 caused the suspension of classes. Although the medical faculties of Oxford and Cambridge grew during the 14th century, Montpellier and then Paris became the foreign sites that trained the most numerous and influential English physicians.[36]

---

[32] Baker, F. (1909, November). The two Sylviuses. An historical study. *Bulletin of the Johns Hopkins Hospital, XX*(224), 329–339.

[33] Friedenwald, H. (1921). On the giving of medical degrees during the Middle Ages by other than academic authorities. *Annals of Medical History, 3*(1), 64–66.

[34] Park, K. (1997). Medicine and the Renaissance. In: *Western medicine, an illustrated history*. London: Irvine/New York: Oxford University Press.

[35] The Salerno school was dissolved by an edict of the Emperor Napoleon I in 1811.

[36] One of the most influential was John of Gaddesden, the model for the "doctour of physic" in Geoffrey Chaucer's *Canterbury Tales*. The persistent influence of astrology and humoral theory of disease are evident in the lines:

Well could he guess the ascending of the star

Wherein his patient's fortunes settled were.

He knew the course of every malady,

Were it of cold or heat or moist or dry.

Despite the spread of secular medical education, the Catholic church still had an influence on this field in France and elsewhere. For example, scholars (including physician-teachers) were required to be celibate: "[A]s a rule, a master who married lost his position, and though married scholars are sometimes mentioned, e.g. at Oxford, they were disqualified for taking degrees."[37] The reason given for prohibition on physician marriage was to lessen the opportunity for licentiousness.[38] The ban in Paris was lifted in 1452.[39]

The Renaissance was the next historical period that substantively influenced medical practice. From this perspective, it is logical to date the start of its changes to the latter half of the 14th century following the bubonic plague pandemic, often called the Black Death. Between its start in 1347 and 1430, many waves of this disease reduced the European population by about 50 percent to 75 percent.[40] For example: "In Britain, for which we have the most accurate demographic data of the period, the population decreased by well over half—from about 5.5 million ... in 1335 to 2.1 million in 1455."[41] The social effects on medical practice were mainly twofold:

1. *Questioning authority*. The church and the medical profession were not able to protect people from the plague's devastation. Perhaps due to this loss of public trust, as well as a feeling of impotence in the face of the disease, physicians began to question existing knowledge and reexamine original sources. For example, prior to the Renaissance, the medical texts (particularly those of Galen) were held sacrosanct and not to be challenged. Anatomist Jacques Dubois (1478–1555), known as Sylvius, highlighted the change in attitude with respect to the study of anatomy: "[I]it is much better that you should learn the manner of cutting by eye and touch than by reading and listening, for reading alone never taught anyone how to sail a ship, to lead an army, nor to compound a medicine, which is done rather by the use of one's own sight and the training of one's own hands."[42]

---

[37] *The law faculty removed the celibacy requirement in 1600.* Retrieved May 22, 2018, from http://www.newadvent.org/cathen/15188a.htm

[38] Physicians are: "at risk by a condition to constantly see persons of the sex, spending their life between the double danger of scandal and very painful continence." D'Aussey, L. Le marriage Des Sept Arts. *Notices et extraits des manuscrits de la Bibliothèque Nationale, 5,* 492. Paris. Year 7 [French Revolutionary calendar corresponding to the Gregorian year September 22, 1798 to September 22, 1799]. Retrieved May 22, 2018 from https://archive.org/details/NoticesEtExtraits5

[39] The ban's lifting was actually the result of international politics. In 1452, Pope Calixtus III, following a petition from the d'Arc family, sought to reverse the ecclesiastic conviction that led to Jeanne d'Arc's burning for heresy in 1431. Since the faculty at the University of Paris was instrumental in bringing her to trial, the Pope needed to "reform" that university before he could take further action. To do so, he appointed Cardinal Guillaume d'Estouteville (1403–1483) as his legate to Paris in 1451. As part of the 1452 "Statuts de Estouteville," the absolute marriage prohibition for the medical faculty was removed, though individuals still needed the legate's permission. By 1456, Jeanne's conviction was annulled. She was canonized in 1920.

[40] Cipolla, C. (1994). *Before the Industrial Revolution: European society and economy, 1000–1700.* New York: W.W. Norton.

[41] Bernstein, W. J. (2008). *A splendid exchange: How trade shaped the world* (p. 145). New York: Atlantic Monthly Press.

[42] Delaboe, F. (Sylvii) (1555). *Introduction to anatomy in Opera Medica.* Amsterdam. The irony of this statement is that Delaboe was a staunch supporter of Galen. When his dissection findings did not match those of Galen, he said it was because of the differences caused by human evolution since ancient times: " ... when Galen reported that the sternum

Many of the revered original sources were Greek medical texts, which came to European physicians through translations via Arabic and/or Hebrew and thence into Latin. Reexamination of the Greek texts often exposed errors in medical practice due to inaccurate translations.

2. *Lessening of the church's interest in and control of medical practice.* Since the plague affected clergy and laity alike, the shortage of clerics at all levels caused the church to focus primarily on religious practices and reduce its secular activities, including monitoring medical practice. The degree of clerical scarcity, even for religious responsibilities, was illustrated in England. "The decision in 1349 that the last rights could be received from the laity when there were no priests around to do the job, although strictly temporary, must already have made inroads into the clergy's absolute monopoly on the sacraments ... Increasingly, salvation seemed a do-it-yourself project."[43] Further, the church had its own internal problems. In 1377, it moved back to Rome from Avignon, where it had been exiled for the previous 70 years. As Norwich[44] points out:

> But the Italy to which it had returned, though in some respects unchanged, in others differed radically from the Italy it had left 70 years before. Unity was as remote a possibility as ever ... and the Black Death had drawn yet another curtain across the past, while exposing the present still more mercilessly to the winds of change. The secular, inquiring spirit which now spread across the land was not in itself new ... But the 14th century had given it a new momentum ... *the papal barriers that had so long blocked its progress had suddenly disappeared* [emphasis added].

These trends cannot be separated from other concurrently sweeping changes in the humanities and technology. The challenges to old doctrines were accompanied by a fascination with temporal matters, particularly interest in the human body; even the church aided in this exploration. We know, for example, that in 1495, the prior of Santo Spirito in Florence supplied Michelangelo with corpses to dissect in its cloisters. Much had changed between 1300, when Boniface VIII issued a bull threatening excommunication for dissection, and 1523, when Clement VII gave permission for that practice for medical instruction.[45]

Of course, knowledge must be disseminated to be of use. The Renaissance invention of an improved, movable-type mechanical printing press[46] by the German printer Johannes Gutenberg (1450) was of significant importance. However, this innovation did not mean everyone owned books. "From 1450 to 1500, between 10,000 and 15,000 titles were

---

had seven segments and Vesalius observes only six, Sylvius concluded, 'it is not an error of Galen, but a change of nature in us.'" Nancy, G., & Siraisi, N. G. (2007). *History, medicine and the traditions of renaissance learning.* Ann Arbor: University of Michigan Press. (He is, in fact, describing the original definition of the word "autopsy" documented in the *Oxford English Dictionary*: "The action or process of seeing with one's own eyes; personal observation, inspection, or experience. Now *rare*.")

[43] Schama, S. (2000). *History of Britain: At the edge of the world? 3500 BC–1603 AD* (pp. 237–238). New York: Hyperion.
[44] Norwich, J. J. (2011). *Absolute monarchs: A history of the papacy* (225–226). New York: Random House.
[45] Newlin, G. (1998). *Understanding a tale of two cities* (p. 217). Westport, CT: Greenwood Press.
[46] Movable type with wood characters was invented about 1040 in China by Sheng Bi.

published in 30–35,000 editions, with an *average printing of 500 copies* [emphasis added]."[47] But only a small portion of those books was on medical topics. Further, the texts that were published tended to be printed versions of older works. As Osler[48] noted:

> The first bit of medical printing known is the Mainz Kalendar for the year 1457. To 1480 at least 46 of these were published in Germany. They were based chiefly on the belief that certain phases of the moon and certain conjunctions of the planets were favorable for bleeding and for the taking of medicines, particularly purges. To 1480 inclusive 182 editions of medical books were printed. These represented 67 authors, viz., Classical 6, Arabian 8, Mediaeval 23, fifteenth century 30. A distribution by countries gave Italy 127 editions, Germany 43, Switzerland and France each 4, Low Countries 3, and Spain 1 (?).

To highlight the slow rate of increase of Western medical book publication even in the 20th century, only 1,666 new books and new editions were published from October 1902 to October 1903.[49]

Still, according to Osler:[50] "The sixteenth and seventeenth centuries did three things in medicine—shattered authority, laid the foundation of an accurate knowledge of the structure of the human body and demonstrated how its functions should be studied intelligently."

It was during the Renaissance that we see the beginnings of true British medicine. Since Great Britain is the immediate source of American medicine, we will start to look at developments there and how they drew on the ancient and continental European traditions. England did not have any medical schools in the Middle Ages, and the Italian tradition of monastery-originated medical education did not exist. Medical training awaited the establishment of universities, particularly Oxford and Cambridge, whose medical faculties were founded in the later 13th century and began to grant medical degrees in the early 14th century.[51] The number of graduates remained small, however, so the practice of medicine was still heavily foreign-influenced. Many prominent physicians attended medical school or pursued additional studies on the continent, and the texts used in England were from such universities as Paris and Montpellier.

Because there were few medical school graduates and the concentration of training was in Oxford and Cambridge, the regulation of medical practice in other places, particularly

---

[47] Zaid, G. (2003). *So many books: Reading and publishing in an age of abundance* (p. 20). Philadelphia: Paul Dry Books.

[48] Osler, W. (1916). Printed Medical Books to 1480. Paper presented at the 21st annual meeting of the bibliographical society of London. January, 2014. In *Transactions of the bibliographical society*, Vol. XIII (October, 1913–March 1915) (pp. 5–6). London: Blades, East & Blades. Retrieved May 22, 2018, from http://www.archive.org/stream/transactions13bibluoft/transactions13bibluoft_djvu.txt The fact that these books were written in Latin was not an impediment for physicians, since they were trained in this language. It did make the writings inaccessible to the common person.

[49] Editorial: A year's medical book production (1903, October 29). *The Boston Medical and Surgical Journal* (Now the *New England Journal of Medicine*), 149(18), 495.

[50] Osler, W. (1921). *The evolution of modern medicine*. New Haven, CT: Yale University Press.

[51] The medical education was patterned after the European model. English medical students completed a bachelor's degree that gave them the right to practice medicine. They might also obtain a doctorate to teach. This system persists today in countries having a British-style medical education system—the initial medical degree is a Bachelor's of Medicine and Surgery, called MBBS. Unlike Italy, women and Jews were excluded from English schools.

such larger cities as London and York, was left to ineffective guilds. However, unlike trade guilds, which trained apprentices, set standards, and maintained quality of the craft, the only purpose of medical guilds was to restrict competition. This situation invites the question: Who was a legitimate practitioner? The answer is problematic since in medieval England:

> No single group of practitioners distinguished itself by force of numbers, by healing skill, or by civic sanction as a dominant medical profession … the vast majority of medics operated independently, and … often part-time. … Brewers who practiced surgery, abbots who delivered babies, friars who wrote medical books, a chancellor of the exchequer who doctored the king, a Cistercian surgeon: all were involved in healing, and all were involved in other pursuits … The limits of proper medical practice, the question of who should be a practitioner, and what he or she could be expected to know were still very much open even in the late fifteenth century.[52]

Except for barber surgeon and apothecary guilds, the organizations of other medical practitioners were not effective in exerting control.

From the Middle Ages through the Renaissance and beyond, this pluralistic approach to practice had several other important consequences.

- *Weak regulation.* Incorporated by charter in 1462 in London, the Barber Surgeons obtained the power to examine and suspend practitioners as well as to inspect drugs. In the third year of Henry VIII's reign (1512), the state's examination authority was reinforced by a decree "that no person within the City of London, nor within seven miles of the same, should take upon him to exercise and occupy as physician or surgeon, except he be first examined, approved, and admitted by the Bishop of London and other, under and upon certain pains and penalties." However, in 1542, Henry issued what has been called the Herbalists' Charter, which rescinded the previous decree and granted rights to herbalists to practice medicine. The king gave as his rationale that

  > the Company and Fellowship of Surgeons of London, minding only their own Lucres and nothing the Profit or ease of the Diseased or Patient, have sued, troubled and vexed divers honest Persons, as well as Men and Women, whom God hath endued [endowed] with the Knowledge of the Nature, Kind and Operation of certain Herbs, Roots and Waters.[53]

  It is also well known that Henry consulted herbalists and kept his own herbal remedies, perhaps contributing another reason for this charter. The effect of the edict was the reinforcement of permissiveness toward diverse practitioners.

- *No requirement for formal university education.* An apprentice-type training program was sufficient for practitioners.

---

[52]Getz, F. (1998). *Medicine in the English Middle Ages.* Princeton, NJ: Princeton University Press.

[53]Law, R. (2012). Observations reality check: Assaulting alternative medicine: worthwhile or witch hunt? *British Medical Journal,* 344, e1075. Retrieved May 22, 2018, from http://www.bmj.com/content/344/bmj.e1075/rr/569321 The author also notes that: "The charter is still in existence to this day, allowing herbalists to help people by providing herbal remedies under English Common Law and, more recently, under Section 12 (1) of the Medicines Act of 1968."

▪ *Separation of physicians and surgeons into two very distinct professional bodies.* As Albutt[54] notes: "[I]n England the division of the house of Medicine into surgery and physic became as deep and more abiding than in France; so deep and abiding that the evil of it is still at work among us."

History of American Medical Care

Since medicine was a lucrative profession in England, physicians had few incentives to establish practices in the new colonies. Many of the early practitioners were, therefore, clergy or sailors (such as ships' captains). For example, despite questionable formal medical training, the first practitioner among the colonists was church deacon Dr. Samuel Fuller, who accompanied the Plymouth settlers in 1620. Davis summarized the situation thusly:

> [A]s a general rule only those physicians who had failed to obtain a practice at home, or were too conscious of their own unfitness to make the attempt, emigrated to America. On the other hand, the great expense attending the education of young men belonging to the colonies, in the medical institutions of Europe, operated as an equal barrier to this source. Thus it was, that while persecution filled the clerical ranks of the colonies with men of the deepest piety, and the most varied learning, and the patronage of the crown induced a full supply of legal talent, the profession of medicine sunk to a comparatively low state.

> In New England, the greater number of those who practiced medicine were priests, whose medical knowledge was chiefly derived from the writings of Hippocrates, Galen. Aretaeus, etc., which they had read during their collegiate education in Europe. Some of the nonconformist clergy, however, who were persecuted or silenced in the Old World, went through with a regular course of medical studies before leaving home and afterwards became exceedingly useful, both as physicians and preachers, among the colonists here.[55]

Formal medical education in the colonies required travel to England or the continent. For example, in 1642, two of the first nine Harvard graduates, Samuel Bellingham and Henry Saltonstall, went to Leyden and Padua, respectively, to obtain their medical degrees. Both stayed in England for the remainder of their careers.[56]

Because of the scarcity and limited skills of physicians in America at that time, it was not unheard of for patients to take a long voyage to England for treatment.[57]

---

[54] Albutt, T. C. (1905). *The historical relations of medicine and surgery to the end of the sixteenth century* (pp. 99–103). New York: MacMillan and company.

[55] Davis, N. S. (1851). *History of medical education and institutions in the United States from the first settlements of the British Colonies to the year 1860; With a chapter on the present condition and wants of the profession and the means necessary for supplying those wants and elevating the character and extending the usefulness of the whole profession* (pp. 17–18). Chicago: S. C. Griggs & Co.

[56] Beinfield, M. S. (1942). The early New England doctor: An adaptation to a provincial environment. *Yale Journal of Biology and Medicine, 15*(1), 99–132.

[57] Thatcher, J. (1828). *American medical biography or memoirs of eminent physicians who have flourished in America.* Boston: Richardson & Lord. The author documents as late as the mid-18th century a patient traveling to London for treatment of a bladder stone.

Perhaps recognizing the varied qualifications of medical practitioners, in 1649, the Massachusetts Bay Colony issued the following law:

Forasmuch as the law of God, Exodus: 20: 13, allows no man to touch the life or limb of any person except in a judicial way, be it hereby ordered and decreed, that no person or person whatsoever that are employed about the bodies of men, women, and children for preservation of life or health, as physicians, surgeon, midwives, or others, shall assume to exercise or in any, way put forth any act contrary to the known rules of art, nor exercise any force, violence, or cruelty upon or towards the bodies of any, whether young or old, — no, not in the most difficult and desperate cases, — without the Order for mid-wives & surgeons advice and consent of such as are skillful in the same art, if such may be had, or at least of the wisest and gravest then present, and consent of the patient or patients, (if they be mentis compotes,) much less contrary to such advice and consent, upon such punishment as the nature of the fact may deserve; this law is not intended to discourage any from a lawful use of their skill, but rather to encourage and direct them in the right use thereof.[58]

In the tradition of clergy-physicians, the first medical publication in the colonies was authored by the founding minister of Old South Church in Boston, the Reverend Thomas Thacher. He came to Boston in the 1630s and published "A Brief Rule to Guide the Common People of New England how to order themselves and theirs in the Small-Pox and Measels" during an epidemic in 1677.

Through the mid-18th century, the public's perception of physicians was cautious, at best. For example, in 1753, an editorial in the *Independent Reflector* (a paper then published in the city of New York) complained:

I believe there is no City in the World, not larger than ours [the population of N.Y. city was about 10,000], that abounds with so many Doctors: We can, at least, boast the Honour of above Forty Gentlemen of the Faculty; ... far the greatest Part of them are meer [*sic*] Pretenders to a Profession, of which they are entirely ignorant.... The very Advertisements they publish of themselves, prove them ignorant of the very Names of their Drugs. It is high Time the Arm of the Magistrate should interpose for relief ... Thousands may be poison'd, and the Doctor pass unpunished.[59]

Two events of note subsequently occurred to remedy this problem of quality care. First, a law was passed regulating who was qualified to practice medicine and the penalties for violation of the statute:

WHEREAS many ignorant and unskilful Persons in Physick and Surgery in order to gain a Subsistence do take upon them-selves to administer Physick and practice Surgery in the City of New York to the endangering of the Lives and Limbs of their Patients; and many poor and

---

[58]Records of the Governor and Company of the Massachusetts Bay, II, p. 217. May 3, 1649. Retrieved May 22, 2018, from https://archive.org/stream/recordsofgoverno03mass/recordsofgoverno03mass_djvu.txt The archaic spellings have been updated by this author.

[59]The Use and Importance of the Practice of PHYSIC; together with the Difficulty of the Science, and the dismal Havock made by Quacks and Pretenders. *The Independent Reflector* (1752–1753), *12* (February 15, 1753), 47.

ignorant Persons inhabiting the said City who have been persuaded to become their Patients have been great Sufferers thereby: ... no Person whatsoever shall practice as a Physician or surgeon in the said City of New York before he shall first have been examined in Physick or Surgery and approved of and admitted by one of His Majesty's Council, the Judges of the Supreme Court, the King's Attorney General, and the Mayor of the City of New York for the time being, or by any three or more of them.... if any Person shall practise in the City of New York as a Physician or Surgeon or both as Physician and Surgeon with-out such Testimonial as aforesaid he shall for every such offence forfeit the sum of five pounds, One half thereof to the use of the Person or Persons who shall sue for the same and the other Moiety to the Church Wardens and Vestrymen of the said City for the use of the Poor thereof.[60]

Unfortunately, this law covered only the city and county of New York. Except for a similar law enacted in the colony of New Jersey in1772, regulation of medical practice prior to the Revolutionary War was nonexistent.[61]

The second event was changes in medical education. Prior to the establishment of formal American medical schools, boys between the ages of 14 and 18 indentured themselves to physicians for 3 to 7 years as apprentices. However, toward the middle of the 18th century, some colonists who studied medicine abroad began to return home with other ideas. Of particular note are Philadelphians John Morgan and William Shippen Jr., who were both graduates of the University of Edinburgh. In 1765, they cofounded the Medical School of the College of Philadelphia (later, the University of Pennsylvania), the first medical school in continuous operation in North America.[62] The first class graduated in 1768.[63] Drawing on the European model, Dr. Morgan detailed the requirements for baccalaureate and doctoral degrees in physic. (Note the similarities to the course of study mentioned earlier for medieval Italian physicians.) For a baccalaureate, students must:

1. [S]atisfy the Trustees and Professors of the College, concerning their knowledge of the Latin tongue, and in such branches of Mathematics, Natural and Experimental Philosophy, as shall be judged requisite to a Medical Education.

---

[60] An Act to regulate the Practice of Physick and Surgery in the City of New York. [Passed, June 10, 1760.] Laws of the Colony of New York 4~55[CHAPTER 1120.] [Chapter 1120, of Van Schaack, and chapter 198 (Volume 2) of Livingstone Smith, where the act is printed in full. Retrieved May 22, 2018, from http://ebooks.library.cornell.edu/cgi/t/text/pageviewer-idx?c=cdl;cc=cdl;idno=cdl182;seq=459 It is noteworthy that the Act was passed because of the support and sponsorship Cadwallader Colden (1689–1776), who was a physician and, at the time, acting colonial governor.

[61] It is not recorded whether the aforementioned 1649 statute survived to pre-Revolutionary times or was ever enforced. Further, these newer laws were more prescriptive with regard to how competence of professionals was to be documented. In 1781, the Massachusetts legislature granted the Massachusetts State Medical Society the right to "examine all Candidates for the Practice of Physic and Surgery ... and if upon such Examination said Candidates shall be found skilled in their Profession, and fitted for the Practice of it, they shall receive the Approbation of the Society." Retrieved May 22, 2018, from http://www.massmed.org/About/History/#.VbE9h3gtznk

[62] L'Universidad Autónoma de Santo Domingo was the first medical school in the Americas, founded in 1538. However, because of wars and occupations it has not been in continuous operation.

[63] John Archer (May 5, 1741–September 28, 1810), later a U.S. congressman from Maryland, is said to be the first medical graduate in America; however, his classmates would claim this distinction was only alphabetical.

2. [T]ake at least one course in Anatomy, Materia Medica [pharmacology], Chemistry, the Theory and Practice of Physic and Clinical Lectures, and shall attend the practice of the Pennsylvania Hospital for one year; and then may be admitted to a public examination for a Bachelor's Degree in Physic, provided that, on previous private examination by the Medical Trustees and Professors, and such other Trustees and Professors as choose to attend, such student shall be judged fit to undergo a public examination.

3. It is further required that each student, previous to obtaining a Bachelor's Degree, shall have served a sufficient apprenticeship to some respectable Practitioner in Physic, and be able to make it appear that he has a general knowledge in Pharmacy.

For a Doctor's Degree in Physic:

It is required that at least three years shall intervene from the time of taking the Bachelor's Degree, and that the candidate be full twenty-four years of age and that he write and defend publicly in college, a Latin Thesis or dissertation on some disease, or other useful medical topic, which shall also be printed at his own expense.[64]

Despite these two trends to *improve* quality, the 18th and 19th centuries experienced two other influences that contravened those efforts; the result was *de*regulation of medical practice. These factors were: "first, the aversion to monopolies and elite fraternities that undermined economic freedom and republican values, and second, the need for free inquiry to advance medical knowledge."[65]

As to the first cause, as early as the mid- to late 1700s, medical societies were granted governmental authority to approve colleagues as qualified for medical practice—the first licensure processes, and ones that reflected the English licensure procedure. However, these societies also set the fees their members should charge patients. In 1769, an anonymous citizen wrote to the *Connecticut Courant* about the conflict of interests of the Litchfield County (Connecticut) Medical Society:

The matter of medicine lies very much in the dark (with regard to the vulgar) and its difficulty for common people to determine whether they are well or ill used in demands made upon them; and a combination of Doctors perhaps gives them a greater advantage to impose on mankind by extravagant demands than if no such combination had been formed.[66]

The editor replied:

[I]n every nation where learning, wisdom and goodness have flourished, there they have always encouraged combination of Doctors, who were countenanced and protected by the

---

[64]The Address and Representation of Dr. John Morgan, of the College of Philadelphia, in behalf of the Seminary, dated 1772 cited in Davis, NS: History of the Medical Profession from the first settlement of the British Colonies in America, to the Year 1783. *North-Western Medical and Surgical Journal, 3(1)*: 11–12, 1850.

[65]Grossman, L. A. (2013). The origins of American Health Libertarianism. *Yale Journal of Health Policy, Law, and Ethics, XIII(1)*, 93.

[66]*The Connecticut Courant,* July 31, 1769, 5. The Litchfield Medical Society was founded in 1764.

legislature ... I presume that there is not a person in this colony ... but who would choose to pay the demands for physical benefits ascertained by the said corporation rather than to leave it to every ignorant and extravagant [practitioner] to set his own prices.

Ultimately, the Connecticut legislature refused to grant the medical society licensing rights.[67] Likewise, according to Blake,[68] the Boston Medical Society was "formed in 1780 chiefly to set up a fee schedule." Stevens[69] comments that this formation "was vigorously opposed by the public, as a potential private monopoly ... [however], public opposition gradually ceased; indeed, in 1800 the legislature voted to withhold the legal power of collecting debts from unrecognized practitioners." The act was repealed in 1842.

The second reason for opposition to licensure was that it tended to lock in old practices and thus stifle competition and innovation. As novel practices and medical theories were emerging, traditional practitioners viewed those who used these new methods or espoused new theories as unfit to practice medicine and so excluded them from medical societies.

In addition to the public's concern mentioned above, some prominent practitioners were also critical of licensure. For example, according to the eminent physician and Declaration of Independence signer Dr. Benjamin Rush: "Conferring exclusive privileges upon Bodies of Physicians, and forbidding men of equal talents and knowledge from practicing medicine within certain districts of cities and countries, are Inquisitions—however sanctioned by ancient charters and names—serving as the bastiles [sic] of our profession."[70]

A principal reason (and many believe the main cause) medical licensure waned after the 1820s was the fight over various theories of medical practice, the most controversial of which was what became known as Thomsonism. It is useful to consider this and other influential movements not only because of their effect on medical practice as a profession but also for the business models used in their spread.

Samuel Thomson (1769–1843) was a self-taught New England practitioner who espoused botanical treatments based on his experience with family, friends, and, subsequently, the public. He described the philosophy of his treatment as follows:

I found, after maturely considering the subject, that all animal bodies are formed of the four elements, earth, air, fire, and water ... That cold, or lessening the power of heat, is the cause of all disease; that to restore heat to its natural state, was the only way by which health could be produced.[71]

---

[67] Shryock, R. H. (1967). *Medical licensing in America, 1650–1965*. Baltimore: Johns Hopkins University Press.
[68] Blake, J. B. (1959). *Public health in the Town of Boston, 1630–1822* (p. 124). London: Oxford University Press.
[69] Stevens, R. (1971). *American medicine in the public interest* (p. 23). Los Angeles: University of California Press.
[70] Rush, B. (1801). "Lecture VI. Upon the causes which have retarded the progress of medicine and the means of promoting its certainty and greater usefulness." In Benjamin Rush, *Six introductory lectures to courses of lectures upon the institutes and practice of medicine*. Philadelphia: John Conrad.
[71] Thomson, S. (1835). *New guide to health: Or botanic family physician. Containing a complete system of practice, on a plan entirely new: With a description of the vegetables made use of, and directions for preparing and administering them, to cure disease. To which is prefixed a narrative of the life and medical discoveries of the author* (p. 15). Printed for the Author, and sold by his General Agent, at the Office of the Boston Investigator. Boston: J. Q. Adams, Printer.

Thomson's treatments depended on serial use of herb preparations, which, he asserted, raised the body's heat.[72] His claims for success angered traditionally trained physicians who were still employing such measures as bleeding, cupping, and purging. These traditional practitioners tried to stop the spread of his approach not only by verbal and written attacks[73] but by having him arrested for murder, for which he was subsequently acquitted.

Thomson developed a business plan that included selling "subscriptions" (the equivalent today of a site license) for $10, which entitled the purchaser to use this method for himself and his family. Further, he crafted a scheme to organize practitioners of his methods, which he called Friendly Botanic Societies. Of note is that women were freely accepted into these societies, marking the first time they were accepted as "legitimate" medical practitioners in America.

These societies were for instruction about Thomson's methods (think about the modern equivalent of user groups) but about which members were to keep secret. The societies' members, however, did not keep the methods private.

Rather than fighting the medical establishment with traditional claims and counterclaims and trying to enforce the confidentiality terms of membership in the societies, Thomson "finally came to the conclusion that there was only one plan for me to pursue with any chance of success; and that was to go on to Washington, and obtain a patent for my discoveries."[74] On March 2, 1813, he was granted patent 1888 for "A specification for preparing and using certain medicines in fevers, colics, dysenteries, and rheumatisms."[75]

In 1822, after he lost a patent challenge in circuit court, Thomson applied for another (substantially similar) patent; it was granted in January 1823 (patent 3646).[76]

During this time, a number of other practice philosophies and schools developed that competed with one another. One reason for this opening of ideas is that experimental science was challenging anecdotal experience as the basis of treatment.[77] The contested issues

---

[72]To view the recipe for this interesting treatment, see: Conducted by Daniel L. M. Peixotto M. D. (1829). *New York Medical and Physical Journal*. Vol. I: New Series (pp. 211–215). New York: Charles S. Francis and Weabe C. Little, Albany.

[73]For example: Butterfield, J. (1842). Case of death from Thomsonism (letter). *Boston Medical and Surgical Journal*, 26216–218, 1842.

[74]Thomson, S., New guide to health: or botanic family physician, op. cit. p. 43.

[75]This type of patent was not unique. The first medication patent in the U.S. (number 111) was issued to Samuel Lee, Jr. on April 30, 1796, for a "Composition of bilious pills." The first medical device patent was issued to Thomas Bruff on July 1, 1797, for a "Device for extracting teeth." Perhaps the broadest early medical patent was granted to John Kunitz on May 7, 1805, (patent 612) for "bleeding with and breeding leaches." This latter patent was for a methodology rather than a product—leeches being an ancient form of treatment; in that respect, it was similar to Thomson's treatment patent. "Most of the patents prior to 1836 [including those of Lee, Kunitz, and Thomson] were lost in the December 1836 Patent Office fire. Only about 2,000 of the approximately 10,000 documents were recovered." (Personal communication, U.S. Patent and Trademark Office. August 10, 2015.)

[76]The 1823 patent was for: "Specification of a Patent granted for a mode of preparing, mixing, compounding, administering, and using, the medicine therein described ... " He also received yet another, essentially similar, patent in May 1836 (9640). Copies of all his patents were lost in the above-mentioned 1836 fire.

[77]Experimental medicine was a hallmark of medical instruction in the Parisian schools, to which increasing numbers of younger physicians were exposed.

dealt with the causes of diseases (was there one cause of all diseases or different causes for each disease?), the roles of different types of treatments (e.g., use of medication derived from plants versus manufactured chemical compounds and treatment using medication versus physical manipulation), and the aggressiveness of treatment (e.g., aggressive bleeding versus watchful waiting for a natural healing process).[78] It is noteworthy that, like botanical medicine, many theories had a champion with whom its movement was associated.

In order to provide a background for how modern medicine was shaped by the beliefs of the past 150 years, brief descriptions of the more prominent movements are presented below.

Homeopathy. This school of thought emerged in the 1790s in Germany, where it was formulated by physician Christian Friedrich Samuel Hahnemann (1755–1843). Like other nontraditional practitioners of that time, Hahnemann thought established measures, such as bleeding, caused more harm than good. He coined the term "allopathy" to describe traditional practitioners who treated patients based on the humoral theory of the ancient Greeks.[79] In experimenting with cinchona tree bark (a malaria treatment), he noticed that it caused the same symptoms as the disease when given to healthy people. This observation, as well as readings from other practitioners, led him to promulgate homeopathy's three principles:

1. "Like treats like." Treat disease with medication that, in higher doses, mimics the symptoms in healthy people (e.g., cinchona for malaria). This principle is the source of the name "homeo" (same or alike) plus "pathy" (in this context, suffering).

2. Because medication in higher doses produces similar symptoms, to be effective in sick persons, it must be greatly diluted.

3. Shaking the active ingredient in water before dilution (succussion) imparts a "memory" of the molecules in the resultant solution. This effect rationalizes the potency of the medication even after the dilution makes it unlikely there are any molecules of the original drug remaining.

Hahnemann first published this homeopathic approach to medicine in the German medical publication *Hufeland's Journal* in 1796 and in 1810 followed with a more expansive work, *Organon of the Medical Art*. Homeopathy was brought to America by Dr. Hans Burch Gram, a Bostonian who studied medicine in Denmark with a student of Hahnemann. Gram opened his homeopathic clinic in New York City in 1825.

A German physician, Dr. Constantine Hering, came to America in 1833 and, in 1835, helped found the first homeopathic medical school in the United States, the North American Academy of the Homeopathic Healing Art (known as the Allentown [Pennsylvania] Academy). Interest in homeopathic medicine was sustained by support from the large

---

[78] See, for example, Bigelow, J. (1835). A discourse on self-limited diseases delivered before the Massachusetts Medical Society, at their annual meeting, May 27, 1835. Boston: N. Hale.

[79] Since treatments were meant to restore a balance of humors by means that were opposed to the cause of illness, he used the terms "allos" (opposite) and "pathos" (suffering). For example, fever was thought to be due to excess blood, hence bleeding cooled the patient. The term "allopathic" has long ceased to be used in this sense; it is now used to distinguish physicians trained in traditional medical schools from osteopathic practitioners.

number of German immigrants who settled in Pennsylvania in the 1820s. The academy flourished until 1843 when it closed, after discovery that its treasurer, Allentown banker John Rice, had embezzled the school's funds.[80]

In 1848, Hering obtained a charter for the Homeopathic Medical College of Pennsylvania in Philadelphia. But in 1867, after he withdrew from the college over his different opinions about the curriculum, he founded Hahnemann Medical College of Philadelphia; the two schools later merged. Hahnemann Medical College[81] canceled its last homeopathy course (an elective) in 1959.

As was the case with Thomsonism, traditional medical practitioners shunned and tried to eliminate homeopathy as a school of medical practice. But unlike Thomson's teachings, homeopathy remained part of American medicine for two reasons: institutionalization in "legitimate" medical schools and popular belief in its effectiveness. The brief story of how organized medicine tried to protect its professional turf and how homeopathy survived is most instructive.

In 1855, the American Medical Association (AMA) required all of its components state societies to adopt its 1847 code of ethics that included this phrase: "[N]o one can be considered as a regular practitioner, or fit associate in consultation, whose practice is based on an exclusive dogma, to the rejection of the accumulated experience of the profession, and of the aids actually furnished by anatomy, physiology, pathology, and organic chemistry."[82]

The purpose of this clause was to forbid members from consulting (essentially associating) with homeopathic practitioners. The Massachusetts Medical Society was the only one that did not expel homeopathic physicians (although no new ones were added). In 1870, the AMA threatened the Massachusetts Medical Society that if it did not expel its homeopaths, it would cease to be a member society.[83] So on November 4, 1871, that society sent eight prominent homeopaths a letter that preferred charges based on "conduct unbecoming and unworthy an honorable physician and member of this Society by practising or professing to practise according to an exclusive theory of dogma, and by belonging to a Society whose purpose is at variance with the principles of, and tends to disorganize, the Massachusetts Medical Society."[84]

The letter instructed these physicians to appear at a trial on November 21, 1871. Proceedings dragged on and, despite the state supreme court's intervention, the society's Board of Trial voted to expel the physicians in May 1873.

---

[80] *Homeopathic Healing Art Plaque*. Retrieved May 22, 2018 from https://www.allentownpa.gov/Play/History/Historical-Allentown

[81] Hahnemann and The Medical College of Pennsylvania (which began in 1850 as the Female Medical College of Pennsylvania) merged after 1993 to become MCP Hahnemann University. In 2002 it was taken over by Drexel University and renamed Drexel University College of Medicine.

[82] The American Medical Association Code of Ethics (1847). Retrieved May 22, 2018, from http://global.oup.com/us/companion.websites/9780199774111/doc/VI.doc

[83] The AMA required "unified membership" until the 1990s; that is, state medical societies were united with the national organization through one dues-paying structure. A physician, therefore, was required to belong to both the state (and often county) medical society and the national organization.

[84] *The Boston Medical and Surgical Journal* (1873), 88, 605.

That expulsion was not the end of homeopathy in Massachusetts but marked a new beginning. In 1848, one of the subsequently expelled physicians, Dr. Israel Tilsdale Talbot, cofounded the Boston Female Medical College (the first medical school for women in the world) whose purpose was to train midwives. By 1850, the college was renamed the New England Female Medical College and offered a full medical curriculum. In 1855, Talbot received a charter for the Massachusetts Homeopathic Hospital and the following year opened the Homeopathic Medical Dispensary. When Talbot and others were expelled from the medical society in 1871, Boston University decided to start a medical school. In 1873, it acquired the New England Female Medical College, its faculty appointed Talbot its first dean, and it made the homeopathic hospital its clinical training facility.[85] Homeopathic courses were taught there until 1918.

Although institutional support for homeopathy was waning (only 15 schools remained by 1910 and currently there are none), homeopathic treatments remain popular among the public. Despite this popularity three important questions remain: Is it safe? Does it work? Who should pay for these treatments?

With regard to safety, since the treatment solutions are so dilute, this issue is not of much importance. As for the latter two questions, perhaps excerpts from an English report[86] offer the final word:

7. … We conclude that the principle of like-cures-like is theoretically weak. It fails to provide a credible physiological mode of action for homeopathic products. We note that this is the settled view of medical science.

8. We consider the notion that ultra-dilutions can maintain an imprint of substances previously dissolved in them to be scientifically implausible …

11. In our view, the systematic reviews and meta-analyses conclusively demonstrate that homeopathic products perform no better than placebos …

14. There has been enough testing of homeopathy and plenty of evidence showing that it is not efficacious …

23. The Government should stop allowing the funding of homeopathy on the NHS [National Health Service].

Osteopathy. Another school of thought that emerged in the 19th century is osteopathic medicine. Its history is instructive because it survives today as a mainstream part of medical practice in the United States.

Like most other movements, this one also had a founder/champion for its philosophy: Dr. Andrew V. Still (1828–1917). Dr. Still studied medicine with his father, a Methodist

---

[85] Though chartered in 1855, the hospital did not accept patients until 1871 when sufficient funds had been raised for its operation. The homeopathic hospital was the forerunner of Boston University Medical Center Hospital.

[86] Science and Technology Committee —Fourth Report. Evidence Check 2: Homeopathy. The policy on NHS funding and provision of homeopathy. Ordered by the House of Commons to be printed 8 February 2010. Retrieved May 22, 2018, from http://www.publications.parliament.uk/pa/cm200910/cmselect/cmsctech/45/4507.htm

minister and physician, and began practicing traditional medicine in 1854. By some accounts, in the early 1860s, he also completed additional coursework at the College of Physicians and Surgeons in Kansas City, Missouri. During the Civil War, he served in the Union Army as a surgeon as well as a military officer in three Kansas regiments.

> In 1864 Still lost two of his own children and one adopted child to an epidemic of spinal meningitis; a month after the epidemic, the daughter born to his second wife, Mary Elvira Turner, died of pneumonia. His inability to save his family, coupled with his grim experiences as a Civil War doctor, led Still to reject most of what he had learned about medicine and search for new and better methods.[87]

Over the next 10 years, he developed another theory of medicine, which was based on massage therapy. Healing massage had been employed in Europe since Hippocratic times[88] but was attracting great interest in the United States in the mid-19th century. In the 1850s, following the principles of the Swedish Gymnastic Movement System developed by the Swedish fencing master Per Henrik Ling (1776–1839), the New York physicians George and Charles Taylor introduced scientific massage therapy in the United States. In 1885, George Taylor, M.D., categorized techniques into "clapping, knockings, stroking, kneading, pulling, shakings and vibrating."

As Still employed more manual techniques of healing, he used fewer and fewer drugs in his practice. Then, on June 22, 1874, he announced he was abandoning traditional therapies. Because of his beliefs, he was censured by his community and forced to relocate from Kansas, eventually settling in Kirksville, Missouri. Since his new home was also traditional in its medical beliefs, he had to make a living as a medical circuit rider, becoming known as a fast bone setter with a congenial personality. The event that gave him his real start was when he cured, by spinal manipulation, a girl who had been unable to walk. Because she was the daughter of the town minister, Still gained acceptance in the community and was able to open a clinic in town in 1875. While considering a name for his therapy, he said "I would start out with the word os (bone) and the word pathology, and then press them into one word—Osteopathy."[89] He further said: "Man is a machine, needing, when diseased, an expert mechanical engineer to adjust its machinery." The rationale for treatment was that disease was caused by organ changes due to the blocked arteries that supplied them; the reason for the blockage was a misplaced bone whose adjustment could restore flow and, hence, restore the patient's health. Still called this explanation "the rule of the artery." Most of the bony lesions occurred in the vertebrae and attached ribs. To explain infections, he said that bacteria thrived in osteopathic lesions and restoration of the flow could be curative. In 1892, he opened the American School of Osteopathy, which granted students the DO (Doctor of

---

[87] http://www.atsu.edu/museum (retrieved May 22, 2018).

[88] "The physician must be experienced in many things, but assuredly also in rubbing ..." Hippocrates. Peri Arthron. (Περί ἀρθρων) [On joints] Littre Vol. iv. (p. 100). In D. Graham (1885). *A practical treatise on massage* (p. 6). New York: William Wood & Co.

[89] Booth, E. R. (1905). *History of osteopathy and twentieth-century medical practice* (p. 65). Cincinnati: Jennings and Graham.

Osteopathy) degree. As with other nontraditional schools of medicine, osteopathy welcomed female students. By 1900, there were more than 10 additional schools of osteopathy in the United States.

Traditional practitioners, seeing the expansion of this alternative treatment method, sought to eliminate competition by prosecuting osteopathic practitioners for practicing medicine without a license. This tactic, however, proved to be ineffective; the courts found that, since osteopathic physicians did not employ drugs and surgery, their methods could not be considered true medical practice.

Osteopathic physicians, however, sought to become more legitimized by lobbying for licensure. After failing to create a licensure path in Missouri in 1895, the American School of Osteopathy added courses in physiology, pathology, histology, chemistry, midwifery, and surgery to its curriculum. In 1897, an osteopathic bill was signed into law by the governor. (In 1896, Vermont was the first state to license osteopathic practitioners.) In that same year, the American Association for the Advancement of Osteopathy was founded; in 1901, it was renamed the American Osteopathic Association (AOA), which today has its headquarters in downtown Chicago.

Many osteopathic practitioners thought the scope of practice needed to be augmented in order to become more acceptable to the public. The first such area was surgery, which required expansion of licensing laws to allow osteopathic physicians to perform such procedures.

Although Still approved of surgery as "but a branch of osteopathy," this practice opened questions about the use of drugs (particularly anesthetics, analgesics and antiseptics), which were anathema to purists of osteopathic practice. As public acceptance of pharmaceuticals grew and state legislatures required a greater scope of training for licensure, many osteopathic physicians began to routinely incorporate drug therapy into their practices. The traditional osteopathic practitioners and those of the newer schools were finally reconciled in 1929 when the AOA approved a resolution calling on all schools to include instruction in drug therapy. Two of Still's major accomplishments were promotion of the practice of preventive medicine and strong advocacy that physicians should focus on treating the whole patient rather than just the disease.

In early 2014, the Accreditation Council for Graduate Medical Education (ACGME), the AOA, and the American Association of Colleges of Osteopathic Medicine (AACOM) approved an agreement to transition to a single accreditation system for graduate medical education (GME) by July 2020. There were about 145,000 osteopathic physicians in the United States in 2019.[90] One in 4 medical students in the United States today attends an osteopathic medical school.

Eclectic Medicine. Originally called reformed medicine, this school of thought was championed by Wooster Beach (1794–1868), who became disenchanted with Thomson's botanical

---

[90] American Osteopathic Association: Osteopathic Medical Profession Report. Retrieved from http://www.osteopathic .org/inside-aoa/about/aoa-annual-statistics/P.s/default.aspx

approach to medicine. Its inaugural institution was established in 1845 in Cincinnati as the Eclectic Medical Institute. The mission for the school stated it

> will be strictly what its name indicates—Eclectic—excluding all such medicines and such remedies as "under the ordinary circumstances of their judicious use, are liable to produce evil consequences, or endanger the future health of the patient," while … draw[ing] from any and every source all such medicine and modes of treating disease, as are found to be valuable, and at the same time, not necessarily attended with bad consequences.[91]

At the institute's first commencement in 1850, 6 students received both eclectic and homeopathic diplomas; however, homeopathy was eliminated from the curriculum later that year. Eclectic schools were the only ones generally open to women.[92] In 1910, the name of the school was changed to the Eclectic Medical College. Because of such pressures as the AMA's efforts to establish uniform requirements for medical colleges, a surge in popularity of allopathic medicine (due in large measure to the discovery of penicillin and other antibiotics), and a general lack of research and progress in the overall field of eclectic medicine, the last class graduated in 1939. The college surrendered its charter in 1942, and the remaining assets of $6,000 were donated to two local hospitals.

Chiropractic Medicine. This branch of treatment was founded by Daniel David Palmer (1845–1913).[93] A Canadian who had tried his hand working in a match factory, at grade school teaching, and in horticulture, Palmer eventually became a healer who employed magnetism in his treatments. The beginning of this school of treatment is often given as September 18, 1895. On that day, a janitor in Palmer's office building in Davenport, Iowa, told him that he had been deaf for 17 years, an occurrence apparently brought on after he felt something "give" in his back. Palmer persuaded the man to let him manipulate the injured spine, which restored his hearing. After this incident, Palmer used vertebral manipulation to treat a patient with "heart trouble," providing "immediate relief." Palmer wrote: "Then I began to reason if two diseases, so dissimilar as deafness and heart trouble, came from impingement, a pressure on nerves, were not other diseases due to a similar cause? Thus the science (knowledge) and art (adjusting) of Chiropractic were formed."[94]

---

[91]Felter, H. W. (1914). Editorial. *Eclectic Medical Journal, 74,* 597.

[92]In 1849, Elizabeth Blackwell (1821–1910) became the first woman in America to graduate from medical school (Geneva Medical College in New York State); however, she was born in Bristol, England, and eventually returned to that country to practice. In 1850, Lydia Folger Fowler (1822–1879) became the first American-born woman to graduate from medical school: Central Medical College (the first co-ed medical school and an eclectic institution). After practicing medicine in New York City, she became the first woman professor in an American medical school by joining the Rochester Eclectic Medical College. See: Rogers, I. (1905). Eclecticism and the woman practitioner. *Transactions of the Ohio State Medical Eclectic Association.* Bellefontaine, OH: Mohr and Carter.

[93]For more information, see: Whorton, J. C. (2002). Innate intelligence: Chiropractic. In *Nature cures.* New York: Oxford University Press; Lawrence, D. J. (1999). Chiropractic medicine. In W. B. Jonas & J. D. Levin (Eds.), *Essentials of complementary and alternative medicine.* Philadelphia: Lippincott Williams & Wilkins.

[94]Singh, S., & Ernst, E. (2008). *Trick or treatment* (p. 158). New York: W.W. Norton & Co. This book is an excellent summary of what has been called "alternative and complementary medicine," that is, nonmainstream treatments. It uses an evidence-based approach to analyze such fields as chiropractic, homeopathy, naturopathy, and acupuncture.

The term "chiropractic" was suggested by a Davenport area minister named Samuel Weed. Palmer had cured him and his daughter and, as payment, Palmer requested a Greek name for his method of treatment; Weed came up with "chiropractic" ("done by hand") in January 1896. Palmer initially tutored disciples in his office and then in 1897 opened the Palmer Chiropractic School & Cure. As was the case with osteopathy, schools rapidly proliferated and, again, unlike traditional medical schools, women were accepted as students.

The general theory that emerged was that the body has great self-regenerative powers, but vertebral misalignments (subluxations) block nerves that help in the healing process. Treatment of disease, therefore, is focused on restoring the spine to normal alignment, with manipulation directed to the portion of the spine that is responsible for causing illness: for example, hearing loss (cervical spine), heart problems (thoracic spine), and bladder (lumbar spine).

This single-cause theory of disease provoked charges of quackery by traditional medical practitioners. These charges gained more credibility as medical science advanced in the 20th century and chiropractic practitioners continued to claim their treatments worked on such varied conditions as autoimmune conditions, asthma, heart disease, and cancers. Most chiropractors now treat only musculoskeletal conditions, particularly back pain.

Despite this narrower focus of care, traditional medical organizations still shunned chiropractic care, claiming it was fraudulent. An important legal case subsequently changed the dynamic. In 1976, Chester A. Wilk and four other chiropractors sued the AMA for anti-competitive behavior. The claim was that the AMA's decades-old campaign was not a science-based rebuttal of chiropractic but a concerted effort to prevent its practitioners from competing with traditional physicians. Such means included prohibiting physicians from associating with or referring patients to chiropractors. (Recall the same tactics the AMA used with homeopathic physicians.) In1987, Judge Susan Getzendanner of the U.S. District Court for the Northern District of Illinois, Eastern Division, found in favor of the chiropractors and issued an injunction prohibiting the AMA from engaging in anti-competitive behavior.[95] As part of this decision, she wrote: "I decline to pronounce chiropractic valid or invalid." The decision was upheld on appeal, and the U.S. Supreme Court rejected the AMA's petition to hear the case in 1990.

Educational Reform. The philosophies described above shaped how medicine was practiced in 19th- and early 20th-century America. In addition to these different beliefs, the quality of medical education was vastly inconsistent, even among those teaching the same theories. Likewise, the preparation for training varied by medical school, ranging from some high school (or, occasionally, none at all) to possession of an undergraduate degree. It was in this setting that early 20th-century medical training was the beneficiary of the efforts of two movements: the advance of science (please see Chapter 4 for some examples) and social reforms to protect the public. (These reforms will be discussed in Chapter 6, "Payers.")

---

[95] Wilk v. American Medical Association, 671 F. Supp. 1465, N.D. Ill. 1987. Of note is that the plaintiffs dropped their original suit for damages and refiled for an injunction only.

With respect to the latter, the singular event leading to wholesale reformation of training was publication in 1910 of *Medical Education in the United States and Canada*,[96] more commonly called the Flexner Report, after its author Abraham Flexner. In the report, Flexner mentioned several exemplary late19th- and early 20th-century medical schools with respect to their admissions requirements, scientific training, and hospital-based clinical experiences (notably the University of Michigan, University of Pennsylvania, Harvard University, and the Johns Hopkins University). Most of the study, however, was a scathing indictment of the overall state of medical education. Flexner was particularly critical of the non-allopathic schools:

> None of the 15 homeopathic schools requires more than a high school education for entrance; only five require so much ... In the year 1900 there were 22 homeopathic colleges in the United States; today there are 15 ... The ebbing vitality of homeopathic schools is a striking demonstration of the incompatibility of science and dogma.

> There are 8 eclectic schools ... Six schools have either nominal requirements or none at all. None of the schools has anything remotely resembling the laboratory equipment which all claim in their catalogues ... five eclectic schools are without exception filthy and almost bare.

> The eight osteopathic schools fairly reek with commercialism. Their catalogues are a mass of hysterical exaggerations, alike of the earning and of the curative power of osteopathy ... [They] now enroll over 1300 students, who pay some $200,000 annually [*sic*] in fees. Instruction furnished for this sum is inexpensive and worthless. Not a single full-time teacher is found in any of them.

Flexner's criticism extended to localities, saying, for example: "The city of Chicago is in respect to medical education the plague spot of the country."

Although direct causation is often difficult to prove, within 20 years after the report's publication, 71 out of the 168 schools Flexner critiqued either closed or merged with universities or other schools.

With this historical background that shaped our current medical system, we now turn to a current perspective.

Current Status of Medical Training

Admissions. In the United States, there are currently two types of medical schools: allopathic and osteopathic. In order for students to be eligible to receive federal loans and for the school to receive federal funding, the medical school must be accredited by an organization approved by the U.S. Department of Education.[97] For allopathic schools (schools that grant the Doctor of Medicine, or MD, degree) that organization is the Liaison Committee on Medical Education (LCME),[98] which is jointly sponsored by the Association of American

---

[96] Flexner, A. (1910). *Medical education in the United States and Canada*. The Carnegie Foundation for the Advancement of Teaching. Bulletin Number 4. D.B. Updike. Boston: The Merrymount Press.

[97] U.S. Department of Education: Accreditation: Universities and Higher Education. Retrieved May 22, 2018 from http://www.ed.gov/accreditation

[98] Retrieved May 22, 2018, from http://lcme.org

Medical Colleges (AAMC)[99] and the American Medical Association.[100] For osteopathic schools (schools that grant the Doctor of Osteopathic Medicine, or DO, degree), accreditation is granted by the Commission on Osteopathic College Accreditation[101] of the American Osteopathic Association.

While specific requirements can vary, typical medical school admissions criteria include a bachelor's degree (or equivalent) from an accredited school; successful completion of certain undergraduate courses in biology, chemistry, physics, and mathematics (often at the calculus level); and completion of the Medical College Admissions Test (MCAT).[102] For the 2017–2018 year, 51,680 applicants each submitted an average of 16 medical school applications.[103] Although 41% eventually matriculated, there was a very large variation in acceptance rates among schools, depending on such factors as academic selectivity and whether they are state-sponsored institutions. Women often outnumber men enrolled in medical schools; nationally, 50.7% of 2017 matriculants were women. In 2017, there were about 210,000 applicants to osteopathic schools.[104] Each submitted an average of nine applications to colleges of osteopathic medicine. The matriculation rate was 35%, of whom 45.3% were women. (Please see the AAMC and AACOMAS references for other characteristics of medical and osteopathic students.)

According to the LCME,[105] it has accredited 147 U.S. MD-granting medical schools, or 22 more than in 2002–2003. The American Osteopathic Association's Commission on Osteopathic College Accreditation (COCA) listed 34 DO-granting schools in 2018, an increase of 10 DO-granting schools since 2002–2003.

Curriculum. Understanding physician training is important for an appreciation of their acculturation into the profession and, hence, practice patterns. According to Levinson et al.,[106] there are three parts to the medical school curriculum.

---

[99] Retrieved May 22, 2018, from www.aamc.org

[100] Retrieved May 22, 2018, from http://www.ama-assn.org/ama

[101] http://www.osteopathic.org/inside-aoa/accreditation/COM-accreditation/P.s/default.aspx

[102] Retrieved May 23, 2018, from https://students-residents.aamc.org/applying-medical-school/taking-mcat-exam/mcat-scores/ In 2015 the test was revamped with a new format. It is a computer-based exam with four sections: Biological and Biochemical Foundations of Living Systems; Chemical and Physical Foundations of Biological Systems; Psychological, Social, and Biological Foundations of Behavior; and Critical Analysis and Reasoning Skills.

[103] AAMC. U.S. Medical School Applications and Matriculants by School, State of Legal Residence, and Sex, 2017–2018. Retrieved May 23, 2018, from https://www.aamc.org/download/321442/data/factstablea1.pdf

[104] 2017 AACOMAS Profile. Applicant and Matriculant Report. Retrieved May 23, 2018, from https://www.aacom.org/docs/default-source/data-and-trends/2017-aacomas-applicant-matriculant-profile-summary-report.pdf?sfvrsn=4f072597_8

[105] AAMC. U.S. Medical School Applications and Matriculants by School, State of Legal Residence, and Sex, 2017–2018, op.cit.

[106] Levinson, W., et al. (2014). The hidden curriculum and professionalism. In W. Levinson, S. Ginsburg, F. W. Hafferty, & C. R. Lucey (Eds.), *Understanding medical professionalism.* New York: McGraw-Hill Education. See also: Hafferty, F. W., & Castellani, B. (2009). The hidden curriculum: A theory of medical education. In C. Brosnan & C. S. Turner (Eds.), *Handbook of the sociology of medical education* (pp. 15–35). New York: Routledge; and Arnold, L., & Stern, D. T. (2006). What is medical professionalism? In D. T. Stern (Ed.), *Measuring medical professionalism.* New York: Oxford University Press.

The first part is the *formal curriculum*, which comes from the school's mission statement and finds form in the course objectives and contents. The formal medical school curriculum traditionally has been divided into preclinical and clinical coursework, each lasting 2 years. The preclinical courses include such basic topics as anatomy, physiology, pathology, biochemistry, immunology, and genetics as well as studies of specific organ systems, such as cardiology (heart), nephrology (kidney), gastroenterology (digestive tract), neurology (nervous system), and hematology (blood). Also included in the first 2 years are courses in physical diagnosis (how to effectively interview patients and perform physical exams). Clinical training involves hands-on patient care experience. Required clinical courses are often completed in the third year of medical school and include internal medicine (care of adults), pediatrics (care of children), family medicine, surgery, psychiatry, and obstetrics/gynecology. The fourth year consists of clinical electives in many of the subspecialties of the above disciplines, such as cardiology, oncology (cancer), and ophthalmology. Students can also study electives that cross the basic disciplines, such as dermatology, anesthesiology, and radiology.

Over the past couple of decades, the formal curriculum has moved clinical experience earlier in the training, so that now most first-year medical students have hands-on patient experience. Also, many of the traditional stand-alone first-year topics have been integrated into courses dealing with organ systems. Further, courses have been added on topics such as medical ethics, epidemiology, and the structure of the U.S. healthcare system. Still largely lacking, however, are formal curricula covering topics related to health law.

An important part of the formal training that is extracurricular is acculturation of the students into the profession of medicine. One of the first such experiences for first-year students is the "white coat ceremony." According to Warren:[107]

> The ritual got started at the University of Chicago in 1989, after a professor complained to Dean of Students Norma F. Wagoner that first-year students were "showing up in shorts and baseball caps for sessions where the patients are pouring their hearts out". Wagoner decided the fix was to create a ceremonial program in which students were given physician coats. The school invited parents and told the students that "for any session where we have patients present, we expect you to look like professionals, wear the white coat and behave appropriately," she said.

In 1993, the Arnold P. Gold Foundation sponsored the first formal white coat ceremony at Columbia University College of Physicians and Surgeons. (Dr. Gold had been a professor of Clinical Neurology and professor of Clinical Pediatrics at the school.) Since that time, the foundation has sponsored ceremonies at almost all medical and some osteopathic schools.[108] At this event, in the presence of friends, family, and faculty, students are welcomed into the

---

[107]Warren, P. (1999, October 18) For new medical students, white coats are a warmup. *LA Times*. Retrieved May 23, 2018, from http://articles.latimes.com/1999/oct/18/local/me-23619

[108]In 2014, the Gold Foundation partnered with the American Association of Colleges of Nursing (AACN) to support a pilot program that has seen 160 nursing schools adopt the Gold-AACN White Coat Ceremony for Nursing. Retrieved May 23, 2018, from http://www.gold-foundation.org/programs/white-coat-ceremony

profession, receive a white coat to wear as a symbol of their expected professionalism, and make pledges that reflect the modern values contained in the Hippocratic Oath. It had been the tradition before this time that students took such an oath at the time of graduation; however, Professor Gold noted that Hippocrates intended that the oath to be taken at the beginning of studies.

It was not until 2002, however, that the medical profession started a formal initiative of introducing professionalism into training. The origin of this agenda came from the observation that patients were being marginalized in the process of healthcare decisions and public policy. In order to remedy the problem, this program started with a Physician Charter[109] that described the nature of professionalism. The charter was based on three fundamental principles: primacy of patient welfare, patient autonomy, and social justice.

To support these principles, the charter asks for commitments to these areas:

- Competence
- Honesty with patients
- Patient confidentiality
- Appropriate relations with patients
- Improving quality of care
- Improving access to care
- Just distribution of finite resources
- Scientific knowledge
- Maintaining trust by managing conflicts of interest
- Professional responsibilities[110]

The second part of medical education is the *informal curriculum*. Levinson et al.[111] describe it as "[t]eaching and learning that occurs outside of the formal curriculum in variety of settings (i.e., ward rounds and bedside) that is unscripted and predominantly ad hoc. This learning can be consistent or inconsistent with the formal curriculum." For example, in a medical clinic, the instructor may say: "I know what the books say, but here is the practical way to approach this problem."

---

[109]From ABIM Foundation (2002). American Board of Internal Medicine; ACP-ASIM Foundation. American College of Physicians-American Society of Internal Medicine; European Federation of Internal Medicine. Medical professionalism in the new millennium: A physician charter. *Annals of Internal Medicine, 136*(3), 243–246.

[110]The first nine commitments are fairly self-explanatory. The charter explains professional responsibilities in this way: "As members of a profession, physicians are expected to work collaboratively to maximize patient care, be respectful of one another, and participate in the processes of self-regulation, including remediation and discipline of members who have failed to meet professional standards. The profession should also define and organize the educational and standard-setting process for current and future members. Physicians have both individual and collective obligations to participate in these processes. These obligations include engaging in internal assessment and accepting external scrutiny of all aspects of their professional performance."

[111]Levinson, W., et al., *Understanding medical professionalism.* op. cit.

The third part is what is now commonly called the *hidden curriculum*. It is not explicitly about learning medicine but finding out the code of behavior and norms that are expected in different situations. In other words, it is more about learning the culture of medicine than its science. The hidden curriculum may clash with the values that the formal acculturation process seeks to instill.[112] For example, Levinson et al.[113] asked fourth-year medical students what lessons they could pass on to entering students. Among this list are several that illustrate the countercultural nature of some informal curricula:

Learn how to act like you know everything, whether or not you do.

It's about surviving, not excelling.

Be good at getting people to like you and know what that means on different rotations.

Politics matter—spend the most time with the most powerful person.

These three parts of the curriculum display the medical school's equivalent of Schein's[114] three parts of culture:

- *Artifacts* are the visible elements in a culture that can be recognized by people not part of the culture. Consider the white coat an artifact.

- *Espoused values* "are the organization's stated values and rules of behavior. It is [*sic*] how the members represent the organization both to themselves and to others. This is often expressed in official philosophies and public statements of identity." Consider the mission and formal curriculum as espoused values.

- *Shared basic assumptions* "are the deeply embedded, taken-for-granted behaviors which are usually unconscious, but constitute the essence of culture." Consider the informal curriculum, but especially the hidden curriculum, as major influences on the shared basic assumptions.

As Schein points out: "Trouble may arise if espoused values by leaders are not in line with the deeper tacit assumptions of the culture."

While the traditional curriculum lasts 4 years, 7 American and 1 Canadian medical schools have implemented an accelerated 3-year program in response to widespread physician shortages (see below) and the enormous debt medical students incur for their

---

[112] A classic example that humorously explains the hidden curriculum is the book *House of God* (Shem, S. [Stephen Bergman] [1978]. *House of God*. New York: Richard Merek). In it, interns learn the "Laws" of the institution, which include:

They can always hurt you more.

The only good admission is a dead admission.

If you don't take a temperature you can't find a fever.

The delivery of good medical care is to do as much nothing as possible.

[113] Levinson, W., et al., *Understanding medical professionalism*. op. cit.

[114] Schein, E. H. (2010). *Organizational culture and leadership* (Chapter 2). San Francisco: Wiley.

education. ("Most students save about $250,000 by eliminating one year of tuition and entering the workforce earlier.")[115]

Cost. The nominal cost of medical school training can vary widely.[116] For public schools, many charge $30,000 to $40,000 per year for tuition and fees for in-state students. For private schools (and for out-of-state public school enrollees), many charge $55,000 to $60,000 per year for tuition and fees. Scholarships and loans from various sources can lower those amounts. In recent years, the Cleveland Clinic Lerner College of Medicine, New York University, and the new Kaiser Permanente Medical School in California offer full scholarships for all students for tuition and fees (the latter only for the first five classes).[117]

Postgraduate Training. In the fourth year of medical school, students apply for postgraduate specialty training positions called residencies. The purpose of these residencies is to give newly graduated physicians an additional opportunity to learn from supervised, direct patient care experience, most often in the hospital setting.[118] The computerized, mathematical algorithm by which applicants are matched with residency positions is run by the National Resident Matching Program (NRMP).[119] Once a match is finalized, it is a binding contract. The length of residencies ranges from 3 years for primary care to 6 years for some surgical specialties (such as neurosurgery).[120] The length and content of each residency is determined by its respective specialty board (see below). Some residencies (such as

---

[115]Warshaw, R. (2015, September). Medical schools form consortium to examine accelerated MD programs. *AAMC Reporter*. Retrieved May 23, 2018, from https://www.aamc.org/newsroom/reporter/september2015/442210/accelerated-programs.html

[116]AAMC (2017). *Medical school graduation questionnaire. All schools summary report*. Retrieved May 23, 2018, from https://www.aamc.org/download/481784/data/2017gqallschoolssummaryreport.pdf

[117]Ibid.

[118]"This bedside method of teaching was in practice in France and England and was introduced to this country from England shortly before the beginning of the 19th-century ... During these early years it was not uncommon for young men—the house physician, the resident physician, or the house pupil (for they had not yet been given the title 'intern') to pay their teachers $50 or $75 for the opportunity to serve in the hospital. It was not until about the time of the Civil War that the term 'intern' came to be used in some institutions ... In spite of the recognized fact that hospital experience was of great value in rounding out the medical education, even as late as the beginning of the 20th century less than one half of all graduates took such training ... The term 'resident' was first applied to young physicians living in the hospital who were augmenting their didactic education with a period of practical training; the word was synonymous with intern. It was not until the opening of Johns Hopkins Hospital in 1889 that the word 'resident' was used to describe the young physicians who, having completed an internship, continued their training in the hospital. The Council on Medical Education and Hospitals of the American Medical Association published its first list of hospitals offering residencies in 1925. This list contains the names of 29 institutions. By 1940, the list had 179 hospitals and affiliated hospitals as offering residencies of two years or longer." *Graduate Medical Education*: Report of the Commission on Graduate Medical Education. University of Chicago Press, Chicago. © 1940.

[119]The algorithm uses the same logic as dating services, though this process predated the latter one. Of note is that, according to the NRMP: "Research on the NRMP algorithm was a basis for awarding the 2012 Nobel Prize in Economic Sciences." Retrieved May 23, 2018, from http://www.nrmp.org/wp-content/uploads/2013/08/The-Sveriges-Riksbank-Prize-in-Economic-Sciences-in-Memory-of-Alfred-Nobel1.pdf

[120]American College of Surgeons. *How many years of postgraduate training do surgical residents undergo?* Retrieved May 23, 2018, from https://www.facs.org/education/resources/medical-students/faq/training

neurology, dermatology and radiology) require 1 year of broader preparation in a primary care specialty or general surgery before starting the other specialty training. Residencies are accredited by the ACGME,[121] a private, nonprofit organization. Founded in 1972 as the Liaison Committee for Graduate Medical Education, it was renamed in 1981. The original ACGME's member organizations were the American Board of Medical Specialties, American Hospital Association, AMA, AAMC, and the Council of Medical Specialty Societies. In 2014, the American Osteopathic Association and American Association of Colleges of Osteopathic Medicine joined the ACGME in order to unify the accreditation process for allopathic and osteopathic programs. This single accreditation started in July 2015. The ACGME accredits 700 institutions that sponsor approximately 9,600 residency and fellowship programs in the United States.

The salaries for these residency positions are about $54,000 for the first year and go up each year thereafter; they vary by geography and year of residency.

In recent years, there has been concern among policy makers, applicants, and residency directors that there will be a shortage of Graduate Medical Education (GME) positions, particularly due to expansion in the number of medical schools (increased supply) and hospital closures (decreased capacity). In 2018, the NRMP reported that "an all-time high 30,232 PGY-1 [first year] positions were offered … the number of registrants reached an all-time high of 43,909, an increase of 752 over 2017."[122]

Expansion of residency positions, however, is expensive; the AAMC estimates it costs about $150,000 per year to educate each resident. To defray costs, residency programs look to the federal government for significant funding to subsidize these positions.[123] According to the Government Accountability Office (GAO):

> Federal agencies and state Medicaid agencies spent over $16.3 billion in 2015 to fund graduate medical education (GME) training for physicians—commonly known as residency training. The federal government spent $14.5 billion through five programs, and 45 state Medicaid agencies spent $1.8 billion. About half of teaching sites that received funding—such as teaching hospitals—received funds from more than one of the five programs.[124]

(Please see Exhibit 5.2.)

The problem is that the Balanced Budget Act of 1997 capped the number of residencies Medicare can fund. Without change in federal law, expansion of residency positions requires states, local governments, and/or the training sites themselves to pick up the extra costs. Given current economic conditions for these institutions, additional GME funding will remain problematic.

---

[121] Accrediting Council for Graduate Medical Education. *What we do.* Retrieved May 23, 2018, from http://www.acgme.org/What-We-Do/Overview

[122] NRMP (2018, April). *Results and data 2018 main residency match.* Retrieved May 23, 2018, from http://www.nrmp.org/wp-content/uploads/2018/04/Main-Match-Result-and-Data-2018.pdf

[123] CMS.gov. *Direct graduate medical education (DGME).* Retrieved May 23, 2018, from https://www.cms.gov/Medicare/Medicare-Fee-for-Service-Payment/AcuteInpatientPPS/DGME.html

[124] GAO (2018, March). *Physician workforce: HHS needs better information to comprehensively evaluate graduate medical education funding.* Retrieved May 23, 2018, from https://www.gao.gov/assets/700/690581.pdf

EXHIBIT 5.2. **Federal Spending on Graduate Medical Education Training, 2015**

Program	Total GME spending (dollars in millions)	Percentage of total spending
HHS programs		
Medicare	10,335	71%
Medicaid (federal share)	2,351	16%
Children's Hospital GME Payment Program	249	2%
Teaching Health Center GME Program	76	1%
VA program	1,499	10%
Total	14,509	100%

Source: GAO (2018, March). *Physician workforce: HHS needs better information to comprehensively evaluate graduate medical education funding.* Retrieved May 23, 2018, from https://www.gao.gov/assets/700/690581.pdf

Fellowships. After completion of residency, physicians who desire competence in a subspecialty (such as cardiology, gastroenterology, gynecologic oncology, etc.) apply to fellowship programs. The applications are processed by the NRMP as described above. Length and content of fellowships are determined by their respective subspecialty boards.

Board Certification. Physicians who successfully complete an approved residency become eligible for certification in their specialty (or subspecialty, after additional fellowship training). This qualification is granted after passing an exam administered by specialty boards formed to evaluate the competencies of applicants. Certification is to be distinguished from licensure; the former is a testament to certain competencies granted by a private professional organization; the latter is a legal grant by a government body allowing practice of a profession. The origin of these specialty boards is explained in Exhibit 5.3.

Licensure

Each state has the right to license professionals practicing in that state. Prior to World War II, each state administered its own exams for physician licensure. After that time, in order to ensure uniformity and ease administrative burdens, national standardized exams were developed. Today, that multipart exam is called the United States Medical Licensing Examination (USMLE).[125] The USMLE is governed by a committee that includes members from the Educational Commission for Foreign Medical Graduates (ECFMG),[126] the Federation of State

---

[125]Retrieved May 23, 2018, from www.usmle.org

[126]International medical graduates (IMGs) must pass an exam (obtain certification) administered by the ECFMG before acceptance into a U.S. residency program. It is also a requirement before IMGs are allowed to take Part 3 of the USMLE. The term "IMG" is now preferred over foreign medical graduate (FMG).

EXHIBIT 5.3. History of Medical Boards

As early as 1908, ophthalmologists discussed the idea of a special examination in certification for their specialty. The reason for this action was to raise barriers of entry into the profession. Two trends made this action necessary. Many physicians were calling themselves ophthalmologists without appropriate training, and growth in optometry provided increasing competition. Thus, in order to strengthen requirements for membership, in 1915 the American Ophthalmological Society recommended 2 years of formal specialty training after medical school graduation. This society joined with the section of ophthalmology of the AMA and the American Academy of Ophthalmology and Otolaryngology to form the American Board of Ophthalmology, which gave its first exam in December 1916.[a]

In 1933, the Advisory Board for Medical Specialties was organized by the then existing specialty boards and representatives from a number of other important medical organizations (e.g., the AMA, American College of Surgeons [which did not have a specialty board equivalent until 1937] and AAMC). The purpose of the Advisory Board was to provide existing and future specialty boards with advice regarding standardization and coordination of their activities. One of the most important standardization recommendations was the requirement that, after 1942, all candidates for certification must have completed a satisfactory 3-year residency or equivalent training. Today, the Advisory Board is called the American Board of Medical Specialties (ABMS).

The ABMS is governed by representatives from the specialty boards[b] and five public members; associate members[c] representing important healthcare organizations are also often consulted. Subspecialty boards also exist in the relevant fields. For example: adult cardiology is part of the American Board of Internal Medicine; pediatric infectious disease is part of the American Board of Pediatrics; and surgery of the hand is part of the American Board of Orthopedics. While new boards must be approved by ABMS, boards set their own qualification criteria, which include successful completion of an approved residency program in that specialty (and fellowship in a subspecialty) as well as passage of written (and sometimes oral) exams. Further, unlike most countries, all U.S. boards require periodic (not longer than 10 years) recertification examinations.

[a] The board was incorporated in May 1917. Other specialty boards formed prior to establishment of the Advisory Board for Medical Specialties (1934) were the American Board of Obstetrics and Gynecology (1930), the American Board of Dermatology (1932), and the American Board of Pediatrics (1933).
[b] For a list of current recognized specialties and subspecialties, see: http://www.abms.org/member-boards/specialty-subspecialty-certificates. Retrieved May 23, 2018.
[c] ABMS Associate Members. Retrieved May 23, 2018, from http://www.abms.org/about-abms/associate-members

Medical Boards (FSMB), the National Board of Medical Examiners (NBME), and public members. While all states accept passage of the exam (in addition to postgraduate training) for initial licensure, many require additional documentation if one wishes to become licensed later in other states.

Changes in medical practice have included increases in telemedicine consultations and physician review of utilization and quality of care in multiple states. Since laws about these practices require licensure in the state where the *patient* resides, the need arose to expedite physician credentialing. In response, the FSMB initiated the Interstate Medical Licensure Compact.[127] As of 2018, 24 states have agreed to cooperate in facilitating reciprocity of medical licensure to other members in the compact.

---

[127] Retrieved May 23, 2018, from http://licenseportability.org

Instead of the USMLE, osteopathic physicians take the three-part Comprehensive Osteopathic Medical Licensing Examination (COMLEX-USA),[128] administered by the National Board of Osteopathic Medical Examiners.

Licensure is not granted for life. States relicense physicians at different intervals, but often about every 3 years. Many states also require proof of varying amounts and types of continuing education activities for relicensure.

Shortage of Physicians

Despite the increase in U.S. medical and osteopathic school graduates, the United States faces a growing shortage of physicians. The AAMC projects that by 2030, this country will have a shortfall of between 42,600 and 121,300 physicians, including between 14,800 and 49,300 for those practicing primary care and between 20,700 and 30,500 for those in surgical specialties.

The causes of the shortages are both decreasing supply (retiring physicians and "declines in physician working hours across all age groups") and increasing demand (aging population and push to achieve population health targets).[129]

The problem is not only shortages in absolute numbers and in certain specialties but also in distribution of physicians. Exhibit 5.4 graphically highlights this maldistribution issue.

Many stakeholders have offered solutions to remedy these shortages, nine of which are listed below. These proposed solutions also touch on many of the trends involving medical practice. What is clear is that it will take implementation of many of these proposals to begin to address this problem.

First, *increase alternate care sites, such as freestanding or pharmacy-based retail clinics.* These centers usually handle common problems (e.g., sore throats, colds, etc.) and can relieve some of the patient volume from primary care offices and emergency rooms. Since they are largely staffed by nurse practitioners, physicians would not be taken away from their practices. However, because of increased convenience, nearly 60% of visits to these clinics are for medical conditions that patients would not otherwise have sought. This increased volume results in about a 20% increase in spending and more than offsets the decreased charges.[130]

Second, *increase non-physician practitioners and expand their scope of practice.* (Please see the Nurses section and the Physician Assistants section later in this chapter.)

Third, *increase efficiency of current and future physicians by offloading nonclinical tasks.* Physicians (and other healthcare professionals) spend a great deal of their time on

[128] Retrieved May 23, 2018, from https://www.nbome.org/exams-assessments/comlex-usa

[129] AAMC (2018). *The complexities of physician supply and demand: Projections from 2016 to 2030. Final report key findings.* Retrieved May 24, 2018, from https://aamc-black.global.ssl.fastly.net/production/media/filer_public/85/d7/85d7b689-f417-4ef0-97fb-ecc129836829/aamc_2018_workforce_projections_update_april_11_2018.pdf

[130] Ashwood, J. S., Gaynor, M., Setodji, C. M., Reid, R. O., Weber, E., & Mehrotra, A. (2016). Retail clinic visits for low-acuity conditions increase utilization and spending. *Health Affairs, 35*(3), 449–455. See also: Cassel, C. (2015). Can retail clinics transform health care? *JAMA, 319*(18), 1855–1856.

EXHIBIT 5.4. **Location Quotients of Physicians and Surgeons, All Other, by State. May 2017**

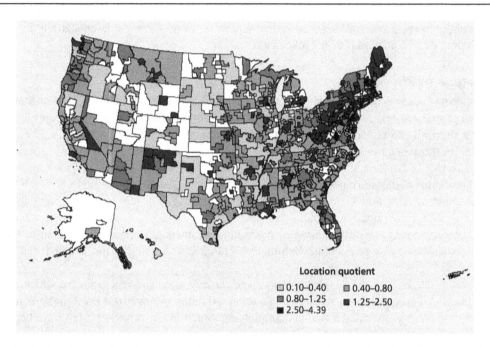

Location quotient
☐ 0.10–0.40   ▥ 0.40–0.80
▨ 0.80–1.25   ■ 1.25–2.50
■ 2.50–4.39

Note: The location quotient is the ratio of the area concentration of occupational employment to the national average concentration. A location quotient greater than 1 indicates the occupation has a higher share of employment than average, and a location quotient less than 1 indicates the occupation is less prevalent in the area than average. Blank areas indicate data not available.

Source: Bureau of Labor Statistics. *Occupational Employment Statistics*. Retrieved from https://www.bls .gov/oes/current/oes291069.htm#(9)

paperwork and administrative tasks, neither of which has been aided by electronic media. The magnitude of this problem is highlighted by the following findings:

- It has been found that primary care physicians spend more than half their workday (nearly 6 hours) interacting with electronic health records during and after office hours.[131]

- Paperwork is "the biggest problem plaguing primary care." According to one study, 79% of respondents ranked it as the top challenge in practice.[132]

[131] Arndt, B. G., Beasley, J. W., Watkinson, M. D., Temte, N. L., Tuan, W.-J., Sinsky, C. A., & Gilchrist, V. J. (2017). Tethered to the EHR: Primary care physician workload assessment using EHR event log data and time-motion observations. *The Annals of Family Medicine, 15*(5), 419–426.

[132] Shyrock, T. (2018, April 25). Drowning in paperwork. *Medical Economics' 89th Physician Report*. Retrieved May 24, 2018, from http://www.medicaleconomics.com/business/drowning-paperwork

▪ The amount of time physicians spend on paperwork and administrative tasks continues to increase, with 70% spending more than 10 hours per week on paperwork, an increase from 57% the previous year.[133]

In order to help alleviate this problem, some individual physicians and healthcare organizations have trained nonclinicians to help with these tasks. For example, a new category of healthcare worker is a "scribe"—someone who takes dictation from the physician to enter information directly into the electronic medical record.[134] While these personnel can save time, they are expensive to use, particularly for primary care physicians.

Fourth, *create compensation incentives and/or debt forgiveness for specialties with shortages.* As mentioned above, in 2017, the median indebtedness for medical students was $180,000. Whether indebtedness affects decisions to pursue medical careers or specialty choices is not completely clear. The following research findings shed some light on this issue.

> The percentage of medical school graduates who said their education debt affected their choice of medical specialty has decreased continuously the past five years. In 2017, nearly fifty-five percent of respondents to the [Medical School Graduation Questionnaire] said that debt had "no influence" on specialty choice. Less than twenty-two percent allowed that debt had either a "strong" (6.2%) or "moderate" (15.3%) influence.[135]

At a time when the proportion of medical students graduating without debt has increased, overall there is a real increase in total debt and it is concentrated among fewer individuals.

> … [C]hanging distributions vary considerably by specialty choice. There is no clear association between specialty-specific proportions of graduates without debt and the income typical of those specialties, but primary care–oriented fields seem to have less of an increase in graduates without debt. The causal associations among debt, specialty choice, and income are challenging to disentangle. Conceptually, debt is likely to be less of a determinant of specialty choice than is future income.[136]

The potential incomes of different specialty choices are displayed in Exhibit 5.5.

Given these income differentials and student debt, it is difficult to separate residency choices from their financial incentives. In an attempt to alleviate indebtedness and help students choose careers in primary care (particularly in shortage areas), the Health Resources and Services Administration (part of the Department of Health and Human Services) has offered scholarship and loan repayment programs.[137] Unfortunately, these programs have not had a significant impact on correcting specialty and geographic imbalances.

---

[133] Kane, L. (2018, April 11). Medscape physician compensation report 2018. Retrieved May 24, 2018, from https://www.medscape.com/slideshow/2018-compensation-overview-6009667#33

[134] Reuben, D. B., Knudson, J., Senelick, W., Glazier, E., & Koretz, B. K. (2014). The effect of a physician partner program on physician efficiency and patient satisfaction. *JAMA Internal Medicine, 174*(7), 1190–1193.

[135] AAMC (2017). *Medical school graduation questionnaire. 2017 all schools summary report.* Retrieved May 24, 2018, from https://www.aamc.org/download/481784/data/2017gqallschoolssummaryreport.pdf

[136] Grischkan, J., George, B. P., Chaiyachati, K., Friedman, A. B., Dorsey, E. R., & Asch, D. A. (2017). Distribution of medical education debt by specialty, 2010–2016. *JAMA Internal Medicine, 177*(10). 1532–1535.

[137] Retrieved May 24, 2018, from https://www.nhsc.hrsa.gov/scholarships/index.html and http://nhsc.hrsa.gov/loanrepayment

EXHIBIT 5.5. Annual Compensation Earned by U.S. Physicians as of 2018, by Specialty (in 1,000 U.S. Dollars)

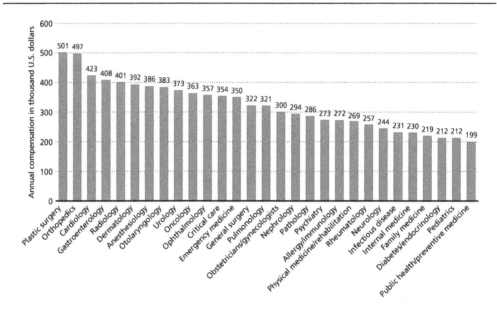

Source: Medscape. United States; November 21, 2017 to February 21, 2018; Survey of 20,329 physicians from 29 specialties © 2018 Statistica. Used with permission.

Fifth, *increase outreach capabilities for practitioners.* One of the media most promoted for this purpose is telemedicine: "[T]he use of medical information exchanged from one site to another via electronic communications to improve a patient's clinical health status."[138] The effectiveness of this mechanism has been shown for a number of conditions.[139] It may, therefore, help solve the problem of geographic shortages when employed to remote areas; however, the time saved for more local visits benefits patients but not physicians. Further, reimbursement for these types of visits is inconsistent, varying by insurance plan and patient location. For example, large companies may pay for televisits to minimize downtime for employees; large insurance companies, however, do not typically pay for such care. Medicare

[138] American Telemedicine Association. *Glossary.* Retrieved May 24, 2018, from https://thesource.americantelemed.org/resources/telemedicine-glossary
[139] Flodgren, G., Rachas, A., Farmer, A. J., Inzitari, M., & Shepperd, S. (2015). Interactive telemedicine: Effects on professional practice and healthcare outcomes. *Cochrane Database of Systematic Reviews, 9.* Art. No.: CD002098. Retrieved May 25, 2018, from http://onlinelibrary.wiley.com/doi/10.1002/14651858.CD002098.pub2/abstract?version=meter+at+0

will pay for telemedicine for rural patients but not for others. This subject is discussed in more detail in Chapter 8, "Information Technology."

Sixth, *reduce demand by increasing opportunities for more self-care* (particularly for those with chronic conditions) and promoting prevention. For example, diabetes is among the most prominent conditions that self-care has benefited. In addition to being able to monitor blood sugar wherever the patient may be, self-care protocols instruct patients about monitoring healthy behavior as well as checking for complications. As an illustration of this recommendation, the Summary of Diabetes Self-Care Activities (SDSCA) "is a brief self-report questionnaire of diabetes self-management that includes items assessing the following aspects of the diabetes regimen: general diet, specific diet, exercise, blood-glucose testing, foot care, and smoking."[140]

Seventh, *increase numbers of domestic- and foreign-trained physicians.* This issue was discussed above with respect to increasing numbers of American medical and osteopathic schools, increased number of student slots, and the need for more residency positions, particularly for international medical graduates. One ethical issue related to this solution is that many countries that can and do supply physicians for the United States (as well as other richer Western nations) have shortages of their own.

Eighth, *increase mentoring opportunities for medical students, particularly in primary care and in underserved areas.* Positive mentoring experiences with exposure to primary care and rural health have been shown to favorably influence student choices of careers in those areas.[141]

Ninth, *enact universal tort reform.* It is controversial whether a state's adverse malpractice climate creates a barrier to recruitment of physicians or an impetus for them to leave (and the opposite with favorable conditions). Predictably, physician groups (such as the AMA) claim tort reform is needed as one tool to cure physician shortages; trial lawyers say such reforms will have no effect on physician numbers. According to a recent comprehensive review:

> [W]hile the effects all point to an increase in the number of physicians in an area in response to the adoption of liability reform, the effects are weak in aggregate and tend to suggest that they are centered in a subset of physicians (e.g., physicians in high risk specialties, older physicians or rural areas). Moreover, the articles typically do not address the experience of specific states . . . . most of the existing multi-state studies use data series ending in the early 2000s, immediately before the latest set of states adopted reforms.[142]

---

[140]Toobert, D. J., Hampson, S. E., & Glasgow, R. E. (2000). The summary of diabetes self-care activities measure. *Diabetes Care, 23,* 943–950. Despite its age, this article is a classic to which others refer for its measurement content and methodology.

[141]Robert Graham Center. American Academy of Family Practice: Specialty and Geographic Distribution of the Physician Workforce: What Influences Medical Student & Resident Choices? Funded by the Josiah Macy, Jr. Foundation 2008. Retrieved May 25, 2018, from http://macyfoundation.org/docs/macy_pubs/pub_grahamcenterstudy.pdf

[142]Robert Graham Center. American Academy of Family Practice: Specialty and Geographic Distribution of the Physician Workforce: What Influences Medical Student & Resident Choices? Funded by the Josiah Macy, Jr. Foundation 2008. Retrieved May 25, 2018, from http://macyfoundation.org/docs/macy_pubs/pub_grahamcenterstudy.pdf

The issue of state-by-state variability is highlighted by another study showing: "Physician supply [in Texas] was not measurably stunted prior to reform, and it did not measurably improve after reform. This is true for all patient care physicians in Texas, high-malpractice-risk specialties, primary care physicians, and rural physicians."[143]

In any case, tort reform will not increase the number of physicians in an area but, at best, will redistribute the existing ones. This debate may become moot very soon, however, as more physicians become employees of health systems, which cover malpractice expenses.

Employment Status

For a number of years, many hospital-based physicians (radiologists, pathologists, emergency physicians, and anesthesiologists) have been employed by the organizations where they practice. A relatively new specialty in this category is a hospitalist. These physicians practice in the hospital and act as the primary care physician used to do—as inpatient coordinator of care. They are either employed by the hospital or contracted through larger local or national organizations.

Regardless of place of practice, more and more physicians have opted to become employees of healthcare systems rather than own their own practices. According to the AMA biennial physician survey:

> 2016 marked the first year in which less than half of practicing physicians owned their own practice—47.1 percent. This was about 6 percentage points lower than in 2012. Similarly, practice size also continued to increase although the shifts in size distribution were small … Hospital ownership of physician practices and direct employment of physicians by hospitals, on the other hand, appears to have stalled after 2014. The percentage of physicians in hospital-owned practices or who were employed directly by a hospital was the same in 2016 as in 2014 (32.8 percent) but higher than in 2012 (29.0 percent).[144]

The reasons for this decline in self-employment vary by age of practitioner. Recent graduates from residency and fellowship programs desire more predictable hours, lower income risk, and freedom from the business aspects of practice. Established practitioners are increasingly selling their practices to: growing reimbursement uncertainties (particularly with a larger part of income coming from value-based incentives); increasing costs due to administrative burdens; and growing information technology requirements. Also, some older physicians are seeking payment for the equity they built over the years but lack buy-out opportunities from younger colleagues. Exhibit 5.6 displays physician characteristics by employment status.

---

[143]Hyman, D. A., Silver, C., Black, B. S., & Paik, M. (2015). Does tort reform affect physician supply? Evidence from Texas. *International Review of Law and Economics, 42,* 203–218.

[144]Kane, C. K. (2017, May). Updated data on physician practice arrangements: Physician ownership drops below 50 percent (AMA Biannual Physician Survey Policy Research Perspectives). Retrieved May 25, 2018, from https://www.ama-assn.org/sites/default/files/media-browser/public/health-policy/PRP-2016-physician-benchmark-survey.pdf

EXHIBIT 5.6. **Characteristics of Employed and Private Practice U.S. Physicians in 2016**

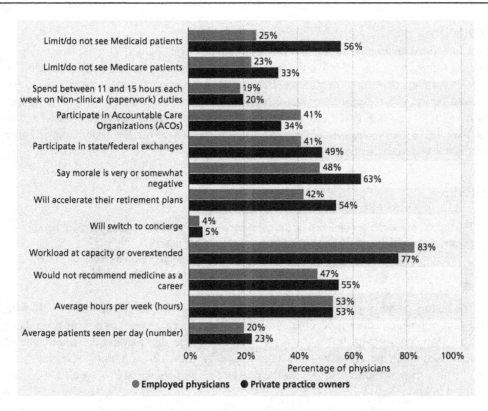

Source: 2018 Survey of America's Physicians Practice Patterns & Perspectives. Survey conducted on behalf of The Physicians Foundation by Merritt Hawkins. Completed September 2018. © 2018, The Physicians Foundation www.physiciansfoundation.org

An important consequence of physician employment by hospitals is increased health-care costs.[145] For example, healthcare services provided in hospital outpatient departments (HOPDs) are reimbursed at higher rates than when provided in physician offices and physicians employed by hospitals perform a higher volume of services in HOPDs than in their offices. Further, when hospitals acquire physician practices, these new employees are

[145] Kacik, A. (2018, March 16). Rapid rise in hospital-employed physicians increases costs. *Modern Healthcare*. Retrieved May 25, 2018, from http://www.modernhealthcare.com/article/20180316/TRANSFORMATION02/180319913

more likely to refer patients to higher-cost facilities within their employer's network.[146] Physician employment resulted in more than $3.1 billion in increased costs from 2012 to 2015.[147]

Summary

Physicians have undergone significant practice changes over many centuries. Beginning as religious figures with few effective therapeutics, physicians have become scientists with an expensive armamentarium of treatments. Because of the training, payment mechanisms, and structure of the U.S. healthcare system, the incentives have caused geographic and specialty maldistributions of practitioners. Solutions to the problems of American medicine will require multiple interventions that, because of failure of the free market system, may require government action to facilitate necessary changes.

NURSES

> The trained nurse has become one of the great blessings of humanity, taking a place beside the physician and the priest, and not inferior to either in her mission.
> —Sir William Osler, Address at Johns Hopkins Hospital (1897);
> later published in *Aequanimitas, and Other Addresses* (1905)

The history of nursing starts at the dawn of humanity with care of the infirm; only with the advent of hospitals does it become a skilled calling. Its emergence as a profession dates from the 19th century with formal theories[148] and practices that parallel the emergence of science-based medicine. (Please see Chapter 4 for a brief history of nursing.) Nurses fulfill many critical responsibilities in the healthcare system. Some general and specific roles are explained below.

Registered Nurses

In order to become a registered nurse (RN), one must graduate from an approved training program and satisfy the licensing requirements of the state where one desires to practice.

Nursing schools have been traditionally divided into three types. *Diploma programs* are hospital-based, usually last 3 years, and training largely comes from direct patient care; they do not grant academic degrees. *Associate degrees* are usually 2 years and are

---

[146]Gaynor, M., Mostashari, F., & Ginsburg, P. B. (2017, April). *Making health care markets work: Competition policy for health care. Actionable policy proposals for the Executive Branch, Congress, and the States*. Retrieved May 25, 2018, from https://www.brookings.edu/wp-content/uploads/2017/04/gaynor-et-al-final-report-v11.pdf Accessed May 25, 2018.

[147]Avalere Health, LLC. (2017, November). *Physicians Advocacy Institute: Implications of hospital employment of physicians on Medicare and beneficiaries*. Retrieved May 25, 2018, from http://www.physiciansadvocacy institute.org/Portals/0/assets/docs/PAI_Medicare Cost Analysis – FINAL 11_9_17.pdf

[148]Nightingale, F. (1860). *Notes on nursing. What it is, and what it is not* (first American ed.). New York: D. Appleton and Company.

based at junior colleges. They combine classroom and bedside teaching and grant associate degrees. *Bachelor degrees* are traditional university-based 4-year curricula that also combine classroom and bedside learning and lead to a Bachelor of Science in Nursing (BSN) degree. The Accreditation Commission for Education in Nursing (ACEN)[149] accredits all of these pathways (as well as masters' and doctoral programs). The other accreditation organization sanctioned by the U.S. Department of Education is the Commission on Collegiate Nursing Education (CCNE),[150] an autonomous arm of American Association of Colleges of Nursing. The latter accredits only bachelors' and masters' programs. The increasing complexity of medical care and preference of employers for nurses possessing a BSN have made this training the preferred one for hospital employers. According to the National League of Nursing, 58% of basic RN programs grant associate degrees, 38% grant baccalaureate degrees, and 4% are diploma schools.[151] "By 2012, more nurses (53 percent) were earning four-year baccalaureate than two-year associate degrees (47 percent)."[152] The number of graduates from U.S. nursing programs has steadily increased from approximately 68,800 in 2001 to nearly 158,000 in 2015.[153]

Once nurses complete formal training, they must pass the National Council Licensure Examination (NCLEX). This test unifies the requirements of all states and is sponsored by the National Council of the State Boards of Nursing (NCSBN). Despite passage of this exam, nurses still must be licensed in each state. The NCSBN is promoting an effort to grant multi-state licensure through the Nurse Licensure Compact (NLC), which allows nurses to practice in both their home state and other compact states. The NLC was changed to an enhanced Nurse Licensure Compact (eNLC) in January 2018.[154]

The "typical" nurse is female (90%), white (75%), and has a bachelor's degree or higher (55%).

The average and median age of RNs is about 45.[155] One of the critical issues of the past several decades has been the availability of RNs to meet the needs of the healthcare system, particularly hospital-based care. Many periods of shortages have been followed by surpluses.

---

[149] Retrieved May 25, 2018, from http://www.acenursing.org/mission-purpose-goals

[150] Retrieved May 25, 2018, from http://www.aacn.nche.edu/ccne-accreditation/about/mission-values-history

[151] National League of Nursing. *Annual survey of schools of nursing, academic year 2013–2014* [This study is the most current on the website]. Retrieved May 25, 2018, from http://www.nln.org/newsroom/nursing-education-statistics/annual-survey-of-schools-of-nursing-academic-year-2013-2014 Of note is that these figures have not changed since 2003.

[152] Robert Wood Johnson Foundation (2015, September 9). *In historic shift, more nurses graduate with bachelor's degrees.* Retrieved May 25, 2018, from https://www.rwjf.org/en/library/articles-and-news/2015/09/more-nurses-with-bachelors-degrees.html

[153] U.S. Department of Health and Human Services Health Resources and Services Administration (HRSA) Bureau of Health Workforce National Center for Health Workforce Analysis (2017). *Supply and demand projections of the nursing workforce: 2014–2030* (July 21). Retrieved May 25, 2018, from https://bhw.hrsa.gov/sites/default/files/bhw/nchwa/projections/NCHWA_HRSA_Nursing_Report.pdf

[154] Retrieved May 25, 2018, from https://www.ncsbn.org/enhanced-nlc-implementation.htm At that date, 29 states participated in this program.

[155] Health Resources and Service Administration (HRSA) (2013, April). *Bureau of Health Professions National Center for Health Workforce Analysis. The U.S. nursing workforce: Trends in supply and education.* Retrieved May 25, 2018, from https://bhw.hrsa.gov/sites/default/files/bhw/nchwa/projections/nursingworkforcetrendsoct2013.pdf

The surpluses were particularly noteworthy during economic downturns, when part-time nurses expanded their hours and "retired" nurses returned to work because their spouses were laid off. The reasons for this expanded workforce often had as much to do with benefits (especially health insurance) as wages. According to the HRSA, the:

> nursing workforce represents a greater problem with distribution across states than magnitude at the national level. Looking at each state's 2030 RN supply minus its 2030 demand reveals both shortages and surpluses in RN workforce in 2030 across the United States. Projected differences between each state's 2030 supply and demand range from a shortage of 44,500 FTEs in California to a surplus of 53,700 FTEs in Florida.[156]

Like most projections, this one is based on current trends in disease patterns and demographics. Changes in the roles of RNs, economic conditions (and jobs that compete with potential applicants) as well as standards of patient care may alter the adequacy of this important resource. A more immediate critical factor in training is the availability of nurse educators, who are in short supply.

At the institutional level, hospitals that can demonstrate a high level of nursing care can achieve magnet status. This designation is awarded by the American Nurses Credentialing Center (ANCC), a subsidiary of the American Nurses Association (ANA), and is based on demonstration of achievements in five areas: Transformational Leadership; Structural Empowerment; Exemplary Professional Practice; New Knowledge, Innovation, & Improvements; and Empirical Quality Results.[157] Magnet hospitals find it easier to recruit highly qualified nurses, and thus shortages are less of a potential problem for them.

Nurse Practitioners

Beyond the initial training for RNs, a number of more specialized career paths are available.

Nurse practitioners (NPs) complete a master's or doctoral degree program and have advanced clinical training beyond their initial nursing preparation. In 2016, there were more than 222,000 NPs licensed in the United States, with about 20,000 graduating programs each year. Their scope of practice varies by the state in which they are licensed; the extent of permitted services usually focuses on the degree to which NPs can practice independent of direct physician supervision. NPs can prescribe medications (including controlled substances) in all 50 states and the District of Columbia. As described by the American Association of Nurse Practitioners (AANP),[158] NPs provide the following services, among others:

- Ordering, performing, and interpreting diagnostic tests such as lab work and X-rays
- Diagnosing and treating acute and chronic conditions such as diabetes, high blood pressure, infections, and injuries
- Prescribing medications and other treatments

---

[156] HRSA Supply and Demand Projections of the Nursing Workforce: 2014–2030.

[157] Retrieved May 25, 2018, from https://www.nursingworld.org/organizational-programs/magnet/magnet-model

[158] AANP. *What's an NP?* Retrieved May 25, 2018, from https://www.aanp.org/all-about-nps/what-is-an-np

- Managing patients' overall care

- Counseling

- Educating patients on disease prevention and positive health and lifestyle choices

Among NPs, 86.6% are certified in an area of primary care, and 77.8% of all NPs deliver primary care.[159]

Nurse Anesthetists

"Nurses were the first professional group to provide anesthesia services in the United States, and nurse anesthesia has since become recognized as the first clinical nursing specialty."[160] These professionals not only administer anesthesia but have been clinical innovators in the field. For example, Dr. Charles Mayo called Alice Magaw (1860–1928) the "Mother of Anesthesia" for her pioneering achievements at what became the Mayo Clinic.[161] These professionals have also provided most of the anesthesia services in military conflicts starting with the Civil War.

Nurse anesthetists have been at the forefront of specialized nursing education. Agnes McGee started the first formal educational program at St. Vincent's Hospital in Portland, Oregon, in 1909; the establishment of additional programs accelerated to meet the needs of World War I. Paralleling medicine's move to specialist accreditation, the first nurse anesthetist certification exam was administered in 1945.

To achieve this specialization, nurses must possess a BSN, graduate from an advanced (masters' or doctoral) degree program (accredited by the Council on Accreditation of Nurse Anesthesia Educational Programs), and pass a national certification exam. Nurses who successfully complete this process are designated Certified Registered Nurse Anesthetists (CRNAs). Continuing education is required for maintenance of certification.

According to the American Association of Nurse Anesthetists (AANA),[162] a

CRNA takes care of a patient's anesthesia needs before, during and after surgery or the delivery of a baby by:

Performing a physical assessment

Participating in preoperative teaching

Preparing for anesthetic management

Administering anesthesia to keep the patient pain free

Maintaining anesthesia intraoperatively

[159] AANP (2018, January 22). *Fact sheet*. Retrieved May 25, 2018, from https://www.aanp.org/all-about-nps/np-fact-sheet

[160] American Association of Nurse Anesthetists. History of Nurse Anesthesia Practice. Retrieved May 25, 2018, from https://www.aana.com/about-us/aana-archives-library/our-history

[161] Magaw, A. (1906). A review of over fourteen thousand anesthesias. *Surgery, Gynecology, and Obstetrics, 3*, 795–799.

[162] Retrieved May 25, 2018, from https://www.aana.com/about-us

Overseeing recovery from anesthesia

Following the patient's postoperative course from recovery room to patient care unit

CRNAs provide services in conjunction with other healthcare professionals such as surgeons, dentists, podiatrists, and anesthesiologists.

Midwives

According to the *Oxford English Dictionary*, the term "midwife" is derived from "someone with" (*mid*) a "woman" (*wife*) during childbirth.[163] The practice of midwifery is obviously of ancient origin: women helping other women during childbirth. Numerous written references include those of biblical origin—the most well known being the midwives commanded by Pharaoh to kill all Hebrew newborn males.[164] The early 19th-century word "obstetrics" is derived from the Latin word *obstetrix*,[165] which means "midwife." For millennia, assistance with childbirth was the province of women with special knowledge. The reasons for exclusion of men include a desire for privacy, absence of a scientific basis for care, and lack of available medical practitioners. This latter reason was particularly important in the United States in colonial times because of physician shortages. It is noteworthy that New York City required licensing of midwives in 1716, 44 years before physicians were licensed. The first formal midwife training program in America was conducted by Dr. William Shippen in 1765, coincident with the founding of the first medical school at what is now the University of Pennsylvania. As mentioned in the section on physicians, in 1848, Dr. Israel Tilsdale Talbot cofounded the Boston Female Medical College (the first medical school for women in the world) whose purpose was to train midwives.[166]

In the late 18th and early 19th centuries, middle-class and wealthier urban populations began to prefer physician attendance at births. By the turn of the 20th century, nearly half of all births were attended by physicians, although only 5% occurred in hospitals. The turning point in the medicalization of obstetrics was due to Dr. Joseph B. DeLee (1869–1942), professor of Obstetrics at Northwestern University, founder of Chicago Lying-in Hospital, and author of an influential textbook on obstetrics.[167] In 1915, he spoke out against midwifery at a meeting of the American Association for the Study and Prevention of Infant Mortality,

---

[163]This section focuses on certified midwives. The other type of midwife is often referred to as lay nurse midwife, traditional midwife, or direct-entry midwife. The difference between them is their training. Certified midwives have formal undergraduate and graduate degrees in nursing/related subjects and midwifery. Lay midwives gain their training from self-study, apprenticeships, or freestanding midwifery schools.

[164]Exodus 1:15–22. While the midwives are named Shiphrah and Puah, one tradition is that they were pseudonyms for Jochevet and Miriam, Moses' mother and sister, respectively.

[165]The word *obstetrix* comes from the Latin word *obstāre*, meaning to stand before (i.e., a woman who stands before another woman during childbirth).

[166]For a more detailed history see: Varney, H., & Thompson, J. B. (2016). *A history of midwifery in the United States: The midwife said fear not.* New York: Springer.

[167]DeLee, J. B. (1914). *The principles and practice of obstetrics.* Philadelphia: W.B. Saunders. (A revised sixth edition was published in 1933.)

saying it inhibited progress in the field of obstetrics. However, DeLee's 1920 paper had the greatest influence. In it, DeLee stated:

> Perhaps laceration, prolapse and all the evils are, in fact, natural to labor and in fact normal ... but, if you believe that a woman after delivery should be as healthy, as well as anatomically perfect as she was before, and that the child should be undamaged, then you will have to agree with me that *labor is pathogenic* [emphasis added], because experience has proved such ideal results exceedingly rare.[168]

Though DeLee began his article by saying that "[t]he time is not yet right for a general recommendation of the procedure to be described in this paper," he advocated that all vaginal deliveries should be performed with episiotomies (cutting, and subsequent suture repair, of the perineum to enlarge the opening for the baby) and routine use of use of forceps (elongated tongs to pull the baby out of the mother by its head). He claimed the former would reduce trauma to the mother, which often caused tears and fistulas. The latter process he said would relieve pressure on the child's skull and thus cause fewer brain injuries.

This proposal, along with a complex anesthesia regimen,[169] made it more certain not only that a physician would perform the delivery but that it would occur in a hospital. Only poorer women or those with strong ethnic preferences would remain as patients of the midwife and deliver at home.[170] After DeLee's recommendations were universally adopted as the standard of care, the results were dramatic. In 1921, 30% to 50% of deliveries were in hospitals; by 1939, the figure increased to 50% overall but was 75% among urban women. In 1960, 97% of births were in hospitals. With this increase in hospital-based care came a decline in attendance by midwives to a low of 1.1% in 1980.[171] In that year, the American Academy of Family Physicians (AAFP) issued a formal statement that "the use of nurse-midwives is not the best interests of quality patient care." Further, the AAFP "does not believe that the midwife can adequately substitute for the physician in obstetrics." It therefore had recommended

> abolishment of midwifery for many years while recommending production of sufficient competently trained family physicians to provide quality obstetrical services. Any trend from competently trained licensed physicians performing quality obstetrics back to midwifery must be considered a regressive step in the delivery of obstetrical service.[172]

The trend back to use of midwives in the 1970s and later is attributable to three factors. First, in the 1970s and 1980s, women's empowerment gained strength, and with it came the

---

[168] DeLee, J. B. (1920). The prophylactic forceps operation. *American Journal of Obstetrics and Gynecology, 1*(1), 34–44. Read at the Forty-fifth Annual Meeting of the American Gynecological Society, Chicago, May 24–26, 1920.

[169] A version of what was called "modified twilight sleep," consisted of morphine and scopolamine for pain relief, then ether administration before application of the forceps.

[170] The newness of hospital births as the norm is highlighted by the fact that in 1924 James Carter was the first future U.S. president born in a hospital.

[171] Feldhusen, A. (2000). *The history of midwifery and childbirth in America: A time line.* Retrieved June 26, 2016, from https://www.midwiferytoday.com/articles/timeline.asp

[172] Rooks, J. P. (1997). *Midwifery & childbirth in America* (p. 83). Philadelphia: Temple University Press.

belief that pregnancy was not a pathologic or mystical process that required physician-only assistance. Further, desire for so-called natural childbirth (such as the use of the Lamaze technique of relaxation and breathing) reduced the absolute expectation of anesthesia. Also, many women wanted to deliver at home. Second, in the 1980s, two important antitrust actions aided midwife practice. After Federal Trade Commission (FTC) intervention in 1983, the State Volunteer Mutual Insurance Corporation (a physician-owned malpractice insurance company in Tennessee) agreed not to unreasonably discriminate against physicians who work with independent nurse midwives.[173] In 1988, the FTC found that the medical staff of Memorial Medical Center "conspired to suppress competition by denying a certified nurse-midwife's application for hospital privileges without a reasonable basis." As a result, the hospital's medical staff was prohibited from denying or restricting "hospital privileges to certified nurse-midwives, unless the staff has a reasonable basis for believing that the restriction would serve the interest of the hospital in providing for the efficient and competent delivery of health care services."[174] Finally, medicine started to embrace evidence-based care; DeLee's recommendations were based on his anecdotal experiences. When, for example, the practice of episiotomy was examined, the data "conclusively determined that the routine use of episiotomy should be abandoned and that perineal trauma is *decreased* [emphasis added] when episiotomy is not performed."[175] Results of trials on use of forceps likewise caused their rapid decline; only 0.57% of all births for 2013–2014 used this method.[176] Since more births did not require procedures performed only by physicians, midwives had the opportunity to participate in more deliveries. On the heels of these changes, midwives were accepted by more obstetricians and family physicians into collaborative practices. Further, these specialists recognized the income that nurse midwives could generate. The result of these trends is that nurse midwives began to deliver more babies. By 2016, certified nurse midwives attended 8.8% of all births in the United States.[177]

Education and Certification

RNs who graduate from a program accredited by the Accreditation Commission for Midwifery Education and pass a national exam administered by the American Midwifery Certification Board are credentialed as certified nurse midwives (CNM). Non-RNs who have a degree in another health-related field but complete the same accredited training and pass the same national exam are credentialed as certified midwives. These professionals must be recertified every 5 years to keep their credentials. Despite this standardized process, each

---

[173] State Volunteer Mutual Insurance Corporation 102 F.T.C. 1232 (1983) (consent order).

[174] Medical Staff of Memorial Medical Center 110 F.T.C. 541 (final order issued June 1, 1988).

[175] Weber, A. M., & Meyn, L. (2002). Episiotomy use in the United States, 1979–1997. *Obstetrics & Gynecology*, 100(6), 1177–1182. Of interest is that women who had episiotomies tended to be younger, white, and insured.

[176] Hamilton, B. E., Martin, J. A., Osteman, M. J. K., Curtin, S. C., & Mathews, T. J. (2015, December 23). *National Vital Statistics Reports*, *64*, 12. Births: Final Data for 2014.

[177] National Vital Statistics Reports, Vol. 67, No. 1 January 31, 2018. Births: Final Data for 2016. Retrieved May 25, 2018, from https://www.cdc.gov/nchs/data/nvsr/nvsr67/nvsr67_01_tables.pdf In 2016, 98.4% of all births in the United States were in hospitals.

state still has its own licensing requirements. According to the American College of Nurse Midwives, current practitioners act as "primary health care providers to women throughout the lifespan. This means that midwives perform physical exams, prescribe medications including contraceptive methods, order laboratory tests as needed, provide prenatal care, gynecological care, labor and birth care, as well as health education and counseling to women of all ages."[178]

As is the case with nurse practitioners, current controversies center on the degree to which these professionals can practice independent of physician supervision.

PHYSICIAN ASSISTANTS

The model for physician assistants[179] originated in the military: the army combat medic and the navy corpsman. The purpose of these soldiers and sailors is to assist physicians (mostly surgeons) with combat-related injuries. Sometimes, as with medics, these persons are at the front lines and are the only available medical care until the patient can be evacuated to a hospital. Because they serve in situations that are, or could become, combat zones, they were originally exclusively men recruited from the ranks of the active military; each branch of the armed forces developed its own training program for these practitioners.

The impetus for training such practitioners in the private sector was a projected physician shortage in the 1960s. Charles H. Hudson, MD (a Cleveland internist and future AMA president) wrote an article in the *Journal of the American Medical Association* calling for training of what he tentatively termed "externs," who would perform technical duties as well as assume some medical responsibilities.[180]

In 1965, Eugene A. Stead Jr., MD, established the first "physician assistant" (PA) educational program at Duke University, enrolling four former navy medical corpsmen who graduated in 1966. In that same year, the first program to train surgical assistants (a category of PA) was begun at the University of Alabama, Birmingham. These origins are important to note because from the beginning, PAs were supported and accepted by the "medical establishment." (Contrast this situation with the one described above for nurse midwives who historically competed with physicians.) Other early milestones demonstrating rapid acceptance include:

- Kaiser Permanente became the first HMO to employ a PA (1970).

- The American Academy of Family Physicians, the American Academy of Pediatrics, the American College of Physicians, the American Society of Internal Medicine, and the

---

[178] Retrieved May 25, 2018, from http://www.midwife.org/Become-a-Midwife

[179] Much of the information in the section come from: The American Association of Physician Assistants, retrieved May 25, 2018, from http://www.aapa.org and the Federal Bureau of Labor Statistics, retrieved May 25, 2018, from http://www.bls.gov/ooh/healthcare/physician-assistants.htm#tab-1

[180] Hudson, C. L. (1961). Expansion of medical professional services with nonprofessional personnel. *JAMA, 176*(10), 839–841.

American Medical Association (AMA) Council on Medical Education all participated in establishing minimum standards for PA program accreditation (1971).

■ The AMA recognized the PA profession and began work on national certification and codification of its practice characteristics (1971), with the first national PA certifying examination administered by the NBME in 1973. (Recall that this organization is the same one that certifies physician specialists.)

Further events facilitated acceptance and growth opportunities for PAs, including the Comprehensive Health Manpower Training Act of 1971, which allocated $4 million for establishment of new PA educational programs; the Balanced Budget Act of 1997, which established a uniform rate of payment for Medicare services that included PAs as covered providers; and the 2000 clarification by the Joint Commission on Accreditation of Healthcare Organizations (now called the Joint Commission) allowing physicians to delegate histories and physical exams to PAs. By 2007, all 50 states and the District of Columbia allowed PAs to prescribe medication.

Education and Certification

The majority of PA programs require undergraduate degrees that contain coursework similar to pre-medical curricula. Prior healthcare experience (about 3 years) is also a prerequisite of many programs and can take the form of actual medical care (as an RN, emergency medical technician, etc.) or related work, such as a Peace Corp volunteer. PA programs are accredited by the Accreditation Review Commission on Education for the Physician Assistant, usually run for 3 academic years, and contain courses in basic sciences, behavioral sciences, and clinical medicine as well as clinical rotations in the basic medical disciplines (i.e., family medicine, internal medicine, obstetrics and gynecology, pediatrics, general surgery, emergency medicine, and psychiatry). After graduation from an accredited program, PAs must pass the PA National Certifying Exam (PANCE) administered by the National Commission on Certification of PAs and obtain a license by the state in which they want to practice. As is the case with NPs, states can vary with respect to the degree of required physician supervision. In order to maintain certification, PAs must pass a recertification exam every 10 years and complete 100 hours of continuing medical education (CME) every 2 years. Employment of PAs is projected to grow 37% from 2016 to 2026, much faster than the average for all occupations. In 2016, there were 106,200 jobs for PAs.

While some PAs engage in general practice, many assist physicians in particular specialties.

According to the American Association of Physician Assistants Physician, PAs:

■ Take or review patients' medical histories

■ Examine patients

■ Order and interpret diagnostic tests, such as X-rays or blood tests

■ Diagnose a patient's injury or illness

■ Give treatment, such as setting broken bones and immunizing patients

- Educate and counsel patients and their families—for example, answering questions about how to care for a child with asthma

- Prescribe medicine

- Assess and record a patient's progress

- Research the latest treatments to ensure the quality of patient care

- Conduct or participate in outreach programs, such as talking to groups about managing diseases and promoting wellness

Physician versus NP/PA Care

Given the projected physician manpower shortages and maldistribution mentioned above, one proposed solution is to increase the supply of nurse practitioners and physician assistants, often collectively called advanced practice clinicians or physician extenders.

In analyzing this shortage, one can draw on many research studies over the past few decades. These studies focus on comparisons with primary care physicians regarding quality of care (such as health status), patient satisfaction, and resource utilization (such as writing prescriptions, ordering lab and radiology tests, and referring for consultations). Results from several large studies are provided below.

Horrocks et al.[181] reviewed 11 trials and 23 observational studies and found that "[p]atients were more satisfied with care by a nurse practitioner ... No differences in health status were found. Nurse practitioners had longer consultations ... and made more investigations ... than did doctors. No differences were found in prescriptions, return consultations, or referrals."

In reviewing the literature from 1966 to 2015, Kurtzman[182] concluded:

Across these studies, NP-delivered primary care has been found to be equivalent or better than PCMD [primary care MD]–delivered care on most processes of care measures (e.g., compliance with diabetes practice guidelines, medication adjustments, timely analgesia), patient outcomes (e.g., mortality, health status, quality of life, adverse events), and measures of cost and utilization (e.g., cost of consultation, emergency department and hospitalization utilization, medication costs, total costs) and consistently better in terms of patient-rated satisfaction.

A more focused study was conducted by Mafi et al.[183] using data from the National Ambulatory Medical Care Survey and National Hospital Ambulatory Medical Care Survey (1997–2011).

[181]Horrocks, S., Anderson, E., & Salisbury, C. (2002). Systematic review of whether nurse practitioners working in primary care can provide equivalent care to doctors. *British Medical Journal, 324,* 819.

[182]Kurtzman, E. (2016, January 31). *Delivery of high quality primary care in community health centers: The role of nurse practitioners and state scope of practice restrictions.* A dissertation submitted to The Faculty of The Columbian College of Arts and Sciences of The George Washington University in partial fulfillment of the requirements for the degree of Doctor of Philosophy. Retrieved May 25, 2018, from https://pqdtopen.proquest.com/doc/1756274772.html?FMT=ABS

[183]Mafi, J. N., Wee, C. C., Davis, R. B., & Landon, B. E. (2016). Comparing use of low-value health care services among U.S. advanced practice clinicians and physicians. *Annals of Internal Medicine, 165*(4), 237–244.

They compared care by physicians with that of PAs and NPs for patients with three common conditions: upper respiratory infections (URIs), back pain, and headache. Instead of beneficial outcomes, they looked for care that did not meet accepted guidelines—for example, antibiotic treatment for URIs and MRI orders for uncomplicated low back pain. The results showed that both groups "provided an equivalent amount of low-value health services"; essentially the study said that neither group was worse than the other.

Aside from these measurable factors, research has shown a great degree of acceptance of these nonphysician practitioners. For example, Dill et al.[184] found that "about half of the respondents preferred to have a physician as their primary care provider. However, when presented with scenarios wherein they could see a physician assistant or a nurse practitioner sooner than a physician, most elected to see one of the other health care professionals instead of waiting."

Of note with these studies is that the conditions for which comparisons are made are straightforward; they do not compare the care of complex cases or patients with multiple systemic problems. Therefore, the evidence supports using PAs or NPs to free-up time the primary care physicians would otherwise spend on more "routine care." The time-saving service they can perform for procedural specialists would be on pre- and postoperative care. The exceptions, of course, are for nurse anesthetists and midwives who can function more independently while working with anesthesiologists and OB/GYNs, respectively. The best way to combine physicians, NPs, and PAs into care teams will require ongoing study, particularly looking at the parameters of available manpower and access to care.

SUMMARY

The healthcare field is a major employer in the United States. (Please see Exhibit 5.7.) Systemic healthcare costs are related not only to the salaries these individuals earn but by the decisions they make about the resources needed to care for patients. How different professionals approach treatment decisions is influenced by their training, which includes the practice philosophies embedded in their histories.

The key issues for ongoing study include how many healthcare professionals we need, what specialties are required, where they should be located, and the best mix of clinician teams that will provide the timeliest and most cost-effective access to care.

---

[184]Dill, M. J, Pankow, S., Erikson, C., & Shipman, S. (2013). Survey shows consumers open to a greater role for physician assistants and nurse practitioners. *Health Affairs, 32*(6), 1135–1142.

EXHIBIT 5.7. **Employment in Private Healthcare Industries as a Percentage of Total Private Employment, 1990–2015 Annual Averages**

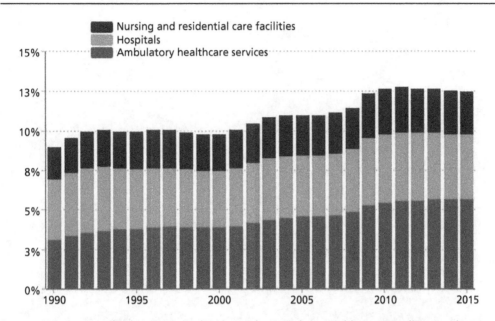

Source: U.S. Bureau of Labor Statistics (2016, June). *A Look at Healthcare Spending, Employment, Pay, Benefits, and Prices.* Retrieved May 25, 2018, from https://www.bls.gov/spotlight/2016/a-look-at-healthcare-spending-employment-pay-benefits-and-prices/pdf/a-look-at-healthcare-spending-employment-pay-benefits-and-prices.pdf

CHAPTER

6

PAYERS

SHYLOCK.

...ships are but boards, sailors but men: there be land-rats and water-rats, water-thieves and land-thieves, I mean pirates, and then there is the peril of waters, winds and rocks...Three thousand ducats; I think I may take his bond.

—William Shakespeare, *Merchant of Venice*, Act 1, Scene 3

This chapter addresses the following questions:

- Who pays for products and services?
- How are payment decisions made?
- What are some of the federal policies that determine payment methods and amounts?
- How did we arrive at the current payment system, and what can it teach us about future trends?

Answering these questions will help the healthcare strategist to:

- Position and price products
- Understand customers' reimbursement environment
- Anticipate and understand the impact of insurer and governmental policy changes

PRINCIPLES OF HEALTH INSURANCE

The concept of insurance derives from commercial finance in ancient Babylonia. Traders (particularly mariners) borrowed money for ventures, promising to repay lenders with interest upon successful completion of their voyages. As part of the cost of these loans, lenders agreed to forgive the amount if borrowers experienced an unexpected loss, like the sinking of the ship or attack by thieves.

Health insurance originated in ancient Greece and Rome in the collegia, precursors to medieval guilds and modern labor unions, which collected fees from members who shared the same profession or craft. If a member (or sometimes a spouse or child) became ill, the organization would provide care and money to support the family during the time of disability. Since the available medical care was primitive, often monies were used to cover funeral expenses.[1] It is important to note that, contrary to current popular belief, health/social welfare insurance as a job-related benefit is an ancient practice.

Private health insurance became prevalent in the United States after World War II; public insurance was widely available only after Medicare and Medicaid began in 1966. (Their histories are explained below.)

---

[1]For an excellent and very readable history of the principles of risk behind insurance and financial instruments see: Bernstein, P. L. (1996). *Against the gods, the remarkable story of risk*. New York: John Wiley & Sons.

Since those times, public debate has centered on such questions as:

- Who is covered by insurance? Who should be covered?
- What benefits should insurance provide?
- How much should insurance cost?
- Who should pay for insurance, for example, employer and/or employee; governments?
- When should insurance cover new technology? (A related question is: When does an experimental technology become a standard of care?)
- What portion of the cost of care should the patient share, that is, deductible, copayment, and coinsurance?
- What are the respective responsibilities of public and private insurers?

In order to start formulating informed answers to questions like these, one must first start with a definition: Insurance is a contract between two or more parties whereby, in exchange for a payment (premium), the insurer protects (indemnifies) the insured against a defined peril or loss by agreeing to pay a specified amount of money and/or provide certain services or products if that loss should occur.

The *Oxford English Dictionary* (*OED*) defines the word "indemnify" as:

1. To preserve, protect, or keep free *from*, secure *against* (any hurt, harm, or loss); to secure against legal responsibility *for* past or future actions or events ...
2. To compensate (a person, etc.) *for* loss suffered, expenses incurred, etc.
3. To compensate *for* disadvantages, annoyances, hardships, etc.

What the insured gains from this contract are protections against catastrophic loss and also the ability to budget for this protection by paying regular premiums. The insurer profits in this relationship in two ways. First, by proper pricing and employment of utilization controls, the insurer seeks to ensure that the collected premiums are more than the amount paid if the loss occurs. In the case of health insurance, we usually consider this loss to be expenses involved in caring for the sick. The healthcare insurance term for this concept is "medical loss ratio"(MLR), defined as the ratio:

$$[\text{Expenses for Medical Care}/\text{Total Revenue}] \times 100$$

(More will be said about this term later.) Second, and more importantly, is that insurers traditionally earn a significant portion of their revenues from investment income. These companies are able to achieve these gains not only because they have large sums to invest but also due to the timing differences between when they collect premiums and when they must pay their bills.

Four circumstances create optimal conditions for an insurance contract:

1. The loss must have some nontrivial value upon which both insured and insurer agree.
2. The peril must occur randomly and be out of the control of the insured.

3. The event must occur neither too frequently nor too rarely.

4. The insurer must be able to write large numbers of contracts indemnifying similar risks.

Consider each of the above statements and how their application creates insurance markets. Because insurance coverage for products and services is often critical to financial success, healthcare strategists must understand where their products or services fit into the spectrum of these conditions. Further, an understanding of these principles is crucial to public policy when structuring health insurance schemes.

The Loss Must Have Some Nontrivial Value Upon Which Both Insured and Insurer Agree

The first condition deals with the value of the event or object insured. Theoretically, *any* object or event is insurable if the insurer and the insured agree on its value and the cost of insurance. If the value is very small, the *insured* would not care about the loss; imagine insuring a paper clip or pencil. Further, the opportunity cost of the time it takes to negotiate and purchase insurance might be greater than the value of the loss itself. From the insurer's perspective, the time and resources incurred in issuing such a policy would require a charge more than the value of the loss.

If the value is very great (or so unique that it cannot be pooled with others having similar risks), the insurer may not want to chance covering it. If the insurer *does* want to write a contract but is still very risk averse, then it has two choices. First, it may form a syndicate with other insurers to spread the jeopardy of loss among them; this arrangement is how firms such as Lloyd's of London operate. The other way to lessen the potential risk is for the insurance company to agree to cover a portion of the loss and buy a policy from another company to cover *its* catastrophic losses. This type of contract is called *reinsurance*. In addition to Lloyd's of London, prominent firms in this sector include Swiss Reinsurance, Munich Reinsurance, and General Re (a subsidiary of Berkshire Hathaway).

The Peril Must Occur Randomly and Be Out of the Control of the Insured

At the individual level, the event must occur at random and be unpredictable; in other words, it must truly be an accident. If a particular event were totally predictable and occurred sometime in the near future, the insurance company would charge the insured a premium based on: nearly the full value of the item being insured; the investment income that would have been earned if the loss occurred at a later date; and an administrative fee for writing the policy. This arrangement does not offer any benefit to the insured, who could save for the loss, not incur the transaction costs, and/or repurchase the lost item at a cost that does not include the insurance premium.

Of course, if the insurer pools large numbers of individuals, each of whom has a random likelihood of loss, there is some *overall* predictability. (Please see below in the fourth condition for insurable contracts.)

An important question raised by this randomness is: Does the presence of insurance have any influence on the probability that the indemnified event will occur? Economists refer to this problem as "moral hazard"; its opposite is "normal hazard," that is, when events truly occur randomly and are unaffected by externalities of insurance. According to the *OED*, the term "moral hazard" was coined by the life insurance industry in 1875 to refer to the situation where the rising premiums that occur with age would cause healthy people to cancel their policies, leaving only the infirm with coverage. According to the late William Safire's column "On Language," the term has taken on a special meaning in healthcare. For example, Safire quotes Princeton economics Professor Burton G. Malkiel, who defines situations involving moral hazard as "cases where the existence of risk insurance alters the behavior of the insured toward taking more risk."[2] Safire further cites Nobel laureate Kenneth J. Arrow's comments about health insurance: "It struck me immediately...that one problem with insurance was that the user (the patient) was not required to pay the full cost (indeed only a relatively small fraction of it). Therefore, according to usual economic principles, the patient would use medical care excessively."

More recently, Nobel laureate Paul Krugman described moral hazard as "any situation in which one person makes the decision about how much risk to take, while someone else bears the cost if things go badly."[3]

Krugman describes a two-party transaction; however, the healthcare setting is much more complicated. For example, an employer may pay most of the premium when it purchases health insurance for an employee. The insurance company then bears the financial risk for services and products the employee will consume, which, in large part, is based on what the healthcare provider recommends.

On a more personal level, consider your answer to the following question: *If you thought about it,* would you be less likely to ski if you knew you were uninsured for a medical accident? Such circumstances also raise the issue of asymmetric information, which, in this case, means the insured knows more than the insurer about the likelihood of the potential loss. Because insurers recognize the inevitability of this asymmetric information, they compensate for it by increasing premiums.

In order to mitigate the effects of moral hazard and asymmetric information, payers have also employed a variety of cost-sharing strategies with consumers. The three most common types of consumer payments are *deductibles, coinsurance*, and *copayments*. The *deductible* is the amount the patient pays before the insurance starts to cover charges. *Coinsurance* is a *percentage* of charges the patient pays; the remainder is the responsibility of the insurance company. A *copayment* is the amount the patient pays at each encounter, whether it is for receiving a service or buying a product (such as medication). (Please see Exhibits 6.1 and 6.2 for examples of how these terms are applied in health insurance.)

---

[2]Safire, W. (1998). On language: Moral hazard. *The New York Times Magazine* (December 20). Retrieved May 25, 2018, from http://www.nytimes.com/1998/12/20/magazine/on-language-moral-hazard.html?scp=11&sq=moral%20hazard&st=cse

[3]Krugman, P. (2009). *The return of depression economics and the crisis of 2008.* New York: W. W. Norton.

EXHIBIT 6.1. **Example of the Application of Out-of-Pocket Expenses to Payment of Healthcare Charges[a]**

Your health plan covers "medically necessary" services and pharmaceuticals. The services are subject to an annual (calendar-year) deductible of $200, 80/20 coinsurance (your insurance pays 80% and you pay 20%), and a maximum out-of-pocket payment (after the deductible is met) of $1,000 per calendar year. (Pharmaceutical benefits are discussed in Exhibit 6.2.) No copayments apply for physician services. Hospital charges are covered in full.

You see a physician at the beginning of the year and are charged $150. It is an acceptable amount, according to a fee schedule upon which the physician and your insurance company have agreed. How much do you pay? First, you determine if you satisfied your annual deductible. Since it is the beginning of a new year and your deductible is $200, you are responsible for the entire bill.

Unfortunately, your physician found a problem that requires a revisit 4 weeks later. After that visit, you have an allowable charge of $100. How much do you now owe? Since you paid $150 of your $200 deductible during your last visit, you first owe an additional $50. Now that your deductible is met, your responsibility is on 20% of the remaining $50 ($100 charge minus $50 left on your deductible = $50). The 20% coinsurance of this amount is $10. For this visit, your out-of-pocket responsibility is: $50 + $10 = $60.

Your doctor now tells you that you need surgery to correct the problem found during the first two visits. You have the surgery and review the physicians' charges (the only part of the bill for which you are responsible). The total of all physicians' charges (surgeon, anesthesiologist, pathologist, and radiologist) is $5,500. Since, as mentioned, you already satisfied your deductible, you would be responsible for 20% of the $5,500 ($1,100). But you are only at risk for the first $1,000 of out-of-pocket expenses after your deductible is met. Since you already paid $10 from the last office visit, you would pay $990.

[a] This example illustrates how out-of-pocket provisions may operate. Plans have diverse provisions. For example, copayments and coinsurance are frequently not the same for all types of services.

Recall the previous explanation of the effect out-of-pocket payments have in reducing utilization (the RAND Health Insurance Experiment discussed in Chapter 2, "Determinants of Utilization of Healthcare Services and Products") and you will understand why these measures are used to address the patient moral hazard issue. At the same time, remember the concept of provider-induced demand and the actions insurers are taking to control it. Combining an appreciation of both these concepts, one can realize a unique feature of health insurance: *The insurer has to contend with moral hazard from both consumer and provider.* One further example concerning provider behavior due to moral hazard concerns trauma care. Delgado et al.[4] found: "Patients with severe injuries initially evaluated at non–trauma center EDs [emergency departments] were less likely to be transferred if insured and were at risk of receiving suboptimal trauma care."[5]

[4] Delgado, M. K., Yokell, M. A., Staudenmayer, K. L., Spain, D. A., Hernandez-Boussard, T., & Wang, N. E. (2014). Factors associated with the disposition of severely injured patients initially seen at non–trauma center emergency departments disparities by insurance status. *JAMA Surgery, 149*(5), 422–430.

[5] Delgado, MK et al.: Factors associated with the disposition of severely injured patients initially seen at non–trauma center emergency departments disparities by insurance status. *JAMA Surgery, 149*(5):422-30, 2014

EXHIBIT 6.2. Example of the Application of Out-of-Pocket Expenses to Payment for Pharmaceuticals[a]

Your insurance plan covers pharmaceuticals that you can take by yourself (self-administered medications, like pills, and simple injections, like insulin). In order to hold down costs, the insurance company has contracted with an independent company (a pharmaceutical benefit management firm [PBM]) to administer these benefits. The PBM classifies the medications into three categories (or tiers) and assigns different copayments to each. The first tier is comprised of all generic drugs, which carry a $10 copayment for a 30-day supply.[b] The second tier is comprised of brand name drugs which do not have a generic equivalent and for which the PBM has negotiated special prices or rebates from the manufacturers. Tier 2 medications have a $25 copayment for a 30-day supply. Tier 3 consists of all other branded medications. The Tier 3 copayment is $40 for a 30-day supply. The list of all these medications, their use, and assigned tier is called a *formulary*.[c] Depending on the plan, these copayments may count toward annual out-of-pocket maximums the individual must pay.

[a] Many different variations exist with respect to pharmaceutical coverage. For example, some plans have more than three tiers, depending on the extent of favorable manufacturer contracts, and others have eliminated copayments and use coinsurance instead. Additionally, some plans may apply annual maximum out-of-pocket cost limits for drugs.

[b] Virtually all plans also provide patients with the opportunity to order 90-day supplies of medication by mail at less than the cost of three copayments.

[c] In addition to U.S. companies, countries that provide pharmaceuticals to their citizens also use formularies and differential cost structures. The difference between the two is that in the United States., the tiers are based on *generic status/medication cost*; other countries (e.g., Italy) assign tiers by *effectiveness*.

The Event Must Occur Neither Too Frequently Nor Too Rarely

If an event occurs too frequently, the insurer will not have time to invest the premium for adequate profits. In this case, in order for the transaction to make financial sense for the insurer, the premium needs to be close to the actual value of the loss *plus* administrative expenses *and* a profit margin to compensate for the lost investment opportunity cost. From the insured's viewpoint, paying a premium that is more than the value of the loss does not make any financial sense. As an extreme example, imagine a driver who frequently (but accidentally) "totals" his car. The value of the loss is known, and the event occurs sporadically, but it happens often. The insurer could insure this driver, but the cost would be greater than that of the vehicle itself.

If the loss occurs very rarely, the insurer would be happy to collect a premium to indemnify against such an event; however, the insured may find that saving for replacement of the loss (by investing what would have been the premium) makes more financial sense. Some people use this financial strategy as the reason for declining to purchase long-term care insurance at younger ages.

Between these two extremes are a variety of possibilities. For example, would there be an insurance market to cover loss from being hit by a falling satellite? You may invoke the rarity principle and answer "no" to this question. Consider, however, that because of the vagaries of space programs, an international convention in 1972 required launchers to take out specified amounts of insurance. This practice became global news on March 23, 2001, when the Mir space station was due to fall out of orbit *somewhere* onto an expected zone of 3,730 square miles in the South Pacific between Australia and South America. The insurance policy cost $200 million. Fortunately, no one was injured.

The Insurer Must Be Able to Write Large Numbers of Contracts to Indemnify Similar Risks

For the insurer, this pooling ensures regular premium inflows for investment as well as the ability to more reliably predict the likelihood of the insured event (the so-called law of large numbers). The benefit for the insured is being in a risk pool with others who will have the events occur at varying frequencies, thus enabling the insurer to charge lower premiums.

***

While these four conditions are the "ideal" for creating an insurance market, in reality, social and cultural imperatives will often come into play. For example, covering such services as immunizations does not, strictly speaking, fall into the scope of insurance. These benefits are offered for social or legal reasons as well as to save costs due to conditions that would occur absent prevention.

As mentioned at the start of this section, these four conditions apply to any type of insurance. With respect to *health insurance* more specifically, people want indemnification against three events: the cost of the care, the unpredictable outcome of such care, and loss of income due to illness.[6] The true purpose of health insurance is to protect against the first peril. Disability insurance can protect against loss of income from illness. In both these cases, the consumer buys the protection. Providers buy malpractice insurance to protect themselves against the unpredictable outcomes of care (whether due to error or lack of scientific knowledge by the field). While the purchase of liability insurance is not unique to healthcare, the fact that another party is paying for care *is* unique and creates perverse incentives. Consider the following scenario. The provider (e.g., physician) buys insurance from a malpractice insurance company (carrier). Since the provider, carrier, and patient do not want any adverse events to occur, the provider may perform a large number of unnecessary tests, for which a fourth party, the patient's health insurance plan, will pay. Further, the provider gains more revenue from additional services that are performed to reduce the likelihood (however remote) of an adverse event. Such provider activity is called "defensive medicine."[7] Another way providers can minimize their malpractice risk is by case selection (refusing to care for high-risk patients).

Once the above conditions are met and a market is created, customer preferences for an ideal health insurance plan can be explored. Most of these features are explained below.

---

[6] Arrow, K. J. (1963). Uncertainty and the welfare economics of medical care. *The American Economic Review*, *53*, 941–973.

[7] For a more comprehensive discussion of this topic, see *Health Affairs*, September 2010 (Vol. 29 No. 9) special issue on Medical Malpractice and Errors.

Access. As mentioned in the section on strategic trade-offs in Chapter 1, "Understanding and Managing Complex Healthcare Systems," access has several dimensions. The first dimension here concerns the ability of the customer to purchase a health insurance policy. Many provisions of the Patient Protection and Affordable Care Act (ACA) of 2010 enable the majority of uninsured Americans to buy health insurance or be enrolled in a public plan.[8] (The ACA will be discussed in more detail below.) For example: Children until age 26 are eligible under their parents' policies; health plans are not able to exclude applicants based on preexisting conditions (nor charge excessive fees for coverage should the applicant have a costly illness); and Medicaid eligibility is expanded (at the discretion of individual states), with the federal government picking up the entire differential cost of new enrollees for a limited time. However, other access issues remain, originating from such problems as shortages of primary care physicians and selected specialists (see Chapter 5, "Healthcare Professionals"), lack of provider participation with certain health plans, and difficulties getting to sites of care (such as inadequate transportation).

Quality Care. While most people will agree that they want their insurance to offer a network of high-quality providers of services and products, with respect to healthcare, customers often assume that quality is a given characteristic. As a result, they often do not ask questions of, or challenge, healthcare providers.[9] This assumption is not unusual in other aspects of our lives that involve potential life-and-death situations. For example, before a flight, how many airline passengers check the carrier's safety record, review the plane's maintenance record, or interview the pilot? (More will be discussed about quality and how consumers use published information in Chapter 9, "Quality.")

Comprehensive Benefits. It is obvious that people want more rather than fewer benefits. The problem is defining what those benefits are and satisfying the disparate needs of different populations, given budget constraints. The ACA requires that health plans provide certain categories of benefits (including screening and prevention). State mandates, discussed below, also set insurance requirements.

Ease of Administration. This feature concerns such customer services as enrollment, eligibility verification, complaint resolution, and claims payment. In addition to company efforts to provide better customer service, there are laws that set requirements in this area. For example, all states and the District of Columbia have enacted legislation requiring "prompt payment" of healthcare claims, with penalties for noncompliance. Likewise, the federal government requires that companies paying Medicare benefits on their behalf (termed Medicare Administrative Contractors) pay interest on overdue provider payments. Further, the ACA requires an enhanced complaint resolution process.

---

[8] *Patient Protection and Affordable Care Act. Public Law 111-148.* (2010, March 23). Retrieved from https://www.gpo.gov/fdsys/pkg/PLAW-111publ148/pdf/PLAW-111publ148.pdf

[9] Landro, L. (2009, March 4). Finding a way to ask doctors tough questions. *The Wall Street Journal* D1.

Despite insurance company claims that they provide policies to as many people as possible, offer the highest-quality providers and products, cover more benefits than competitors, and are "user friendly" with regard to administrative issues, by and large, health plans do not substantially differ with respect to these attributes. For example, in a given geographic area, there is considerable overlap among plans in provider networks. As well, at the local level, all plans must provide the benefits the marketplace demands and state laws require.

Low Premiums, First-Dollar Coverage, and Freedom to Choose Providers. In order to position their products and meet customers' specific demands, these plans principally distinguish themselves from one another by variations in how they design their payment terms to offer: low premiums, first-dollar coverage, and freedom to choose providers. Ideally, customers do not want to pay a lot for health insurance (low premiums); when they do access the healthcare system for services or products, they do not want to pay much (or anything) out of pocket (deductibles, coinsurance, and/or copayments); and they want to be able to see any provider wherever and whenever they choose. However, *these three features are inextricably linked, so that if customers want to maximize one of them, one or both of the other two need to be reduced.* This customization is costly to price and administer. Since government-sponsored policies are one-size-fits-all, the argument that its administrative costs are much cheaper than private insurance is, therefore, not completely accurate.[10]

The reason for this trade-off stems from an insurance company's need to control for moral hazard: Premiums and out-of-pocket expenses concern patient utilization, while limiting the network addresses provider induced demand. Consider two examples that illustrate the trade-offs customers may make among these three features. First is a mother who believes that she and her family are, by and large, healthy. When they do need healthcare, however, she wants her family to get "the best care" and not have the insurance company dictate where they can go. What she seeks, therefore, are low premiums and freedom of choice of providers. The trade-off is that when a family member does need healthcare, the out-of-pocket expenses may be substantial. Another example is a low-wage employee with chronic health problems who cannot afford high premiums or out-of-pocket expenses for doctor visits or pharmaceutical purchases. This worker might be willing to give up some freedom of choice of providers for the desired economic benefits of lower premiums and lower out-of-pocket costs. The first type of plan mentioned is a preferred provider organization (PPO); the second example is characteristic of a health maintenance organization (HMO). These plans will be discussed in the section on Managed Care below.

---

[10]For a summary of this issue, see Litow, M. (2006). Medicare versus private health insurance: The cost of administration. *Health Watch Newsletter. (52)*, 28-30. Retrieved May 25, 2018 from https://www.soa.org/Library/Newsletters/Health-Watch-Newsletter/2006/May/hwn-2006-iss52-litow.aspx

BACKGROUND AND CURRENT STATUS OF HEALTH INSURANCE IN THE UNITED STATES

Private Health Insurance

Overview. Given the above background, this topic examines the status and structure of the health insurance sector in the United States. First, consider the current insurance coverage of the U.S. population in Exhibit 6.3. The exact percentages in each category are difficult to discern, since large numbers of people are eligible in more than one category. For example, workers over 65 are eligible for Medicare, though they may be receiving benefits from their employer; working veterans may have private coverage as well as government benefits; and 11.7 million people are enrolled in both Medicare and Medicaid.[11]

EXHIBIT 6.3. **Percentage of People by Type of Health Insurance Coverage—2016**

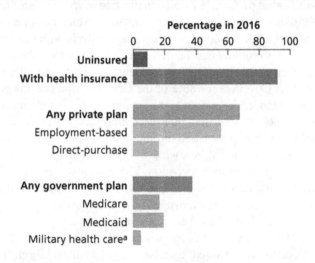

[a] Military healthcare includes TRICARE and CHAMPVA (Civilian Health and Medical Program of the Department of Veterans Affairs), as well as care provided by the Department of Veterans Affairs and the military.

Source: Barnett, J. C., & Berchick, E. R. (2017, September). *Health insurance coverage in the United States: 2016 U.S. Census Bureau current population reports.* Retrieved May 25, 2018, from https://www.census.gov/content/dam/Census/library/publications/2017/demo/p60-260.pdf

---

[11]CMS. (2018, February). *People enrolled in Medicare and Medicaid. Fact sheet.* Retrieved May 25, 2018, from https://www.cms.gov/Medicare-Medicaid-Coordination/Medicare-and-Medicaid-Coordination/Medicare-Medicaid-Coordination-Office/Downloads/MMCO_Factsheet.pdf

Of particular concern are the *number* and *percentage* of uninsured, which rose dramatically prior to the ACA's implementation in 2014. After this law became operational, the number of uninsured decreased, but it has risen again (though not to the extent before the law). More will be said about this effect below. One must offer a caution in interpreting the data on the uninsured: Figures are often only for those who did not have *any* coverage *during the entire year*; the number would be much larger if it included persons who were uninsured for only part of a year. Figures also do not include others who are "underinsured" (i.e., those who have insurance coverage with benefits or dollar limits that are not sufficient for their healthcare needs). While the ACA is designed to reduce these numbers, it is unclear how it is addressing the adequacy of benefits.

In order to make sense of this complex "system," all of these categories of insurance are discussed below. Each section will begin with its historical development in order to: (a) explain why the current system is structured and operates as it does; (b) discuss what has been tried and why it succeeded or failed; and (c) perhaps most importantly, highlight that healthcare changes, like other social movements, are part of larger trends in the social, political and economic arenas.

Origins and Current Status of Private Health Insurance in the United States

Development of Employer-Sponsored Health Insurance. Since most people in the United States are insured through their employer, we begin our analysis with this sector. Many consider the prevalence of this employment-based health insurance to be both a unique feature of the American healthcare system as well as a recent (and undesirable) arrangement. Neither is true. For example: Coverage for 88% of the German population is provided through private sickness funds financed by workers and employers;[12] Canadian coverage for non-governmental benefits (such as outpatient pharmaceuticals) is often provided by employers; and Argentine benefits are largely provided through the workplace but are union rather than employer sponsored. As mentioned above, work-based social welfare schemes originated in ancient times and were organized by occupation. These arrangements developed further in the Middle Ages when guilds provided medical, disability, and social support to members and their families when an illness, injury, disability, or death occurred.[13]

This private support took hold in America in the 19th century, when social benefits began to be provided by such groups as mutual benefit associations and fraternal benefit societies. These organizations charged members regular dues in return for providing benefits and were usually established according to nationality and religious affiliation. (This history accounts for the starting point of many hospitals named "Swedish-American," "Norwegian-American," "French," etc., as well as ones named after religions and religious orders.) By the late 19th century, similar associations developed in the workplace and were sponsored by employees, employees *and* employers, and (rarely) solely by employers. Initially, the main purpose of these associations was to provide cash payments for disability

---

[12]OECD. *State of health in the EU: Germany. Country health profile, 2017.* Retrieved May 26, 2018, from https://ec.europa.eu/health/sites/health/files/state/docs/chp_de_english.pdf

[13]For more examples and a deeper understanding of the development of the U.S. healthcare system see Starr, P. (1982). *The social transformation of American medicine.* New York: Basic Books.

and death; rarely were medical benefits provided. When medical benefits began to be offered, these associations hired physicians to care for members (usually on a prepaid/capitated basis) and to provide advice and certification of disability. An early example of this type of plan was the Pacific Railway Beneficial Association, founded in 1882. When labor unions became more prominent and powerful in the late 19th century, they started to provide death and disability benefits for their members; health benefits came decades later.

The first employer-sponsored group health policy is generally considered to date from 1912, when Montgomery Ward & Co. purchased such coverage from the Equitable Life Assurance Society of the United States, now part of AXA Equitable. (Actually, Equitable sold the first policy the previous year to the Pantasote Leather Company.) The concept was adopted by other companies so rapidly that, in the same year, the National Convention of Insurance Commissioners (now the National Association of Insurance Commissioners [NAIC]) was formed to provide guidance to states about regulating health insurance. At this point it is pertinent to recognize the general climate of this country that brought about these changes. Recall that the first two decades of the 20th century were times of rapid economic growth and intense social reform. Examples of significant events included:

- Ida Tarbell published a series of articles in *McClure's* magazine (subsequently complied as "The History of the Standard Oil Company") to expose the corruption and greed of the Standard Oil Monopoly (1902–1904).

- Upton Sinclair published *The Jungle* (1906), exposing problems in the meat-packing industry. The resultant social uproar was responsible for passage of the Pure Food and Drugs Act (1906) and the Meat Inspection Act (1906). It also ushered in the era of what President Theodore Roosevelt called "muckraking" journalism.

- President Taft used the Sherman Antitrust Act to break up the Standard Oil trust and American Tobacco Company (1911).

- The International Ladies Garment Workers Union (ILGWU) provided the first union-based medical services (1913).

- Congress passed the Clayton Antitrust Act to supplement the Sherman Act (1914).

- The federal government established the Federal Trade Commission (1914).

These events highlight the nurturing and protective climate that allowed healthcare changes to occur and take root. The successful healthcare strategist needs to be able to read the current social climate and assess the need a particular product or service will fill and whether the market is ready to embrace the changes.

Origins of Blue Cross/Blue Shield Plans. The next major innovation in healthcare coverage occurred in 1929. In order to reduce bad debt, Baylor Hospital, in Dallas, offered the city's school teachers a prepaid health plan consisting of 21 days of in-hospital care for 50 cents per month. The stock market crash in October of 1929, with its resulting unemployment and bankruptcies, provided further impetus for the spread of such plans; by implementing prepaid insurance schemes, hospitals tried to avoid potential bad debts.

Several features of this plan are noteworthy. First, a hospital was dealing directly with customers, instead of through an insurance intermediary. Second, the mechanism was pre-payment (i.e., the hospital got paid whether or not the customer was admitted). Third, this arrangement is generally considered to be the birth of Blue Cross plans, as will be described below.

While such an arrangement seems like a good idea for both hospitals and customers, two issues arose that transformed these plans. The first was practical: The health contract was between the purchaser and a *particular* hospital. If the insured customers became ill and needed care out of that hospital's service area, they would not be covered. Second, since these contracts were a form of health insurance, they were subject to regulation by state insurance commissions. In order to deal with these issues, hospitals came together in each state to form nonprofit companies (frequently sponsored by state hospital associations) that were regulated by the respective state's insurance department. In return for the benefits of nonprofit status, the insurance departments required open enrollment (whereby members were free to sign up on a rolling basis without screening) and community rating. *Community rating* means that within a specified locale, all are charged the same premium for insurance, regardless of health status; the opposite method is called individual (or risk rating), where persons are charged based on their health history or risk. The states' insurance departments regulated premiums in a manner like utility rate control boards. In 1931, these plans negotiated the first hospital discounts. By 1933, there were 16 hospital-sponsored plans nationwide that covered 35,000 members. Today, Blue Cross and Blue Shield plans comprise about 36 independent companies that cover more than 100 million people in all 50 states, the District of Columbia, and Puerto Rico.

In order to enhance chances for success, all these state-based plans recognized the need to brand the product. According to the Blue Cross/Blue Shield Association:[14]

> In 1934, E.A. van Steenwyk, executive secretary with the forerunner to Blue Cross and Blue Shield of Minnesota, identified his hospital care program with a solid blue Greek cross design. The symbol began to show up in other parts of the country and soon, as one historian has written, the Blue Cross "perpetuated itself as a unifying force" among the newly emerging Plans.

The brand symbol was adapted from the logo of the American Hospital Association (AHA). (In fact, it incorporated the AHA logo in its center until 1973.) By linking this symbol with the trusted hospital sector, these plans were able to inspire customer confidence. In an example of shared branding, in 1939, the AHA began using the Blue Cross symbol to identify health plans across the country that met certain standards. The AHA continued to administer the use of the symbol until the Blue Cross Association was founded in 1960.

---

[14]Lichtenstein, M. *Health insurance from invention to innovation: A history of the Blue Cross and Blue Shield companies.* Retrieved May 26, 2018, from https://www.bcbs.com/the-health-of-america/articles/health-insurance-invention-innovation-history-blue-cross-and-blue

The association's purpose is to: evaluate and grant franchises to insurers to use the Blue Cross (and subsequently also Blue Shield) brand; provide technical support to member plans; coordinate national accounts (employers who have employees for whom they purchase health insurance and are located in multiple states); and conduct and evaluate health services and policy research.

Shortly after these hospital plans began forming, similar ones came into being to cover benefits for physician services. The first such physician plans were prepaid systems in the lumber and mining camps of the Pacific Northwest. Another early example was the California Physicians Service Incorporated (the forerunner of Blue Shield of California), which, in 1939, charged members $1.20 to $1.70 per month.[15] The plans that covered physician services also pursued a branding strategy. Again, according to the Blue Cross/Blue Shield Association:[16]

> The Blue Shield symbol was devised in Buffalo, New York. Carl Metzger, an early pioneer in the Blue movement, wanted a design that would distinguish the new medical service plan. He also wanted to make sure that there was an obvious link to the companion hospital plan. It soon flourished among the growing number of Blue Shield Plans.

The well-known logo that resulted was a shield with the staff of Aesculapius (Greek god of healing and symbol of the American Medical Association) in its center. The blue color linked these plans to their hospital counterparts, though they were separate legal entities. (The associations of these plans formally merged in 1982.) (Please see Exhibit 6.4.)

EXHIBIT 6.4. Evolution of Blue Cross and Blue Shield Logos

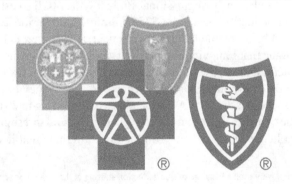

---

[15]Recall that the original Baylor Hospital plan only cost 50 cents per month. To explain this discrepancy, you should understand that most care at that time was delivered in settings outside of the hospital and, thus, total insurance expenses for these services could be higher than those for hospital care. While most care is still delivered outside the hospital, overall costs, excluding pharmaceutical expenses, are now higher for hospital care.

[16]Lichtenstein, M. *Health insurance from invention to innovation* op. cit.

It is important to note that when nonprofit corporations replaced direct hospital and physician organization contracts with patients, the financial arrangement changed from pre-payment to one of discount fee-for-service (FFS). That is, providers were no longer collecting prepaid fees but were paid according to a discounted fee schedule after they rendered services to patients.

Tax-exempt Status of Health Insurance. From 1939 to 1949, the social, political, and economic changes that affected our country profoundly altered the health insurance industry in ways that are still with us. The first transforming event was passage of the Revenue Act of 1939 (Section 104) that granted tax-exempt status to employees for compensation they received from workers' compensation or accident or *health insurance* as a result of injury and/or sickness. Employers were also able to deduct these costs as business expenses.[17] However, this exemption applied only to large companies, not small businesses.[18] Since these smaller firms and their owner-employees need the financial subsidy more than large corporations, the stage was set early on for health insurance to be unaffordable for them.

The tax treatment of health insurance is so important that its significance requires further explanation. Since employers are able to deduct health insurance premiums as expenses, and since these benefits are not taxable to employees (as are wages and other benefits, such as tuition reimbursement), many policy analysts believe this situation results in excessive employee demands for coverage and discourages employers from prudent purchasing. For example, while the average family coverage in 2009 cost $13,375, managing directors and top executives at Goldman Sachs received a package estimated at about $40,000.[19] In fact, employers prefer to offer more health benefits instead of higher salaries. The reason for this preference is that higher salaries result in greater expenses for such items as unemployment taxes, the employer portion of Medicare taxes, and possibly salary-based employer contributions to retirement funds. The Congressional Budget Office (CBO) estimates that the lost revenue from this tax deductibility will be $757 billion for the period 2019 to 2028.[20] It is the largest single tax subsidy by the federal government. (Please see Exhibit 6.5.)

Policy makers argue that removing this subsidy would encourage more prudent purchasing of insurance policies and the use of healthcare services. Further, tax revenues that would result from elimination of the subsidy could create a pool of money to finance care for the uninsured. To address these issues, the ACA mandates that, starting in 2018, a 40% tax[21] will be levied on the value of health plans that exceed specified federal threshold amounts for individual and family policies. One problem with the tax formula is that it was not adequately

---

[17] Of note is that, while employers took advantage of this deduction starting at that time, it was only officially sanctioned by the Revenue Act of 1954 (Sec. 106).

[18] For example, "IRS Publication 15-B (2018), Employer's Tax Guide to Fringe Benefits" instructs that owners of a 2% or greater share in a Subchapter S corporation cannot deduct such fringe benefits as healthcare. Retrieved from https://www.irs.gov/pub/irs-pdf/p15b.pdf.Retrieved

[19] Abelson, R. (2009, September 21). A tax on Cadillac health plans may slso hit the Chevys. *New York Times*, A17.

[20] CBO, *The budget and economic outlook: 2018 to 2028*. Retrieved May 26, 2018, from https://www.cbo.gov/system/files/115th-congress-2017-2018/reports/53651-outlook.pdf

[21] The tax was postponed until 2020.

EXHIBIT 6.5. Largest Tax Expenditures in 2017

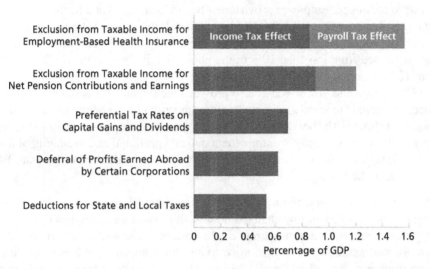

Source: CBO (2017, March). *Tax expenditures*. Retrieved May 26, 2018, from https://www.cbo.gov/publication/52493

indexed to account for inflation and rising healthcare costs. Opponents of this measure point out that the designated amounts will, therefore, increasingly include more of the middle class and make insurance more expensive for them. Unlike similar taxes on luxury items and "gas-guzzler" autos, where the purchaser pays the tariff, the assessment is on the *issuer* of the health insurance policy, which in the case of a self-insured plan is the employer.

Acceleration of Employer-Sponsored Insurance. The labor situation that resulted from America's entry into World War II also accelerated changes in the availability and spread of employer-sponsored health insurance. Four events, in particular, contributed to these changes.

1. The men drafted into the military left families behind who did not have health insurance.[22]

2. In order to replace these men, women entered the workforce in unprecedented numbers and performed jobs traditionally done by them.

3. With wartime unemployment at a low of 1.2%, employers were competing for employees.

4. In order to prevent inflation, the War Board imposed a wage and price freeze but exempted fringe benefits, such as health insurance.

[22]Coverage for military families only became law in 1956 with passage of the Dependents Medical Care Act.

Given these circumstances, healthcare benefits became one of the methods by which employers competed for workers. When men returned to the workforce after the war, these benefits were continued. Employer provision of health insurance got a further boost in 1949 when the U.S. Supreme Court upheld a National Labor Relations Board ruling that employee benefits are subject to collective bargaining. As a result of all these changes, health insurance coverage increased from less than 10% of the population in 1940 to nearly 70% in 1955, a rise from 12.3 million to over 100 million people.[23]

The Depression and World War II also provided the impetus for another form of health insurance, the prepaid medical group model (forerunner of current health maintenance organizations, or HMOs).[24] The best known, and still largest, of these plans is Kaiser-Permanente. The story of this plan is a study in entrepreneurship and profound understanding of the marketplace.[25] Today more than 8.6 million people are covered by Kaiser-Permanente. We will discuss HMOs in the Managed Care section below.

Regulation of Insurance and the McCarran-Ferguson Act. In this same period, a Supreme Court ruling and subsequent law changed how health insurance is regulated. In 1944, the federal government brought suit against South-Eastern Underwriters under the Sherman Antitrust Act for, among other things, price fixing; the company had a 90% market share of the fire insurance and "allied lines" in the six states from where the suit originated. The case made its way to the Supreme Court, where Justice Hugo Black wrote for the majority. Because of the importance of this decision for regulation of health insurance, the opinion will be quoted at length:

> For seventy-five years this Court has held, whenever the question has been presented, that the Commerce Clause of the Constitution does not deprive the individual states of power to regulate and tax specific activities of foreign insurance companies which sell policies within their territories. Each state has been held to have this power even though negotiation and execution of the companies' policy contracts involved communications of information and movements of persons, moneys, and papers across state lines. Not one of all these cases, however, has involved an Act of Congress which required the Court to decide the issue of whether the Commerce Clause grants to Congress the power to regulate insurance transactions stretching across state lines. Today for the first time in the history of the Court that issue is squarely presented and must be decided...

> The kind of interference with the free play of competitive forces with which the appellees are charged is exactly the type of conduct which the Sherman Act has outlawed for American "trade or commerce" among the states. Appellees have not argued otherwise. Their ... defense ... has been that they are not required to conform to the standards of business conduct established by the Sherman Act because "the business of fire insurance

---

[23]Thomasson, M. A. (2002). From sickness to health: The twentieth-century development of U.S. Health Insurance. *Explorations in Economic History, 39*, 233–253

[24]Mayer, T. R., & Mayer, G. G. (1985). HMOs: origins and development. *The New England Journal of Medicine, 312*, 590–594.

[25]Kaiser Permanente. *Our history*. Retrieved May 26, 2018, from http://xnet.kp.org/newscenter/aboutkp/historyofkp.html

is not commerce..." [P]ower to govern intercourse among the states remains where the Constitution placed it. That power, as held by this Court from the beginning, is vested in the Congress, available to be exercised for the national welfare as Congress shall deem necessary. No commercial enterprise of any kind which conducts its activities across state lines has been held to be wholly beyond the regulatory power of Congress under the Commerce Clause. We cannot make an exception of the business of insurance...

Having power to enact the Sherman Act, Congress did so; if exceptions are to be written into the Act, they must come from the Congress, not this Court.[26]

This decision, therefore, established Congress's ability to regulate insurance, unless it decides to delegate this power to the states—which it subsequently did. On the heels of this ruling, Senators Pat McCarran (D-NV) and Homer Ferguson (R-MI) sponsored such a bill. Enacted on March 9, 1945, Public Law 79–15 (called the McCarran-Ferguson Act) states:

the Congress hereby declares that the continued regulation and taxation by the several States of the business of insurance is in the public interest, and that silence on the part of the Congress shall not be construed to impose any barrier to the regulation or taxation of such business by the several States.

SEC 2.

(a)   The business of insurance, and every person engaged therein, shall be subject to the laws of the several States which relate to the regulation or taxation of such business.

(b)   No Act of Congress shall be construed to invalidate, impair, or supersede any law enacted by any State for the purpose of regulating the business of insurance, or which imposes a fee or tax upon such business, unless such Act specifically relates to the business of insurance:

> *Provided*, That after January 1, 1948, the Act of July 2, 1890, as amended, known as the Sherman Act, and the Act of October 15, 1914, as amended, known as the Clayton Act, and the Act of September 26, 1914, known as the Federal Trade Commission Act, as amended, shall be applicable to the business of insurance to the extent that such business is not regulated by State law...

Nothing contained in this Act shall render the said Sherman Act inapplicable to any agreement to boycott, coerce, or intimidate, or act of boycott, coercion, or intimidation.

Specifically, the act provides *limited* exemption for insurance companies from the federal antitrust legislation that applies to most businesses (such as certain information sharing) and allows states to regulate, tax, and license insurance.

Employee Retirement and Income Security Act. As employer-sponsored insurance became more prevalent in the 1950s and 1960s, and the costs of this benefit began to rise, companies investigated other ways to provide coverage. In 1968, Firestone Tire and Rubber Co. started

---

[26] United States v. South-Eastern Underwriters, 322 U.S. 533 (1944). Retrieved May 26, 2018, from https://supreme.justia .com/cases/federal/us/322/533/case.html

to self-fund health benefits; instead of paying premiums to an insurance company, the firm decided to pay for healthcare out of current income and reserves. This self-funding movement accelerated after passage of the Employee Retirement and Income Security Act (ERISA) of 1974. (Please see Exhibit 6.6 for a brief description of this very important act.)

While the main purpose of ERISA is to ensure that employees receive the benefits to which they are entitled and that they are administered in a fiscally responsible manner, one portion of the law (Section 514) provides incentives for companies to self-fund health insurance benefits. Before explaining these incentives, recall that health insurance is established by laws of each state and is regulated by states' respective departments of insurance. Since ERISA is a *federal law*, companies that set up health plans under *its* terms are exempt from many state laws and regulations. It should be noted that the ACA amended title I of ERISA, by adding a new Section 715, which makes these plans subject to provisions in the Act (explained below).

Even given the new ACA requirements, the advantages to self-insurance persist and include:[27]

- *No state tax on insurance premiums.* These taxes are incorporated in the prices health insurance plans charge companies and can be 2% to 3% of their cost.

- *Exemption from state financial reserve requirements.* Insurance companies must set aside certain liquid financial reserves. Since these reserves may not earn as much as those invested for a longer time, the insurance company has lost potential income. This potential loss is passed along to the customer in the form of higher premiums. Self-insured

EXHIBIT 6.6. ERISA

The goal of Title I of ERISA is to protect the interests of participants and their beneficiaries in employee benefit plans. Among other things, ERISA requires that sponsors of private employee benefit plans provide participants and beneficiaries with adequate information regarding their plans. Also, those individuals who manage plans (and other fiduciaries) must meet certain standards of conduct, derived from the common law of trusts and made applicable (with certain modifications) to all fiduciaries. The law also contains detailed provisions for reporting to the government and disclosure to participants. Furthermore, there are civil enforcement provisions aimed at assuring that plan funds are protected and that participants who qualify receive their benefits.

ERISA covers pension plans and welfare benefit plans (e.g., employment-based medical and hospitalization benefits, apprenticeship plans, and other plans described in Section 3(1) of Title I). Plan sponsors must design and administer their plans in accordance with ERISA. Title II of ERISA contains standards that must be met by employee pension benefit plans in order to qualify for favorable tax treatment. Noncompliance with these tax qualification requirements of ERISA may result in disqualification of a plan and/or other penalties.

Source: Employee Benefit Security Administration. U.S. Department of Labor. *History of EBSA and ERISA*. Retrieved May 26, 2018, from https://www.dol.gov/agencies/ebsa/about-ebsa/about-us/history-of-ebsa-and-erisa

---

[27]Brown, RE: Access to health insurance in the US Medical Care Review *46*:349-385, 1989.

businesses are not subject to the same reserve requirements, though they must display Department of Labor–defined fiduciary responsibility in administering these funds.[28]

■ *Exemption from contribution to state risk pools*. States typically require insurance plans to make contributions to two special funds. One fund is maintained by the state in order to pay creditors of any plan that becomes insolvent. Prior to the ACA, the second contribution subsidized state-sponsored health insurance for those who could not obtain or afford private coverage because of a debilitating preexisting condition (e.g., diabetes, heart disease, cancer, or HIV/AIDS). (These plans are often called Catastrophic Health Insurance Plans, or CHIPs; they are not to be confused with the *federally* sponsored Children's Health Insurance Program, formerly called S-CHIP, described below. The ACA has provisions for expanding these catastrophic plans.) Since insurance companies must contribute to these pools, they pass along the costs to their customers. Self-insured plans do not have the obligation to contribute to these funds.

■ *Full access to claims data*. One of the major complaints that employers have had with health insurance companies is that they do not provide enough data about the healthcare costs/utilization of their employees. Of course, insurance companies are reluctant to give too much information because of the proprietary nature of their provider contracts; also, disclosing costs may work against them when they negotiate employer premiums and provider payment rates. In addition to cost savings gained by better information, when employers self-insure they are caught between the risk of invading individual employee privacy and their interest in improving the health status of all workers. Self-insurance increases risk of the former but also facilitates the latter.

■ *Ability to pay claims after they are received*. Businesses pay insurance premiums in advance of the period of coverage. The insurance company then invests the money until claims must be paid. If a company is self-insured, it can hold the money it would have paid for premiums and keep the investment income until claims payments are due.

■ *No broker commissions*. Many insurance companies sell policies through brokers, who receive commissions of several percentage points on sale of the account and bonuses on renewals. If companies self-insure, they avoid these fees that the insurance plans must include in their premiums.

■ *Exemption from state-mandated benefits*.[29] This feature is, perhaps, the most important and most often cited benefit of self-insurance. The three mandate categories are: benefit mandates (requiring the plans to provide certain benefits, like behavioral health

---

[28] United States Department of Labor: Fiduciary Responsibilities. Retrieved May 26, 2018 from http://www.dol.gov/dol/topic/retirement/fiduciaryresp.htm

[29] References: National Conference of State Legislatures' Health Policy Tracking Service in *Healthcare Financial Management* 57: 14(2), 2003; Bunce, V. C., & Wieske, J. P. (2012). Health insurance mandates in the states 2011 (monograph) prepared for the Council for Affordable Health Insurance (now America's Health Insurance Plans); Jensen, G. A. & Morrisey, M. A. (1999). Mandated benefit laws and employer-sponsored health insurance. (Monograph). Prepared for the Health Insurance Association of America (now America's Health Insurance Plans).

services); provider mandates (requiring the plans to include certain classes of providers in its approved network, e.g., chiropractors and nurse midwives); and process mandates (requiring the plans to do certain things, like pay claims within a specified time period or allow women to stay in the hospital for 48 hours after delivery).[30] Insurance plans can and do charge their clients extra for these benefits. For the 50 states and District of Columbia, the most popular mandates (and how many states/DC require them) are: breast reconstruction after mastectomy for cancer (51), minimum hospital stay after childbirth (50), mammography (50), diabetic supplies (47), and alcoholism treatment (47). Parenthetically, mandatory coverage for prostate cancer and cervical cancer screening are required in only 36 and 31 states, respectively. At the other end of the spectrum is compulsory coverage for treatments and products that do not meet the definition of insurable conditions and resulted from special interest lobbying. For example, coverage for: "hair prostheses" (i.e., wigs) for chemotherapy patients (11) and athletic trainers (3). Depending on the number and type of these mandates, they can add several percentage points to the cost of premiums. Self-insured companies can design their own benefit package, free from these state mandate requirements; but, as mentioned, they are subject to ACA requirements for coverage of "Essential Health Benefits" (discussed below) and nondiscrimination laws. Regarding the latter, while firms can exclude non–federally required benefits, they cannot illegally discriminate against individuals or classes of people. For example, in 1988, the convenience store chain Circle K was sued when it decided to exclude healthcare benefits related to alcohol, drugs, and HIV infection for new employees. Since the plan was organized under ERISA and applied to *all* employees, the court decided these exclusions were permissible. (Public pressure subsequently forced the company to rescind these restrictions.)

▪ *Standardize benefits for national companies.* Companies with a national presence find it easier to administer standard benefits (not just what is covered but terms of coverage, like out-of-pocket expenses) for all employees, particularly if there is a labor union contract. This standardization is very difficult if companies must buy local policies subject to numerous state mandates.

Most companies do not have the wherewithal to contract with a provider network, manage benefits, pay claims, or purchase reinsurance to cover a catastrophically costly illness. In order to be able to set up a self-funded program, they contract with healthcare businesses (usually traditional health insurance companies) to help them manage these functions. Such contracts are called administrative service only (ASO) agreements, and the businesses that manage them are termed third-party administrators (TPAs). The difference between traditional insurance and ASO contracts is that in the former, insurance companies bear the financial risk, while with the latter, the employers are held accountable. Please see Exhibit 6.7 and note that the majority of all firms (60%) in the United States have a self-insurance program, with participation significantly higher among businesses with more than 1,000 employees.

---

[30]Bunce, V. C. (2011). Council for Affordable Health Insurance: Health insurance mandates in the states. Retrieved May 26, 2018, from https://lintvwpri.files.wordpress.com/2013/10/mandatesinthestates2011execsumm.pdf

EXHIBIT 6.7. **Percentage of Covered Workers in Partially or Completely Self-Funded Plans, by Firm Size, 2017**

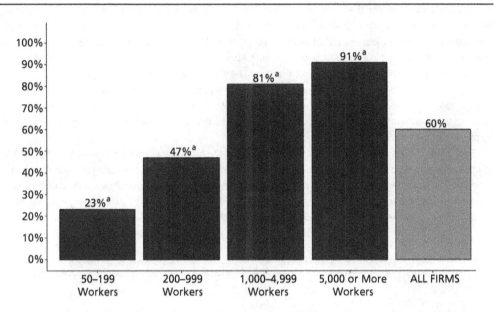

[a] Estimate is statistically different from estimate for the previous year shown ($p <.05$).

Source: Kaiser Family Foundation (2017). *Employer health benefits survey. Section 10: Plan funding.* Retrieved May 26, 2018, from https://www.kff.org/report-section/ehbs-2017-section-10-plan-funding/#figure101

Consider the important implications of ERISA plans for costs in the open health insurance marketplace. When providers, suppliers, and potential patients lobby at the state level for passage of laws that will add insurance mandates, these laws apply only to those who purchase insurance policies (i.e., mostly small companies and individuals). Since those purchasers are the ones who can least afford insurance, such laws exacerbate affordability problems in what is termed the "small group market."

Consolidated Omnibus Reconciliation Act. Despite rising healthcare costs and fluctuations in the economy in the 1980s, most employers continued employee healthcare coverage. The public policy question that took on increased significance was this: What do you do if you are no longer eligible to receive employer-sponsored health insurance? This predicament was addressed by laws that were passed decades apart: the Consolidated Omnibus Reconciliation Act (COBRA-1985), the Health Insurance Portability and Accountability Act (HIPAA-1996), and ACA (2010). (Please see Exhibit 6.8 for basic descriptions of the former two laws.) COBRA can help an employee and his/her dependents obtain health insurance if the insured is fired, laid off, or dies. The problem for the insured is that the employer is no longer required to pay for its share of the premiums and can charge the employee or dependents up to 102% of the cost of the policy. This amount is often out of the financial reach of families whose breadwinner just lost a job or died. To address this problem during the

EXHIBIT 6.8. COBRA and HIPAA (Insurance Provisions)

The COBRA gives workers and their families who lose their health benefits the right to choose to continue group health benefits provided by their group health plan for limited periods of time under certain circumstances such as voluntary or involuntary job loss, reduction in the hours worked, transition between jobs, death, divorce, and other life events. Qualified individuals may be required to pay the entire premium for coverage up to 102% of the cost to the plan. COBRA generally requires that group health plans sponsored by employers with 20 or more employees in the prior year offer employees and their families the opportunity for a temporary extension of health coverage (called continuation coverage) in certain instances where coverage under the plan would otherwise end. COBRA outlines how employees and family members may elect continuation coverage. It also requires employers and plans to provide notice.

The HIPAA provides rights and protections for participants and beneficiaries in group health plans. The HIPAA includes protections for coverage under group health plans that limit exclusions for preexisting conditions; prohibit discrimination against employees and dependents based on their health status; and allow a special opportunity to enroll in a new plan to individuals in certain circumstances. The HIPAA may also furnish the right to purchase individual coverage if the employee has no group health plan coverage available and has exhausted COBRA or other continuation coverage.

Source: United States Department of Labor. Retrieved May 26, 2018, from https://www.dol.gov/agencies/ebsa/workers-and-families/changing-jobs-and-job-loss and https://www.dol.gov/agencies/ebsa/about-ebsa/our-activities/resource-center/faqs/hipaa-consumer

economic downturn in 2009, the federal government provided funds to specified persons for a limited time that covered 65% of COBRA premiums. Of note is that many believe COBRA became irrelevant with implementation of the ACA; however, anecdotal reports indicate that COBRA may provide better benefits at a lower cost than the ACA's insurance Exchanges. The reason is that large companies often negotiate very favorable financial terms with insurance companies, and former employees can take advantage of these deals. The drawbacks are that COBRA's benefits are time-limited, and beneficiaries are locked into the last plan they had before leaving their employer.

Health Insurance Portability and Accountability Act. The Health Insurance Portability and Accountability Act (HIPAA) was passed, in part, to help solve another problem: an employee's inability to transfer insurance coverage between jobs. For example, under HIPAA, if an employer has a waiting period for the start of insurance benefits and the new employee satisfied this requirement during a prior job, the wait is waived. This law was supposed to diminish circumstances of "job lock," where an employee feared losing benefits in a change of employment. The problem with this act is that the new employer did not need to offer any health insurance or may have had a different benefit package from the one the employee enjoyed at the prior job.

The provisions of the ACA that deal with coverage for those without employer benefits are discussed below; in particular, they involve the requirement of certain employers to furnish health insurance for their employees.

Personal Healthcare Spending Accounts. Another form of insurance was made possible by the HIPAA: Medical Savings Accounts (MSAs). Because of the strong backing of Bill Archer, then the chairman of the House Ways and Means Committee, the plans are called Archer MSAs. While MSAs existed for a number of years in some states, HIPAA established federal parameters for setting up these accounts and the conditions for funding them with pretax income.

Before describing MSAs further, it should be noted that prior to the existence of such plans, the only other tax-exempt arrangement available to employees were Flexible Spending Accounts (FSAs). These accounts, funded by employees using pretax money pledged before the start of a given calendar year, are used to pay for eligible expenses that occur in the successive calendar year. The federal government determines the maximum amount that can be put aside tax-free as well as what can be paid from the account. Eligible reimbursements include amounts due from coinsurance and deductibles and certain items not covered under insurance benefits (such as eyeglasses). The problem with such accounts is that if one does not use the savings in the designated year, the money does not carry over into the following one; any excess amounts go to the federal government. Likewise, if one changes jobs during the calendar year, any unused funds do not follow to the next employer. The federal government allows a choice of two extensions to the "use it or lose it" rule: Employers can offer the option to carry over up to $500 from the previous year into the next year's FSA or can extend the period for which funds can be used by 2 ½ months beyond the close of the plan year (March 15 if the FSA plan is on a calendar year).

Businesses that provide products or services eligible under FSAs but not covered by traditional insurance should develop a marketing strategy timed to when employees make their allocation decisions. Unlike the situation with impulse buying, marketing in this category must begin in the year *prior* to anticipated use, since that is when the potential customer will decide to set aside funds. One such example is orthodontics. However, impulse buying does occur at the end of the year when employees find unspent funds that "must" be used. For example, eyeglass sellers can have an increase in business at year's end.

MSAs are very different from FSAs in a number of respects. MSAs started as an experiment to see whether making individuals more accountable for their health expenses reduced the overall costs of care. This goal was to be accomplished by having individuals save their own money (in a savings account) and use it to cover a large deductible before their insurance started to pay. Recall this issue from the prior discussion of the RAND Health Insurance Experiment: As a person's out-of-pocket expenses increase (in this case through high deductibles), overall utilization and spending are reduced. The first MSAs had limited eligibility: self-employed persons and workers in companies with 50 or fewer employees. The key operational feature of MSAs is the requirement that the coverage has to be by a High Deductible Health Plan (HDHP). (Please see Exhibit 6.9 for terms of this and other personal spending schemes.) Once this plan is established, the employer or employee (but not both in a given year) can contribute money to the MSA. Like FSAs, there are limits on the amount of the contribution; unlike the FSA, however, contributions can be made any time prior to when the previous year's income tax is due (exclusive of extensions), and *all* remaining funds can

EXHIBIT 6.9. Personal Healthcare Spending Accounts

Type of Plan / Characteristics	Flexible Spending Account (FSA) IRC § 125	Medical Savings Account (MSA) IRC § 220(b) and (c) AKA "Archer" MSA	Health Reimbursement Arrangement (HRA) IRC § 105(h), 419	Health Savings Account (HSA) IRC § 223(c)(2)(A)
Who is eligible?	Anyone who works for an employer having such a plan	Self-employed and those working for employers with ≤50 employees	Any self-employed person or employer group, regardless of size	Any self-employed person or employer group, regardless of size; cannot be a dependent on another's tax return, e.g., children or spouses
Who funds the account?	Usually employee	Employer or employee (but not both in a given year)	Employer	Employer and/or employee
What are the annual financial requirements for contribution or nature of the underlying insurance?	For 2019: Health Care Flexible Spending Account (HCFSA) maximum/minimum $2700/$0 per employee regardless of the number of dependents covered. Covers eligible expenses not covered by health insurance. A "Limited HCFSA" can be set up by those with an HSA to reimburse dental and vision expenses not covered by the plan. Generally, contributed amounts that are not spent by the end of the plan year are forfeited	Employee must have a "high deductible" plan; minimum and maximum limits and out of pocket limits subject to federal regulation. For 2019: the deductibles must be a minimum/maximum of $2350/$3500 for individual coverage and $4650/$7000 for family; the out-of-pocket maximum is $4650 for individual coverage and $8550 for family coverage.	None.	Employee must have a "high deductible" plan; For calendar year 2019: a "high deductible health plan" is defined as a health plan with an annual deductible that is not less than $1350 for self-only coverage or $2700 for family coverage, and the annual out-of-pocket expenses (deductibles, copayments, and other amounts, but not premiums) do not exceed $6750 for self-only coverage or $13,500 for family coverage.

Are contributions federally tax exempt if used for "qualified" expenses?	Yes	Yes	Yes	Yes
Can the unused contributions be carried into the next year?	No	Yes	Yes	Yes
Can the employee take the unused contributions to a new job?	No	Yes	No	Yes
The annual limitation on tax deductions is $3500 for self-only coverage and $7000 for family coverage. (Plus "catch up" of $1000 for those over 55.)				

For annual amounts and limits, check www.irs.gov.

be rolled over to the new year. Also, unlike FSAs, MSAs are the property of the insured and can be transferred to another job or maintained if the beneficiary is unemployed. (If the new employer does not have an MSA, the beneficiary cannot continue to contribute but can spend down the accumulated amount or roll the funds over into an eligible Health Savings Account [HSA], described below). The MSA contributions can be used to pay expenses similar to those allowed for FSAs. While funds cannot usually be used to cover premiums, they can be used to buy coverage under COBRA, qualified long-term care insurance, and/or traditional health insurance (if the person is unemployed). Although the HIPAA provision authorizing MSAs was extended by the Consolidated Appropriations Act of 2001 (passed in 2000), the U.S. Treasury Department did not extend authorization for new accounts after December 31, 2008. MSA participants can continue their contributions and use of such plans or roll them over into an HSA.

In 2002, a variant of FSAs emerged called Health Reimbursement Arrangements (or Accounts) (HRAs). These plans are funded solely by the employer from general revenues and have no funding requirements. Like MSAs, funds not used in a given year can be rolled over into the next year; used to reimburse employees for qualified medical expenses; and pay for health coverage for current employees and retirees or for those who qualify under COBRA. Unlike MSAs, however, accumulated amounts are not held in trust for the employee and therefore cannot be transferred with job changes.

The Medicare Prescription Drug, Improvement, and Modernization Act of 2003 (MMA) expanded the opportunity for enrollment in HDHPs. These plans are called Health Savings (or, sometimes, Spending) Accounts (HSAs). Both MSAs and HSAs have large front-end deductibles designed to make their owners more cost-conscious about healthcare purchases. Because of this feature, they are often called Consumer Directed Health Plans (CDHPs). The experiences that lent credibility to this concept were the RAND Health Insurance Experiment (discussed above) and the MSA experience in South Africa. (Please see Exhibit 6.10.)

Since MSAs and HSAs are true savings accounts that can accumulate earnings, health plans that administer them have developed relationships with banks and investment companies to provide traditional financial services for their owners. In a further trend, some health companies have even integrated a banking function into their insurance product. For example, starting in 2006, UnitedHealth Group's OptumHealth Bank and OptumHealth Financial Services[31] have provided customers with a variety of investment instruments, including mutual funds. Investment income in these accounts accumulates tax free.

About a quarter of all employers offer an HSA-like option, which covers about 30% of employees. Estimates of persons covered under these plans (employees and dependents) in 2017 range from 21.4 million to 33.7 million.[32]

As Exhibit 6.11 demonstrates, these plans have grown rapidly since inception as their members seek to trade lower premiums for higher (future) out-of-pocket payments.

---

[31] These organizations operated under the name Exante until 2008.

[32] EBRI. (2018, February). Has Enrollment in HSA-Eligible Health Plans Stalled? Issue Brief #441. Retrieved May 26, 2018, from https://www.ebri.org/publications/ib/index.cfm?fa=ibDisp&content_id=3547

EXHIBIT 6.10. Medical Savings Accounts—Experience in South Africa

MSAs were started in South Africa in 1994 and by 2002 captured half the 7-million-person health insurance market. For the MSA product in South Africa, nondiscretionary services do not incur out-of-pocket expenses. For example, hospitalizations and medications for chronic conditions are not counted against the individual's annual deductible. Based on this experience, Discovery Health (an MSA) found that:

- "On average, discretionary spending (primarily outpatient spending) is 47 percent lower for those enrolled in Medical Savings Account plans."

- "[N]o evidence suggests that members of MSA plans are shifting costs to a hospital setting where the insurer would foot the entire bill."

- "Patients using their MSAs also were much more likely to purchase a generic equivalent . . . use of the brand-name drug [Prozac in this case] jumped 45 percent when patients were spending insurance company money."

- Patients do not skimp on necessary chronic medications when paying for drugs from an MSA. (This conclusion was reached comparing use of osteoporosis treatment medications before enrollment in a chronic disease program—when the medication costs came out of the MSA—with costs after enrollment—when the medication was free. There was no statistical difference in prescription filling between the two groups.)

Source: Matisson, S. (2002, August). Medical savings accounts and prescription drugs: Evidence from South Africa. National Center for Policy Analysis Policy Report No. 254. Retrieved May 26, 2018, from http://www.ncpathinktank.org/pub/st254?pg=5

EXHIBIT 6.11. For Firms Offering Health Benefits, Percentage that Offer an HDHP/HRA and/or an HSA-Qualified HDHP, 2005–2017

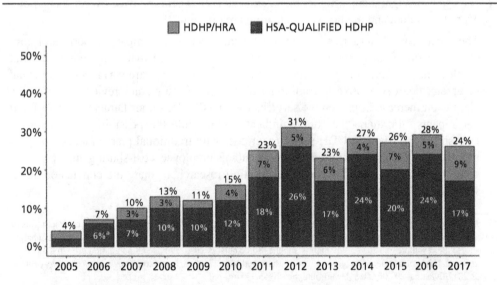

[a] Estimate is statistically different from estimate for the previous year shown (*p* < .05).

Note: Among all firms that offer health benefits, 2.3% offer both an HDHP/HRA and an HSA-qualified HDHP. Adding the percentage of firms offering HDHP/HRA-Qualified HDHPs may not sum to the percentage of firms offering HDHP/SOs [Savings Options] because some firms offered both.

Source: Kaiser Family Foundation (2017, September 19). *2017 Employer health benefits survey. Section 8: High-deductible health plans with savings option*. Retrieved May 26, 2018, from https://www.kff.org/report-section/ehbs-2017-section-8-high-deductible-health-plans-with-savings-option/

Proponents contend that if enough people enroll in these plans and exhibit prudent purchasing behavior, many costs would be lower. They also speculate that providers will be more attuned to consumer cost concerns and alter their behavior accordingly. It should be noted that empirical observations from managed care settings indicate that a tipping point for this latter change is at least 30% of a physician's practice; that is, at least 30% of a physician's patients must belong to such plans before behavior will be substantially affected.

Because high-deductible plans aim to reduce costs by making care more price-sensitive, it is important to assess their performance. (Please also see Chapter 2 for studies on the effect of out-of-pocket costs and utilization.) Unfortunately, the results are not always consistent, since data originates from health plans that may use different calculations and assumptions. The following examples illustrate what has been reported.

- Aetna[33] compared results from 2002 to 2008 for customers who changed from PPOs (discount fee-for-service plans described below) to their HSA/HRA plan, called Aetna Health Fund (AHF). The study group comprised 1.6 million PPO members and 436,000 AHF members. *Cost*: The average plan sponsor saved nearly $9 million per 10,000 members when an AHF HRA or HSA was offered as a plan option. (This figure decreased to $8.6 million in 2017.)[34] Medical costs for HSA members were more than 10% lower than for PPO members. Compared to PPO members, these members accessed the same or higher levels of preventive services, had a 5–10% lower rate of non-urgent emergency room use, had a higher generic drug use, and participated more frequently in health assessment screens.

- CIGNA found similar utilization patterns with its Choice Fund product. Cumulative Cost savings were significantly higher than Aetna at $7,900 per employee over 5 years; however, the product and method of calculation are different.[35]

- The Academy of Actuaries[36] analyzed several insurance company reports and concluded reports that, generally, "all of the studies indicated that cost savings did not result from avoidance of appropriate care and that necessary care was received in equal or greater degrees relative to traditional plans. All of the studies reviewed reported a significant increase in preventive services for CDHP [Consumer Directed Health Plan] participants." Further, "the studies indicated that while the possibility for employer cost-shifting exists with CDH plans, (as it does with traditional plans) most employers are not doing so, and might even be reducing employee cost-sharing under certain circumstances." It should be noted that not all researchers share the conclusion about what type of care was avoided.

[33] *Sixth Annual Aetna HealthFund Study 2010*. Retrieved May 27, 2018, from http://www.aetna.com/aetna-press/document-library/Aetna_HealthFund_2009_Study_Results_NA_Sell_Sheet.pdf. Note: Not all of these studies analyze member use. For example, the 2017 study mainly supplies some cursory cost-savings and population growth data.

[34] *Results of the 12th Annual Aetna HealthFund Study*. Retrieved May 27, 2018, from https://news.aetna.com/wp-content/uploads/2017/09/aetna_29738_2016_Healthfund_broch_v5c_hi-res.pdf

[35] *8th Annual Cigna Choice Fund Experience Study* (2014, April). Retrieved May 27, 2018, from https://www.cigna.com/static/www-cigna-com/docs/employers-brokers/874630-executivesummary-final.pdf

[36] *Emerging data on consumer-driven health plans. A public policy Monograph*. (2009, May). American Academy of Actuaries Consumer-Driven Health Plans Work Group.

- RAND's[37] review of this subject led to the following conclusions:
  - Based on strong evidence from the literature, we expect that increased cost sharing will result in some reductions in health spending.
  - Multiple studies confirm that individuals use less when faced with health plans requiring higher cost sharing, such as HDHPs.
  - Health savings accounts in conjunction with HDHPs may blunt the decreases in health spending associated with higher cost sharing in health plans.
  - Lower spending observed in HDHPs may be the result of favorable selection, that is, may attract a higher proportion of healthier enrollees.

The above conclusions must be tempered by consideration of whether the population is self-selected. For example, perhaps these health plan members use fewer medical services and access preventive measures more because they are healthier and more health-conscious than are those in the comparison group. Two research studies provide further insight. Naessens et al. noted:

> As the number of chronic co morbidities among family members increased, the probability of choosing a high-premium option also increased. Seventy-two percent of employees with at least 1 family member with co morbidity chose the high-cost option versus 54.7% of employees with no co morbidities. High-premium and low-premium plans seem to subdivide population into discrete risk categories, which may adversely affect the future stability of the insurance plan options.[38]

Recall that high-premium plans mean the patient has relatively lower out-of-pocket payments when seeking care.

The other study, by the EBRI, found that:

> CDHP premiums may be lower than non-CDHP premiums simply because the CDHP population is healthier, and there is some evidence of this. One study found that while actual savings ranged from a high of 15.5 percent to a low of −4.7 percent, and average savings were 4.8 percent, most of the savings were due to fact that younger, healthier workers choose CDHPs; the study concluded that once typical risk- and benefit-adjustment factors were taken into account, CDHPs saved only 1.5 percent on premium costs.[39]

Critics continue to argue that as more people join these plans, those who remain in traditional insurance products will be sicker, causing premiums for this latter population to rapidly rise.

---

[37] RAND Corporation. *Analysis of high-deductible health plans.* Retrieved May 27, 2018, from https://www.rand.org/pubs/technical_reports/TR562z4/analysis-of-high-deductible-health-plans.html

[38] Naessens, J. R., Khan, M., Shah, N. D., Wagie, A., Paultz, R. A., Campbell, C. R. (2008, October). Effect of premium, copayments, and health status on the choice of health plans. *Medical Care, 46*(10), 1033–1040.

[39] Fronstin, P. (2010, August). What Do We Really Know About Consumer-Driven Health Plans? Employee Benefit Research Institute Issue Brief, No. 345. Retrieved from www.ebri.org

Voluntary Employee Beneficiary Association. With the economic downturn that started in 2008, many firms and government agencies began to seriously worry about future financial commitments to retirees. In addition to pension plans, these organizations found themselves with large future healthcare liabilities. The change in accounting for these liabilities had begun a number of years before. In December 1990, the Financial Accounting Standards Board (FASB) issued Statement No. 106, which mandated that companies show future liabilities on their current balance sheets rather than the amounts they owe in the current year.[40] Likewise, the Government Accounting Standards Board issued Statement No. 45 in June 2004, requiring government entities to account for these liabilities in the same fashion. At the time of a 2007 study, it was estimated that the states owed $558 billion and local governments had commitments of $951 billion.[41] New York City alone set up a Retiree Health Benefits Trust Fund in fiscal year 2006 by contributing $1 billion. One of the ways that corporations have addressed this liability is by establishing voluntary employee beneficiary associations (VEBAs). (Please see Exhibits 6.12 and 6.13 for more information about this type of plan.)

EXHIBIT 6.12. VEBA Example

In 2007, the "Big Three" U.S. automakers were in trouble—again. One of their complaints was that their cost structure did not allow them to compete with foreign competitors. A major component of that cost structure was the healthcare benefits for 800,000 retired workers and their families that had been negotiated over the years by the United Auto Workers (UAW) union. At that time, the future liability for these benefits was estimated at more than $100 billion. In order to maintain financial liability and honor their commitments for these benefits, in 2008, the auto companies helped the union set up the UAW Retiree Medical Benefits Trust, which officially began operations January 1, 2010. This trust was established under a decades-old law enabling the establishment of VEBAs. Under this arrangement, the companies agreed to provide, over time, $57 billion to the trust, which would then assume responsibility for managing the healthcare benefits for its members. In return, the UAW agreed to concessions on some wage and cost-of-living increases. Initially GM contributed $23.6 billion, Ford supplied $15 billion, and Chrysler gave $6.8 billion. While the remainder was supposed to be cash, the VEBA subsequently accepted equity shares in these companies. In March 2010, it sold its Ford holdings for a significant profit, but as of June 2010, it still owned common stock accounting for 68% of Chrysler and 17.5% of GM (plus warrants for an additional 2.5%). In March 2018, it sold 40 million of its shares in GM worth $1.6 billion, retaining 100.15 million shares. The sale may bring the plan below an ownership threshold guaranteeing it a seat on GM's board.

Sources: Dolan, M. (June 15, 2010). UAW fund: $45 billion for investing. *Wall Street Journal.* http://online.wsj.com/article/SB10001424052748704324304575306921536410884.html?KEYWORDS=VEBA; Maynard, M., & Chapman, M. (2007, October 6). G.M. Pact calls for a push for health care reform. *New York Times.* Retrieved from https://www.nytimes.com/2007/10/06/business/06auto.html; and Naughton, N. (2018, March 5). UAW trust sells $1.6B worth of GM stock. *Detroit News.* Retrieved from https://www.detroitnews.com/story/business/autos/general-motors/2018/03/05/uaw-veba-stock-sale/111124700/. All retrieved May 27, 2018.

---

[40]Fernstrom, S. C., & Chen, N. Y. (1991). Coping with FASB statement No. 106—"Accounting for post-retirement benefits other than pensions." *Benefits Quarterly, 7*(2), 13–17.

[41]Zion, D., & Varshney, A. (2007, March 22). You dropped a bomb on me, GASB. *Credit Suisse.* Retrieve May 27, 2018, from http://online.wsj.com/public/resources/documents/DroppedB.pdf

EXHIBIT 6.13. **VEBA Regulation**

A voluntary employees' beneficiary association (VEBA) under Internal Revenue Code section 501(c)(9) is an organization organized to pay life, sick, accident, and similar benefits to members or their dependents, or designated beneficiaries if no part of the net earnings of the association inures to the benefit of any private shareholder or individual. The organization must meet the following requirements:

1. It must be a voluntary association of employees;

2. The organization must provide for payment of life, sick, accident, or other similar benefits to members or their dependents or designated beneficiaries and substantially all of its operations are for this purpose; and

3. Its earnings may not inure to the benefit of any private individual or shareholder other than through the payment of benefits described in (2) above.

Membership of a section 501(c) (9) organization must consist of individuals who are employees who have an employment-related common bond. This common bond may be a common employer (or affiliated employers), coverage under one or more collective bargaining agreements, membership in a labor union, or membership in one or more locals of a national or international labor union. An organization that is part of a plan will not be exempt unless the plan meets certain nondiscrimination requirements. However, if the organization is part of a plan maintained under a collective bargaining agreement between employee representatives and employers, and such plan was the subject of good faith bargaining between such employee representatives and employers, the plan need not meet such nondiscrimination requirements for the organization to qualify as tax exempt.

Source: Internal Revenue Service. *Selected problems of voluntary employees' beneficiary associations (VEBAs)*. Retrieved May 27, 2018, from https://www.irs.gov/pub/irs-tege/eotopicf84.pdf

The reasons employees (or their unions) accepted these arrangements are twofold. First, they realized that many of their employers could no longer remain going concerns without some concessions and restructuring. Second, from the perspective of health insurance, employees highly value these benefits and wanted to maintain them. The value of these benefits is sometimes perceived to be more than they are actually worth to the employer. Further, employers (or large groups, like VEBAs) can get better health insurance prices than employees negotiating individually, since they are able to negotiate more favorable insurance contracts and realize the cost savings of self-insured plans. Additionally, individuals are not able to take advantage of the tax exemption large employers enjoy.

Patient Protection and Affordable Care Act. The most significant law to affect the current American healthcare landscape is the Patient Protection and Affordable Care Act (ACA, P.L. 111–148), which was signed by President Obama on March 23, 2010. In order to reconcile the House of Representatives and Senate versions, a modification of this act called the Health Care and Education Reconciliation Act of 2010 (P.L. 111–152) was signed on March 30, 2010. Much has been written about the legislative process that preceded enactment, but the following observation epitomizes what transpired: "Never in modern memory has a major piece of legislation passed without a single Republican vote. Even President Lyndon B. Johnson got just shy of half of Republicans in the House to vote for Medicare in 1965, a piece of legislation that was denounced with many of the same words used to oppose this one."[42]

The act touches every part of the U.S. healthcare system. Some of its features have been mentioned above; others (such as implications for Medicare, Medicaid, and quality) will be explained in other sections. In this section, only those portions primarily affecting the private health insurance sector will be considered. Since the ACA is detailed in 906 pages,[43] the considerations here contain only selected highlights. More detailed summaries are available elsewhere, and include features and dates of implementation of the different provisions.[44]

The principle purposes of the ACA are ensuring that more Americans have health insurance available and that coverage is more affordable. Sources such as the U.S. Census Bureau estimated that without this law, there would continue to be between 45 and 50 million uninsured in the United States.

At the time of the ACA's passage, the CBO and other organizations estimated that the law would cost approximately $1 trillion from 2010 to 2019; however, predictions were that it would reduce the federal deficit by $143 billion over the same time period.[45] It is noteworthy that *cost estimates included the number of uninsured who were to be covered but not their health status or the nature of the benefits*. These factors will be discussed below.

Knowledge of the sources for funding the ACA is important since each group represents a distinct stakeholder with its own political and economic agendas.

At the time the Act was passed these sources were:

- $1 billion from the treasury for administration

- $498 billion from reduction in Medicare and Medicaid spending

    About $282 billion was to come from a physician pay freeze over 10 years (starting in 2010), and much of the rest from institutions such as hospitals (about $113 billion).

---

[42] Sanger, D. E. (2010, March 21). Big win for Obama, but at what cost? *The New York Times,* A1.

[43] *Public Law 111-148 Patient Protection and Affordable Care Act*: Retrieved from https://www.gpo.gov/fdsys/pkg/PLAW-111publ148/html/PLAW-111publ148.htm *and Public Law 111-152 Health Care and Education Reconciliation Act of 2010*: Retrieved from https://www.gpo.gov/fdsys/pkg/PLAW-111publ152/pdf/PLAW-111publ152.pdf

[44] Kaiser Family Foundation. (2013, April 25) *Summary of the Affordable Care Act*. Retrieved May 27, 2018, from https://www.kff.org/health-reform/fact-sheet/summary-of-the-affordable-care-act/

[45] Note: Some figures are estimates, such as levies of increased percentages on taxes; other amounts are precise numbers set in law, such as dollars owed by health insurance and pharmaceutical companies. Also, the amounts are nominal and not in present dollars. See also: Elmendorf, D. W. [CBO Director] March 20, 2010 letter to Nancy Pelosi [Speaker of the House of Representatives] regarding "an estimate of the direct spending and revenue effects of an amendment in the nature of a substitute to H.R. 4872, the Reconciliation Act of 2010." Retrieved May 28, 2018, from https://www.cbo.gov/sites/default/files/111th-congress-2009-2010/costestimate/amendreconprop.pdf

It is noteworthy that the federal government was *also* counting on these savings to prolong the viability of the Medicare program (i.e., the savings were being "double counted").

- $420 billion from new tax revenues[46] coming from such sources as:

  - The pharmaceutical industry: $25.5 billion (2012–2019 in unequal annual amounts and $2.8 billion each year thereafter). Payments would be based on market share of each company.

  - The "manufacturer, producer or importer" of medical devices would be subject to a 2.3% tax on the sales price of those devices. Excluded are such items as eyeglasses, contact lenses, hearing aids, and "any other medical device determined by the Secretary [of HHS] to be of a type which is generally purchased by the general public at retail for individual use." Based on 2009 revenues of the top 57 device companies, the tax would have generated about $1.87 billion that year. Projections were therefore that this sector would generate $20 billion over 10 years (starting in 2103).[47]

  - Private insurers: $58.8 billion (2014–2018 in unequal increasing amounts) based on market share of each company. Thereafter, the tax would increase based on the rate of premium growth.

  - Tanning salons: 10% tax. (Originally this tax was on cosmetic surgery, but physician lobbying changed the source of funding.)

  - Increased Medicare Hospital Insurance tax of 0.9% for individuals earning more than $200,000 or couples earning more than $250,000. A tax of 3.8% also applies to *unearned* (passive) income for these higher income people. (This tax is *in addition to* the 2.9% tax on earned income used to fund Medicare Part A [see below].) This method is a major departure from the way Medicare Part A is funded; in the past, a fixed tax of 2.9% applied only to earned income.

  - Increased taxes resulting from new limits on exemptions. For example: FSA limits were capped at $2,500 per year; the ability to itemize health expenses for federal tax deductibility was changed to 10% of adjusted gross income from 7.5%; non-prescribed, over-the-counter (OTC) drugs could no longer be paid from an HSA or

---

[46]The insurance company tax was suspended in 2017 and current plans are for a suspension in 2019. Congress also eliminated the individual mandate (and penalty) starting in 2019 and delayed the "Cadillac tax" (see below) and 2.3% excise tax on the sale of medical devices for two years. The only tax currently in effect is the employer mandate. See Luthi, S. (2018, May 24). House lawmakers look to delay health insurance tax until 2021. *Modern Healthcare*. Retrieved May 28, 2018, from http://www.modernhealthcare.com/article/20180524/NEWS/180529953

[47]Medical device tax would mostly hit the biggest firms. *Med City News*. (2010, March 24). Retrieved May 28, 2018, from http://www.medcitynews.com/2010/03/medical-device-tax-would-mostly-target-the-biggest-companies/

count toward total healthcare expenses; and health insurance company tax deductions for executive and employee compensation were to be limited to $500,000 per individual.

- Elimination of the tax deduction for Medicare Part D retiree subsidy payments to employers.
- $167 billion from employer and employee penalties, such as failure to enroll in, sponsor, or pay for a qualified plan. Also included taxes on *health plans* that offer high-cost options providing benefits greater than a specified amount, viz. 40% of the benefit that exceeds $10,200 per individual and $27,500 per family from 2018 to 2020, indexed to the Consumer Price Index for urban consumers thereafter. This charge has been called the "Cadillac tax."

Just as important as cost is how the ACA changed the operational features of the private health insurance industry. Some of the most significant aspects are listed below. The ACA:

- Couples the requirement for individuals to carry health insurance (or face penalty payments) with the obligation of insurance companies to issue policies (called guaranteed issue). The individual requirement is called mandatory enrollment; more will be said about this feature below. Companies cannot exclude an applicant because of a preexisting condition. Policies likewise must be renewable and cannot be canceled because of a past medical condition. (This latter practice is called rescission.)
- Allows insurance companies to vary their rating based only on age (limited to a 3 to 1 ratio), premium rating area, family composition (number of members), and tobacco use (limited to a 1.5 to 1 ratio). In other words, plans cannot charge more based on the health status of the population. This requirement applies to the individual/small group market as well as the state-sponsored Exchanges (explained below).
- Prohibits lifetime and annual limits.
- Requires coverage of dependents up to age 26.
- Requires companies with more than 50 employees to purchase insurance for their employees.
- Requires qualified health plans[48] to provide, *without out-of-pocket charges*, preventive services (rated A or B by the U.S. Preventive Services Task Force); recommended immunizations and preventive care for infants, children, and adolescents; and additional preventive care and screenings for women.
- Requires health plans to report the proportion of premium dollars spent on clinical services, quality, and other costs (see MLR, above). The federal government delegated the

---

[48] See Section 1301 of the ACA for a definition and features of such plans.

responsibility for the definition of what goes into this calculation to the NAIC.[49] If the MLR is less than 85% for plans in the large-group market and 80% for plans in the individual/small-group markets, the plans must provide rebates to policy holders.

- Requires insurers to submit to the Secretary of HHS and relevant state regulators "justification for an unreasonable premium increase prior to the implementation of the increase" (Section 2794).

- Sets annual out-of-pocket limits for individuals and families at the same amounts as HSAs.

- Applies, as mentioned, to ERISA plans.

Since many of the uninsured did not have access to affordable insurance plans, the ACA provided resources to set up Health Benefit Exchanges[50] in each state. Such Exchanges must be run by either the state government or a nonprofit organization. (If the state does not set an exchange up, the federal government has the authority to do so.) Initially (starting in 2014), these Exchanges were available to individuals and small businesses with up to 100 employees; by 2017, businesses with more than 100 employees were permitted to buy coverage from this source. All plans in the Exchanges must offer what the HHS Secretary defines as Essential Health Benefits (EHBs) and include, at a minimum, the following items (see Section 1302 of the ACA):

1. Ambulatory patient services
2. Emergency services
3. Hospitalization
4. Maternity and newborn care
5. Mental health and substance use disorder services, including behavioral health treatment
6. Prescription drugs
7. Rehabilitative and habilitative services and devices
8. Laboratory services
9. Preventive and wellness services and chronic disease management
10. Pediatric services, including oral and vision care

---

[49] National Association of Insurance Commissioners. (2018). *Medical loss ratio* (February 14). Retrieved May 28, 2018, from http://www.naic.org/cipr_topics/topic_med_loss_ratio.htm Of note is that physician credentialing and accreditation fees are not eligible to be counted as quality initiatives as part of the MLR.

[50] The term "Health Benefit Exchanges" was the original, official designation. Other terms that have been used are Health Insurance Exchanges (or HIEs, not to be confused with the same term for Health Information Exchanges), Health Plan Exchanges, or simply Exchanges (understood in context). For brevity, the term Exchanges will be used here.

Despite this apparent specificity, the *extent* of these benefits was yet to be determined (e.g., how many days/visits are covered). In fact, as seen below, this list is remarkably similar to the requirements for Medicaid services.

In order to construct the insurance products in the Exchanges, actuaries used the mandated conditions and benefits described above and calculated the cost for a plan in which patients had no cost sharing; such a plan was given an "actuarial value" of 1.0. Based on this valuation, the ACA allows Exchanges to offer four different types of benefit packages, depending on how much the individual/family has to contribute out of pocket (as mentioned above, subject to the limits specified for HSAs). The four types of packages are categorized by the actuarial value of the plan compared to the one without any cost sharing:

Bronze: Actuarial value of 0.60 (i.e., covers 60% of the plan's benefit costs)

Silver: Actuarial value of 0.70 (i.e., covers 70% of the plan's benefit costs)

Gold: Actuarial value of 0.80 (i.e., covers 80% of the plan's benefit costs)

Platinum: Actuarial value of 0.90 (i.e., covers 90% of the plan's benefit costs)

From the previous discussion about different types of out-of-pocket expenses, it should be obvious that for a given premium at each level, the number of combinations of trade-offs among copays, coinsurance, and deductibles is enormous.

A fifth type of plan termed "catastrophic" was made available to individuals up to age 30 who are exempt from the individual responsibility requirement because coverage is unaffordable to them or because of a hardship. It must include the basic benefits but requires cost sharing up to the annual individual HSA limit.

After passage of the ACA, legal challenges led to a Supreme Court ruling.[51] On June 28, 2012, the Court decided that the ACA was constitutional based on the fact that Congress has the right to levy taxes and the penalty for not having insurance (see below) was a tax. A second part of the ruling concerned the mandatory Medicaid expansion for all states. (Please see Medicaid section below.) In this matter, the Court ruled that the penalty for a state's refusal to participate (withholding Medicaid funds) was coercive; therefore, the Medicaid extension was to be voluntary.

The next major ACA-related milestone was January 1, 2014, when the Exchanges began operation. Before that date, however, a number of questions remained:

1.   How Are the Exchanges to Be Set Up?

Each state has two types of Exchanges—an individual exchange and a small business health options program (SHOP) exchange. An individual exchange is where individuals can purchase nongroup insurance and apply for premium and cost-sharing subsidies [see below for

---

[51] National Federation of Independent Business et al. v. Sebelius, Secretary of Health and Human Services, et al. Certiorari to the U.S. Court of Appeals for the Eleventh Circuit. No. 11–393. Argued March 26, 27, 28, 2012—Decided June 28, 2012.

an explanation of these features]. A SHOP exchange is where small businesses can purchase small-group insurance and apply for small business health insurance tax credits. These Exchanges may be operated under the same or separate governing structures.[52]

The federal government offered grants to states to establish their own state-based Exchanges (SBEs). These grants lasted until January 1, 2015, after which these organizations were expected to be self-sufficient, for example, by charging member plans a fee. If states refused to set up their own exchange (as happened in most Republican-controlled states), the Secretary of Health and Human Services was empowered to establish a federally facilitated exchange (FFE). FFEs could be run exclusively by the federal government or in partnership with states. (Please see Exhibit 6.14 for a distribution of such plans.) Once the exchange was established, it was tasked with certifying the Qualified Health Plans (QHPs) to be offered. QHPs must meet certain requirements, particularly offering EHBs and complying with certain financial terms (such as out-of-pocket limits).

EXHIBIT 6.14. **State Health Insurance Marketplace Types, 2018**

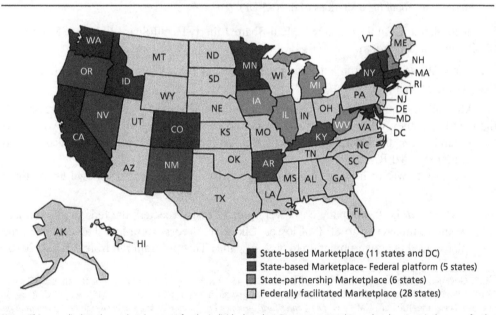

- State-based Marketplace (11 states and DC)
- State-based Marketplace- Federal platform (5 states)
- State-partnership Marketplace (6 states)
- Federally facilitated Marketplace (28 states)

Notes: This map displays the marketplace type for the individual market. For most states, the marketplace type is the same for the small business, or SHOP, marketplace; however, AR, MS, NM, and UT operate state-based SHOP Marketplaces.

Source: *State Health Insurance Marketplace Types, 2018*. KFF State Health Facts. Retrieved May 28, 2018, from https://www.kff .org/health-reform/slide/state-decisions-for-creating-health-insurance-exchanges/

---

[52]Namrata, K., Uberoi, N. K. [for the Congressional Research Service] (2016, July 1). *Overview of health insurance exchanges*. Retrieved May 28, 2018, from https://fas.org/sgp/crs/misc/R44065.pdf

The question remained, however: What exactly were the EHBs that plans needed to offer? The ACA set the broad categories, but coming up with details in each area was much more difficult. Rather than face political pressure, the federal government decided to let the states determine these details. In February 2013, the Exchanges were given a mandate to choose one plan that would serve as a benchmark for the insurance benefits offered by all *in that state*.[53]

One further type of plan should be mentioned. The ACA established eligibility and funding for Consumer Operated and Oriented Plans (CO-OPs), which were to be nonprofit, member-run health insurance companies. The purpose of these plans was to create local (statewide), nonprofit competition to the large, established insurers that were expected to participate in the Exchanges. According to the Congressional Research Service:[54]

> The Centers for Medicare & Medicaid Services (CMS), which administers the CO-OP program, has awarded loans to 24 CO-OPs since 2012. One of the 24 was unable to secure a state license to operate and was dropped from the program prior to offering coverage. CMS awarded about $2.4 billion to the remaining 23 CO-OPs. Eleven of the 23 are offering health plans in 2016. The other 12 are not offering health plans in 2016 and have either ceased operations or are in various stages of winding down operations. The fact that about half of the CO-OPs have failed has prompted questions about the program's design, administration, and funding and about the operations of the CO-OPs.

In 2018, four CO-OPs remained: Medi-Share, Liberty HealthShare, Christian Healthcare Ministries, and Samaritan.

2. How Was the Government Going to Entice Insurance Companies to Participate on These Exchanges?

After all, these firms faced a business prospect where their premiums were reviewed, the population they were covering had an unknown cost history, their benefits were now being mandated by the federal government (not just the states), and profitability was capped according to the MLR.

The answer was to limit insurance company risk by what became known as the three R's:[55]

a. *Risk corridors.* If company costs were greater than expected, the federal government would reimburse up to 80% of losses. Likewise, if costs were less than expected, the plans owed the government up to 80% of gains. This program ran from 2014 to 2016.

---

[53]U.S. Government Publishing Office. (2013, February 25). 45 CFR 156.100 State Selection of Benchmark [Source: 78 FR 12866]. Retrieved May 28, 2018, from https://www.gpo.gov/fdsys/pkg/CFR-2014-title45-vol1/pdf/CFR-2014-title45-vol1-sec156-100.pdf ; CMS.gov. *The Center for Consumer Information & Insurance Oversight. Information on Essential Health Benefits (EHB) Benchmark Plans.* Retrieved from https://www.cms.gov/cciio/resources/data-resources/ehb.html#review%20benchmarks

[54]Mach, A. L., & Driessen, G. A. [for the Congressional Research Service] (2016, March 11). *Consumer Operated and Oriented Plan (CO-OP) Program: Frequently asked questions.* Retrieved May 29, 2018, from https://fas.org/sgp/crs/misc/R44414.pdf

[55]American Academy of Actuaries. (2013, December 4). *ACA-fact sheet on risk-sharing mechanisms.* Retrieved from http://www.actuary.org/files/ACA_Risk_Share_Fact_Sheet_FINAL120413.pdf and CMS Center for Consumer Information and Insurance Oversight (2012, March). *Reinsurance, risk corridors, and risk adjustment: Final rule.* Retrieved May 28, 2018, from http://www.cms.gov/cciio/resources/files/downloads/3rs-final-rule.pdf

b. *Reinsurance*. In 2014, the federal government collected $10 billion from health plans, to be used to pay insurers in the individual market 80% of expenses if an individual's claims were between $60,000 and $250,000 in a given year. This program was budget neutral (viz., reinsurance payments were adjusted so as not to exceed contributions collected from health plans). This program also ran from 2014 to 2016.

c. *Risk adjustment*. The permanent risk-adjustment program aims to reduce incentives for health insurance plans to avoid enrolling people with higher-than-average costs; it does so by shifting money among them based on the risks of the people they enroll. Insurers with higher shares of low-cost enrollees contribute to a fund that will make payments to insurers with larger shares of high-cost enrollees. The risk-adjustment program is designed to be revenue neutral (i.e., no effect on the federal budget).

Based on these assurances, many insurance companies participated in the Exchanges. However, the protections did not work out as expected because the amount of money from profitable plans was much lower than projected. As a result, for the risk corridor program alone, the federal government owed $12.3 billion for 2014 to 2016. As of the end of 2017, only $100 million from 2014 losses were paid.[56]

As a result of these losses and perceived risks going forward (as well as other factors to be described), several plans went out of business, including some CO-OPs, and others decided not to continue to participate. By the start of 2018, the Trump administration estimated that there were "only 700 issuers in the individual and small group markets, which is down from 2,400 in an earlier estimate,"[57] and the CBO said that "about 26 percent of the population lives in counties with only one insurer in the marketplace in 2018, up from 19 percent in 2017."[58] (Please see Exhibit 6.15.) Because of this lack of promised payments, the federal government was the target of 36 lawsuits, including a class action involving about 150 insurers.

3. How Was the Federal Government Going to Make Sure Individuals Signed Up, Even Though Enrollment Was Mandated?

Three methods were established to encourage and assist enrollment: incentives, penalties, and federal government help with questions and enrollment.

a. *Incentives*. Two types of incentives were offered to people meeting certain financial criteria.[59] First, the Obama administration promised and paid out-of-pocket expenses (e.g., deductibles and copayments) over certain limits, a process called cost sharing

---

[56]Livingston, S. (2017, November 14). Feds owe health insurers $12.3 billion in unpaid risk-corridor payments. *Modern Healthcare*. Retrieved May 28, 2018, from http://www.modernhealthcare.com/article/20171114/NEWS/171119935

[57]Dickson, V. (2018). Estimated number of health plans on federal exchange plummets by two-thirds. *Modern Healthcare* (January 10). Retrieved May 28, 2018, from http://www.modernhealthcare.com/article/20180110/NEWS/180119985

[58]CBO. (2018, May). *Federal subsidies for health insurance coverage for people under age 65: 2018–2028*. Retrieved from https://www.cbo.gov/system/files/115th-congress-2017-2018/reports/53826-healthinsurancecoverage.pdf

[59]For personal calculations, see Kaiser Family Foundation: Health Insurance Marketplace Calculator. Financial Help for Health Insurance Coverage through Marketplaces. November 3, 2017 (Updated for 2018 plans). Retrieved May 28, 2018, from https://www.kff.org/interactive/subsidy-calculator/

EXHIBIT 6.15. Average Annual Premiums for Single and Family Coverage, 2014–2017

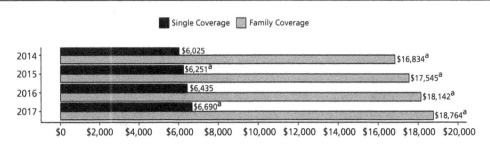

■ Single Coverage   ▨ Family Coverage

Year	Single Coverage	Family Coverage
2014	$6,025	$16,834[a]
2015	$6,251[a]	$17,545[a]
2016	$6,435	$18,142[a]
2017	$6,690[a]	$18,764[a]

[a] Estimate is statistically different from estimate for the previous year shown ($p < .05$).

Source: Kaiser Family Foundation (2017, September 19). *2017 employer health benefits survey*. Retrieved May 29, 2019, from https://www.kff.org/report-section/ehbs-2017-summary-of-findings/

reduction (CSR). In 2018, 6.3 million people (54% of exchange enrollees) were eligible for CSR subsidies.

The legal problem with CSRs is that they were never included in the ACA and Congress never appropriated money for them. When political control over the House of Representatives (where funding originates) went to the Republicans, investigations into use of unauthorized funds led to filing of a lawsuit on November 21, 2014: *U.S. House of Representatives v. Burwell* (the HHS Secretary at the time). The suit continued through successor HHS Secretaries and was put on hold several times.[60] Despite previous CSR funding, President Trump decided to stop it in 2018.

The second incentive for enrollment is premium subsidies, which are written into the ACA. Eligible enrollees must join a silver-level plan to get this benefit. In 2018, 83% of exchange members received these subsidies.[61] When President Trump announced the elimination of CSRs for 2018, health plans significantly raised their premiums for that year. (Recall that if out of pocket payments decrease, premiums increase.) Since the ACA required premium subsidies, federal payments shifted from CSRs to the subsidies. Because of these premium increases, however, the number of people buying exchange plans at full price dropped by about 20%, or 1.3 million, from 2016 to 2017.[62]

---

[60]U.S. Health Policy Gateway. U.S. House of Representatives v. Burwell (U.S. District Court, District of Columbia). Retrieved May 29, 2018, from http://ushealthpolicygateway.com/vii-key-policy-issues-regulation-and-reform/patient-protection-and-affordable-care-act-ppaca/ppaca-repeal/pending-legalconstitutional-challenges/u-s-house-of-representatives-v-burwell-u-s-district-court-district-of-columbia/#Overview

[61]Norris, L. (2018). *The ACA's cost-sharing subsidies*. Retrieved May 29, 2018, from https://www.healthinsurance.org/obamacare/the-acas-cost-sharing-subsidies

[62]Sanger-Katz, M. (2018, July 3). *When health insurance prices rose last year, around a million Americans dropped coverage*. Retrieved July 3, 2018, from https://www.nytimes.com/2018/07/03/upshot/when-health-insurance-prices-rose-last-year-around-a-million-americans-dropped-coverage.html

b. *Penalties*. The penalties for being unable to prove enrollment in a QHP started low—1% of adjusted gross income or $93 per person, whichever was greater. Amounts were to be paid when filing federal income tax. In 2017 (for taxes paid in April 2018), the penalty was the greater of: 2.5% of adjusted gross household income or $695 per adult and $347.50 per child under 18, subject to a maximum of $2,085 per household or the total yearly premium for the national average price of a Bronze plan sold on the Exchanges. The reason for giving these details is that, by comparison, paying the penalty can seem cheaper than purchasing insurance, even with the subsidies. (Please see Exhibit 6.15 for the average premiums for the years of exchange existence.) As a result, many people, particularly those who are younger and healthier, did not sign up for the plans. More recently, the tax reform bill passed in December 2017 eliminated the penalty for not having insurance starting in 2019.[63] While it is unclear what the effect this change will have, the action may be moot, since the government website has offered this advice: "What happens if I do not pay the fee? The IRS will hold back the amount of the fee from any future tax refunds. *There are no liens, levies, or criminal penalties for failing to pay the fee* [emphasis added]."[64]

c. *Assistance*. In order to facilitate enrollment, HHS set up a portal (http://Healthcare.gov) and phone lines to help potential enrollees. When open enrollment for the Exchanges started in October 2013, the technology did not work as planned,[65] causing the deadline for sign-ups to be extended several times until the final cutoff on March 31, 2014.[66] In addition to enrollee frustration, this delay caused a significant instability in the insurance marketplace. Because this previously uninsured or underinsured population did not have a history of utilization or cost data, insurance companies had to guess about their future costs. The first year was a complete estimate, but companies hoped that their experience in 2014 would inform better decisions about plan structures for 2015. However, the delayed enrollment removed this ability and the plans had to guess again about their projections. A further problem was that the enrollment deadline postponement encouraged healthy people to delay buying plans until the last minute. Enrollment in 2015 was also delayed, though not as much. By 2016, the sign-up process went more smoothly. In 2017, the Trump administration cut funding for enrollment education and assistance. Though the process went smoothly despite these cuts, fewer people enrolled.

---

[63] Public Law No: 115-97: H.R.1—An Act to provide for reconciliation pursuant to titles II and V of the concurrent resolution on the budget for fiscal year 2018. Part VIII Sec.11081 "This section repeals the penalty for individuals who fail to maintain minimum essential health coverage as required by the Patient Protection and Affordable Care Act (commonly referred to as the individual mandate."

[64] Healthcare.gov. *The fee for not having health insurance*. Retrieved May 29, 2018, from https://www.healthcare.gov/fees/fee-for-not-being-covered/

[65] Becker's HealthIT and CIO Report. (2015, March 5). *What went wrong with HealthCare.gov: 10 things to know*. Retrieved May 29, 2018, from https://www.beckershospitalreview.com/healthcare-information-technology/what-went-wrong-with-healthcare-gov-10-things-to-know.html This article is a summary of the findings of the Government Accountability Office investigation into what caused the errors. The report, requested by Congress, was released March 5, 2015.

[66] Nather, D., & Levine, S. (2014, March 25). *A brief history of Obamacare delays. Politico*. Retrieved May 29, 2018, from https://www.politico.com/story/2014/03/obamacare-affordable-care-act-105036

EXHIBIT 6.16. **Average Second Quarter Individual Market, Medical Loss Ratios, 2011–2018**

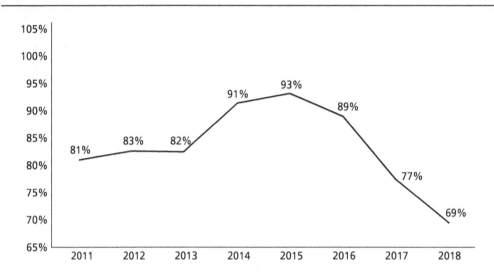

Note: Figures represent simple loss ratios and differ from the definition of MLR in the Affordable Care Act.

Source: Kaiser Family Foundation: Individual Insurance Market Performance in Mid-2018. Oct 05, 2018. https://www.kff.org/health-reform/issue-brief/individual-insurance-market-performance-in-mid-2018/ Retrieved January 4, 2019.

4.   Where Does Exchange-Provided Coverage Now Stand and What Are the Future Prospects?

The enrollment process has stabilized and the remaining plans are now finding exchange participation, by and large, profitable. (For example, please see Exhibit 6.16.)

More people were uninsured in 2018 than in the previous 2 years. According to the Commonwealth Fund: "The uninsured rate among working-age people—that is, those who are between 19 and 64—is at 15.5 percent, up from 12.7 percent in 2016, meaning an estimated 4 million people lost coverage."[67] (Please see Exhibit 6.17.) One reason given for this increase in the number of uninsured persons is that despite subsidies, premiums have increased significantly for many who are not eligible to receive them. Further, the out-of-pocket expenses have grown beyond the affordability of many families.

The Exchanges are facing future financial instability. This prediction is based on three observations.

---

[67]Collins, S. R. (2018, May 1). *First look at health insurance coverage in 2018 finds ACA gains beginning to reverse Commonwealth Fund*. Retrieved May 30, 2018, from http://www.commonwealthfund.org/publications/blog/2018/apr/health-coverage-erosion

EXHIBIT 6.17. **Plan Selections During the 2014–2018 Open Enrollment Periods**

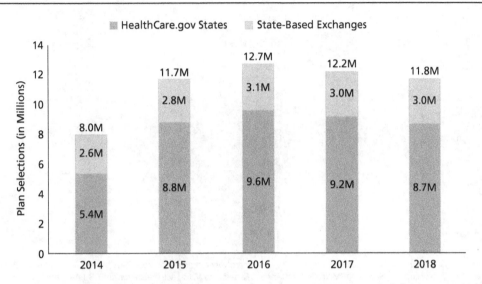

Source: CMS. (2018). *Health insurance exchanges 2018 open enrollment period final report* (April 3). Retrieved May 28, 2018, from https://www.cms.gov/Newsroom/MediaReleaseDatabase/Fact-sheets/2018-Fact-sheets-items/2018-04-03.html

1. Removal of penalties for non-enrollment may remove the healthiest people from the insurance pool, leading to higher insurance costs and further increases in premiums and out-of-pocket expenses.

2. Current Republican proposals would allow people to substitute "short-term policies" for exchange plans. The alternate plans do not need to comply with EHB requirements and thus would be much cheaper. For example, a young, single male could buy a policy that excluded pregnancy benefits. If these plans are approved, it would further exacerbate the financial instability.

3. The demographic makeup of the current exchange plans may not be sustainable. Original ACA projections were based on a greater number of younger and healthier enrollees than has been the case. (Please see Exhibit 6.18.)

In summary, the viability of the ACA's commercial insurance provisions is still in flux, due to both the flaws in its (Democratic) construction and Republican measures to cripple it. Its final place in the history of the U.S. insurance market has yet to be determined

EXHIBIT 6.18. **Demographic and Plan Characteristics of Consumers, 2018**

Age	Number	% of Total
0 to 17	1,003,325	9
18 to 34	3,073,716	26
35 to 54	4,231,303	36
55+	3,359,533	29
Metal Level		
Catastrophic	93,389	1
Bronze	3,358,073	29
Silver	7,353,570	63
Gold	833,026	7
Platinum	110,893	1

Source: CMS. (2018). *Health insurance exchanges 2018 open enrollment period final report* (April 3). Retrieved May 28, 2018, from https://www.cms.gov/Newsroom/MediaReleaseDatabase/Fact-sheets/2018-Fact-sheets-items/2018-04-03.html

Medicare

Overview and Eligible Populations. In 2018, the approximately 59.18 million[68] Americans eligible for Medicare came from two groups. The first group (85%) comprised those 65 years of age or older, provided they or their spouse made payroll tax contributions for 10 years and were eligible for Social Security payments. The other group (15%) consisted of those younger than 65 years old who have been permanently and continuously disabled for 24 months and were eligible to receive Social Security Disability Payments. Within these groups are those who are eligible for the Medicare Savings Programs, which help low-income individuals pay for their Medicare Part A and/or Part B copays and deductibles. As well, these programs also subsidize Part D expenses (including premiums). The four Medicare Savings programs are paid jointly from state and federal funds administered by state Medicaid agencies.[69]

Structure, Governance, and Funds Flow. Medicare (as well as Medicaid) is administered by the Centers for Medicare and Medicaid Services (CMS), which is part of the Department of Health and Human Services. (From 1977 to 2001, CMS was called the Healthcare Financing Administration, or HCFA.) Please see Exhibit 6.19 for an organizational chart that shows

---

[68]Medicare.gov. *Medicare enrollment dashboard*. Retrieved May 31, 2018, from https://www.cms.gov/Research-Statistics-Data-and-Systems/Statistics-Trends-and-Reports/Dashboard/Medicare-Enrollment/Enrollment%20Dashboard.html

[69]The Medicare Payment Advisory Commission. Retrieved May 31, 2018 from http://medpac.gov/

EXHIBIT 6.19. Organizational Chart for Medicare: Policy and Financial Flows

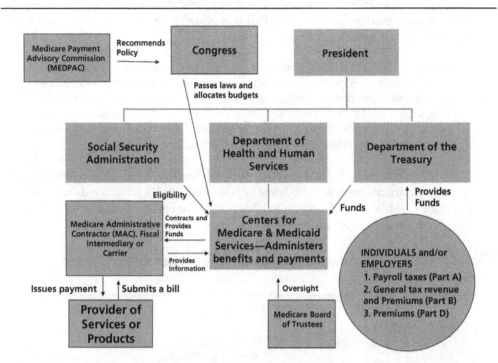

how funds and decisions flow for Medicare. Of note are three organizations not familiar to most people:

1. In 1997, the Balanced Budget Act (BBA) created the *Medicare Payment Advisory Commission* (MedPAC)[70] to advise Congress about such issues as payment amounts and methods, access to and quality of care, and other governance issues that might arise for this program. MedPAC is an independent body whose appointees are not government employees.

2. Medicare also has a *Board of Trustees* comprised of five government representatives (Secretaries of Treasury, Labor, and HHS; commissioner of Social Security; and CMS administrator) and two public members.[71]

3. Providers and suppliers do not submit claims directly to CMS for payment. Rather, the government set up a system of private payers that act on its behalf. The reason for this process is that when Medicare was passed into law in 1965, public fears of government intervention into the provision of services caused legislators to separate the source of

---

[70]The Medicare Payment Advisory Commission. Retrieved May 31, 2018, from http://medpac.gov/
[71]CMS.gov. *Trustees report & trust funds*. Retrieved May 31, 2018, from https://www.cms.gov/ReportsTrustFunds/ Accessed

funds (federal government) from the adjudication and payment of claims. The latter function was outsourced to businesses called fiscal intermediaries (in the case of Part A providers) and carriers (in the case of Part B providers). The reason for this separation comes from the first section of the Medicare Act:

> Sec. 1801. [42 U.S.C. 1,395] Nothing in this title shall be construed to authorize any Federal officer or employee to exercise any supervision or control over the practice of medicine or the manner in which medical services are provided, or over the selection, tenure, or compensation of any officer or employee of any institution, agency, or person providing health services; or to exercise any supervision or control over the administration or operation of any such institution, agency, or person.[72]

The Medicare Modernization Act of 2003 mandated that CMS consolidate intermediaries and carriers into single, regional organizations called *Medicare Administrative Contractors* (MACs).[73] (Please see Exhibit 6.20. Different MACs and covered regions exist for durable medical equipment as well as for home health and hospice.)

EXHIBIT 6.20. **Medicare Administrative Contractors for Parts A and B (October 2017)**

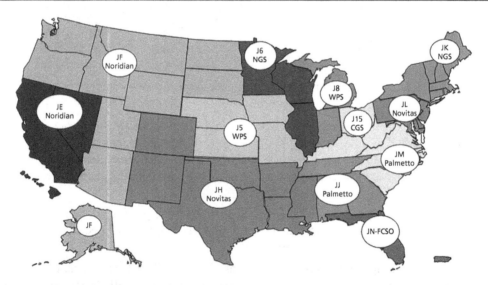

Source: CMS.gov. *What is an MAC?* Retrieved May 31, 2018, from https://www.cms.gov/Medicare/Medicare-Contracting/Medicare-Administrative-Contractors/What-is-a-MAC.html

---

[72] Social Security Administration. *Prohibition against any federal interference.* Retrieved May 31, 2018, from http://www.ssa.gov/OP_Home/ssact/title18/1801.htm

[73] CMS.gov. *What is an MAC?* Retrieved May 31, 2018, from https://www.cms.gov/Medicare/Medicare-Contracting/Medicare-Administrative-Contractors/What-is-a-MAC.html

The MACs (usually insurance companies) contract with CMS under a competitive bidding process. CMS supplies the money for claims payment as well as administrative fees. These contracted payers receive bills (claims) from providers (such as hospitals and physicians), determine patient eligibility and whether services are covered benefits, apply Medicare's fee schedule to the claim, deduct any amounts that are patient responsibility (deductibles and coinsurance), and then issue payment to the provider. These functions must be accomplished in a timely fashion; otherwise, interest on the claim must be paid to the provider. (The timing and interest rate can vary, but the claim is usually paid within 60 days; the federal government sets the interest rate penalties at its discretion.)

Since Medicare recipients can be subject to large out-of-pocket expenses (e.g., 20% coinsurance with no upper limit for Medicare Part B), the great majority of recipients who are eligible for both Parts A and B purchase supplemental (Medigap) insurance to cover what Medicare does not pay. In order to facilitate comparison of these supplements and minimize opportunities for fraud, the federal government approves a standardized list of eligible plans. These plans must fit into specified categories labeled by letters. Please see Exhibit 6.21 for a summary of the category characteristics. (The missing letters are categories of products that have been eliminated.) Since there are no pricing requirements, plans can compete on this dimension. Companies are able to provide "select" products within each category, which cover the same benefits but use a narrower network and, thus, charge lower premiums.

The types of services that Medicare covers and distributions of payments are displayed in Exhibit 6.22.

EXHIBIT 6.21. Medigap Policy Descriptions

Medigap Benefits	Medigap Plans									
	A	B	C	D	F[a]	G	K	L	M	N
Part A coinsurance and hospital costs up to an additional 365 days after Medicare benefits are used up	Yes	Yes	Yes	Yes	Yes	Yes	Yes	Yes	Yes	Yes
Part B coinsurance or copayment	Yes	Yes	Yes	Yes	Yes	Yes	50%	75%	Yes	Yes[b]
Blood (first 3 pints)	Yes	Yes	Yes	Yes	Yes	Yes	50%	75%	Yes	Yes
Part A hospice care coinsurance or copayment	Yes	Yes	Yes	Yes	Yes	Yes	50%	75%	Yes	Yes
Skilled nursing facility care coinsurance	No	No	Yes	Yes	Yes	Yes	50%	75%	Yes	Yes
Part A deductible	No	Yes	Yes	Yes	Yes	Yes	50%	75%	50%	Yes
Part B deductible	No	No	Yes	No	Yes	No	No	No	No	No

Part B *excess charge*	No	No	No	No	Yes	Yes	No	No	No	No
Foreign travel exchange (up to plan limits)	No	No	80%	80%	80%	80%	No	No	80%	80%
Out-of-pocket limit[c]	N/A	N/A	N/A	N/A	N/A	N/A	$5,120	$2,560	N/A	N/A

[a] Plan F also offers a high-deductible plan. If you choose this option, this means you must pay for Medicare-covered costs up to the deductible amount of $2,200 in 2017 before your Medigap plan pays anything.

[b] Plan N pays 100% of the Part B coinsurance, except for a copayment of up to $20 for some office visits and up to a $50 copayment for emergency room visits that don't result in inpatient admission.

[c] After you meet your out-of-pocket yearly limit and your yearly Part B deductible, the Medigap plan pays 100% of covered services for the rest of the calendar year.

Yes = the plan covers 100% of this benefit

No = the policy does not cover that benefit

% = the plan covers that percentage of this benefit

N/A = not applicable

Source: Medicare.gov. *How to compare Medigap policies*. Retrieved May 31, 2018, from https://www.medicare.gov/supplement-other-insurance/compare-medigap/compare-medigap.html

EXHIBIT 6.22. Medicare Benefit Payments by Type of Service, 2016

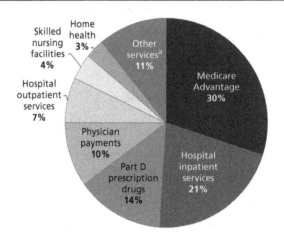

Total Medicare Benefit Payments, 2016: $675 billion

[a] Consists of Medicare benefit spending on hospice, durable medical equipment, Part B drugs, outpatient dialysis, outpatient therapy, ambulance, lab, community mental health center, rural health clinic, federally qualified health center, and other Part B services.

Source: Kaiser Family Foundation (2017, November 22). *A review of Medicare*. Retrieved May 31, 2018, from https://www.kff.org/medicare/issue-brief/an-overview-of-medicare/

Medicare has four parts (A to D) as well as a special program for persons with chronic kidney disease (end-stage renal disease program [ESRD]). These programs will be discussed separately below, since their funding sources and benefits are, by and large, different.

Medicare Part A. Part A, sometimes called the Hospital Insurance (HI) program, was established to pay for "reasonable and necessary" costs of inpatient hospital and skilled nursing facility care, home health services, and, later, hospice (a program for the terminally ill). The vague terms "reasonable and necessary" were not defined, which is one reason for constant cost overruns.

People who are eligible to receive Part A benefits get them automatically and cannot disenroll, even if they have other insurance. The funds used to support Part A come from payroll taxes of 1.45% that *both* employer and employee contribute (self-employed persons contribute 2.9%). As mentioned above, the ACA mandates an extra 0.9% on marginal income for higher earners and makes unearned income also subject to the tax. The tax on earned income appears on paychecks as FICA (Federal Income Contributions Act) Medicare. Unlike the Social Security deduction, there is no income limit to which the Medicare FICA is applied. These payroll taxes are paid to the U.S. Treasury, which then allocates them to the Medicare Part A Hospital Insurance Trust Fund. This fund is not an account per se but a bookkeeping obligation to pay for Medicare Part A services. Since current workers are paying into a fund that benefits the existing elderly, and since this fund exists merely on paper, it is analogous to what are called unfunded pension plans. The solvency of this account therefore depends on: the number of persons eligible to work (a function of demography); the actual number of employed people (a function of the overall economy); the number of Medicare eligibles—both in total and relative to those paying payroll taxes (also a function of demography); and the cost of services provided to those eligibles (as stated in Chapter 1, a function of price, volume, and intensity of services). According to MedPAC: "The number of taxpaying workers per Medicare beneficiary has declined from 4.6 during the early years of the program to 3.1 today; by 2030, this number is projected by the Medicare Trustees to be 2.3."[74] Given current economic and demographic conditions, Medicare's trustees predict the Part A trust fund will be solvent only until 2026 (3 years

---

[74]MedPAC. (2015, June). *Report to Congress. Chapter 2: The next generation of Medicare beneficiaries.* Retrieved May 31, 2018, from http://www.medpac.gov/docs/default-source/reports/chapter-2-the-next-generation-of-medicare-beneficiaries-june-2015-report-.pdf?sfvrsn=0 These figures are the most recent through the 2018 MedPAC Report to Congress.

earlier than the previous year's prediction).[75] Strategies to delay or prevent insolvency include:

▪ Reduce benefits.

▪ Raise taxes.

▪ Delay age of eligibility.

▪ Increase out-of-pocket payments by those who use the services.

▪ Impose means-tested costs on recipients (those with higher incomes from earned or unearned income would pay more for the benefit).

▪ Encourage more enrollment in managed care plans.

▪ Encourage the establishment of HSAs (as has been successfully implemented for this type of population in Singapore).

▪ Shift responsibility for certain services away from Part A (as was done by the balanced Budget Act of 1997 when many home healthcare services were moved from Part A to Part B).

▪ Change the amount and method of provider payments (as was done with implementation of Prospective Payment Systems [PPS]).

▪ Exert more government buying power over providers by soliciting bids for regionalized, high-cost, nonemergency services (e.g., transplantation, elective invasive cardiac procedures, and cancer treatments).

All of these proposals are fraught with political difficulties that make any short-term program changes challenging.

As mentioned, CMS determines annual beneficiary out-of-pocket responsibilities for Part A services. For 2019, the charges[76] were:

Hospital Stay

▪ $1,364 deductible per benefit period

▪ $0 for the first 60 days of each benefit period

▪ $341 per day for days 61–90 of each benefit period

▪ $682 per "lifetime reserve day" after day 90 of each benefit period (up to a maximum of 60 days over your lifetime)

---

[75]2018 Annual Report of the Boards of Trustees of the Federal Hospital Insurance and Federal Supplementary Medical Insurance Trust Funds. Published June 5, 2018. Retrieved from https://www.cms.gov/Research-Statistics-Data-and-Systems/Statistics-Trends-and-Reports/ReportsTrustFunds/Downloads/TR2018.pdf?wpisrc=nl_health202&wpmm=1. Of note is that the MedPAC: Report to the Congress: Medicare Payment Policy I March 2018 projected a 2029 insolvency date. Retrieved June 6, 2018, from http://www.medpac.gov/docs/default-source/reports/mar18_medpac_entirereport_sec_rev_0518.pdf?sfvrsn=0 This discrepancy is not only practically important but highlights how much results can vary between agencies that use different assumptions.

[76]CMS: 2019 Medicare Parts A & B Premiums and Deductibles https://www.cms.gov/newsroom/fact-sheets/2019-medicare-parts-b-premiums-anddeductibles Retrieved January 4, 2019.

Skilled Nursing Facility Stay

In 2018, patients paid:

- $0 for the first 20 days of each benefit period
- $170.50 per day for days 21–100 of each benefit period
- All costs for each day after day 100 of the benefit period

Given this overview, the history of the development of Medicare (particularly Part A) illustrates how the federal government typically acts and reacts to address cost overrun problems. Having an appreciation of these events will help the healthcare strategist, and those who seek to influence policy, to understand and anticipate governmental regulatory actions.

After the initial Medicare legislation was passed in 1965, President Lyndon Johnson was afraid that pent-up demand from the previously uninsured elderly would cause hospital overcrowding when the program started operating the following year. He was further concerned that, since hospital participation was voluntary, if sufficient numbers did not join the program, this bed shortage would be exacerbated.[77] In order to entice hospitals to participate, the federal government told them to track all costs for the care of these beneficiaries, *including allocated capital costs, such as depreciation and interest expenses on buildings and equipment.* (Hospitals must still maintain this accounting in order to file an annual Medicare Cost Report with CMS.) The government then promised to reimburse hospitals for these costs, plus an added 2%. As a further inducement to participate, hospitals received regular disbursements based on historical payment amounts; the actual accounting (over or under those payments) would be periodically reconciled. Under this system (termed "periodic interim payments"), hospitals were thus assured of a generous stream of cash flows. Because this compensation method was "cost plus," hospitals lacked incentives to reduce expenses. It is also noteworthy that, since payments included a portion of interest on bond issues, hospitals took advantage of this windfall subsidy to expand their building programs, thus further contributing to the costs of the system.[78]

As might be expected from such a scheme, "[m]ore than a dozen times between 1970 and 1997 the [Medicare] trustees reported the HI Trust Fund would be depleted in 10 or fewer years."[79] In order to address these solvency crises, the government implemented a variety of reimbursement changes. In 1969, the 2% bonus was eliminated; however, because there were no national cost standards, and each hospital's costs were defined only by its own experience, no incentives existed to operate efficiently. Costs continued to rise. In 1974, Medicare started to limit individual hospital reimbursements by using peer-group comparisons. Initially, costs could not be more than 120% of the mean of this group; gradually the amount was lowered to 108%. It is obvious that it was never in any hospital's best interest to be under the 108%.

---

[77]Wilbur Cohen, personal communication to J. Shalowitz, March 1987.

[78]An amusing article prompted by this payment system was: Fisher, G. R. (1979). The hospital that ate Chicago. *The New England Journal of Medicine, 301,* 56–57.

[79]Patashnik, E., & Zelizer, J. (2001). Paying for Medicare: Benefits, budgets, and Wilbur Mills's policy legacy. *Journal of Health Politics, Policy and Law, 26,* 7–36.

Since all hospitals targeted the maximum reimbursement level, the *peer-group means* also rose. Further, because capital costs and ancillary services (such as laboratory) were exempt from these caps, Medicare expenditures rose even further.

To address these continuing cost escalations, in 1982, Congress passed the Tax Equity and Fiscal Responsibility Act (TEFRA) and turned to a new method to pay hospitals: the Diagnosis Related Group (DRG). This method was derived from research performed by Yale professors John Thompson and Robert Fetter over the previous decade and was phased in over several years, starting on October 1, 1983.[80] This technique combines similar diagnoses into groupings based on resource use. Each diagnosis within a DRG is paid at the same rate. DRG designations were set not only by the diagnoses they included but also by such factors as: whether surgery was performed, patient age (if <17), if a comorbidity or complication occurred during the hospital stay, and discharge status (e.g., if the patient needed further skilled care). Because these payment rates are determined in advance, the DRG method is also called a Prospective Payment System (PPS). In order to more accurately pay for conditions based on the patient's clinical condition, in 2008, CMS began to use a system of Medicare Severity DRGs (called MS-DRGs). This methodology was also attractive to state governments and the private sector. For example, in 1987, the state of New York passed legislation instituting a DRG-based prospective payment system for all non-Medicare patients; the measure was particularly directed at the New York State Department of Health. The idea was to control costs for very expensive patients, viz. neonates and those with HIV/AIDS. To accomplish this goal, the Department of Health contracted with the 3M Company to make the necessary modifications in definitions and software. The result was the development of what is now known as All Patient DRGs (AP-DRGs). Subsequently, this method was further developed into All-Patient-Refined DRGs (APR-DRGs).[81] In order to prevent hospitals from using separately paid outpatient care to add to DRG costs, on June 25, 2010, President Obama signed into law the Preservation of Access to Care for Medicare Beneficiaries and Pension Relief Act of 2010, Pub. L. 111–192. In order to protect Medicare and the beneficiary from paying separately for services that should be included in the hospital stay, Section 102 of the law made some reimbursement changes. Diagnostic services and most admission-related nondiagnostic services provided in the hospital outpatient department (HOPD) are to be included in the DRG payment if they are performed on the day of admission or during the three calendar days before admission. This policy is known as the 3-day (or 1-day) payment window.[82]

The PPS system represented a major departure from the FFS scheme it replaced. The significant changes affecting hospitals that resulted from the TEFRA are explained next.

---

[80] See, for example, Thompson, J. D.. (1975) Case mix and resource use. *Inquiry, 12*, 300–312.

[81] Goldfield, N. (2010). The evolution of diagnosis-related groups (DRGs): From its beginnings in case-mix and resource use theory, to its implementation for payment and now for its current utilization for quality within and outside the hospital. *Quality Management in Health Care*, 19, 3–16.

[82] CMS.gov. *Three-day payment window*. Retrieved May 31, 2018, from https://www.cms.gov/Medicare/Medicare-Fee-for-Service-Payment/AcuteInpatientPPS/Three_Day_Payment_Window.html

1. *With the implementation of the PPS, the periodic interim payments ceased.* This latter method gave hospitals a steady cash flow, with reconciliations occurring quarterly. Under the PPS, hospitals receive payments only after they submit claims for services on an individual case basis, thus slowing collections.

2. *Implementation of the DRG System also caused an increase in tension between physicians and hospitals in three areas.*

   a) In order to determine appropriate DRGs for billing purposes and expedite reimbursement, hospitals must make sure that physicians complete their charting accurately and promptly. Physicians have no economic incentive to do so since their billing is separate from that of the hospital.

   b) Another area of conflict between hospitals and physicians deals with the opposing reimbursement incentives. Under the PPS, hospitals achieve maximum profitability from patients who have shorter stays using only those resources that are medically necessary. Physicians, in contrast, often get paid by the visit or by the level of technology they bring to diagnosis and/or treatment of illness. While utilization review procedures have mitigated this conflict somewhat, these opposing incentives still remain.

   c) A further source of conflict is potential malpractice suits. In some cases, physicians may order more services in order to protect themselves against possible future legal action. This protection costs them nothing since the hospital pays the bill for these services from its DRG payments.

3. *Implementation of the DRG system led hospitals to fear reduced Medicare revenues.* In order to preserve profitability, they increased charges to private payers in a process commonly called "cost shifting." Since private insurance companies found themselves paying higher hospital charges, they increased their premiums. In the face of these double-digit increases, employer groups increasingly turned to self-insurance plans and/or purchased services from managed care companies.

4. The TEFRA required formation of two organizations to oversee hospital and physician payment mechanisms and amounts. These organizations were, respectively, the Physician Payment Review Commission (PPRC) and Prospective Payment Assessment Commission (ProPAC). The Balanced Budget Act of 1997 merged these two groups into the Medicare Payment Assessment Commission (MedPAC).

Since hospitals became concerned about their finances once this new payment system was in place, many systems coded patient stays at a higher level of intensity. Researchers who studied this practice found it to be widespread, referring to it as "DRG creep." To highlight the resiliency of hospitals' anticipation and responses to this new payment system, "in the first year of PPS, hospital PPS revenues per case increased almost 19 percent over the average cost-based payment per case in the previous year. This unanticipated, large increase in revenues undoubtedly was due primarily to case-mix index increases."[83] Further: "This DRG 'creep' improperly increased net reimbursement [in 1985] by 1.9%, +$308 million when projected nationally."[84]

In response to these still-increasing costs, the federal government implemented two strategies. First, it required physicians to sign an "attestation statement," in which they certified that the diagnoses they specified as the reasons patients were hospitalized were accurate. (This requirement is no longer in effect because of physician protests.) The tactic was aimed at physician-hospital collusion to maximize hospital revenue. Second, peer review organizations (PROs), set up under the TEFRA to monitor physician utilization and quality, increased their scrutiny of DRG coding. These approaches were so successful that, by 1988, "hospitals did not receive a significant overreimbursement."[85] However, since MedPAC recommended DRG payments based on *charges* (as reported in hospitals' Medicare Cost Reports), payment for DRGs could continue to increase. With implementation of MS-DRGs in 2008, CMS addressed this issue by changing the basis of DRG payments from a *charge-based* system to a *cost-based* method. Still, hospitals are free to use different methods to allocate indirect costs in order to maximize expenses in their Medicare cost reports.

In addition to DRG creep, after inpatient PPS was put in place, hospitals adopted another strategy for increasing revenues: shifting more services to the out-of-hospital sectors that were still paid on a FFS basis. Subsequently, expenditures for hospital-based ambulatory care services (such as outpatient surgery), home healthcare, and skilled nursing facility care dramatically increased. In responding to this shift in services, CMS enacted separate prospective payment schemes for outpatient hospital services, home health services, hospice, skilled nursing facilities, inpatient psychiatric facilities, inpatient rehabilitation facilities, and long-term care hospitals. Hospitals that provided specialty care in the latter three categories previously had been exempt from DRG payments for those services.

In order to better understand formation of governmental health policy in response to rising DRG-related costs, we will consider how Congress dealt with outpatient hospital services, skilled nursing facility care, and home healthcare. Note that all the different types of PPSs that the federal government developed use different units of analysis, ranging from per-day (per-diem) payments (for hospice and skilled nursing facilities) to global payments based on an episode of care or diagnosis (for hospitals for inpatient and ambulatory services).

Addressing the hospital-based ambulatory care cost escalation, Congress passed provisions in the Omnibus Budget Reconciliation Act (OBRA) of 1986 that required Medicare to develop ambulatory patient groups, analogous to the in-patient DRGs. Subsequently, some

---

[83] Steinwald, B., & Dummit, L. A. (1989). Hospital case-mix change: Sicker patients or DRG creep? *Health Affairs, 8,* 35–47.

[84] Hsia, D. C., Ahern, C. A., Ritchie, B. P., Moscoe, L. M., & Krushat, W. M. (1992). Medicare reimbursement accuracy under the prospective payment system, 1985 to 1988. *JAMA, 268,* 896–899.

[85] Ibid.

EXHIBIT 6.23. Example of APC Methodology

A 78-year-old man comes to the emergency room with a cough and fever. After examination by the emergency room physician, the patient has a chest X-ray and blood tests. The tests show a pneumonia and mild dehydration. The patient was healthy before this episode and has good social support and a regular primary care physician for follow-up. He prefers to be treated at home for this illness. The emergency room personnel administer intravenous fluids to correct his dehydration and administer ceftriaxone (an antibiotic) intravenously. He is discharged home with appropriate follow-up instructions.

Service	Codes	# of units	APC payment[a]
Emergency Room (APC 5024)	99284	1	$355.53
Blood Count (SI: Q4)	85025	1	0
Basal Metabolic Panel (SI: Q4)	80048	1	0
Chest X-Ray (TC) (APC 5521)	71046	1	62.12
Intravenous Fluids (SI: N)	J7042	4	0
Potassium Chloride (SI: N)	J3480	20	0
Ceftriaxone (SI: N)	J0696	4	0
			$417.53

[a] Payments are for 2018. Medicare Charge for facility fee is APC payment. Amounts are for hospital-only payment. Professional charges are additional.

Source: CMS.gov (2018, April). *Hospital outpatient PPS. Addendum B*. Retrieved May 31, 2018, from https://www.cms.gov/Medicare/Medicare-Fee-for-Service-Payment/HospitalOutpatientPPS/Addendum-A-and-Addendum-B-Updates.html

private insurers (such as Blue Shield of California) and states (such as Iowa, Maryland, Massachusetts, and Washington) also required payment based on this method. It was not until passage of the Balanced Budget Act of 1997 that this system was mandated for Medicare payments; it was finally put into operation on August 1, 2000. (Note the length of time between these events before a corrective measure was implemented.) CMS refers to this program as the Outpatient Prospective Payment System (or OPPS), and reimbursement is by Ambulatory Payment Categories (APCs). (Please see Exhibit 6.23 for an example of how these APCs are applied to hospital emergency room services.)[86] Note that if you are the supplier of intravenous fluids, laboratory reagents, or antibiotics, your customer will not be able to bill separately for those items. Medical imaging companies, however, have successfully lobbied for additional payments to hospitals on top of the APC payments.

[86]For a current list of APC codes and payment amounts, see http://www.cms.gov/HospitalOutpatientPPS/AU/list.asp#TopOfPage Retrieved May 31, 2018. Choose Addendum A and Addendum B Updates tab.

Of additional note is that since 2008, ambulatory (sometimes called same-day surgery) surgical centers have been paid according to the OPPS methodology.[87] The rates apply to both hospital-based centers and freestanding facilities.

As previously mentioned, after implementation of DRGs, skilled nursing facility costs were also rising rapidly. As a result, provisions of the Balanced Budget Act of 1997 mandated that Medicare also pay *these* facilities using a PPS. It is noteworthy that this PPS was based on a methodology (developed as early as the 1970s) that states used to pay nursing homes for Medicaid services. This procedure is explained below.

In order to be eligible for payment for Medicare Skilled Nursing Facility (SNF) care, the following conditions must be met:

1. Beneficiary must be eligible for Medicare Part A.

2. Beneficiary must have days available to use (limited to 100 days per benefit period).

3. Beneficiary must have had a 3-day qualifying hospital stay within 30 days of admission to the SNF.

4. The reason for admission to the SNF must be related to the reason the beneficiary was hospitalized.

5. Beneficiary must require and be able to receive daily medically necessary, skilled care. This care must be under direct supervision of a registered nurse or licensed rehabilitation professional (i.e., speech, occupational, and/or physical therapist).

6. On admission, each patient must undergo a comprehensive evaluation that determines the resources needed to care for that patient, including medical diagnosis, cognitive status, behavioral problems, nursing needs, and activities of daily living (ADL) impairments. (The basic ADLs are being able to perform the following activities unassisted: eating, bathing, dressing, toileting, and transferring from bed to chair.)

7. Starting October 1, 2019, a new methodology that uses this evaluation, called the Patient-Driven Payment Model, will be used to group patients into cost groups that will determine per-diem payments.[88]

8. Excluded from this PPS are costs for chemotherapy, radiation therapy, and customized prostheses. It should be noted that *all other items required for care, including diagnostic tests and intravenous medications, are covered under the global payment.* In this respect, SNFs have a financial interest to transfer the patient to the hospital whenever

---

[87] CMS. *Ambulatory surgical center payment system.* Retrieved June 2, 2018, from https://www.cms.gov/Outreach-and-Education/Medicare-Learning-Network-MLN/MLNProducts/downloads/AmbSurgCtrFeepymtfctsht508-09.pdf

[88] Acumen. (2018, April). *Skilled nursing facilities patient-driven payment model technical report.* Retrieved June 2, 2018, from https://www.cms.gov/Medicare/Medicare-Fee-for-Service-Payment/SNFPPS/Downloads/PDPM_Technical_Report_508.pdf Acumen developed the methodology under contract with CMS. This report provides background and details of this payment method. See also Federal Register: Medicare Program; Prospective Payment System and Consolidated Billing for Skilled Nursing Facilities (SNF) Proposed Rule for FY 2019, SNF Value-Based Purchasing Program, and SNF Quality Reporting Program (2018, May 8). Retrieved from https://www.federalregister.gov/documents/2018/05/08/2018-09015/medicare-program-prospective-payment-system-and-consolidated-billing-for-skilled-nursing-facilities

care becomes very expensive (e.g., if an MRI or other expensive diagnostics need to be performed).

9. Beneficiaries pay a daily copayment for days 21 to 100, after which benefits expire. (No copayment is required for days 1–20.)

The final PPS we will consider is for home healthcare. These services also increased significantly after DRG implementation. To qualify for Medicare benefits, a beneficiary must:

- Be homebound (unable to leave home under normal conditions).

- Require intermittent skilled nursing care (other than blood draws), physical or speech therapy, or continuing occupational therapy. Note the word "intermittent"; it means *daily* skilled care is not reimbursable.

- Have care provided per a written physician's plan of care.

Other services, such as a home health aide, are also covered if the beneficiary also receives the skilled services described above. Excluded from these benefits are drugs and biologicals (except injectable calcitonin [used to treat osteoporosis], which the home health agency bills separately), transportation, and prosthetics. Included in payments are costs for routine medical supplies, including catheters and ostomy bags, and durable medical equipment.[89]

Upon admission to skilled home healthcare, a nurse or therapist performs a patient assessment using the Outcome and Assessment Information Set (OASIS). This assessment describes the patient's medical needs and clinical condition, factoring in an adjustment for geographic wage differences. The patients are then classified into one of about 80 Home Health Resource Groups (HHRG). Each group will determine how much the home health agency (HHA) will receive for a 60-day episode of care. As soon as the care plan is processed and the HHRG is validated, the HHA receives half of the amount it is due; the other half is paid at the close of the 60-day period. Unlike SNF care, as long as the above criteria are met, there is no limit to the number of 60-day periods a beneficiary can receive. Also, there are no out-of-pocket expenses for home care (copays, deductibles, or coinsurance). To further complicate the issue, in order to relieve some of the financial burden on the Hospital Insurance Trust Fund, the Balanced Budget Act of 1997 changed the source of some of the funding for HHAs. Medicare Part A is responsible only for the first 100 *visits* after a hospitalization; the other eligible services are paid by Part B. In addition to these global 60-day payments, home health providers are subject to quality evaluations through the Home Health Consumer Assessment of Healthcare Providers (HHCAHPS) survey. Patients are able to search evaluations of these providers on the federally sponsored website: Home Health Compare.[90]

The prospective payment systems described above are summarized in Exhibit 6.24. In order to evaluate these policy changes, some sample outcomes are summarized in Exhibit 6.25.

---

[89]CMS. (2018, March). *Home health prospective payment system*. Retrieved June 2, 2018, from https://www.cms .gov/Outreach-and-Education/Medicare-Learning-Network-MLN/MLNProducts/Downloads/Home-Health-PPS-Fact-Sheet-ICN006816.pdf

[90]CMS.gov. Home health compare. Retrieved June 2, 2018, from https://www.medicare.gov/homehealthcompare/search .html

EXHIBIT 6.24. **Prospective Payment Systems for Medicare Part A**

Place of Service	Payment Method
Inpatient Hospital	International Classification of Disease (ICD)-10 coding that determines a Diagnosis Related Group (DRG). Global amount paid per hospital stay.
Outpatient Hospital	Ambulatory Payment Category (APC) Outpatient Prospective Payment System (OPPS) based on Current Procedural Terminology (CPT)-4 and Healthcare Common Procedural Coding System (HCPCS). Global amount paid per type of care (e.g., emergency room visit or chemotherapy visit). May have more than one APC per encounter.
Ambulatory Surgicenter	After 2008, new rates were phased in linked to the APC methodology.
Skilled Nursing Facility	SNF Patient Driven Payment Model (PDPM).Pays on per-diem basis. (Starts October 1, 2019.)
Home Healthcare	Outcome and Assessment Information Set (OASIS) Home Health Resource Groups (HHRG). Pays global amount for each 60-day episode of care (adjusted downward for increments <60 days).

EXHIBIT 6.25. **Sample Effects of PPS Changes on Cost and Utilization of Healthcare Services**

Site of Care	Post-DRG (1983) Changes	Post-PPS (1998) Changes
Inpatient Hospital	Just prior to BBA of 1997, costs increased 5.3% per year.	Total hospital payments flat for first 3 years, then increased again.
Outpatient Hospital	Payments rose 12% per year: 1983–1997.	Continued decline in hospital Medicare outpatient margins after OPPS implemented in 2000 (–17% in 1998 to –8.1% in 2002).
Skilled Nursing Facility	Payments rose 19% per year: 1989–1996.	Charges for rehab (most expensive RUG-III category) dropped by 44.6%.
Home Healthcare	Payments rose 31% per year: 1988–1996.	By 1999, payments dropped by about half and 14% of HHAs closed.

Note: RUG (Resource Utilization Group) was the payment method for SNFs prior to the Patient Driven Payment Model.

The importance of prospective pay schemes for suppliers of goods and services should be obvious: Their customers cannot pass along *their* costs to the payer since they are "bundled" in a global payment. For long-standing products and services, there is not as much of a problem, since costs have been incorporated into the prospectively determined rates. However, new offerings may pose reimbursement problems, since overall costs may be greater than the payments received.

In order to add value in that setting, one can apply two strategies. First, CMS can be petitioned for extra payment to the global amount. If successful, this tactic can result in additional revenue if CMS: (a) pays more for an existing DRG, (b) reclassifies DRG codes to include some with higher payments (as was done in the past with some cardiovascular services), or (c) in the case of APCs, grants what are termed "transitional pass through payments." These latter payments are time-limited additions (e.g., 3 years) to the prospective payments to which they apply. A product or service company must petition CMS for this exception. To qualify, the applicant must demonstrate that the technology:

1. is new—that is, generally, that it has been commercially available for no more that 2 to 3 years prior to the year for which the additional payment is sought;

2. is high cost relative to other cases in the relevant MS-DRG(s); and

3. offers substantial clinical improvement over existing services or technologies for the Medicare patient population.[91]

The second method for adding value for customers in a PPS is introducing a product or service that saves money. For example, introduction of laparoscopic surgery has reduced inpatient stays dramatically; for a customer who is paid on a prospective basis, this shortened time translates into using fewer resources and results in higher margins (at least until CMS catches up to the new use of the cost-saving technology). The new-product strategist must therefore consider reimbursement issues *during the product development stage* by asking such questions as: What is the setting in which the new product or service will be used (e.g., inpatient or hospital-based ambulatory care); who determines the reimbursement (e.g., CMS); is there a new code that must be established to capture the product or service for reimbursement purposes; and what is the approval time cycle for new code and price setting? Since the latter process may take over 2 years, managers must address these questions concurrent with considering issues of safety and efficacy that determine product regulatory approval.

***

One can learn four policy lessons from the above Medicare history.

1. When implementing new programs, the government tends to make financial terms very generous in order to entice private-sector participation. This precept is true for sectors ranging from healthcare to defense.

---

[91] CMS.gov: Pass-Through Payment Status and New Technology Ambulatory Payment Classification (APC). Retrieved June 2, 2018 from https://www.cms.gov/Medicare/Medicare-Fee-for-Service-Payment/HospitalOutpatientPPS/passthrough_payment.html

2. When costs get out of control, the government reacts slowly and incrementally at first and then makes major structural changes.

3. When these major changes occur, they tend to be implemented rapidly and the market responds promptly.

4. The private sector often (but not always) adopts successful federal cost containment strategies (e.g., APCs and DRGs), making these methods universal.

Medicare Part B. Part B, also called Supplementary Medical Insurance (SMI), covers physician services; physical, occupational and speech therapies; hospital outpatient services; some home healthcare (see above); and durable medical equipment that is not provided as part of skilled home healthcare. An important part of the physician payments is coverage for non-self-administered medication (e.g., chemotherapy and immune system modulators). (Pills are paid under Part D, discussed later.) Beneficiaries are eligible to receive Part B benefits on becoming eligible for Medicare. Unlike Part A, beneficiaries can decline Part B and reenroll at a later time. The reason they may choose to do so is that Medicare Part B requires a premium, so if they are still working and receiving full coverage from their employer, there is no need for duplicate insurance. Beneficiaries who delay enrollment because they are employed may reenroll without penalty when they are no longer covered by their employer. It is important to note that with both Parts A and B, if an individual has employer-sponsored insurance, this private insurance is the primary coverage for those workers who are also eligible for Medicare (i.e., providers and suppliers must bill the private insurance first, before billing Medicare). This process is the opposite of what is done if the beneficiary has Medicare and a private Medigap policy.

Part B differs from Part A in the methods to calculate most payments. As mentioned above, hospital payments are made using *diagnoses* that determine the DRG designation. Professional fees, in contrast, are paid based on *service* codes. The different codes used for billing purposes are reviewed in Chapter 8, "Information Technology." The main difference is that physicians largely bill on a fee-for-service basis using Current Procedural Terminology-Version 4 (CPT-4) codes.[92]

The sources of funding for Part B are also very different from those of Part A. By design, about 75% of the program's cost is supposed to come from general tax revenues; the remaining approximately 25% should come from premiums the beneficiaries either pay directly or have the Treasury Department automatically deduct from their Social Security checks. In practice, the former payments have exceeded that limit while the latter percentage has been less than target. Exhibit 6.26 lists the premiums for Part B. Means testing for premiums began in 2007 as a result of the Medicare Modernization Act (MMA).

Finally, in addition to the premiums, Part B out-of-pocket expenses greatly differ from those of Part A. Part B recipients have to meet an annual deductible ($185 for 2019), after

---

[92]CPT codes are copyrighted and licensed for use by the American Medical Association.

EXHIBIT 6.26. **Medicare Premiums for 2019**

If your yearly income in 2017 (for what you pay in 2019) was			You pay each month (in 2019)
File individual tax return	File joint tax return	File married & separate tax return	
$85,000 or less	$170,000 or less	$85,000 or less	$135.50
above $85,000 up to $107,000	above $170,000 up to $214,000	Not applicable	$189.60
above $107,000 up to $133,500	above $214,000 up to $267,000	Not applicable	$270.90
above $133,500 up to $160,000	above $267,000 up to $320,000	Not applicable	$352.20
above $160,000 and less than $500,000	above $320,000 and less than $750,000	above $85,000 and less than $415,000	$433.40
$500,000 or above	$750,000 and above	$415,000 and above	$460.50

Source: CMS: 2019 Medicare Parts A & B Premiums and Deductibles. Retrieved from https://www.medicare.gov/Pubs/pdf/11579-Medicare-Costs.pdf.

which there is an unlimited 20% coinsurance on physician charges (except laboratory) and durable medical equipment. These potentially devastating liabilities are another reason beneficiaries need the supplemental insurance described above.

The payment flows are, however, analogous to Part A. The general revenues and premiums that pay for Part B are put into its own "trust fund," which is also merely a bookkeeping entry. Because the sources of funding are more diverse and do not depend solely on payroll taxes and number of employed (as with Part A), this fund is a bit more secure than its counterpart. However, Part B pays a significant and growing amount of money to providers. Please see Exhibit 6.27 for where these increases are occurring.

A number of strategies to hold down these costs have been implemented, including:

- Raising the individual premium contribution to the intended 25% level.

- Increasing the annual deductible (at inception in 1966, this payment was $50, so it has hardly kept pace with general inflation).

- Implementing means-tested premiums (again, see Exhibit 6.26; income brackets and charges are adjusted annually).

- Changing the methods and amounts paid to providers. For example, in 2018, MedPAC recommended that physicians be paid at the same rate for office visits whether the service is provided in their offices or Hospital Out Patients Departments (HOPDs). (HOPD rates are much higher.) In making this recommendation, the committee noted: "[W]e estimate

EXHIBIT 6.27. **Growth in the Volume of Clinician Services, 2000–2017**

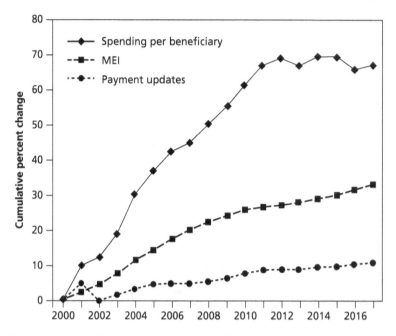

Note: MEI (Medicare Economic Index). The MEI measures the change in clinician input prices. Spending per beneficiary includes only services paid under the fee schedule for physicians and other health professionals and excludes services paid under the clinical laboratory fee schedule.

Source: MedPAC. *Report to the Congress: Medicare payment policy*. Chapter 4: Physicians and other professional services. March 2019. Retrieved April 12, 2019. http://www.med pac.gov/docs/defaultsource/reports/mar19_medpac_ch4_sec.pdf?sfvrsn=0

that the Medicare program spent $1.8 billion more in 2016 than it would have if payment rates for E&M office visits in HOPDs were the same as freestanding office rates. In addition, beneficiaries' cost sharing for E&M office visits in HOPDs was $460 million higher in 2016 than it would have been had payment rates been the same in both settings."[93]

Despite the fact that Part B payments have been escalating largely due to increases in volume of services (and to some degree use of technology, particularly new medications), the government's response has been to adjust *fees*, particularly for physician-administered pharmaceuticals and professional payments. These two measures are discussed in detail below.

[93]MedPAC. (2018, March). *Report to the Congress: Medicare payment policy* (p. 111). Retrieved June 2, 2018, from http://www.medpac.gov/docs/default-source/reports/mar18_medpac_entirereport_sec.pdf?sfvrsn=0

With respect to injectable pharmaceuticals administered in the doctor's office, prior to 2005, pharmaceutical companies sold injectable drugs (such as chemotherapy) to physicians at one price and simultaneously published a much higher Average Wholesale Price (AWP). Physicians would then bill Medicare carriers (and private insurers) based on a percentage of this latter inflated amount. Despite periodic outrages at the large markups, all payers (including CMS) were fully aware of this practice. Due to cost escalations, the Medicare Modernization Act mandated that, starting in 2005, the payment method for these items would be changed to an Average *Sales* Price (ASP), plus 6% (i.e., the federal government averages the national sales prices for individual drugs to all customers, netted for rebates, and 6% is added to payments).[94] This change raised two important issues. First, since the ASP is based on *national* figures, physicians could theoretically lose money because of market distortions. In some places acquisition costs could be more than ASP plus 6%. To address the concerns of physicians (particularly oncologists) who purchase these high-cost medications, CMS established a Competitive Acquisition Program (CAP). Under this scheme, physicians could buy drugs directly from several large wholesalers, which, by being able to purchase large quantities at best national rates, would be better able to bear the financial responsibility of acquiring and billing for the medication. However, because the sale of these medications is so profitable for physicians, the demand for CAP organizations was extremely low; by 2009, the program was functionally dead. Second, since this ASP strategy uses a cost-plus method, it is not likely to hold down expenditures in the long run and will continue to encourage physicians to use higher-cost medications.[95] Also, consider that the more pharmaceutical companies charge physicians, the more the latter will make in their 6% markups.

The other fee control tactic involves changing direct physician payments. The method of payment Medicare uses to compensate physicians and other professionals for their services is called the Resource Based Relative Value Scale (RBRVS). Details are summarized in Exhibit 6.28. Understanding this fee schedule is important since private payers have also adopted it as the basis of FFS payments. We will begin with some background on how and why it was developed.

In 1987, Hsiao and colleagues[96] published their landmark article explaining the methodology to be used to formulate an RBRVS. This new system promised to remedy the payment inequities between cognitive specialists (such as primary care physicians) and procedural specialists (such as surgeons) and set fees based on resource use rather than arbitrary physician-determined charges. While intended to replace the compensation system only for Medicare Part B providers, just 2 years after its implementation, it was quickly

---

[94] As a result of Congressional action in 2011 aimed at lowering government expense (called the budget sequester), starting in 2012 the drug reimbursement rate was cut to ASP plus 4.3 percent.

[95] See, for example: Jacobson, M., Earle, C. C., Price, M., & Newhouse, J. P. (2010). How medicare's payment cuts for cancer chemotherapy drugs changed patterns of treatment. *Health Affairs, 29,* 1391–1399.

[96] Hsiao, W. C., Braun, P., Becker, E. R., & Thomas, S. R. (1987). The resource-based relative value scale: Toward the development of an alternative physician payment system. *Journal of the American Medical Association, 258,* 799–802.

EXHIBIT 6.28. **Summary of Features of the Resource Based Relative Value Scale**

Origin:

1988—Harvard study under W. Hsiao that completed first phase of methodology research

1989—Omnibus Budget Reconciliation Act mandated use of methodology

January 1, 1992—RBRVS implemented

Covers:

Professional services of physicians, nurse practitioners, physician assistants, clinical psychologists, social workers, and certified nurse anesthetists and midwives.

Diagnostic tests except clinical laboratory tests, which are paid on a separate schedule. Professional fees of a pathologist for clinical lab tests are covered in the RBRVS.

Outpatient therapies, such as physical, occupational, and speech.

Radiology services, including professional and facility.

Supplies and services that are provided "incident to" physicians' professional services.

Calculation of rates:

Relative Value Units (RVUs) are determined for each service using the following categories:

Work—incorporates time and difficulty of service

Practice Expense—incorporates the cost of running a practice using geographic adjustments

Malpractice Expense—the cost of liability insurance (smallest component, implemented after 2000)

After each of these categories is adjusted for geographic differences, the RVUs are then added and a total is obtained.

The RVU for a given service is multiplied by a conversion factor in dollars. This factor applies to all services covered by the RBRVS. By federal law, the conversion factor was set annually; there is no regular time specified for RVU updates.

becoming the benchmark for most private and public physician payments.[97] (These payers often base their reimbursement on a percentage at, above, or below the Medicare rates.) More than two decades later, payment parity among specialties had not occurred and, in many cases, was worse.[98]

---

[97] McCormack, L.A., & Burge, R. T. (1994). The diffusion of RBRVS. *AHSR FHSR Annual Meeting Abstract Book, 11*, 130–131.

[98] Bodenheimer, T., Berenson, R. A., & Rudolf, P. (2007). The primary care-specialty income gap: Why it matters. *Annals of Internal Medicine, 146*, 301–306.

Prior to full RBRVS implementation in 1992, Medicare paid physicians based on a fee schedule termed Customary, Prevailing, and Reasonable (corresponding to the Usual, Customary, and Reasonable schedules in the private sector). Customary fees were a particular physician's typical charge for a specific service. Prevailing fees were set as a percentile (e.g., 75th percentile) of the range of charges by physicians in a particular specialty and geographic area for a specified service. The Reasonable category was established for services that were unusual or new. Most payments were made based on the lower of Customary or Prevailing charges. At least three problems existed with that system:

1. Physicians could arbitrarily increase their charges, resulting in a spiraling increase in local prevailing fees.[99]

2. Coding for services was not standardized. In fact, physicians could write a description of what they did and leave it up to the carrier to figure out how to pay.

3. Because the coding was not standardized and computerized systems were still several years away, many bills were "unbundled" (i.e., a global procedure was broken into its component parts). For example, imagine a bill for removing the appendix. Normally it would be one charge. Unbundling would mean the surgeon would bill for opening the abdomen, exploring (essentially "looking around"), removing the appendix, and, finally, closing the abdomen. Billing all the components individually would result in a bill much larger than the correct global charge.

All these problems contributed to cost escalations and a desire by CMS (then called the Health Care Financing Administration [HCFA]) to develop a new payment method. Price control was important *then* because, prior to RBRVS implementation, half of the increase in Medicare expenditures for physicians was due to rising fees.[100]

This history is significant because the expenditures that resulted from this inefficient system were those that served as the starting point for payments under the new RBRVS that is explained below. In other words, the new system, while providing a new calculus for payments, picked up the payment levels where the old system left off.

In searching for another method for payment, CMS chose a relative value methodology. The idea is that all medical services are ranked according to values relative to one another and multiplied by a dollar amount in order to obtain an actual payment for a particular service. (Specifics of current relative value units, or RVUs, are further explained below.) Differences among services were distinguished by *the amount of provider work*, which includes the time, risk, and skill necessary to deliver it. Frequently a common service, like gallbladder surgery (cholecystectomy), was selected to act as an index procedure (reference point) to compare relative values. For example, cardiac bypass surgery (CABG) takes more time, is riskier, and requires more skill than does a routine cholecystectomy. An office exam for a sore throat is less work than a cholecystectomy. How *much* greater or less, however, is subject to some

---

[99]Roe, B. B. (1981). The UCR boondoggle: A death knell for private practice? *The New England Journal of Medicine, 305*(1), 41–45.
[100]Physician Payment Review Commission. (1988, March). *Annual report to Congress.*

debate. Further, the *actual relative values* assigned depend on the chosen index procedure. For example, choosing an appendectomy as the index procedure, rather than cholecystectomy, will give a different value to CABG surgery. The method that CMS finally chose was based on the *relative resources* used to deliver each service, including, but not limited to, the work component.

While CMS wanted to involve physicians in the process of formulating the new payment method, it was concerned that antitrust issues precluded direct contracting with organizations like the American Medical Association (AMA). A compromise was to involve a third party: CMS, with AMA approval, chose William Hsiao and colleagues at the Harvard University School of Public Health. Work began in December 1985. According to the AMA: "Under terms from its subcontract form Harvard, the AMA's major role in the RBRVS study was to serve as a liaison between the Harvard researchers, organized medicine, and practicing physicians."[101] The AMA provided names of physicians for Technical Consulting Groups as well as representative practicing physicians. Hsiao and colleagues issued their final research reports on their methods and conclusions in a special issue of the *Journal of the American Medical Association* on October 28, 1988.

In their report, the investigators divided the resource cost of work into three parts. Each part relates to the resources used to perform a particular service, identified by a unique CPT (service procedure) code. The first and most important part is service-specific work (work RVU). This element is "a function of four dimensions: time [pre-service, intraservice and post service], mental effort and judgment, technical skill and physical effort, and stress."[102] Although the AMA had an arm's-length relationship in the *development* of the RBRVS, it is currently very much involved in determining fees for each specialty in two ways. *First*, the Relative Value Scale Update Committee (RUC) of the AMA reevaluates the work RVUs every 5 years. Of committee members representing specialty societies, only about 20% are primary care physicians.[103]

Since CMS accepts 95% of RUC recommendations,[104] it should come as no surprise that while many specialty RVU changes have been made over the past decade, office visit RVUs have not increased substantially. This process is one reason physicians who do procedures are paid more for their time than cognitive specialists, like primary care physicians. The AMA's *second* major input in this process is that it holds the copyright to the CPT; it can, therefore, add or delete codes.

Determination of work units (and hence payment amounts) largely by procedural specialists is only one problem with this system. Another problem is that the work component does not always change to account for higher volumes, greater individual experience, and

[101] Smith, S. L. (2008). *Medicare RBRVS 2008, The physician's guide*. Chicago: The American Medical Association.

[102] Hsiao, W. C., Braun, P., Dunn, D., Becker, E. R., DeNocola, M., & Ketcham, T. R. (1988). Results and policy implications of the resource-based relative-value study. *The New England Journal of Medicine, 319*, 881–888.

[103] American Medical Association. (2018). *Composition of the RVS update committee (RUC)*. Retrieved June 3, 2018, from https://www.ama-assn.org/about/composition-rvs-update-committee-ruc

[104] American Medical Association. (2018). *RBRVS: Resource-based relative value scale*. Retrieved June 3, 2018, from www.ama-assn.org/go/rbrvs

more professionals trained to perform the services. For example, Hayes et al.[105] found that "for cardiovascular services with high rates of volume growth . . . work RVUs for these services have tended to stay the same or—in the case of the echo exam of the heart—go up." In other words, medical care does not display the same cost-lowering behavior as do other products and services that are subject to a learning curve. Further, while older technology costs may not decrease, newer technologies are paid at relatively higher rates, even if they do not provide additional benefits. Comparative effectiveness research provisions in the ACA will probably not solve these problems, since cost cannot be considered in making implementation recommendations.

This process has also resulted in some unusually irrational rules. As an example of work component inequalities that do not make sense, consider a lesion removal. A surgeon or dermatologist removes a suspicious skin lesion that measures <0.5 cm (including excised skin). Assume the surgery is performed in a hospital where a pathologist examines the specimen while the surgeon waits for the results. If the lesion is benign or malignant and the margins (edges of the removed lesion) are free of cancer, the physician is "done" with that procedure. Regardless of the nature of the lesion, the same work was performed for the patient. However, if the lesion is benign, the physician bills 11400; if malignant, the CPT code is 11600. The latter code is paid at a higher rate than the former. This logic is not consistently applied for other procedures. For example, if a surgeon suspects a patient has appendicitis and removes the appendix, he or she does not get paid less if the appendix proves to be normal upon subsequent pathological examination. Another example of these questionable payment difference is exemplified by removal of colon polyps. This procedure has several codes depending on the *method* used to remove the lesions: for example, 45333 (removal by hot forceps or cautery), 45338 (removal by snare), and 45339 (removal by other methods). The reimbursement rates are all different. By contrast, a primary care physician who removes a wart would code 17110, regardless if it was accomplished by laser, liquid nitrogen, or surgical excision.

Although the work component is the first and most important determinant of payment, two other factors are included. The second RVU component is practice expense (PE). Briefly, in 2010, a 4-year transition began to change from an AMA-generated top-down process to one calculated by CMS that is a bottom-up approach, using information from a Physician Practice Information (PPI) survey. According to the November 1, 2005, CMS Final Rule:[106] "The bottom up approach would be simple to understand—we merely sum the costs of the . . . staff, supply and equipment inputs that are assigned to each service." This "simple" process is documented elsewhere and consists of *19 steps*![107]

---

[105] Hayes, K. J. (2007). Getting the price right: Medicare payment rates for cardiovascular services. *Health Affairs, 26*, 124–136.

[106] CMS.gov. *Medicare efforts to improve the accuracy of payment for physician practice expenses.* Retrieved June 3, 2018, from https://www.cms.gov/Newsroom/MediaReleaseDatabase/Fact-sheets/2005-Fact-sheets-items/2005-11-026 .html

[107] For a detailed explanation of determination of the practice expense component, see Federal Register: Rules and Regulations. 74 (226): 61742–61,756, 2009 (Wednesday, November 25, 2009).

The third component Hsiao et al. included was the financial opportunity cost of training, amortized over the physician's estimated practice lifetime. This portion was subsequently dropped.

The current third contributing factor is the relative value of professional liability insurance (PLI).[108] The PLI RVU assigned to a CPT service code is determined by:

1. Calculating a national average PLI premium for each specialty,

2. Normalizing specialty premiums to create a specialty-specific risk factor,

3. Calculating unadjusted PLI RVUs for each service based on the relative volumes of practitioners in each specialty who perform a service, and

4. Adjusting the RVUs for budget neutrality.

Medicare requires the PLI RVUs to be updated every 5 years.

In addition to these RVUs, CMS recognizes that the cost of delivering medical care varies by geographic location due to factors that may be out of the physician's control. These adjustments are called Geographic Practice Cost Indices (GPCIs), and each component has its own method for calculating its respective GPCI.

The work component GPCI is based on a cost-of-living factor determined by the U.S. decennial census for seven categories of professional occupations: architecture and engineering; computer, mathematical and natural sciences; social scientists, social workers and lawyers; education, library and training; registered nurses; pharmacists; writers, artists, and editors.

This factor takes into account physician preferences for living and practicing in certain areas, knowing that the costs of living and working are different. In this respect, the GPCI of the work component is also difficult to justify. Zuckerman[109] offers a rationale for geographic adjustments in payment for the time component of physician services and includes an explanation based on professional preference to locate. Recalling the issue of local area variations, however, it would seem just as appropriate to geographically adjust payment rates for physician-driven overutilization of services.

The practice expense GPCI reflects *differences* of resource input costs among different locales. The rent portion employs *apartment* data from the Department of Housing and Urban Development. Employee wage inputs use the decennial census data for clerical workers, nurses, and healthcare technicians. CMS does not adjust equipment and supply costs for geographic differences, believing that these items constitute commodities with more or less similar national prices.

---

[108] For more details, see Acumen, LLC (Prepared for CMS). *Interim report on the malpractice relative value units for the CY 2018 Medicare physician fee schedule.* Retrieved June 3, 2018, from https://www.cms.gov/Medicare/Medicare-Fee-for-Service-Payment/PhysicianFeeSched/Downloads/CY2018-PFS-NPRM-MP-RVU.pdf

[109] Zuckerman, S. (2002). *Just why do we adjust Medicare physician fees for geographic practice cost differences? Testimony before the Committee on Ways and Means / Subcommittee on Health.* Retrieved June 3, 2018, from http://www.urban.org/url.cfm?ID=900540

The GPCI for malpractice uses actual premium data; however, this data lags actual costs since, as mentioned, it may be updated only every 5 years.

The resultant formula for a specific service (listed as a CPT code) is therefore:

$$[\text{Work RVU} \times \text{Work GPCI}] + [\text{PE RVU} \times \text{PE GPCI}] + [\text{PLI RVU} \times \text{PLI GPCI}]$$
$$= \text{Total RVU}$$

Currently the overall Medicare RBRVS costs are weighted as follows: Physician Work: 51%; Practice Expense: 45%; and Professional Liability 4%.[110]

Once the RVU is determined for a particular service, it needs to be multiplied by a single, dollar-denominated conversion factor to give the actual payment amount. For 2019, the conversion factor is $36.05. After a dollar amount is determined for each service code for each CMS-designated geographic region (usually by county), further adjustments are made to individual payment rates based on three factors:

1. Does the physician accept the Medicare fee schedule as the basis for billing, or will she bill the patient and the MAC at a higher rate? Agreeing to accept the Medicare fee schedule is called "accepting assignment."

2. Where is the service provided (i.e., in the office or hospital-based facility)?

3. What is the physician's performance on quality activities?

The latter adjustment is determined by evolving regulations under the Medicare Access and CHIP Reauthorization Act of 2015. Because a large part of MACRA is tied to quality performance measures, this payment method is discussed in Chapter 9, "Quality."

The systems in place to control costs prior to MACRA are explained in Exhibit 6.29. Understanding how they failed is an instructive policy lesson.

Understanding the flaws in the RBRVS is important to fully appreciating newer Medicare payment initiatives. All of these programs use payment calculations based on RBRVS-determined fees; therefore, it is important that the system is fixed before other costs can be assessed. The backgrounds of three of these programs are discussed briefly below.

- *Global rates/bundled payments for care.* A number of demonstration projects showed that a single fee for a global episode of care can lower costs.[111] One often-cited example is the Heart Bypass Center Demonstration (1991–1996). In this seven-hospital study, "the Medicare program saved $42.3 million on bypass patients treated in the demonstration hospitals. The average discount amounted to roughly 10% on the $438 million in expected spending on bypass patients, including a 90-day post-discharge period. In

[110]American Medical Association. *RBRVS overview*. Retrieved June 3, 2018, from https://www.ama-assn.org/rbrvs-overview

[111]AHA Committee on Research: Bundled Payment: AHA Synthesis Report. May 20, 2010. Retrieved June 5, 2018 from http://www.hret.org/resources/1360004236

EXHIBIT 6.29. Brief History of Medicare's Volume and Spending Target Payment Methods

As mentioned earlier in this book, long before the RBRVS, it was well known that fee controls can cause physicians to compensate for lost revenue by increasing the volume and intensity of services.[a] In order to address this potential problem, Congress enacted a Medicare Volume Performance Standard (MVPS), under which physician payments were to be lowered if volume targets were exceeded. When the RBRVS was implemented, CMS maintained the MVPS spending target, but manipulated the dollar multiplier to control costs. Beginning in 1992, CMS set three different multipliers for: primary care, surgical specialties, and "other nonsurgical" specialties (such as radiology). This method changed in 1997 with passage of the Balanced Budget Act, which replaced the MVPS adjustment method by calculation of a Sustainable Growth Rate (SGR). (Starting in 1998, this law also mandated that a single conversion factor apply to all specialties.) According to CMS,[b] like the MVPS, the SGR targets were not direct limits on expenditures; rather they were used to update the next year's fees schedule. If expenditures for the current year exceeded the target, the update was reduced; if expenditures were less than the target, the update was increased. These calculations started April 1, 1996. In every year but one, physician reimbursement always exceeded targets; however, CMS never reduced payments but increased them in each year. A further problem was that CMS was using fee reductions as a tool to lower costs when most of the problem was with volume and intensity. According to the CBO, since 1997, the increase in spending for services paid under the physician fee schedule increased an average of 6.5% per year. *Fee increases accounted for 2%, and volume and intensity accounted for 4.5%.* As early as 2006, the CBO recognized "that the decline in payment rates will be slightly more than offset by increases in enrollment and growth in the volume and intensity of services being delivered."[c] As a result of these flaws, the deficit used for the fee reduction calculation continued to accumulate. For example, by 2010, the cumulative deficit was estimated at $12 billion; to zero the account, CMS would have had to cut physician Medicare payments by about 30%.

Because the SGR reconciliation consistently threatened payment reductions, physician groups (most prominently the AMA) lobbied for many years for elimination of the SGR. It was finally repealed with passage of the MACRA; years of deficits were wiped away, but much smaller increases in physician payment rates were planned.[d]

[a] One of the earliest publications on this subject was: Fuchs, V. R. (1978). The supply of surgeons and the demand for operations. *Journal of Human Resources, 13* (Supplement), 35–56.

[b] CMS.gov. Sustainable Growth Rates & Conversion Factors. Retrieved June 5, 2018 from http://www.cms.gov/Sustainable GRatesConFact/

[c] Marron, D. B. (2006, July 25). Testimony before the Subcommittee on Health, Committee on Energy and Commerce. Retrieved June 5, 2018, from https://www.cbo.gov/sites/default/files/109th-congress-2005-2006/reports/07-25-sgr.pdf

[d] From the second half of 2015 through 2019, the rates will be increased by 0.5% annually. The rates are then frozen from 2020 to 2025. Thereafter, the rates will be increased by either 0.25% annually for providers participating in the Merit-Based Incentive Payment System or by 0.75% annually for providers participating in Alternative Payment Models.

addition, beneficiaries (and their insurers) saved another $7.9 million in Part B coinsurance payments, so total Medicare savings were estimated as $50.3 million in 5 years."[112]

Building on these trials, on January 1, 2009, CMS started Acute Care Episode (ACE)

---

[112] Health Care Financing Administration [HCFA—now called CMS]. (1998, September). *Medicare Participating Heart Bypass Center Demonstration.* Retrieved June 6, 2018, from https://www.cms.gov/Research-Statistics-Data-and-Systems/Statistics-Trends-and-Reports/Reports/downloads/oregon2_1998_3.pdf

demonstrations in Texas, Colorado, New Mexico, and Oklahoma to pay hospitals and physicians global rates for certain orthopedic and cardiovascular procedures.[113] The global rate was less than the sum of all the individual components for a particular service (e.g., hospital and surgeon fees for CABG surgery). Under this arrangement, physicians and hospitals shared the financial rewards for providing care at less than the global payment. Further, CMS shared 50% of *its* savings with the patient. The results of this project yielded net per-episode savings of $319 and total net savings of approximately $4 million. Of note is that *savings on the procedures and inpatient care were offset in large part by increased post-acute care expenses.*[114] As a result, several types of bundled payments have been considered to include the entire episode of care. More recently, CMS has proposed the Bundled Payments for Care Improvement Advanced (BPCI Advanced) as a voluntary program for a 90-day episode of care.[115] More will be discussed about bundled payments in the Managed Care discussion and in Chapter 9.

■ *Medical homes.*[116] In this model, patients are assigned to a primary care physician who is responsible for coordinating all care across a continuum of health-related services. While bonus payments have been offered to encourage these doctors to sign up, given their voluntary nature and based on similar programs in France,[117] it is unlikely that much of an impact will be made without an increase in primary care fees or a government mandate for implementation. A precedent exists in Japan. Although there is a national fee schedule that pays all physicians the same for the same service, a higher differential payment was implemented for pediatricians because of a shortage in that specialty. This suggestion would require a return to significantly differential RBRVS multipliers for different specialties, as existed prior to 1997. Despite these caveats, CMS implemented a 4-year medical home project that expired in 2016. "Most medical home models incurred net costs to Medicare after accounting for care management fees . . . net Medicare spending totaled $51 million in its fourth and final year."[118] Currently, MACRA allowed creation of a CPC+ (Comprehensive Primary Care Plus) model; results are not yet available. More will be said about this model in Chapter 9.

[113]Centers for Medicare and Medicaid Services. (2008). *Medicare Acute Care Episode (ACE) Demonstration. CR 6001 rescinds and fully replaces CR 5767.* Retrieved 2008 from http://www.cms.hhs.gov/MLNMattersArticles/downloads/MM6001.pdf

[114]Health Care Financing Administration [HCFA, now called CMS]. (1998, September). *Medicare Participating Heart Bypass Center Demonstration.* Retrieved June 6, 2018, from https://www.cms.gov/Research-Statistics-Data-and-Systems/Statistics-Trends-and-Reports/Reports/downloads/oregon2_1998_3.pdf

[115]CMS.gov. (2018, May 31). *BPCI advanced.* Retrieved June 6, 2018, from https://innovation.cms.gov/initiatives/bpci-advanced

[116]While medical homes are an essential core of ACOs (explained in Chapter 4, "Hospitals"), these models are free-standing.

[117]Sandier, S., Paris, V., & Ploton, D. (2004). Healthcare systems in transition: France. Copenhagen: WHO Regional Office for Europe, on behalf of the European Observatory on Health Systems and Policies. Retrieved June 6, 2018, from www.euro.who.int/document/e83126.pdf

[118]Kaiser Family Foundation. *Medicare delivery system reform: The evidence link: The latest facts and results on Medicare ACO, medical home, and bundled payment models.* Retrieved June 6, 2018, from https://www.kff.org/faqs-medicare-medical-home-models/

▪ *Pay for performance/use.* This subject will also be discussed in Chapter 9. As mentioned, it is important to note that these incentive programs are based on fees calculated using the RBRVS methodology; making sure they truly achieve their desired purposes will require fee reforms.

In summary, the CMS physician reimbursement system (as well as that for the private sector) is complex and in need of major repairs. In considering the alternatives to maintaining current practices, two principles should be kept in mind:

1. As long as the majority of payment increases are due to volume and intensity, paying attention to price alone will never solve the problem of rapidly rising costs.

2. As long as there is no payment equity for primary care, we will continue to have problems staffing medical homes and coordinating comprehensive global payment programs.

Medicare Part C. Medicare Part C (called Medicare Advantage [MA]) is a program whereby beneficiaries enroll in a governmentally approved private health insurance plan that is largely funded by CMS. These plan types are explained below, but it is important to note that one insurance company can offer many different types of plans; the discussion here considers each of these plans as a stand-alone product.

The Medicare Parts A and B trust funds provide most of the financing for Part C (i.e., Part C does not have its own funding source). The additional funding comes from enrollees' premiums. Plans with which Medicare contracts must generally include all Medicare Part A and Part B benefits (except hospice) and offer an option that includes a Part D drug benefit. CMS allows the plans to offer "supplemental healthcare benefits," which are "(1) not covered by Original Medicare, (2) that is primarily health related, and (3) for which the Medicare Advantage plan must incur a direct medical cost."[119] Examples include extending skilled nursing home coverage beyond Medicare's 100-day limit and providing an eyeglass benefit, for which Medicare does not usually pay. One reason stricter limitations existed in the past was to prevent plans from providing illegal inducements to join them. In 2018, CMS relaxed criteria for supplemental benefits "if they are used to diagnose, prevent, or treat an illness or injury, compensate for physical impairments, act to ameliorate the functional/psychological impact of injuries or health conditions, or reduce avoidable emergency and healthcare utilization."[120]

The advantage to the enrollee for joining such plans is that, compared to traditional Medicare, the costs are less and the benefits are better. A typical Medicare beneficiary who has Parts A and B buys a supplemental (Medigap) policy as well as a Part D plan (which pays for self-administered medication). If that beneficiary enrolls in a Medicare Advantage plan, for a small or no additional premium than that for Medicare Part B, Medigap benefits and the

---

[119] *2019 Medicare Advantage and Part D Rate Announcement and Call Letter.* (2018, April 2). Retrieved June 6, 2018, from https://www.cms.gov/Newsroom/MediaReleaseDatabase/Fact-sheets/2018-Fact-sheets-items/2018-04-02-2.html.
[120] Ibid.

option for a no- or low-cost Part D plan are included. The disadvantage is that these plans have more focused networks. Recall that the trade-off for lower premiums and out-of-pocket expenses is a reduction of provider choice.

The historical development of these plans and their operational features are explained in the following sections. Again, history is instructive as it informs future policy decisions.

After Medicare became operational in 1966, the government experimented with several different types of private contracts.[121] The easiest method was contracting with established prepaid group practices called healthcare prepayment plans (HCPPs) to furnish only Part B services.[122] Other contracts were mostly on a "reasonable" cost reimbursement basis, though some risk plans were also in place. Then, as now, in order to join these private plans, beneficiaries were required to be eligible for both Parts A and B. If they chose such coverage, they signed up directly with a private insurer. The insurer then notified the Social Security Administration (SSA) about the change from traditional Medicare; SSA, in turn, informed CMS. Despite their existence, these plans were never really popular until, in 1982, the TEFRA expanded both the rules for contracting with CMS and the allowable methods of payment. Specifically, the act mandated that CMS add contracts with qualified private HMOs to offer coverage on a capitated *risk* basis (i.e., CMS would pay the HMO a fixed, monthly amount for each beneficiary in return for which the insurer would accept full financial risk for care).

TEFRA set the health plan capitation at 95% of what was called the Average Adjusted Per Capita Cost (AAPCC); that is, for *each* enrollee, CMS paid the HMO 95% of the calculated average cost of caring for a Medicare recipient of the same age and sex in that geographic area; a further, higher, adjustment was made for nursing home residents, those who also received Medicaid benefits (called dual eligibles), and/or those in the ESRD program. These Medicare HMOs were also allowed to charge premiums with CMS approval. In return for capitation, the plan not only had to provide all Medicare A and B services, but, as mentioned above, additional benefits which the company could choose.

Because of the incentives capitation may create, critics had two major concerns. First, they worried that those who enrolled in these plans would be healthier than the Medicare fee-for-service population, either because of self-selection or due to plan tactics to enroll healthier members. Second, once enrolled, there was a worry that those who were sick would not receive adequate care, forcing them to disenroll and rejoin traditional Medicare. The result of any of these events would be that CMS was overpaying. Research studies yielded mixed results in attempting to clarify if favorable selection or differential service use were, indeed, occurring.[123] Because of these concerns, a new payment methodology was mandated by the Balanced Budget Act of 1997 (BBA), which renamed these organizations

---

[121] Gruber, L. R. (1988). From movement to industry: The growth of HMOs. *Health Affairs*, 7(3), 197–208.

[122] HCPPs have been subject to numerous subsequent regulations. See, for example, 2002 (10/1/02 Edition) Code of Federal Regulations (CFR) Title 42: 417.800 Payment to HCPPs: Definitions and basic rules. Retrieved June 6, 2018, from https://www.gpo.gov/fdsys/pkg/CFR-2014-title42-vol3/pdf/CFR-2014-title42-vol3-part417.pdf

[123] Morgan, R. O., Virnig, B. A., DeVito, C. A., & Persily, N. A. (1997). The medicare-HMO revolving door—The healthy go in and the sick go out. *The New England Journal of Medicine*, *337*, 169–175; DeVito, C. A. (1997). Use of veterans affairs medical care by enrollees in medicare HMOs. *The New England Journal of Medicine*, 337, 1013–1014.

Medicare+Choice (pronounced "Medicare plus Choice") plans. After 2000, CMS began to pay plans *risk-adjusted* capitation based on Principle Inpatient Diagnostic Code Groups (PIP-DCGs). The hope was that by paying plans more to care for sicker patients, they would not try to (illegally) attract healthier enrollees or stint on patient care. Because this method incorporated hospital data only, ambulatory diagnoses were subsequently added. This adjustment scheme uses a list of diagnoses called the Centers for Medicare & Medicaid Services-Hierarchical Condition Categories (CMS-HCC). (Please see Exhibit 6.30 for a sample list.)

EXHIBIT 6.30. Sample of CMS Hierarchical Condition Categories

HCC1	HIV/AIDS
HCC2	Septicemia, Sepsis, Systemic Inflammatory Response Syndrome/Shock
HCC6	Opportunistic Infections
HCC8	Metastatic Cancer and Acute Leukemia
HCC9	Lung and Other Severe Cancers
HCC10	Lymphoma and Other Cancers
HCC11	Colorectal, Bladder, and Other Cancers
HCC12	Breast, Prostate, and Other Cancers and Tumors
HCC17	Diabetes with Acute Complications
HCC18	Diabetes with Chronic Complications
HCC19	Diabetes without Complication
HCC21	Protein-Calorie Malnutrition
HCC22	Morbid Obesity
HCC23	Other Significant Endocrine and Metabolic Disorders
HCC27	End-Stage Liver Disease
HCC28	Cirrhosis of Liver
HCC29	Chronic Hepatitis
HCC33	Intestinal Obstruction/Perforation
HCC34	Chronic Pancreatitis
HCC35	Inflammatory Bowel Disease
HCC39	Bone/Joint/Muscle Infections/Necrosis
HCC40	Rheumatoid Arthritis and Inflammatory Connective Tissue Disease

HCC46	Severe Hematological Disorders
HCC47	Disorders of Immunity
HCC48	Coagulation Defects and Other Specified Hematological Disorders
HCC54	Drug/Alcohol Psychosis
HCC55	Drug/Alcohol Dependence, or Abuse/Use with Complications
HCC56	Drug Abuse, Uncomplicated, Except Cannabis
HCC57	Schizophrenia
HCC58	Reactive and Unspecified Psychosis
HCC59	Major Depressive, Bipolar, and Paranoid Disorders
HCC60	Personality Disorders
HCC70	Quadriplegia
HCC71	Paraplegia
HCC72	Spinal Cord Disorders/Injuries

Source: CMS (2017, December 17). Note to: Medicare Advantage Organizations, Prescription Drug Plan Sponsors, and Other Interested Parties. Subject: Advance Notice of Methodological Changes for Calendar Year (CY) 2019 for the Medicare Advantage (MA) CMS-HCC Risk Adjustment Model. Retrieved June 6, 2018, from https://www.cms.gov/Medicare/Health-Plans/MedicareAdvtgSpecRateStats/Downloads/Advance2019Part1.pdf

In order to determine proper payment, plans submit utilization and diagnostic data for each member on an ongoing basis. Every 6 months, CMS performs an analysis of these codes and adjusts payments (retroactively) according to the individual's severity of illness. Note that these conditions are ones that substantively affect future anticipated healthcare expenditures. Acute, episodic illnesses and treatments, like appendectomy and gallbladder removal, usually do not influence future payments and thus are not included.

Another provision of the BBA of 1997 enabled CMS to contract with private PPOs. The law also created three new categories of health plans (which will be briefly explained below): Private Fee-For-Service (PFFS), Provider Sponsored Organizations (PSOs),[124] and the Program of All-inclusive Care for the Elderly (PACE).[125]

Unlike HMOs, PFFS plans were not required to have a contracted network and could charge Medicare beneficiaries a premium for costs in excess of the actuarial value of traditional Medicare Parts A and B. The fees they negotiated with providers needed to be at least equal to Medicare rates. The advantage to Medicare beneficiaries was that they could choose any participating Medicare provider, potentially receive extra services not covered

---

[124]Brock, T. H. (1998). New HCFA regulations clarify PSO requirements. *Healthcare Financial Management, 52,* 45–47.
[125]Retrieved from http://www.npaonline.org/website/article.asp?id=12

by traditional Medicare, and not have to pay an extra premium for a supplement. (The latter benefit is true of all MA plans.) In 2008, CMS announced that, starting in 2011, these plans needed to contract with a network of providers, thus reducing a major marketing advantage for them. As a result of this announcement, in 2009 two major participants, Coventry and WellCare, withdrew their participation in this product, requiring 500,000 Medicare members to seek other coverage. Many other participants followed suit in 2010, including many Blue Cross plans, CIGNA, and Harvard Pilgrim.

The requirements for a PSO were somewhat stricter than for PFFS plans. CMS (then HCFA) paid PSOs capitation and mandated that:

1. They are established, organized, and operated by a healthcare provider or a group of "affiliated" providers. The term "affiliated" generally referred to members with a common ownership or who, in the process of organizing, agreed to "share substantial risk."

2. They must provide a "substantial" portion of the services covered under Medicare (70% of the services through affiliated providers in urban areas; 60% in rural setting).

3. They enroll at least 1,500 members if they are an urban plan or 500 if a rural one.

4. They must be state-licensed as an insurer or meet certain federally established capitalization and liquidity requirements.

Note that these plans share similar organizational and financial risk features with ACOs.

PACE began as a community effort in San Francisco in 1970 and, 3 years later, became the On Lok program.[126] The aim was to provide comprehensive *social and medical* services for the frail elderly in order to enable them to continue living at home. Though initially locally funded, by 1990 it received Medicare and Medicaid waivers to operate with federal funds. With On Lok support, in 1994 the National PACE Association was formed, enabling 11 organizations in 9 states to become operational. The BBA of 1997 recognized the PACE model as a permanent plan type for both Medicare and Medicaid. "Currently, there are 124 PACE programs operating 255 PACE centers in 31 states serving over 45,000 participants."[127] Please see Exhibit 6.31 for details about this type of plan.

Under the Medicare program, the monthly capitation rate paid by CMS to the PACE provider is a blend of two formulas: (a) the county rate multiplied by a uniform PACE frailty adjuster and (b) a risk-adjusted payment methodology. This blend will transition to 100% risk adjustment in the coming years. Under the Medicaid program, the monthly capitation rate is negotiated between the PACE provider and the state Medicaid agency. Unlike Medicare HMOs, for which CMS retroactively adjusts payments based on the HCCs (see above), the capitation rate for PACE plans is fixed during the contract year regardless of changes in

---

[126]Hollander, M. J., Chappell, N. L., Prince, M. J., & Shapiro, E. (2007). Providing care and support for an aging population: Briefing notes on key policy issues. *Healthcare Quarterly*, *10*, 34–45; Bodenheimer, T. (1999). Long-term care for Frail Elderly People—The On Lok model. *The New England Journal of Medicine*, *341*, 1324–1328.

[127]National PACE Association. *Find a PACE program in your neighborhood*. Retrieved June 6, 2018, from https://www.npaonline.org/pace-you/find-pace-program-your-neighborhood

EXHIBIT 6.31. **PACE Organizations**

A PACE organization is a not-for-profit private or public entity that is primarily engaged in providing comprehensive medical and social services for frail elderly in a defined service area on a capitated basis. The PACE program delivers these services through an interdisciplinary team approach in an adult day health center that is supplemented by in-home and referral services in accordance with participants' needs.

Participants must be: age 55 or older; meet a skilled nursing facility level of care; and live in the PACE organization service area. A potential PACE enrollee *may* be, *but is not required* to be, any or all of the following: (a) entitled to Medicare Part A; (b) enrolled under Medicare Part B; or (c) eligible for Medicaid. The Omnibus Appropriations Act of 1998 permits states to cover non-Medicare/Medicaid PACE enrollees under institutional groups and rules similar to those that apply under home- and community-based services waivers; therefore, states can elect to cover PACE enrollees under the special income level group (also known as the 300% group). States can also apply other institutional rules to PACE enrollees, such as spousal impoverishment and posteligibility treatment of income.

PACE services are delivered at an adult day health center, home, and/or inpatient facilities and include, but are not limited to, all Medicare and Medicaid services, including a Part D benefit (and OTC medications if they are authorized by the PACE interdisciplinary team and are included in the participant's plan of care). Minimum services that must be provided in the PACE center include primary care, social services, restorative therapies, personal care and supportive services, nutritional counseling, recreational therapy, and meals. Hospice care is also covered unless the member chooses to opt out for the separate Medicare hospice program.

Source: CMS (2017, December). *Quick facts about Programs of All-Inclusive Care for the Elderly (PACE)*. Retrieved June 6, 2018, from https://www.medicare.gov/pubs/pdf/11341-PACE.pdf

---

the participant's health status. Beneficiary payments depend on the program that qualified them for PACE. If the individual qualifies for Medicare, all Medicare-covered services are paid for by Medicare. If a beneficiary also qualifies for the Medicaid program, he or she will either have a small monthly payment or pay nothing for the long-term care portion of the PACE benefit. If a beneficiary does not qualify for Medicaid, he or she will be charged a monthly premium to cover the long-term care portion of the PACE benefit and a premium for Medicare Part D drugs. However, in PACE, there is never a deductible or copayment for any drug, service, or care approved by the PACE team.

Similar to the PACE concept was one phased-out model that should be noted for its valuable lessons: the Social HMO (S/HMO). These demonstration projects, which began in 1984, were developed to coordinate acute, chronic, and long-term care for healthy Medicare beneficiaries as well as those who were eligible for skilled nursing home care. By limiting enrollment numbers and controlling for the health status of its members, plans were allowed to mirror the characteristics of the general Medicare population. Early versions (S/HMO I plans) focused on case management; second-generation plans, begun after 1996 (S/HMO II plans), intensified the case management and added comprehensive geriatric care. Depending on the beneficiary's characteristics (see above adjustments for Medicare HMOs), plans were paid capitation of *at least* 105% of what Medicare fee for service would pay for the same person. In addition to traditional Medicare services, S/HMOs also typically covered help with home-making activities and household chores, personal care, transportation to medical appointments, adult day care, respite care, limited nursing home services, eyeglasses, and (sometimes) pharmaceuticals.

Since CMS was paying more than its usual rates to these plans, it authorized two studies over their years of operation to assess cost savings and quality. These evaluations found that S/HMOs did not consistently reduce hospital or long-term nursing facility use, nor did they improve physical, cognitive, or emotional health of members. As a result, MedPAC recommended in April 2003 that S/HMOs be converted to Medicare +Choice plans starting on December 31, 2003. In January 2004, there were only about 120,000 members in the four remaining plans.[128]

The next major changes to this part of Medicare came in 2003 with passage of the Medicare Prescription Drug, Improvement, and Modernization Act (MMA). The act allowed most private plan options in the Medicare program under the term "Part C"[129] and changed the Medicare+Choice name to Medicare Advantage (MA). The act further expanded the types of private plans with which CMS could contract.[130] The current types of plans are discussed next.

- *Health maintenance organizations* (HMOs). Enrollees pick a primary care physician who coordinates all care in a narrower network than original Medicare. Plans are paid according to risk-adjusted capitation for each enrollee. More will be explained about HMOs in the Managed Care section.

- *Private fee-for-service (PFFS) plans.* Please see the above explanation.

- *Medical Savings Account (MSA) plans.* Except for covering Medicare beneficiaries, these plans are structured and function the same as those previously described.

- *Regional Preferred Provider Organizations* (RPPOs) and *Local Preferred Provider Organizations.* MA plans can define their service areas when applying for federal approval. When the MMA allowed PPOs, CMS established defined service areas where the plan is required to enroll all beneficiaries who apply and ensure appropriate access to care. For example, regional plans can serve a state while local plans can cover one or several counties. In other respects, they operate like PPOs (see the Managed Care section below).

- *Employer Group Waiver plans (EGWPs).*[131] As the name implies, these plans are customized exclusively for employer and union groups. Since 70% of enrollees in this

---

[128] Social Health Maintenance Organization (S/HMO). (2003, August). *Recommendations for the future of the demonstration. MedPAC.* Retrieved June 6, 2018, from https://permanent.access.gpo.gov/websites/www.medpac.gov/www .medpac.gov/publications/congressional_reports/Aug03_SHMO%20Report.pdf Congressional Budget Office. (2004, April). Financing long-term care for the elderly. Appendix B: Recent policy initiatives affecting long-term care financing. Retrieved from https://www.cbo.gov/sites/default/files/108th-congress-2003-2004/reports/04-26-longtermcare.pdf

[129] It is interesting to note that the term *Part C* was used for many years for a proposed Medicare long-term care plan.

[130] For contractual obligations, see CMS. (2019). *Part C—Medicare Advantage and 1876 Cost Plan Expansion Application.* Retrieved June 6, 2018, from https://www.cms.gov/Medicare/Medicare-Advantage/MedicareAdvantageApps/ Downloads/CY-19-Application.pdf

[131] AHIP. *Medicare Advantage, Employer Group Waiver Plans: What you need to know.* Retrieved June 6, 2018, from https://www.ahip.org/wp-content/uploads/2017/03/MA_EGWPs_FINAL_324.pdf

category belong to local PPO models, statistics about this type of plan often appear under that other category. In 2017, 3.7 million Medicare beneficiaries were in EGWPs, representing 20% of MA enrollees. Companies and unions are interested in these plans to control healthcare costs for retirees for whom they are often contractually obligated to furnish much more expensive non-MA private plans.

■ *Special Needs Plans (SNPs).* SNPs consolidated other existing programs to cover only certain targeted populations, including those who are eligible to receive both Medicare and Medicaid benefits (dual eligibles), the institutionalized (or those who would otherwise require care in those settings), and beneficiaries with specified severe or disabling chronic conditions. SNPs function and are paid like other MA plans, but they must provide a Medicare Part D drug benefit. Further modifications were made to this type of plan by the Medicare Improvements for Patients and Providers Act of 2008 (MIPPA).

Exhibit 6.32 summarizes some key differences among these plans. Exhibits 6.33 and 6.34 provide overviews of the growth of MA plans and their relative importance, respectively.

Despite risk-adjusted payments, several years after passage of the MMA, CMS was again worried that it was paying MA plans too much. This concern arose from several observations. First, as before, there was some evidence that MA enrollees were healthier than Medicare fee-for-service beneficiaries. Second, MA plans learned to code more accurately to capture additional payment offered by the HCC-adjusted compensation. Finally, after several years of decline, enrollment in Medicare HMOs started to increase again as Medicare beneficiaries recognized the advantages mentioned above while overall Medicare eligibility grew.

For those reasons, starting in 2006, payments to MA plans were based on a new system, called competitive bids. Unlike other competitive bidding systems in which the government engages, this one does not result in a "winner." Instead, plans submit their bids to CMS based on cost estimates to care for enrollees with Medicare Parts A and B benefits. CMS accepts *all* bids as long as they meet certain requirements (such as covered benefits). Each bid is then compared to a benchmark amount set by a statutory formula which varies by county (or region, in the case of regional PPOs). The benchmarks are the maximum amounts Medicare will pay a plan in a given area. If a plan's bid is higher than the benchmark, enrollees pay the difference in the form of a monthly premium (i.e., in addition to the Medicare Part B premium). If the bid is lower than the benchmark, the plan receives a rebate of up to 70% of the difference between those amounts. The plan is expected to use this rebate for such purposes as subsidizing Part D premiums or providing extra benefits. If the plan offers a Part D benefit, it submits a separate bid for that portion; CMS will then calculate payment as if the plan were offering a stand-alone Part D package. Part D is discussed in more detail below.

Following this bidding process, payments are adjusted by three additional factors. First, as previously explained, individual payments are changed depending on risk profiles determined by the CMS-HCCs and patient demographics.[132]

---

[132]For more detail about how the calculations are carried out, see CMS. (2017, October). Medicare Advantage Program Payment System. Retrieved June 6, 2018, from http://medpac.gov/docs/default-source/payment-basics/medpac_payment_basics_17_ma_finalc1a311adfa9c665e80adff00009edf9c.pdf?sfvrsn=0

EXHIBIT 6.32. **Different Requirements and Provisions Apply to Different Types of MA Plans**

	PFFS	Medical Savings Account	HMO/Local PPO	Regional PPO	SNP
Must build networks of providers[a]			✓	✓	✓
Must report quality measures			✓	✓	✓
Must have bids reviewed and negotiated by CMS			✓	✓	✓
Must return to the trust funds 25 percent of the difference between bid and benchmark[b]	✓		✓	✓	✓
Must offer Part D coverage[c]			✓	✓	✓
Must have an out-of-pocket limit on enrollee expenditures		✓		✓	
Can limit enrollment to targeted beneficiaries[d]					✓
Must offer individual MA plan if offering employer group plan[e]			✓	✓	✓

MA = Medicare Advantage, PFFS = private fee for service, PPO = preferred provider organization, SNP = special needs plan
Note: These features are as of 2008. Features can change annually but usually the basic structure is the same.

[a] PFFS plans are exempted from other MA plans' network adequacy requirements if they pay providers Medicare fee-for-service rates.

[b] This provision applies when bids are under the benchmark. For regional PPO plans, one half of the 25% amount is retained, and the remainder is included in the stabilization fund that, as of 2013, may be used to retain or attract such plans.

[c] Medical savings account plans are prohibited from offering Part D coverage. PFFS plans may offer Part D coverage, but special rules apply to such plans (e.g., it is not required that they receive drugs at a discounted rate when the deductible applies or the person is in the Part D coverage gap).

[d] MA plans must allow all Medicare beneficiaries in their service area to enroll with few exceptions (e.g., beneficiaries with end-stage renal disease). Other exceptions apply to medical savings account plans (e.g., Medicaid beneficiaries may not enroll in such plans). SNPs are permitted to limit their enrollment to their targeted beneficiary population (i.e., dual eligibles, beneficiaries who reside in an institution, or those with a chronic or disabling condition). SNPs can be local or regional coordinated care plans. They cannot be medical savings account or PFFS plans.

[e] Only nonnetwork PFFS plans can operate exclusively as plans limited to employer group enrollees.

Source: *Private fee-for-service plans in Medicare Advantage*, Medicare Payment Advisory Commission, Statement of Mark E. Miller, Ph.D., Executive Director, Before the Committee on Finance, U.S. Senate (January 30, 2008), p. 11. Retrieved June 6, 2018, from http://67.59.137.244/documents/MedPAC_Jan08_testimony_PFFS.pdf

Second is the quality score each plan receives. (For example, the quality score can change the percentage of the rebate calculation mentioned above.) In a process called "Star Rating Measures," plans are evaluated and assigned grades from one (low) to five (high) stars. According to CMS, evaluations are done in five broad categories:

1. Outcomes: Outcome measures reflect improvements in a beneficiary's health and are central to assessing quality of care.

EXHIBIT 6.33. Total Medicare Private Health Plan Enrollment, 1999–2018

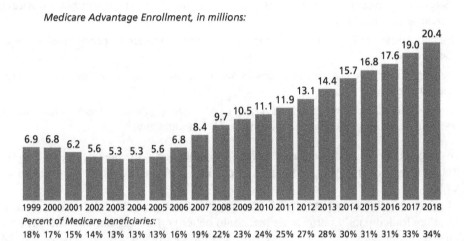

Medicare Advantage Enrollment, in millions:

Percent of Medicare beneficiaries:
18% 17% 15% 14% 13% 13% 13% 16% 19% 22% 23% 24% 25% 27% 28% 30% 31% 31% 33% 34%

Note: Includes Medicare Advantage plans and cost plans

Source: Kaiser Family Foundation: An Overview of Medicare. February 13, 2019. https://www.kff.org/medicare/issue-brief/an-overview-of-medicare/ Retrieved April 12, 2019.

EXHIBIT 6.34. Number of Medicare Advantage plans available by plan type, 2007–2019

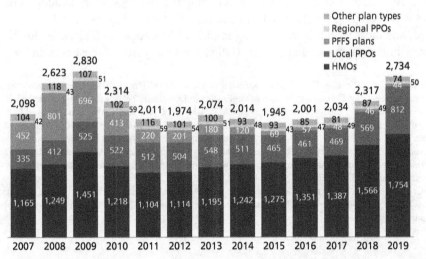

More Medicare Advantage plans are available in 2019 than in any year since 2009

Note: Excludes SNPs, employer-sponsored (i.e., group) plans, demonstrations, HCPPs, PACE plans, and plans for special populations. Other category includes cost plans and Medicare MSAs.

Source: Kaiser Family Foundation: Medicare Advantage 2019 Data Spotlight: First Look October 2018. https://www.kff.org/report-section/medicare-advantage-2019-spotlight-first-look-data-note/ Retrieved April 12, 2019.

2. Intermediate outcomes: Intermediate outcome measures reflect actions taken which can assist in improving a beneficiary's health status. Controlling Blood Pressure is an example of an intermediate outcome measure where the related outcome of interest would be better health status for beneficiaries with hypertension.

3. Patient experience: Patient experience measures reflect beneficiaries' perspectives of the care they received.

4. Access: Access measures reflect processes and issues that could create barriers to receiving needed care . . .

5. Process: Process measures capture the health care services provided to beneficiaries which can assist in maintaining, monitoring, or improving their health status.[133]

The specific metrics that are used depend on whether or not the plan has a Part D option. Star Rating Measures are also used for stand-alone Part D plans (i.e., those not affiliated with a MA plan).

Of concern is that insurance companies that own these plans found a way to game the process; they folded poorly performing plans into better performing ones to take advantage of higher payment rates.[134] "Since 2013, over 4 million enrollees—over 20 percent of MA enrollees—have been moved among contracts to secure bonus payments that would not otherwise be payable. Thus, while over 70 percent of MA enrollees are classified as being in plans rated 4 stars or higher, taking into account the enrollees who are in bonus-status plans because of consolidations, the actual share could be as low as 50 percent."[135]

In response, MedPAC recommended that starting in 2018, companies should be required to report quality measures using the geographic reporting units and definitions as they existed prior to consolidation, and the star ratings should be calculated as though the consolidations had not occurred; the pre-consolidation reporting units should be maintained until new geographic reporting units are implemented.[136] Subsequent to that recommendation, Congress passed the Bipartisan Budget Act of 2018, directing the HHS Secretary to address the consolidations by averaging the star results of contracts that are being combined.

Third, and most recent, is that starting in 2017, CMS began to include health disparity differences in the payment calculations. Called the Categorical Adjustment Index (CAI),

---

[133]CMS. Medicare 2018 Part C & D star ratings technical notes. Retrieved June 6, 2018, from https://www.cms.gov/Medicare/Prescription-Drug-Coverage/PrescriptionDrugCovGenIn/Downloads/2018-Star-Ratings-Technical-Notes-2017_09_06.pdf The specific measures can be found at: CMS: 2018 Part C & D Rating Measures, retrieved from https://www.cms.gov/Medicare/Prescription-Drug-Coverage/PrescriptionDrugCovGenIn/Downloads/2018MeasureList.pdf

[134]Mathews, A. W., & Weaver, C. (2018, March 11). Insurers game medicare system to boost federal bonus payments: Humana, Aetna, and other providers enhance revenue by shuffling customers among privately managed plans. *The Wall Street Journal*. Retrieved June 6, 2018, from https://www.wsj.com/articles/insurers-game-medicare-system-to-boost-federal-bonus-payments-1520788658

[135]MedPAC. (2018, March). Report to the Congress: Medicare Payment Policy. Chapter 13: The Medicare Advantage Program: Status Report. Retrieved June 6, 2018, from http://www.medpac.gov/docs/default-source/reports/mar18_medpac_ch13_sec.pdf?sfvrsn=0

[136]Ibid.

it "is a factor that is added to or subtracted from a contract's overall and/or summary Star Ratings to adjust for the average within-contract disparity in performance associated with a contract's percentages of beneficiaries with Low Income Subsidy/Dual Eligible (LIS/DE) and disability status. The value of the CAI varies by a contract's percentages of beneficiaries with Low Income Subsidy/Dual Eligible (LIS/DE) and disability status."[137] With the exception of Medicaid, *this adjustment is noteworthy because it is the first time that these characteristics have been used in any payment formula in the public or private sector.*

Despite these measures, costs for MA plans continued to rise.

To correct this persistent problem, the ACA (2010) contained the following provisions to revise the methodology:

1. *Change the benchmarks.* First, Medicare reimbursements to hospitals have included what is called "indirect medical education" payments (i.e., subsidies to cover some of the training costs for residents). The ACA scheduled their removal from the benchmark calculations. Second, starting in 2012, benchmark reductions were phased in to make all payments closer to the fee-for-service portion of Medicare. In its first move, CMS divided all benchmarked areas into quartiles, based on their per-capita cost to deliver care to Medicare beneficiaries. Plans in areas in the highest quartile—that is, with the highest costs (such as Miami-Dade County, FL, and Orange County, CA)—would have the fee-for-service-determined benchmark multiplied by 95%; plans in counties in the second quartile would be paid at 100% of the benchmark; those in counties in the third quartile would be paid at 107.5% of the benchmark; and those in counties in the lowest quartile (e.g., Boise and Honolulu) would be paid 115% of the benchmark.

2. *Alter the rebate amount and method.* Instead of keeping the lower bid rebates at 75% for all, plans would have this percentage determined by quality scores based on the Star Rating Measures described above. The shares of the rebates were to be: <3.5 stars: 50%; 3.5–4.0 stars: 65%; and 4.5–5.0: 70%. Further, CMS was to pay bonuses to plans achieving scores of at least 4.0 stars that started at 1.5% in 2012, increased to 3% in 2013, and were 5% in 2014 and thereafter.[138]

3. *Apply a Medical Loss Ratio.* Beginning in 2014, plans must maintain a MLR of at least 85%, consistent with the ACA requirement for large group plans.

4. *Change the risk adjustment calculation.* Because much of the payment increases to MA plans came from risk adjustments, CMS started to reduce the risk scores in 2010. The ACA extended CMS authority to lower these scores. In 2011, rates were reduced by 3.41%, with plans to reduce them by at least 5.7% in 2019 and thereafter.

---

[137] CMS.gov. *2017 star ratings.* Retrieved June 6, 2018, from https://www.cms.gov/Newsroom/MediaReleaseDatabase/Fact-sheets/2016-Fact-sheets-items/2016-10-12.html#_ftn6

[138] See ACA Section 1102. Medicare Advantage Plans for other details on fee adjustments.

Results of these changes are mixed. According to MedPAC:[139]

> Lower benchmarks have led to more competitive bids from plans: Bids have dropped from roughly 100 percent of FFS before the Patient Protection and Affordable Care Act of 2010 to 90 percent of FFS in 2018. For 2018, about 70 percent of plans, accounting for 77 percent of projected MA enrollment, have bids below FFS spending.
>
> On average, quality bonuses in 2018 will add 4 percent to the average plan's base benchmark and will add 3 percent to plan payments. The base benchmarks (that is, excluding the quality bonuses) are expected to average 103 percent of FFS spending in 2018, an increase from 102 percent in 2017, due to demographic changes in the Medicare population . . .
>
> Our updated analysis for 2016 shows that higher diagnosis coding intensity resulted in MA risk scores that were 8 percent higher than scores for similar FFS beneficiaries.

As is evident from the above history, these plans continue to evolve and federal efforts are directed at further reducing costs while increasing Star ratings.

Medicare Part D. The Medicare Catastrophic Coverage Act of 1988 was the first law to contain provisions for payment for self-administered medications for Medicare beneficiaries. While seniors wanted this benefit, it was never made clear to them that it came with an extra premium and that those with higher incomes would have to pay a proportionately greater amount. This law was, therefore, also the first time that any means testing was applied to Medicare. When seniors became aware of this extra charge, they publicly demonstrated their disapproval, which included the famous attack on the car of Dan Rostenkowski (D-IL), then the chair of the House Ways and Means Committee. The repeal of the law in 1989 was unprecedented; no previous piece of social legislation of this nature had ever been withdrawn.

The Medicare Modernization Act (MMA) of 2003 authorized the resurrection of a plan to provide pharmaceuticals to this group. This time, however, the environment was different from the situation in 1988. First, with the MMA, seniors were more involved in requesting the legislation. Second, the structure of the benefits is much more complicated under the MMA, and complaints about this complexity and difficulty understanding the plan diverted some initial attention from the premium amounts. Third, the MMA plan was not initially means tested; this portion was phased in over time, and seniors, by and large, were not aware of this feature. A discussion of some of Part D's characteristics follows.

Persons eligible for Part D must also qualify for Medicare. Participation is strictly voluntary, but unlike Part B, one must enroll in a particular plan; coverage is not automatic. (The exception is that those eligible for Medicare *and* Medicaid are automatically enrolled and assigned to a particular plan, though they also can voluntarily disenroll.) Also, individuals who qualify for a Medicare Savings program (mentioned above) automatically qualify for Part D, as do those under the Low Income Subsidy (LIS) program. The SSA annually

---

[139]MedPAC. (2018, March). Report to the Congress: Medicare Payment Policy. Chapter 13: The Medicare Advantage Program: Status Report, op. cit.

determines eligibility for these latter programs. The LIS helps qualified individuals pay all or part of their Part D premiums and out-of-pocket expenses. Further, some states (22 in 2018)[140] fund their own State Pharmacy Assistance Program to help the elderly and/or disabled. Details of these programs vary from state to state, but federal law allows them to subsidize Part D expenses for eligible individuals.

After someone becomes eligible to join Medicare, he or she has 6 months to enroll in Part D without paying a higher premium; this mechanism discourages members from buying the insurance only when they need it the most. The premium penalty is calculated at 1% per month on an annually determined amount based on the average national premium ($41[141] in 2018, but with a large variation by state).[142] Exceptions to late enrollment penalties are granted to individuals who had "creditable coverage" prior to enrollment (such as private insurance through an employer) or were covered under the LIS program.[143] In order to facilitate enrollment in Part D, an innovative, web-based program (www.medicare.gov) allows Medicare eligibles to sign up for the plan that best meets their needs. After entering their Social Security numbers and dates of Medicare (A and B) eligibility, the website prompts individuals for their zip codes and medication names, with doses, preferences for generics (if available), and frequency of use. The resulting list ranks plans by total expected annual cost (including premiums, copayments, and deductibles) for these specified medications. Individuals can enroll in a plan online and choose to have premiums deducted from their Social Security payments.

The federal government chose to neither administer the Part D plan directly nor be involved in negotiations with pharmaceutical companies. Instead, in 2005, CMS began to issue annual requests for proposals from companies wanting to participate as Part D insurance plans. Two types of plans can participate: Medicare Advantage (MA) plans and freestanding companies, called Prescription Drug Plans (PDPs).

> In 2018, 43 million of the 60 million people with Medicare have prescription drug coverage under a Medicare Part D plan; most (58%) are covered under a stand-alone prescription drug plan (PDP) but a growing share (42% in 2018) are in Medicare Advantage prescription drug plans (MA-PDs), which also provide other Medicare-covered benefits. More than 12 million Part D enrollees receive premium and cost-sharing assistance through the Part D Low-Income Subsidy (LIS) program.[144]

---

[140]Medicare.gov. *State pharmaceutical assistance programs*. Retrieved June 6, 2018, from https://www.medicare.gov/pharmaceutical-assistance-program/state-programs.aspx?varstate=ID

[141]Cubanski, J. (2018, May 17). *Medicare Part D in 2018: The latest on enrollment, premiums, and cost sharing*. Retrieved June 6, 2018, from https://www.kff.org/medicare/issue-brief/medicare-part-d-in-2018-the-latest-on-enrollment-premiums-and-cost-sharing/

[142]As an example, if an individual were eligible January 1, 2018, and waited 6 months to enroll, the penalty would be 6% × 41 = $2.46 per month *for life*. The exception is if eligibility was due to disability; in that case the base starts at zero again when the individual turns 65.

[143]Exceptions have also been granted to victims of natural disasters, such as hurricanes, where enrollment delays are caused because of these events.

[144]Cubanski, J. et al.: Medicare Part D in 2018: The Latest on Enrollment, Premiums, and Cost Sharing, op. cit.

EXHIBIT 6.35. Medicare Part D Standard Benefit Design in 2019

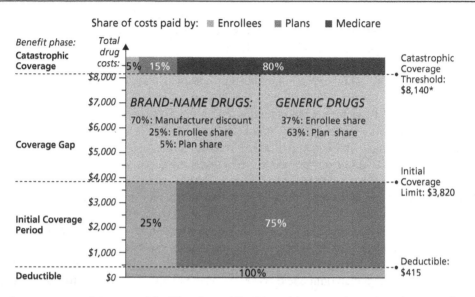

Share of costs paid by: ▨ Enrollees ▨ Plans ▨ Medicare

Benefit phase:	Total drug costs:		
Catastrophic Coverage		5% 15% 80%	Catastrophic Coverage Threshold: $8,140*
Coverage Gap	$8,000 / $7,000 / $6,000 / $5,000 / $4,000	*BRAND-NAME DRUGS:* 70%: Manufacturer discount / 25%: Enrollee share / 5%: Plan share — *GENERIC DRUGS* 37%: Enrollee share / 63%: Plan share	Initial Coverage Limit: $3,820
Initial Coverage Period	$3,000 / $2,000	25% 75%	
Deductible	$1,000 / $0	100%	Deductible: $415

Note: Some amounts rounded to nearest dollar. "The estimate of $8,140 in total drug costs corresponds to a $5,100 out-of-pocket threshold for catastrophic coverage in 2019.

Source: Kaiser Family Foundation: An Overview of the Medicare Part D Prescription Drug Benefit October 12, 2018 https://www.kff.org/medicare/fact-sheet/an-overview-of-the-medicare-part-d-prescriptiondrug-benefit/ Retrieved April 12, 2019.

Each year CMS sets parameters for the actuarial basis for PDPs' premium calculation. (Please see Exhibit 6.35 for 2019.) Given this basis, plans can offer actuarially equivalent benefits by altering the beneficiary's expenses (i.e., using different copayments, premiums, and deductibles). Further, Part D sponsors can offer products with enhanced benefits (like lower out-of-pocket expenses or payment for noncovered products) for an extra premium. The plans must offer at least two medications in each therapeutic category but can exclude such drugs as OTC medications, weight modification treatments, vitamins (except prenatal), barbiturates, benzodiazepines, cosmetic pharmaceuticals (such as to enhance hair growth), and drugs used for erectile dysfunction.

The plan then submits an annual bid to CMS for each state where it wishes to do business. Since inception, the process has worked in this way:[145] After receipt of these bids, CMS calculates a national weighted averaged benchmark premium; about 75% of the benchmark premium comes from CMS while the remaining 25% is paid by the beneficiary. The lower

[145]MedPAC. (2017, October). *Part D payment system.* Retrieved June 9, 2018, from http://www.medpac.gov/docs/default-source/payment-basics/medpac_payment_basics_17_partd_final86a411adfa9c665e80adff00009edf9c.pdf?sfvrsn=0

the plan bid, the less the beneficiary pays in premiums. Starting in 2011, individual premiums have been based on adjusted gross incomes (similar to those for Medicare Part B) and can be lowered by additional government payments. Please see Exhibit 6.36 for these income-based amounts. In addition to those calculations, CMS employs a formula using Prescription Drug Hierarchical Condition Categories (RxHCCs). These categories are based on higher drug use in patients with certain diagnoses (combined with age, sex, and disability information); payment is adjusted three times a year for changes in health status. The system is now in transition from a Risk Adjustment Processing System (RAPS) where calculations are inferred to one relying on encounter data.[146]

The covered drugs are contained in formularies, which are lists of pharmaceuticals, their uses, generic status, and out-of-pocket costs for patients. These costs are usually copayments, though coinsurance is starting to be used more commonly. Drugs are classified according to payment tiers. The lowest payments are for generic drugs. The next tier is for branded drugs for which the supplier has a favorable contract either with the pharmaceutical company or through a wholesaler. (Please see Chapter 7, Healthcare Technology, Exhibit 7.11 for the flow of goods.) Finally, if there is no contract with the manufacturer or wholesaler, or if the price is higher than an equivalent drug, the patient pays a still-higher rate.

EXHIBIT 6.36. Medicare Part D Costs 2019

Monthly premium costs determined by 2017 tax filing

Individual Tax Return	File Joint Tax Return	File Married & Separate Tax Return	You Pay Each Month (in 2019)
$85,000 or less	$170,000 or less	$85,000 or less	Your plan premium
above $85,000 up to $107,000	above $170,000 up to $214,000	not applicable	$12.40 + your plan premium
above $107,000 up to $133,500	above $214,000 up to $267,000	not applicable	$31.90 + your plan premium
above $133,500 up to $160,000	above $267,000 up to $320,000	not applicable	$51.40 + your plan premium
above $160,000 and less than $500,000	above $320,000 and less than $750,000	above $85,000 and less than $415,000	$70.90 + your plan premium
$500,000 or above	$750,000 and above	$415,000 and above	$77.40 + your plan premium

Source: Medicare.gov: Monthly premiums for drug plans. https://www.medicare.gov/drug-coverage-part-d/costs-for-medicare-drugcoverage/monthly-premium-for-drug-plans Retrieved April 12, 2019.

---

[146]Clark, A., & Koenig, D. (Milliman Whitepaper). *Risk score impacts of the Medicare Advantage 2018 RxHCC risk score model update. How does this model update affect plan risk scores?* Retrieved June 8, 2018, from http://us.milliman.com/uploadedFiles/insight/2017/risk-score-impacts-Medicare-Advantage-2018.pdf

One little-appreciated fact is that before enactment of the MMA, about 75% of Medicare recipients had some form of drug coverage: through work (active workers or retirees with this benefit), private individual coverage (such as Medigap policies), or Medicaid. The current system covers more people but is costlier. For example, between 2007 and 2016, "Part D program spending on an incurred basis increased from $46 billion to $79 billion (an average annual growth rate of about 6 percent)."[147] One strategy to lower costs has been a proposal for CMS to directly negotiate drug costs with the manufacturers instead of leaving the process to the drug plans. However, CBO analyses have not shown large potential savings.[148] Interestingly, Democrats have advocated this policy for a number of years, but more recently it has been raised by Republicans.

Outpatient End Stage Renal Dialysis Program (ESRD). The ESRD of Medicare covers beneficiaries for outpatient dialysis services, drugs, and equipment.[149] It is the only disease-specific government-funded plan, and Medicare is by far the single largest payer for these services. "In 2016, more than 390,000 beneficiaries with ESRD on dialysis were covered under fee-for-service (FFS) Medicare and received dialysis from more than 6,700 dialysis facilities... Compared with all Medicare FFS beneficiaries, dialysis beneficiaries are disproportionately young, male, and African American."[150] Services are provided by few private companies; for example, in 2017, Fresenius and DaVita provided dialysis for about 86% of all patients (public and private) and owned about 82% of all facilities.[151] Consolidation is continuing and is being closely followed by the Federal Trade Commission.

In order to fully understand this program's funding and health policy implications, presented below is the background of relevant technology and how the program came into existence.

Among other functions, the kidney filters waste products (excreting them into the urine); produces erythropoietin, a hormone that stimulates red blood cell production; helps the body produce vitamin D (which is essential for calcium regulation and bone formation); and aids in blood pressure regulation. When the kidneys fail, waste accumulates in the blood (largely in the form of urea, a protein metabolite), red blood cell production drops and anemia develops, calcium metabolism is faulty (bones can lose calcium and become

---

[147]MedPAC: Chapter 14: The Medicare prescription drug program (Part D): Status report. March 2018. Retrieved June 6, 2018 from http://www.medpac.gov/docs/default-source/reports/mar18_medpac_ch14_sec.pdf For a current accounting and future projections of Part D as well as other parts of Medicare, see 2018 Annual Report of the Boards of Trustees, Federal Hospital Insurance and Federal Supplementary Medical Insurance Trust Funds (June 5, 2018). Retrieved June 9, 2018, from https://www.cms.gov/Research-Statistics-Data-and-Systems/Statistics-Trends-and-Reports/ReportsTrustFunds/Downloads/TR2018.pdf

[148]Cubanski, J., & Neuman, T. (2018, April 26). *Searching for savings in Medicare drug price negotiations.* Retrieved June 9, 2018, from https://www.kff.org/medicare/issue-brief/searching-for-savings-in-medicare-drug-price-negotiations/

[149]Medicare inpatient services are paid by DRGs. Dialysis is, therefore, covered by that method.

[150]MedPAC. (2018, March). Chapter 6: Outpatient dialysis services. Report to the Congress: Medicare Payment Policy. Retrieved June 9, 2018, from http://www.medpac.gov/docs/default-source/reports/mar18_medpac_ch6_sec.pdf?sfvrsn=0

[151]Nephrology News and Issues (2017, July 16). Retrieved June 9, 2018, from https://www.healio.com/nephrology/practice-management/news/online/%7Bd894132b-b577-435e-8dec-401cd89d1b1e%7D/the-largest-dialysis-providers-in-2017-more-jump-on-integrated-care-bandwagon

weaker), and blood pressure can increase. Failure can come from a variety of causes, including complications from diabetes, long-standing high blood pressure, infections, and autoimmune conditions, like lupus. Medications can help treat all but the first problem (i.e., accumulation of urea). Two techniques are available to remove this waste. The first is hemodialysis, which works by pumping a patient's blood on one side of a semipermeable membrane while a fluid similar in content to the blood (but without the urea) flows in the opposite direction on the other side; the waste products diffuse from the blood through the membrane and into the other fluid, which is then discarded. (Please see Exhibit 6.37.)

While this concept is very simple to understand, applying it to a working dialysis machine requires: (a) knowledge that urea is a major toxin in kidney failure; (b) commercial availability of an appropriate semipermeable membrane; and (c) the ability to reliably prevent blood from clotting so that it can flow out of the body, past the membrane, and back into the body. Technologies to apply all of these concepts started in the 1830s, but it was only about 1937 that the latter two were available to treat humans. World War II impaired the spread of further technological developments and the ability to mass replicate any devices. After the war, the clinical application of hemodialysis resumed; however, it was only used for *acute* cases of kidney failure, where the patient was expected to recover in a relatively short amount of time. Experts thought it clinically and financially impracticable to apply this technology to chronically ill patients. Further breakthroughs came in the early 1960s, primarily with better devices and techniques for easily getting the blood from the body to the machine (where urea was removed) and back into the patient without clotting. One such device (usually placed in the arm) was an external shunt, a Teflon tube in a U-shape with one end in an artery and the other in a vein. Blood traveled out from the arterial end into the tube from where it was diverted into the dialysis machine, filtered of wastes, and returned to the body via the venous part of the loop. Because these devices enabled physicians to dialyze the blood repeatedly with minimal patient trauma, they were well suited for chronic treatment. The problem was that since these devices are outside the skin, they predispose the patient to infection. The next development was a surgical technique connecting an artery directly to a vein *inside* the body; the resulting configuration is called an arteriovenous fistula or arteriovenous shunt. Using this internal shunt, physicians needed to access the vessels and puncture the skin only for dialysis, thus reducing the potential for infection. (It should be noted that shunts and fistulas were not new, but techniques were perfected and disseminated during this time. For example, the first artery to vein connection for dialysis was performed in 1924.)

The second technique for removing waste is called peritoneal dialysis (PD). Fluid is introduced into the abdominal cavity (peritoneum) and left for a time to accumulate the wastes that diffuse from the blood vessels. The fluid is then drained and discarded. The advantages of PD over hemodialysis are that it can be accomplished more easily by the patient at home, can be done in the evening or while the patient sleeps (rather than at set hours in a dialysis facility), and is less costly overall. "The lower cost is primarily related to the fact that in PD, the patient or family member administers the dialysis, whereas in hemodialysis, it is performed by a relatively expensive trained staff. Also, there are much greater capital costs in setting up a hemodialysis as compared with a PD unit. PD does require expensive sterile solutions and disposable tubing, but the end result is that the total cost of delivering

EXHIBIT 6.37. **Hemodialysis and Arteriovenous Graft**

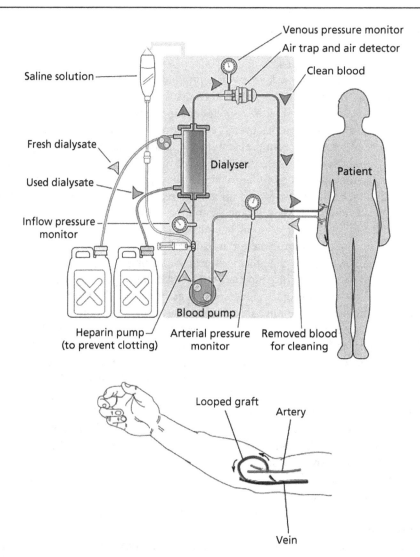

PD is 50% to 70% of the cost of delivering hemodialysis."[152] PD also compares very favorably to hemodialysis with respect to outcomes when adjusted for patients with diabetes and cardiovascular disease (who do better with the latter method).[153] Since physicians are not involved with every session, it is less profitable for them to supervise this type of treatment. Hemodialysis remains the predominant method for dialysis. (Please see Exhibit 6.38 for a schematic of peritoneal dialysis.)

The legislative history behind the ESRD Program (passed as Section 299I of the Social Security Amendments of 1972 [Public Law 92-603]) is a lesson in public advocacy and good fortune that has been well described by firsthand participants.[154] While the technology for hemo- and peritoneal dialysis developed roughly simultaneously, legislative activities were mainly directed at the former, more expensive, treatment. The following initiatives were all important and cumulatively accounted for the success of the amendment's passage:

EXHIBIT 6.38. Peritoneal Dialysis

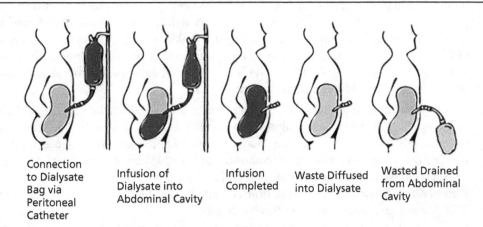

Connection to Dialysate Bag via Peritoneal Catheter

Infusion of Dialysate into Abdominal Cavity

Infusion Completed

Waste Diffused into Dialysate

Wasted Drained from Abdominal Cavity

Source: Wikipedia contributors. Peritoneal dialysis. In *Wikipedia, The Free Encyclopedia*. Retrieved from https://en.wikipedia.org/w/index.php?title=Peritoneal_dialysis&oldid=883641927

[152]Sharma, A., & Blake, P.G. (2007). Peritoneal dialysis (Chapter 59). In Brenner: *Brenner and Rector's The kidney* (8th ed.). Philadelphia: W.B. Saunders.

[153]Weinhandl, E. D., Foley, R. N., Gilbertson, D. T., Arneson, T. J., Snyder, J. J., & Collins, A. J. (2010). Propensity-matched mortality comparison of incident hemodialysis and peritoneal dialysis patients. *Journal of the American Society of Nephrology, 21*(3), 499–506; Vonesh, E. F., Snyder, J. J., Foley, R. N., & Collins, A. J. (2006). Mortality studies comparing peritoneal dialysis and hemodialysis: What do they tell us? *Kidney International, 70*, S3–S11.

[154]Plante, C. L. (2000, April). 1971 Medicare amendment: Reflections on the passage of the end-stage renal disease medicare program. *American Journal of Kidney Diseases, 35*(4), Supplement 1, S45–S48; Schreiner, G. E. (1997). How ESRD-medicare developed. *Seminars in Nephrology, 17*, 152–159.

- Strong and persistent advocacy by the National Kidney Foundation (NKF) from 1967 to 1972.

- The inclusion of the NKF in the federal government's Combined Federal Campaign (CFC), allowing federal employees to donate to select charities using payroll deductions. Funds thus raised allowed the NKF to finance a prolonged lobbying campaign.

- National media touted the life-saving technology hemodialysis could offer. Of particular note was a January 1, 1964, *Life Magazine* article about a patient on home dialysis and his wife who helped him with the procedure.

- Numerous public awareness campaigns at the local level. For example, because of the lack of consistent monetary resources in the 1960s, people held fundraisers for specific dialysis patients. Such activities included bake and candy sales, collecting coupons (e.g., from Kool cigarettes and Betty Crocker products), running marathons, playing bridge, and so on.

- Concurrent with the development of dialysis technologies were advances in organ transplantation capabilities. Due in part to the publicity of the first human heart transplantation by Dr. Christian Barnard in 1967, states passed enabling laws that set the terms for all potential organ transplants.[155] Because the states had different laws that needed harmonization if regional programs were to succeed, in 1968, the first Uniform Anatomical Gift Act was passed. The publicity from these legal efforts, as well as from individuals who signed donor cards, raised the public's knowledge about kidney transplantation and the plight of chronic kidney disease patients.

- Along with federal initiatives, several states enacted or considered legislation to help cover a portion of the costs of dialysis. It became clear to all concerned that individual states simply did not have the deep pockets to provide the kind of financial support needed. Out of this situation came the horror stories of selection committees deciding who should live and who should die and of the impoverishment of ESRD patients and their families. Some patients moved from so-called poor support states to rich states (in ESRD coverage terms) in order to receive treatment.

- In 1971, both the UAW and United Steel Workers unions negotiated dialysis coverage as part of their health insurance benefits.

Due to all these initiatives and public pressures, in 1972, members of Congress introduced more than 100 bills dealing with dialysis funding. When the House and Senate versions of what was to become P.L. 92-603 came to conference committee, the Senate version contained not only an ESRD benefit provision but also language that called for prescription drug funding for Medicare beneficiaries. The House members opposed these cost-increasing measures; the compromise was to drop the drug coverage in return for keeping the ESRD benefits. It should be noted that advocates for other diseases protested special use of resources for this

---

[155]National Anatomic Gift Act (2006). Retrieved June 12, 2011, from http://uniformlaws.org/ActSummary.aspx?title=Anatomical Gift Act

one condition; however, funding was justified by focusing on specific high-cost treatments (dialysis and transplantation).

After implementation of the ESRD law, costs for those services rose dramatically. Efforts to rein in expenses began in 1981 with the OBRA, which mandated "that each facility would receive a payment rate per dialysis treatment ('composite rate') that is adjusted for geographic differences in area wage levels for the treatment furnished in the facility or at home."[156] The intent of that change, which became effective August 1, 1983, was to include some routinely provided drugs, laboratory tests, and supplies, along with the usual dialysis services, in a global payment. Over time, however, some of the bundled items were excluded from the composite rate, particularly erythropoiesis-stimulating agents (ESAs) that replace the lost erythropoietin-producing ability of the kidney and vitamin D supplements.

Despite this effort, costs continued to rise. As a result, Congress and governmental agencies made many additional attempts to bundle these separately billable items, since they were largely responsible for the rapid cost escalations; by 2010, they comprised about 40% of the cost of outpatient maintenance dialysis.

It was only with passage of the MIPPA in 2008 that this bundling goal was accomplished. As a result of this law, since 2011 "Medicare has paid for outpatient dialysis services using a prospective payment system (PPS) that is based on a bundle of services. The bundle includes certain dialysis drugs and ESRD-related clinical laboratory tests that were previously paid separately. In 2016, Medicare expenditures for outpatient dialysis services were $11.4 billion, a 2 percent increase compared with 2015 expenditures."[157] Like other prospective payment programs, this one is calculated using baseline payment projections adjusted for individual patient characteristics and includes quality adjustments. Although Medicare Part D covers self-administered drugs, this new payment system also includes oral forms of injectable medications (even if available in the future) and oral medications that are strictly related to chronic kidney failure. (The oral drug coverage began in 2014.) Please see Exhibit 6.39 for a summary of payment features.

Payments are still made based on an episode of dialysis; for hemodialysis, they are capped at an amount equal to 3 dialysis sessions per week. They do not include physician fees. Even though PD is less costly, for those over age 18 the reimbursement is the same per session as hemodialysis.

The payment method for home hemodialysis is the same as that for facility-based outpatient services. The option to get supplies directly from a durable medical equipment (DME) provider for home dialysis no longer exists. Also, Medicare pays for teaching sessions for those who want to self-administer their dialysis. With either facility or home-based treatments, the beneficiary is still responsible for the annual Medicare deductible and 20% coinsurance.

---

[156] August 12, 2010, Federal Register Part II Vol. 75, No. 155. 42 CFR Parts 410, 413, and 414 Medicare Program; End-Stage Renal Disease Prospective Payment System; Final Rule and Proposed Rule.

[157] MedPAC. Chapter 6: Outpatient dialysis services, op. cit.

EXHIBIT 6.39. Key Features of the ESRD Prospective Payment Program

Payment Method Feature	Details
Payment bundle	▪ Composite rate services
	▪ Separately billable (Part B) injectable dialysis drugs and their oral equivalents
	▪ ESRD-related laboratory tests
	▪ Selected ESRD Part D drugs
	▪ Self-dialysis training services
Unit of payment	Single dialysis treatment
Add-on payment to the composite rate	None
Self-dialysis training services adjustment	Yes
Beneficiary-level adjustments	▪ For adults: age, dialysis onset, body surface, body mass, specific acute (pericarditis; gastrointestinal tract bleeding or hemorrhage) and chronic (hereditary hemolytic or sickle cell anemias; myelodysplastic syndrome) patient comorbidities
	▪ For pediatric patients: age, dialysis method
Facility-level adjustments	▪ Wage index
	▪ Low-volume adjustment
	▪ Adjustment for rural location
Outlier policy	Applies to the portion of the broader payment bundle composed of the drugs and services that were previously separately billable
Quality incentive program	For 2018, 11 outcome measures and 5 process measures

ESRD = end-stage renal disease.
Note: The low-volume adjustment does not apply to pediatric patients.

Source: MedPAC (2017, October). *Outpatient dialysis services payment program*. Retrieved June 9, 2018, from http://www.medpac .gov/docs/default-source/payment-basics/medpac_payment_basics_17_dialysis_finald8a311adfa9c665e80adff00009edf9c.pdf? sfvrsn=0

In addition to changing the payment method for episodes of dialysis, MIPPA also mandated an ESRD Quality Improvement Program (QIP) for facility payments. Since the prospective payment system bundles facility costs, it puts providers at higher financial risk than an FFS system. The QIP program is in place to evaluate the adequacy of the dialysis process in removing waste from the blood, making sure that adequate medication is administered (particularly erythropoietin drugs), and keeping complication rates to a minimum. The QIP extends public reporting of dialysis center outcomes that was started in 2001 and appears on the Dialysis Facility Compare website.[158] The new initiative affected payments on or after January 1, 2012, and is based on quality performance measures that are set by CMS. For the 2018 payment year, the ESRD quality incentive program included 16 measures:[159]

- Four outcome measures that assess dialysis adequacy (i.e., the extent to which dialysis is removing enough wastes and fluid from the body).

- Two outcome measures that assess hemodialysis vascular access—use of autogenous AV fistulas and intravenous catheters.

- An outcome measure that assesses the ratio of the number of observed unplanned 30-day hospital readmissions to the number of expected unplanned 30-day hospital readmissions.

- An outcome measure that assesses the ratio of observed red blood cell transfusions to the number of expected transfusions.

- An outcome measure, the National Healthcare Safety Network bloodstream infection measure, that assesses the number of hemodialysis outpatients with positive blood cultures per 100 hemodialysis patient-months.

- An outcome measure that assesses the proportion of patients with hypercalcemia, an indicator of the management of bone mineral metabolism and disease.

- An outcome measure that uses the in-center hemodialysis Consumer Assessment of Healthcare Providers and Systems Survey instrument to measure, from the perspective of in-center hemodialysis patients, the quality of dialysis care they receive from their nephrologist and from the staff of the dialysis facility.

- A process measure that assesses the percentage of patients with documentation of a pain assessment using a standardized tool and documentation of follow-up when pain is present.

- A process measure that assesses the percentage of patients screened for clinical depression using a standardized tool and documentation of a follow-up plan when necessary.

- A process measure that assesses the percentage of a facility's health personnel who received an influenza vaccination, had a medical contraindication to vaccination, declined vaccination, or were of an unknown vaccination status.

- A process measure that assesses the number of months for which facilities report the dosage of ESAs (as applicable) and hemoglobin/hematocrit of dialysis beneficiaries.

- A process measure that assesses the number of months for which facilities report patients' serum phosphorus levels (another indicator of bone mineral metabolism and disease).

---

[158] CMS.gov. (2018). *Dialysis facility compare*. Retrieved June 9, 2018, from www.medicare.gov/dialysis
[159] MedPAC. (2017, October). *Outpatient dialysis services payment program*. Op. cit.

The success of prospective payment implementation in 2011 to reduce excessive medication use and costs is demonstrated in Exhibits 6.40 to 6.43.

Transplantation. Once a person is chronically dependent on dialysis (and otherwise meets certain medical criteria), he or she is a candidate for transplantation. According to MedPAC:[160]

> Kidney transplantation is widely regarded as a better ESRD treatment option than dialysis in terms of patients' clinical and quality of life outcomes . . . transplantation results in lower Medicare spending; in 2015, average Medicare spending for patients who had a functioning kidney transplant or received a kidney transplant was less than half the spending for dialysis patients ($36,389 vs. $93,064, respectively). However, demand for kidney transplantation exceeds supply.

After surgery, patients are placed on lifelong medications to lessen the likelihood of rejecting the transplant. If a beneficiary is eligible only because of the kidney failure,

EXHIBIT 6.40. **Use of Dialysis Drugs Before and After Prospective Payment System Implementation in 2011**

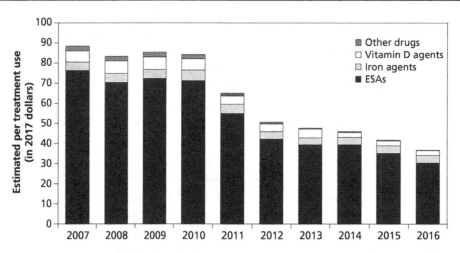

Note: Dollars per treatment are calculated by multiplying drug units reported on claims by the 2017 average sales price. Drugs included are epoetin alfa, epoetin beta, darbepoetin (ESAs); iron sucrose, sodium ferric gluconate, ferumoxytol, ferric carboxymaltose (iron agents); calcitriol, doxercalciferol, paricalcitol (vitamin D agents); daptomycin, vancomycin, alteplase, levocarnitine (all other drugs).

ESA = erythropoietin-stimulating agent.

Source: MedPAC (2017, October). *Outpatient dialysis services payment program.* Chapter 6, Outpatient dialysis services. Retrieved June 9, 2018, from http://www.medpac.gov/docs/default-source/payment-basics/medpac_payment_basics_17_dialysis_finald8a311adfa9c665e80adff00009edf9c.pdf?sfvrsn=0

---

[160]MedPAC. Chapter 6: Outpatient dialysis services, op. cit.

EXHIBIT 6.41. Total spending per year by modality for ESRD beneficiaries

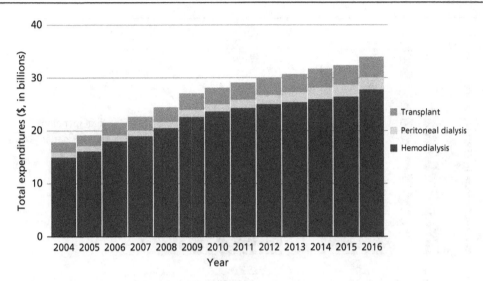

Note: In 1988, the National Institute of Diabetes and Digestive and Kidney Diseases of the National Institutes of Health established the United States Renal Data System.

Source: United States Renal Data System: Chapter 9: Healthcare Expenditures for Persons with ESRD. October 24, 2018. https://www.usrds.org/20 18/view/v2_09.aspx Retrieved April 12, 2019.

EXHIBIT 6.42. Total Medicare ESRD Expenditures, by Modality, 2004–2015

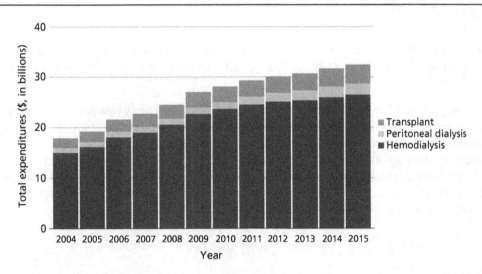

Note: In 1988, the National Institute of Diabetes and Digestive and Kidney Diseases of the National Institutes of Health established the United States Renal Data System.

Source: United States Renal Data System. *2017 Annual Data Report. Volume 2: End-stage renal disease in the United States. Chapter 9: Healthcare expenditures for persons with ESRD.* Retrieved from https://www.usrds.org/2017/view/v2_09.aspx

EXHIBIT 6.43. Annual Percentage Change in Medicare ESRD Spending, 2004–2016

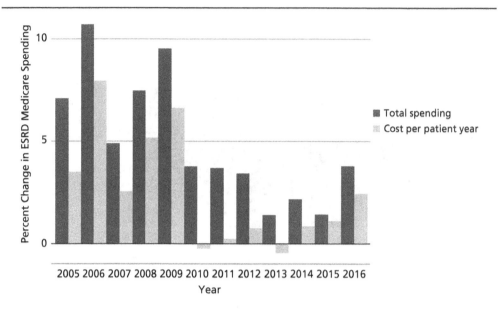

Note: In 1988, the National Institute of Diabetes and Digestive and Kidney Diseases of the National Institutes of Health established the United States Renal Data System.

Source: United States Renal Data System: Chapter 9: Healthcare Expenditures for Persons with ESRD. October 24, 2018. https://www.usrds.org/2018/view/v2_09.aspx Retrieved April 12, 2019.

then CMS will cover the cost of these medications for 36 months. If the beneficiary is also over age 65 or is eligible because of chronic disability, then medications are covered indefinitely.

Summary. While Medicare is often called a single-payer system, its various parts, sources of funding, and reasons for existence make it subject to very different financial and policy concerns. Without understanding this complexity, the public and lawmakers tend to prefer simplistic solutions that may only make the system worse. The one exception that has worked is prospective payment methods; however, they must apply to the entire system to avoid passing cost and quality problems downstream as patients receive care. Please see summaries of Medicare sources and spending of funding in Exhibits 6.44 and 6.45.

EXHIBIT 6.44. Sources of Medicare Revenue, 2017

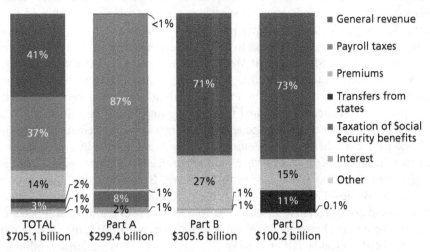

				Legend
41%	<1%			■ General revenue
	87%	71%	73%	■ Payroll taxes
37%				▨ Premiums
				■ Transfers from states
14% ⌐2%		27%	15%	■ Taxation of Social Security benefits
⌐1%	8% ⌐1%			▨ Interest
3% ⌐1%	2% ⌐1%	⌐1% ⌐1%	11% ⌐0.1%	▨ Other
TOTAL $705.1 billion	**Part A** $299.4 billion	**Part B** $305.6 billion	**Part D** $100.2 billion	

Note: Data are for the calendar year

Source: Kaiser Family Foundation: The Facts on Medicare Spending and Financing. June 22, 2018 https://www.kff.org/medicare/issue-brief/the-facts-on-medicare-spending-andfinancing/ Accessed April 12, 2019.

EXHIBIT 6.45. Medicare Benefit Payments by Type of Service, 2016

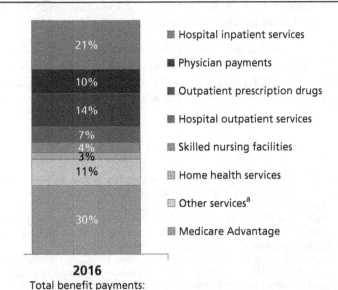

	Legend
21%	▨ Hospital inpatient services
10%	■ Physician payments
14%	■ Outpatient prescription drugs
7%	■ Hospital outpatient services
4%	▨ Skilled nursing facilities
3%	
11%	▨ Home health services
	▨ Other services[a]
30%	▨ Medicare Advantage

2016
Total benefit payments:
$675 billion

[a] Consists of Medicare benefit spending on hospice, durable medical equipment, Part B drugs, outpatient dialysis, ambulance, lab services, and other Part B services. Current web address: http:files.kff.org/attachment/Issue-Brief-The-Facts-on-Medicare-Spending-and-Financing

Source: Cubanski, J., & Neuman, T. (2017, July 18). *The facts on Medicare spending and financing*. Retrieved June 9, 2018, from https://www.kff.org/medicare/issue-brief/the-facts-on-medicare-spending-and-financing/

Medicaid

Background. Medicaid, the single largest healthcare program in the United States, was implemented along with Medicare in 1966[161] and covers about one fifth of the U.S. population. Although all states currently participate in Medicaid, it is not mandatory for them to do so. (Arizona was the last state to join the Medicaid program in 1982.) Several key differences exist between Medicare and Medicaid. The former is a strictly federally funded program with uniform national benefits. Most Medicare beneficiaries are categorically eligible based on age; therefore, the number of current and future recipients is known with great precision. Medicaid has shared federal-state funding for benefits that are largely determined at the state level. Despite federal requirements for participation, the *extent* of coverage and payment schemes for specific services varies dramatically from state to state, making generalizations unfeasible. Further, individuals need to apply for benefits rather than qualifying automatically, as is the case with Medicare. Because of this latter feature, the exact number of Medicaid *eligibles* is impossible to determine. Also, since individuals and families go on and off Medicaid rolls with great frequency, the exact number of beneficiaries nationwide is constantly changing. For example, as of December 2018, the average monthly enrollment for Medicaid and CHIP was about 72.5 million.[162] However, many millions more are enrolled for one or more months during the year. Beginning in 2014, the ACA expanded federally sponsored Medicaid eligibility to cover nearly all nonelderly Americans with incomes below 138% of the federal poverty level (FPL) (about $34,000 for a family of four in 2018),[163] or about 16.3 million additional people to date. Not all states have participated in this voluntary expansion; Republican-controlled states usually did not participate, despite federal promises to initially cover 100% of the costs of expansion and 90% on an ongoing basis. (Please see Exhibit 6.46 for a map of expansion states.)

Eligibility. Prior to 1996, Medicaid eligibility was linked to welfare benefits; that is, those eligible for the program of Aid to Families with Dependent Children (AFDC) were automatically entitled to Medicaid. With passage of the Personal Responsibility and Work Opportunity Reconciliation Act of 1996 (P.L. 104-193), this link was severed. AFDC was replaced by

---

[161] For a history of Medicaid and CHIP legislation, see Medicaid and CHIP Payment and Access Commission (MACPAC). *Federal legislative milestones in Medicaid and CHIP*. Retrieved June 17, 2018, from https://www.macpac.gov/federal-legislative-milestones-in-medicaid-and-chip/

[162] Kaiser Family Foundation: Total Monthly Medicaid and CHIP Enrollment. https://www.kff.org/health-reform/state-indicator/total-monthly-medicaidand-chip-enrollment/?currentTimeframe=0&sortModel=%7B%22colId%22:%22 Location%22,%22sort%22:%22asc%22%7D Retrieved April 12, 2019.

[163] The ACA changed the calculation to determine eligibility with respect to the FPL. The new method is called the Modified Adjusted Gross Income (MAGI). MAGI is adjusted gross income (AGI) plus: untaxed foreign income, nontaxable Social Security benefits, and tax-exempt interest. It excludes Supplemental Security Income (SSI).

EXHIBIT 6.46. Status of State Medicaid Expansion Decisions as of February 2019

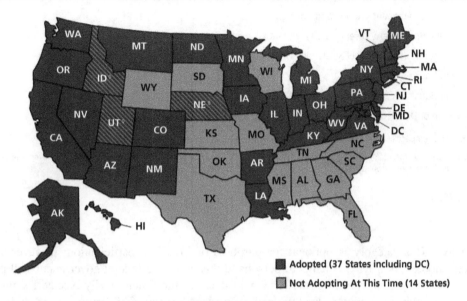

Adopted (37 States including DC)

Not Adopting At This Time (14 States)

Notes: Current status for each state is based on KFF tracking and analysis of state activity. ᐃExpansion is adopted but not yet implemented in ID, NE, and UT. (See link below for additional state-specific notes).

Source: "Status of State Action on the Medicaid Expansion Decision," KFF State Health Facts, updated February 13, 2019. https://www.kff.org/health-reform/state-indicator/state-activity-around-expanding-medicaid-under-the-affordable-care-act/   Retrieved April 12, 2019.

Temporary Assistance for Needy Families (TANF), which put time limits on welfare benefits. In order to preserve health insurance for those whose welfare benefits expired, Medicaid set up separate eligibility criteria; for families with children, the criteria initially were those existing under AFDC.

In order to receive federal funding, states can include three populations eligible for public healthcare assistance. First, if a state wishes to obtain any federal contributions, it must cover persons who are classified as "Categorically Needy." (Please see Exhibit 6.47 for examples in this group.) Changes in the criteria for this and other categories are frequently linked to income percentiles based on the FPL for individuals and families. The eligibility for the second and third categories described below requires that the beneficiary is first eligible for the Categorically Needy group. The second group is called "Medically

EXHIBIT 6.47. **Mandatory Categorically Needy Examples**

Low Income Families

Qualified Pregnant Women and Children

Mandatory Poverty Level Related Pregnant Women

Mandatory Poverty Level Related Infants, Children Aged 1–5 and Children Aged 6–18

Individuals Receiving SSI

Individuals Receiving Mandatory State Supplements

Blind or Disabled Individuals Eligible in 1973

Note: For a complete list of mandatory and optional needy as well as medically needy, see Medicaid.gov.

Source: *List of Medicaid eligibility groups*. Retrieved June 15, 2018, from https://www.medicaid.gov/medicaid-chip-programinformation/by-topics/waivers/1115/downloads/list-of-eligibility-groups.pdf.

Needy." This category is optional for purposes of Medicaid participation; however, if a state chooses to provide benefits to persons in this class, the federal government will provide matching funds on the same basis as it does for the Categorically Needy. Examples in this category include Medically Needy: Pregnant Women; Children under 18 and Age 18 through 20 (separate age categories); Parents and Other Caretaker Relatives; and Aged, Blind, and Disabled. A third category are those with "Special Needs." The largest group in this category (12 million in 2017)[164] are those persons who are eligible for both Medicare (over 65 and/or permanently disabled) *and* Medicaid (low income); they are called *dual eligibles*.[165] Medicare is the primary insurance for this group, and Medicaid pays for what is not covered (e.g., deductibles and coinsurance). Further, Medicaid pays Medicare premiums, including those for Medicare Advantage plans and Medicare Parts B and D. Medicaid also pays for benefits not covered by Medicare (e.g., long-term care; certain behavioral health services; hearing, vision, and dental costs). In addition to the Medicare Advantage plans

---

[164]CMS: People Dually Eligible for Medicare and Medicaid. Fact Sheet March 2019. https://www.cms.gov/Medicare-Medicaid-Coordination/Medicare-and-Medicaid-Coordination/Medicare-Medicaid-Coordination-Office/Downloads/MMCO_Factsheet.pdf Retrieved April 12, 2019.

[165]Medicaid and CHIP Payment and Access Commission (MACPAC). *Beneficiaries dually eligible for Medicare and Medicaid*. Retrieved June 15, 2018, from https://www.macpac.gov/wp-content/uploads/2017/09/Beneficiaries-dually-eligible-for-Medicare-and-Medicaid.pdf

described above, a special category exists for this group called a dual eligible special needs plan (D-SNP).[166]

Other special needs categories also exist. Two examples are noteworthy. The first program is the Qualified Disabled and Working Individuals (QDWI) Program for working disabled persons under 65 who lost premium-free Part A when they went back to work, are not receiving state medical assistance, and meet the income and resource limits required by their state. The Medicaid program can help them pay Part A premiums.[167] The second program was established by the Breast and Cervical Cancer Prevention and Treatment Act of 2000 (P.L. 106–354). It allows states to provide time-limited Medicaid coverage with federal matching funds to uninsured women—regardless of their income or resources—who are screened by the Centers for Disease Control and Prevention's National Breast and Cervical Cancer Early Detection Program and found to need treatment for breast or cervical cancer. These women can receive all Medicaid-eligible services, not only those related to their cancers.[168]

One further category of Medicaid coverage is for those persons who do not qualify for Medicaid benefits but are allowed by their state to buy into the program.

> Under a Medicaid buy-in proposal, the core target population would typically be those who are purchasing insurance using advanced premium tax credits (APTCs), or who are eligible for APTCs but uninsured. States have the flexibility to specify either a broader or narrower target group. A Medicaid buy-in may allow individuals not eligible for commercial group coverage to purchase a Medicaid-like plan. This type of proposal may allow a state to replace or augment the current insurance marketplace and ACA premium assistance structure under federal waiver authorities.[169]

---

[166]Lester, R. S., & Chelminsky, D. [Mathematica Policy Research] (2018, March 27). *Using CMS data to understand D-SNP market trends and performance, dual eligible characteristics, and state Medicaid managed care programs.* Retrieved June 17, 2018, https://www.google.com/url?sa=t&rct=j&q=&esrc=s&source=web&cd=1&cad=rja&uact=8& ved=0ahUKEwjFjIy9wNvbAhUK5YMKHaU0AIIQFggpMAA&url=https%3A%2F%2Fwww.mathematica-mpr.com %2Four-publications-and-findings%2Fpublications%2Fusing-cms-data-to-understand-d-snp-market-trends-and-performance-dual-eligible-characteristics&usg=AOvVaw1wnCasXkRaFT1aCIE_boQU; Two other Medicare Advantage Special Needs Plan (SNP) categories are Chronic Condition (C-SNP) and Institutional (I-SNP). See CMS.gov. *Special Needs Plans.* Retrieved June 17, 2018, from https://www.cms.gov/Medicare/Health-Plans/SpecialNeedsPlans/ index.html

[167]Benefits.gov. *Qualified disabled and working individuals (QDWI) program.* Retrieved June 17, 2018, from https:// www.benefits.gov/benefits/benefit-details/6180

[168]For one example (Connecticut) of this program, see Connecticut 211: *Breast and cervical cancer Medicaid coverage group / BCC Medicaid coverage group* (2018, April). Retrieved June 16, 2018, from http://uwc.211ct.org/breast-and-cervical-cancer-medicaid-coverage-group-bcc-medicaid-coverage-group/

[169]Houchens, P., Mytelka, C. M., & Phillip, S. [Milliman White Paper] (2018, May). *Medicaid buy-in: Section 1332 innovation waivers, state options, and top ten considerations.* Retrieved June 17, 2018, from http://www.milliman.com/ uploadedFiles/insight/2018/medicaid-buy-in-section-1332.pdf

States can use their own funds for this program but can also get federal funding if they qualify for a State Innovation Waiver (called a Section 1332 Waiver).

The financial criteria for Medicaid eligibility vary greatly from state to state and also depend on the eligible group to which a person belongs—Children in Medicaid/CHIP, Pregnant women, Parents, and "other adults."[170]

Exhibit 6.48 summarizes Medicaid coverage for population categories.

EXHIBIT 6.48. Percentage of Populations Covered by Medicaid

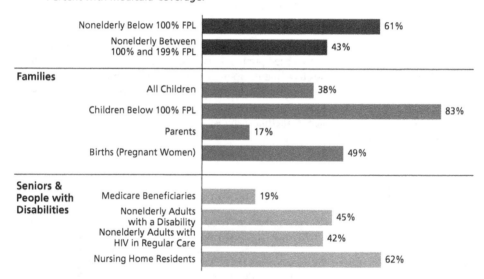

Medicaid plays a key role for selected populations.

Percent with Medicaid Coverage:

Population	Percent
Nonelderly Below 100% FPL	61%
Nonelderly Between 100% and 199% FPL	43%
Families	
All Children	38%
Children Below 100% FPL	83%
Parents	17%
Births (Pregnant Women)	49%
Seniors & People with Disabilities	
Medicare Beneficiaries	19%
Nonelderly Adults with a Disability	45%
Nonelderly Adults with HIV in Regular Care	42%
Nursing Home Residents	62%

FPL = Federal Poverty Level.

Note: The U.S. Census Bureau's poverty threshold for a family with two adults and one child was $20.420 in 2017.

Source: Kaiser Family Foundation: 10 Things to Know about Medicaid: Setting the Facts Straight. March 6, 2019 https://www.kff.org/medicaid/issue-brief/10-things-to-know-about-medicaid-setting-thefacts-straight/ Retrieved April 12, 2019.

---

[170]To appreciate this extreme variability, see Kaiser Family Foundation. (2018, March 28). *Where are states today? Medicaid and CHIP eligibility levels for children, pregnant women, and adults.* Retrieved June 17, 2018, from https://www.kff.org/medicaid/fact-sheet/where-are-states-today-medicaid-and-chip/

Benefits. CMS sets general benefit categories that states must offer in order to qualify for federal funding. However, these Mandatory Benefits vary greatly from state to state in their nature and extent. For example, while states must offer inpatient care and physician services, they can limit the number of days and visits per year, respectively. Of particular note is Early and Periodic Screening, Diagnostic, and Treatment Services (EPSDT). This benefit is the core of services for children. Its purpose is to screen for conditions of childhood that can be detected and treated early. As a result, states must provide: medical assessments that focus on developmental issues and age-appropriate immunizations; vision and hearing screens (providing eye glasses and hearing aids, if needed); and dental exams (with restorative surgery, if necessary). This benefit also covers other diagnostic and treatment services for acute and chronic physical and mental health conditions.

States may also offer Optional Benefits to which federal funding can contribute. Of note in this latter category are pharmaceuticals; although optional, all states offer this benefit since its absence would increase overall costs substantially. (Please see Exhibit 6.49 for a list of Mandatory and Optional benefits.)

Funding and Expenditures. Medicaid spending grew 2.9% to $581.9 billion in 2017, or 17 percent of total national health expenditures.[171] As stated above, the source of funding for this program comes from two sources: state and federal contributions. As described above, overall funding is based on the number of eligibles and the services the state will provide between mandatory and optional offerings. The federal contribution is determined by a statutory formula called the Federal Medical Assistance Percentage (FMAP). According to the Federal Research Service:

> The FMAP formula compares each state's per capita income relative to U.S. per capita income. The formula provides higher reimbursement to states with lower incomes (with a statutory maximum of 83%) and lower reimbursement to states with higher incomes (with a statutory minimum of 50%). The formula for a given state is:

$$\text{FMAP state} = 1 - ((\text{Per capita income state})^2 / (\text{Per capita income U.S.})^2 \times 0.45)$$

> The use of the 0.45 factor in the formula is designed to ensure that a state with per capita income equal to the U.S. average receives an FMAP rate of 55% (i.e., state share of 45%). In addition, the formula's squaring of income provides higher FMAP rates to states with below-average incomes (and vice versa, subject to the 50% minimum).[172]

---

[171]CMS.gov: NHE Fact Sheet. 02/20/2019 https://www.cms.gov/research-statistics-data-and-system s/statistics-trends-and-reports/nationalhealthexpenddata/nhe-fact-sheet.html Retrieved April 12, 2019.

[172]Mitchell, A. (Congressional Research Service) (2018, April 25). *Medicaid's federal medical assistance percentage (FMAP)*. Retrieved June 28, 2018, from https://fas.org/sgp/crs/misc/R43847.pdf

EXHIBIT 6.49. **Medicaid Mandatory and Optional Benefits**

Mandatory Benefits

- Inpatient hospital services
- Outpatient hospital services
- EPSDT: Early and Periodic Screening, Diagnostic, and Treatment Services (for children)
- Nursing Facility Services
- Home health services
- Physician services
- Rural health clinic services
- Federally qualified health center (FQHC) services
- Laboratory and X-ray services
- Family planning services
- Nurse Midwife services
- Certified Pediatric and Family Nurse Practitioner services
- Freestanding Birth Center services (when licensed or otherwise recognized by the state)
- Transportation to medical care
- Tobacco cessation counseling for pregnant women

Optional Benefits

- Prescription drugs
- Clinic services
- Physical therapy
- Occupational therapy
- Speech, hearing, and language disorder services
- Respiratory care services
- Other diagnostic, screening, preventive, and rehabilitative services
- Podiatry services
- Optometry services
- Dental services
- Dentures
- Prosthetics
- Eyeglasses
- Chiropractic services

- Other practitioner services

- Private duty nursing services

- Personal care

- Hospice

- Case management

- Services for individuals age 65 or older in an institution for mental disease (IMD)

- Services in an intermediate care facility for individuals with intellectual disability

- State plan home and community-based services—1915(i)

- Self-directed personal assistance services—1915(j)

- Community First Choice Option—1915(k)

- TB related services

- Inpatient psychiatric services for individuals under age 21

- Other services approved by the Secretary[a]

- Health Homes for Enrollees with Chronic Conditions—Section 1945

[a] This item includes services rendered in a religious nonmedical healthcare institution, emergency hospital services by a non-Medicare certified hospital, and critical access hospitals (CAHs)

Source: Medicaid.gov. *List of Medicaid benefits*. Retrieved June 17, 2018, from https://www.medicaid.gov/medicaid/benefits/list-of-benefits/index.html

The inputs to this formula are calculated annually. (Please see Exhibit 6.50 for the FMAP for fiscal year 2019.)

Since benefits and payment rates vary significantly, one must use caution in interpreting the national average percentages by service and eligible population in Exhibit 6.51.

An important breakdown of these payments is displayed in Exhibit 6.52, which shows that although about three quarters of all eligibles are children and poor adults, more than half of expenditures are for long-term care for the elderly and the disabled. In fact, Medicaid is the single largest payer of long-term care in the United States. Although this inequity has been long appreciated, it has not been corrected. One can speculate that it persists because the stakeholders most affected (children and their advocates as well as poor adults) are not politically as well organized as are the disabled and elderly. The former groups also cannot or do not vote in as high proportion as do the latter ones.

Further, as mentioned above, while the federal government sets the *types* of services the states must offer to receive matching funds, each state determines the *extent* and *duration* of services as well as the *amounts* it will pay and when it will pay; each state administers its own program. For example, while the federal government requires hospital care benefits, states often put annual limits on the number of days per year per beneficiary. (For a state-by-state comparison of hospital payment differences for Medicaid see: Kaiser Family Foundation: Medicaid Benefits: Inpatient Hospital Services, other than in an Institution for Mental

EXHIBIT 6.50. **Federal Medical Assistance Percentage (FMAP), Fiscal Year 2019**

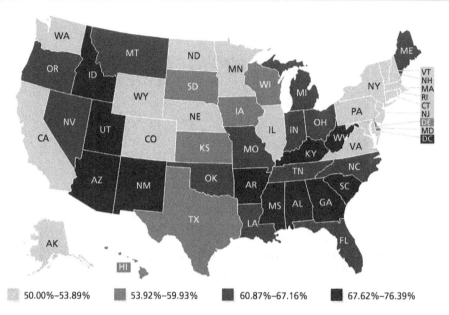

Source: Kaiser Family Foundation. *Federal medical assistance percentage (FMAP) for Medicaid and Multiplier, FY 2019*. Retrieved June 18, 2018, from https://www.kff.org/medicaid/state-indicator/federal-matching-rate-and-multiplier/?activeTab=map&currentTimeframe=0&selectedDistributions=fmap-percentage&sortModel=%7B%22colId%22:%22Location%22,%22sort%22:%22asc%22%7D

Diseases 2018. https://www.kff.org/medicaid/stateindicator/inpatient-hospital-services-other-than-in-an-institution-for-mental-diseases/?currentTimeframe=0&sortModel=%7B%22col Id%22:%22Location%22,%22sort%22:%22asc%22%7D Retrieved April 12, 2019.)

The current Medicaid outpatient pharmaceutical pricing structure—what has come to be known as the 340B Drug Pricing Program—was created by the Omnibus Budget Reconciliation Act of 1990 (OBRA'90), which mandated pharmaceutical companies sell their products at lowest prices to Medicaid programs. In order to compensate for these reductions, drug manufacturers raised prices for the Veterans Administration and certain federally funded clinics and public hospitals. As a result, Congress passed the Veterans Health Care Act of 1992 (VHCA; P.L. 102–585). The VHCA amended the Public Health Service (PHS) Act with Section 340B[173] that required drug manufacturers to enter into another pricing agreement

---

[173]HRSA.gov. Sec. 340B Public Health Service Act. Limitation on Prices of Drugs Purchased by Covered Entities. Retrieved June 18, 2018, from http://www.hrsa.gov/opa/programrequirements/phsactsection340b.pdf

EXHIBIT 6.51. Distribution of Medicaid Benefit Spending by Eligibility Group and Service Category

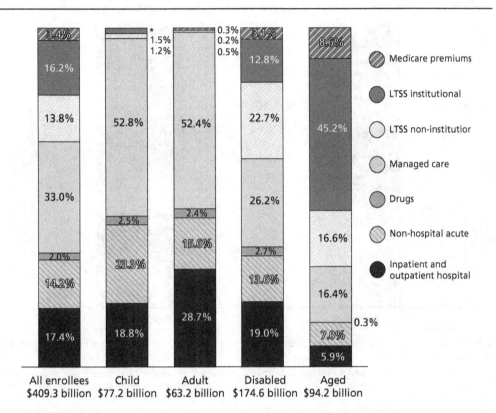

| | Medicare premiums |
| LTSS institutional |
| LTSS non-institutior |
| Managed care |
| Drugs |
| Non-hospital acute |
| Inpatient and outpatient hospital |

All enrollees — $409.3 billion
Child — $77.2 billion
Adult — $63.2 billion
Disabled — $174.6 billion
Aged — $94.2 billion

LTSS = long-term services and supports. Notes: Includes federal and state funds. Excludes spending for administration, the territories, and Medicaid-expansion CHIP enrollees. Amounts are fee for service unless otherwise noted. Values less than 0.1% are not shown.

Source: MACPAC. MACStats: Medicaid and CHIP Data Book. December 2018. https://www.macpac.gov/wp-content/uploads/2018/12/December-2018-MACStats-Data-Book.pdf Retrieved April 12, 2019.

with HHS called the Section 340B Drug Pricing Program.[174] The outpatient medications covered by this program generally include FDA-approved prescription drugs, OTC drugs written on a prescription, biological products that can be dispensed only by a prescription (other than vaccines), and FDA-approved insulin.[175]

In order to participate in the federal funding of outpatient drugs dispensed to Medicaid patients, drug manufacturers must enter into pharmaceutical pricing agreements (PPAs) with

---

[174] Further modifications were made by the Deficit Reduction Act (DRA) of 2005 and the ACA.

[175] Apexus. 340B Price/Covered Outpatient Drugs. Retrieved June 19, 2018, from https://www.340bpvp.com/resource-center/faqs/340b-pricing--covered-outpatient-drugs/

EXHIBIT 6.52. **Estimated Medicaid Enrollment and Expenditures by Enrollment Group, as Share of Total, Fiscal Year 2016**

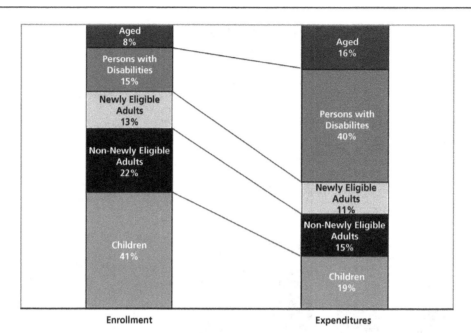

| Enrollment | Expenditures |

Note: Totals and components exclude DSH expenditure, Territorial enrollees and expenditures, and adjustments. Totals may not add to 100% due to rounding.

Source: Office of the Actuary, Centers for Medicare & Medicaid Services Report to Congress. 2016 Actuarial Report on the Financial Outlook for Medicaid. Retrieved June 18, 2018, from https://www.cms.gov/Research-Statistics-Data-and-Systems/Research/ActuarialStudies/Downloads/MedicaidReport2016.pdf As of this date, 2016 is the latest reported data.

the Secretary of HHS to sell their products at a discount to certain healthcare providers, known as covered entities. A covered entity is statutorily defined and includes various types of health centers, HIV/AIDS program grantees, and specialized clinics, including FQHCs, FQHC Look-Alikes, Native Hawaiian Health Centers, Tribal/Urban Indian Health Centers, Ryan White HIV/AIDS Program Grantees, Black Lung Clinics, Comprehensive Hemophilia Diagnostic Treatment Centers, Sexually Transmitted Disease Clinics, Tuberculosis Clinics, and Title X Family Planning Clinics.[176] The drug rebate program is administered by the CMS's Center for Medicaid and State Operations (CMSO). This latter program is managed by the Office of Pharmacy Affairs (OPA) of the Health Resources and Services Administration (HRSA), a unit of the DHHS.

---

[176]HRSA. *340 B eligibility.* Retrieved June 19, 2018, from https://www.hrsa.gov/opa/eligibility-and-registration/index.html

The purpose of the pricing is to set a maximum drug companies can charge covered entities for their products. Its statutory formula follows:

> HRSA calculates the ceiling price for each 340B drug as the difference between the drug's average manufacturer price (AMP) and its unit rebate amount (URA), obtaining both the AMP and URA from the Centers for Medicare and Medicaid Services (CMS) as part of quarterly reporting for the Medicaid Drug Rebate Program. AMP is defined as the average price paid to manufacturers by wholesalers for drugs distributed to retail community pharmacies and retail community pharmacies that purchase drugs directly from the manufacturer. The URA is based on the formula used to calculate Medicaid drug rebates as specified in Section 1927 of the Social Security Act. Currently, the Medicaid Drug Rebate Program rebate is 23.1 percent for single-source and innovator drugs and 13 percent for generic drugs. Occasionally, the formula results in a negative price for a 340B drug. In these cases, HRSA has instructed manufacturers to set the price for that drug at a penny for that quarter—referred to as HRSA's penny pricing policy.[177]

According to the OPA, "Participation in the Program results in significant savings estimated to be 20% to 50% on the cost of pharmaceuticals for safety-net providers."[178] "It is estimated that discounted drug purchases made by covered entities under the 340B program totaled more than $16 billion in 2016—a more than 30% increase in 340B program purchases in just one year. As of October 1, 2017, 12,722 covered entities were participating in the program; as of January 2, 2018, 743 pharmaceutical manufacturers were participating in the program."[179]

Covered entities find this program so attractive not only because it helps them to afford providing medication for their needy patients but also because they can sell these discounted drugs at market rates for other patients, thus gaining significant profits. The reason for this latter benefit is that the HRSA definition of a patient[180] is not limited to those who are low income, uninsured, or underinsured. Pharmaceutical companies have naturally become angry at this use because it can cut into their profitability. The problem with its resolution is that HRSA does not have regulatory authority to clarify the definition of an eligible patient; therefore, Congress must pass legislation refining this meaning. Hospital groups have strongly lobbied to keep the program intact, since they claim its profits subsidize

---

[177]House Energy and Commerce Committee. (2018, January 8). *Review of the 340B drug pricing program.* Retrieved from https://energycommerce.house.gov/wp-content/uploads/2018/01/20180110Review_of_the_340B_Drug_Pricing_Program.pdf For additional information, see also United States Government Accountability Office (2018). Statement of Debra A. Draper (Director, Health Care) before the Committee on Health, Education, Labor & Pensions, U.S. Senate: Drug Discount Program, Status of Agency Efforts to Improve 340B Program Oversight (May 15). Retrieved June 19, 2018, from https://www.gao.gov/assets/700/691742.pdf

[178]HRSA. (2018). *340B Office of Pharmacy Affairs information system.* Retrieved June 19, 2018, from https://www.hrsa.gov/opa/340b-opais/index.html

[179]House Energy and Commerce Committee: Review of the 340B Drug Pricing Program, op. cit.

[180]Apexus. *Patient definition.* Retrieved June 19, 2018, from https://www.340bpvp.com/resource-center/faqs/patient-definition

other, underpaid, activities. Until Congress clarifies the role of this program, certain major problems remain:

> The 340B statute does not require covered entities to report the level of charity care provided. As a result, there is a lack of data on how much charity care is provided by covered entities. Further, because there is no universally accepted definition of charity care, drawing a fair comparison of charity care provided across covered entities is difficult, if not impossible. Finally, while charity care spending often exceeds program savings, charity care levels have been on the decline at some hospitals, even as program savings increase.

> There is a financial incentive for 340B hospitals to prescribe more, and/or more expensive drugs to Medicare Part B beneficiaries, and prescribing trends indicate that 340B hospitals do prescribe more and more expensive drugs to Medicare Part B beneficiaries as compared to non-340B hospitals.

> There has been a marked increase in consolidation of private oncology practices, which, in some instances, negatively impacts the quality of patient care and can result in increased patient cost.[181]

Cost Control Initiatives. Despite states' attempts to control expenses by limiting payment amounts and extent of benefits, costs have continued to rise. States have, therefore, looked to creatively design their own programs. Three amendments to the Social Security Act have given states some flexibility in this regard. Section 1115 allows states to request a federal waiver to modify the content of benefits offered to eligible Medicaid beneficiaries. Section 1915 allows states to request a federal waiver so they can require Medicaid beneficiaries be assigned to a managed care organization, such as an HMO. The Balanced Budget Act of 1997 created an additional option whereby states could require managed care enrollment without the need to obtain a federal waiver (Section 1932).

Despite the fact that the majority of states have used these amendments to modify their programs, costs *still* escalated. (Please see Exhibit 6.53.) As a result, governors asked for federal law changes to allow them even more flexibility without having to apply for a waiver. Complying with this request, Congress passed provisions in the Deficit Reduction Act of 2005 (refined in early 2006), allowing states to charge beneficiaries extra sums for premiums, copayments, and coinsurance. The results of these additional charges reduced Medicaid costs, but at the price of coverage. For example, in 2003, the Oregon Health Plan (the state's Medicaid program that is on a federal waiver) instituted income-based premiums for those below 100% of the FPL. Over the next 8 months, enrollment dropped by about 45,000 to almost half the pre-premium number. Most of this decline was due to drop-outs, but there was also a component of nonenrollers.

When the ACA's Medicaid expansion started in 2014, enrollment and costs again increased significantly. (Again, please see Exhibit 6.53.) As a result, in 2017, several

---

[181] House Energy and Commerce Committee: Review of the 340B Drug Pricing Program, op. cit.

EXHIBIT 6.53. **Annual Percentage Changes in Total Medicaid Enrollment and Spending Changes, Fiscal Years 1998–2019**

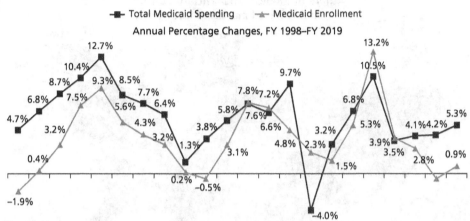

Note: Spending growth percentages refer to state fiscal year (FY).

Source: Kaiser Family Foundation: Medicaid Enrollment & Spending Growth: FY 2018 & 2019. October 25, 2018 https://www.kff .org/medicaid/issue-brief/medicaid-enrollment-spending-growth-fy-2018-2019/ Retrieved April 12, 2019.

Republican proposals to restructure Medicaid and repeal and replace the ACA were crafted; none passed congressional vote. The Medicaid reform ideas, however, were not new and were part of a portfolio of changes that have been proposed over the years to address increasing costs. Some of the more prominent recommendations[182] are briefly explained next.

1. The result of the waivers mentioned above is that two-thirds of Medicaid beneficiaries belong to Managed Care Organizations that have assumed financial risk for their care. (Please see Exhibit 6.54 for state-by-state membership variation.) The success of this strategy has been variable state-to-state.

2. States still continue to have premiums and cost sharing arrangements; however, as mentioned, research shows that cost savings are largely due to lower participation.

3. On the heels of the Medicare ACO offerings, Medicaid ACO demonstration plans have also been tried. After 4 years, the evaluation concluded that although care coordination improved for most of the Value-based Payment Models (VPMs), these improvements generally did not result in fewer emergency department visits or hospitalizations, lower expenditures, or improved quality of care for patients served by VPM-participating

---

[182] See, for example: Wiener, J. M. (2017, June). Strategies to Reduce Medicaid Spending: Findings from a Literature Review. Kaiser Family Foundation Issue Brief (June). Retrieved June 19, 2018, from http://files.kff.org/attachment/Issue-Brief-Strategies-to-Reduce-Medicaid-Spending-Findings-from-a-Literature-Review

EXHIBIT 6.54. **Medicaid Risk-Based Managed Care Enrollment by State**

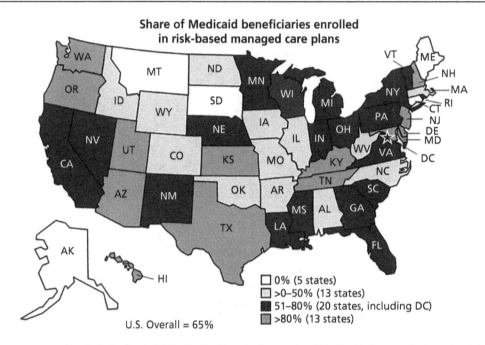

Share of Medicaid beneficiaries enrolled
in risk-based managed care plans

□ 0% (5 states)
□ >0–50% (13 states)
■ 51–80% (20 states, including DC)
▨ >80% (13 states)

U.S. Overall = 65%

Source: Rudowitz, R., & Garfield, R. (2018). *10 Things to Know about Medicaid: Setting the Facts Straight,* op. cit.

providers during the early State Innovation Models (SIM) test period.[183] Results have not been much better for "complex case management" (i.e., clinical programs directed at patients with multiple and/or serious medical problems for whom care is very costly).

4. The success of incentives to encourage wellness program participation has been inconsistent in the private sector, and specific Medicaid evidence is not available.

Congress has also considered changing the method of payment to states. One method is Per Capita Caps, whereby federal payments would be based on the number of Medicaid enrollees up to a fixed amount per person. The other method that is often mentioned is block grants to states, whereby federal payments would be made in fixed lump sums to states based on a fixed formula that does not explicitly include number of Medicaid enrollees. These models were proposed in 2017 in both houses of the Republican-controlled Congress. One reason neither passed was because the

---

[183]RTI International (prepared for CMS). (2018, March). State Innovation Models (SIM) Initiative Evaluation. Model Test Year Four, Annual Report. Retrieved June 19, 2018, from https://downloads.cms.gov/files/cmmi/sim-rd1-mt-fourthannrpt.pdf

"Congressional Budget Office (CBO) estimates that the House bill would reduce federal outlays for Medicaid by $834 billion and that the Senate bill would reduce outlays by $772 billion over the 2017–2026 period.... [B]oth bills would also result in lower Medicaid enrollment (14 million under the House bill and 15 million under the Senate bill by 2026), although such reductions also reflect the effects of other provisions such as eliminating the enhanced matching rate for the new adult group."[184]

At the time of this writing, several states have initiated or are planning work requirements as conditions of Medicaid eligibility. So far the courts have invalidated these provisions but appeals are expected (retrieved April 12, 2019, from Hackman, M: Third Lawsuit Filed Over Medicaid Work Requirements. *The Wall Street Journal* March 20, 2019, https://www.wsj.com/articles/third-lawsuit-filed-overmedicaid-workrequirements-11553120783).

Children's Health Insurance Program: Social Security Title XXI

After the Clinton health plan failed in 1993, Democrats were looking for other programs that could garner bipartisan support to cover some of the uninsured. In 1997, drawing on a pilot program in his home state of Massachusetts, Democratic Senator Edward Kennedy, in partnership with Republican Senator Orrin Hatch, proposed legislation that would extend Medicaid benefits and create other opportunities to cover uninsured children. The law that resulted from this collaboration was part of the Balanced Budget Act of 1997 and became Title XXI of the Social Security Act: State Child Health Plans (S-CHIP). Its purpose is "to provide funds to States to enable them to initiate and expand the provision of child health assistance to uninsured, low-income children in an effective and efficient manner that is coordinated with other sources of health benefits coverage for children."[185] From 2007 to 2009, Congress overrode presidential vetoes to keep the program funded. At the end of that period, the CHIP Reauthorization Act of 2009 (CHIPRA; the program is now called CHIP) was passed, extending new funding through fiscal year 2013. Funding continued to be precarious as Congress passed a number of short extensions. As the most recent funding expired, Congress passed the budget extension law P.L. 155–120 (January 22, 2018): Division C Healthy Kids Act, which extended funding through 2023. Shortly thereafter, the Bipartisan Budget Act of 2018, P.L. 115–123 (February 9, 2018), made some Medicaid and CHIP programmatic changes and extended funding to 2027.

CHIP funding is intended for uninsured children up to age 19 whose families have too much income to qualify for Medicaid but too little to afford private insurance. About 9.5 million children were enrolled in the program at any time during fiscal year 2017.[186]

---

[184]MACPAC. (2017, July). Issue Brief. Design Issues in Medicaid Per Capita Caps: An Update. Retrieved June 19, 2018, from https://www.macpac.gov/wp-content/uploads/2017/07/Design-Issues-in-Medicaid-Per-Capita-Caps-An-Update.pdf

[185]Social Security Administration. Purpose; State Child Health Plans Sec. 2101. [42 U.S.C. 1397aa]. Retrieved June 19, 2018, from https://www.ssa.gov/OP_Home/ssact/title21/2101.htm

[186]Statistical Enrollment Data System (SEDS). (2018). Combined CHIP enrollment total report and form CMS-64.EC (May 30). Retrieved June 19, 2018, from https://www.medicaid.gov/chip/downloads/fy-2017-childrens-enrollment-report.pdf

As with Medicaid, states set their own eligibility cutoffs and administer their own programs. Within limits on certain services and enrollees, states can also impose premiums and cost sharing arrangements as long as costs do not exceed 5% of the family's annual income. States can use federal money to extend their Medicaid coverage, create new programs, or implement a combination of both extensions. As with Medicaid, non-Medicaid programs are also subject to minimum benefit criteria. The formula for federal contributions is based on the FMAP described above with an added 15%; its designation is enhanced FMAP (E-FMAP).[187] The ACA increased the enhancement to 23%; P.L. 155–120 maintains that rate through 2019, reduces it to 11.5% in 2020, and eliminates the enhancement thereafter. With the 23% enhancement, on average, the federal government pays 93% of the formula's calculations, which are determined annually; after 2019, payments will drop to FMAP rates. Unlike Medicaid, however, federal matching payments are limited by national and state-specific "allotments," or annual limits on federal funding. If the state does not use its annual allotments, it has up to 2 years to spend it before any excess was redistributed to the other states.

While the above discussions about Medicaid and CHIP have focused on structure, policy, and payment aspects, it is noteworthy that *federal* data on the quality of care in these programs is severely lacking. Under the ACA, research studies have shown that "expansion was associated with increases in coverage, service use, quality of care, and Medicaid spending. Furthermore, very few studies reported that Medicaid expansion was associated with negative consequences, such as increased wait times for appointments."[188] However, CMS published its first Medicaid and CHIP quality scorecard only in June 2018.[189] The evaluations[190] are based on six performance areas from data collected in 2016:

1. Promoting communication and care coordination

2. Reducing harm in care delivery

3. Promoting prevention and treatment of chronic diseases

4. Strengthening engagement in care

5. Making care affordable

6. Working with communities to promote healthy living

Clearly more work needs to be done to evaluate whether Medicaid and CHIP are getting value for their expenditures.

---

[187]Mitchell, A. (Congressional Research Service) (2018, May 23). *Federal financing for the State Children's Health Insurance Program (CHIP)*. Retrieved June 19, 2018, from https://fas.org/sgp/crs/misc/R43949.pdf

[188]Mazurenko, O., Balio, C. P., Agarwal, R., Carroll, A. E., & Menachemi, N. (2018). The effects of medicaid expansion under the ACA: A systematic review. *Health Affairs, 37*(6), 944–950..

[189]The Advisory Board. (2018, June 5). *CMS releases first-ever scorecard for Medicaid and CHIP*. Retrieved June 19, 2018, from https://www.advisory.com/daily-briefing/2018/06/05/cms-scorecard

[190]Medicaid.gov. *State health system performance*. Retrieved June 19, 2018, from https://www.medicaid.gov/state-overviews/scorecard/state-health-system-performance/index.html

Other Federally Sponsored Programs

Veterans Healthcare System. Understanding the healthcare system for veterans is important for two reasons. First, although its providers collect some outside payments from private sources, the system is primarily described as a single payer/provider; therefore, it is held up as a model of what a universal healthcare system would look like in this country. Second, because of its size (in the federal government, only the Defense Department has more employees), contracting with this entity provides extraordinary opportunities and challenges for private businesses.[191] In addition to the large number of employees, approximately 9 million people are currently receiving benefits; in addition to veterans,[192] people potentially eligible for benefits and services include their family members or survivors. The time scope of eligibility is highlighted by the fact that the last dependent of a Revolutionary War veteran died in 1911, while as recently as 2006, three children of Civil War veterans were still receiving VA benefits.

History. The history of veterans' healthcare benefits follows that of health insurance in general, starting with compensation only for death and disability and evolving into provision of medical care as resources and technology evolved. Attention to veterans' benefits began with a 1636 law enacted in Plymouth Colony granting compensation to those who were disabled defending against Pequot Indian attacks. Similar stipends were granted to disabled veterans by the Continental Congress in 1776; however, financial responsibility for those payments rested with the states until the federal government took responsibility in 1789 upon ratification of the U.S. Constitution. The beginnings of medical care for veterans can be dated to the establishment of the Naval Home in Philadelphia in 1812, which provided services to disabled veterans. However, over 40 years later, only two other facilities had been built: the Soldiers' Home in 1853 and St. Elizabeth's Hospital in 1855, both in Washington, DC. The sizable number of veterans who were disabled in the Civil War resulted in a much-enlarged program of government-sponsored medical care. In 1865, in his second inaugural address, President Lincoln called upon Congress "to care for him who shall have borne the battle and for his widow, and his orphan."[193] Subsequently, in March 1865, he signed legislation creating the National Asylum for Disabled Volunteer Soldiers. (The name was changed to the National Home for Disabled Volunteer Soldiers in 1873.) The National Asylum was not a building but a vehicle for establishing regional facilities (called branches) to care for disabled veterans. Decisions about where to locate and maintain these structures were then, as now, based on a highly politicized process overseen by a board of managers. In 1866, the federal government purchased the first branch for $50,000 from owners of a defunct

---

[191]The Veterans Administration provides a wide range of benefits to eligible beneficiaries; however, only healthcare-related items are discussed here.

[192]Those eligible for full-time service benefits can have served in the Army, Navy, Air Force, Marine Corps, Coast Guard, or as a commissioned officer of the Public Health Service, the Environmental Services Administration, or the National Oceanic and Atmospheric Administration. Members of the National Guard may be entitled to some VA benefits depending on the nature of their service.

[193]The Veterans Administration subsequently adopted this statement as its motto.

hotel in Togus, Maine. Branches provided not only room and board to disabled and indigent veterans but also medical care, regardless of whether disabilities were service-related. As a result of the Consolidation Act of 1873, disabled veterans could also receive compensation to hire a nurse or housekeeper. Most of the higher-level medical care was provided in armed services hospitals, though some was delivered at a few facilities operated by the Public Health Service (PHS).

As a result of U.S. entry into World War I, the War Risk Insurance Act Amendments of 1917 (and subsequently the Vocational Rehabilitation Act of 1918) authorized rehabilitation and vocational training for veterans with dismemberment, loss of sight or hearing, or other permanent disabilities. This commitment led to pioneering rehabilitation research, especially in the area of prosthetics. In 1919, the PHS was put in charge of veterans' medical care, and some military hospitals were transferred to PHS control. Despite authorization to build new hospitals, these facilities could not keep up with demand. As a result, the law that transferred veterans' care to the PHS permitted the continued use of contracted private hospitals. This historical allowance is significant because, in recent years, there have been proposals to privatize all or a large portion of veterans' medical services.[194] (More will be said about this issue below.) Additionally, proposals have periodically surfaced to open underutilized VA[195] hospitals to the general population (particularly in rural areas).

By 1921, Congress consolidated three veterans' programs (including the PHS hospitals that cared for this population) into the Veterans' Bureau. On July 21, 1930, the bureau was merged with the Bureau of Pensions of the Interior Department and the National Homes for Disabled Volunteer Soldiers to form the Veterans Administration (VA). World War II accelerated the development of rehabilitative and vocational services, particularly furnishing artificial limbs. In 1946, VA hospitals started clinical programs to train residents and fellows and implemented a policy to affiliate with medical schools.[196] Seventy years later, the VA had affiliations with more than 1,800 educational institutions; more than 70% of all doctors in the United States received training in the VA healthcare system.[197] Since the VA was competing with the private sector to recruit health professionals, physicians were removed from Civil Service rules. Because of the complexity of benefits and further influx of Korean War veterans, in 1953, the VA was further reorganized into three services: medical care, financial assistance to veterans, and insurance.

To meet the needs of a growing number of aging veterans, in 1975 the VA began training teams of interdisciplinary geriatric health specialists. In 1980, Congress formalized and

---

[194]This concept is working in Australia, where veterans have access to private hospitals. See Australian Government, Department of Veterans Affairs. *Program 2.2: Veterans' Hospital Services.* Retrieved June 20, 2018, from https://www.dva.gov.au/about-dva/accountability-and-reporting/annual-reports/annual-reports-2012-13/department-veterans-11

[195]While the organization responsible for veterans is officially called the U.S. Department of Veterans Affairs, the abbreviation VA (dating from when it was known as the Veterans Administration) is commonly used.

[196]The first such affiliation was Hines hospital in Maywood, IL, with Northwestern University and the University of Illinois. The hospital was named after General Frank T. Hines, who was Bureau and VA administrator for 22 years. It is now affiliated with Loyola University's Strich School of Medicine.

[197]U.S. Department of Veterans Affairs (2016, February 12). *VA celebrates 70 years of partnering with medical schools.* Retrieved June 20, 2018, from https://www.va.gov/opa/pressrel/pressrelease.cfm?id=2747

funded this commitment by authorizing Geriatric Research, Education and Clinical Centers (GRECCs).

In addition to the problems of aging, the medical needs of veterans changed significantly as a result of the Vietnam War. Medical advances in early evacuation and treatment led to an increased proportion of veterans who survived combat but were disabled. Due to the great need for outpatient treatment for these veterans, the Veterans Health Care Amendments Act of 1979 helped establish a network of freestanding Vet Centers[198] across the country. The act also created a program to treat veterans for alcohol and drug dependence in community facilities. Subsequent legislation in 1991 and 1996 opened Vet Center services to all those who served in combat or danger zones from World War II and later.

From the time veterans' benefits began, policy and laws expanded eligibility and benefits. Despite the strong military/veterans lobby, however, during economic downturns the VA has not been immune to changes. Bowing to the financial pressures in the 1980s, Congress started to streamline some benefits. First, a minimum service requirement of 2 years (or the full period of their initial service obligation) was introduced for those who enlisted after September 7, 1980, and officers commissioned or who entered active military service after October 16, 1981.[199] Next, in 1986, Congress set means testing as a criterion for free medical care. Those with higher incomes could still receive services but had to pay for a portion of their care. Along with those restrictions, however, Congress expanded some benefits to special groups of veterans, such as former prisoners of war, veterans exposed to herbicides (particularly Agent Orange) and ionizing radiation, and veterans of World War I.

Because of the increasing number of persons eligible for VA benefits, in 1988, President Reagan signed legislation to change the VA to the Department of Veterans Affairs and granted it cabinet status effective March 15, 1989. The newly reorganized department included three main divisions: the Veterans Health Administration, the Veterans Benefits Administration, and the National Cemetery System.

In recognition of the growing number of women serving in the military, a number of laws and programs in the 1990s addressed gender-specific issues. These programs began with the Veterans Healthcare Act (VHCA) (1992), continued with institution of the Center for Women Veterans (1994), and culminated with establishment of the Women Veterans Health Program Office in the Office of Public Health and Environmental Hazards (1997).

In 1995, the VA restructured into Veterans Integrated Service Networks (VISNs, called "Visions") in order to meet the further expanding need for more ambulatory care services, enhance operational efficiency, coordinate care across different types of services, and improve quality. (Please see Exhibit 6.55.) Each VISN comprises about 7 to 10 hospitals, 25 to 30 ambulatory clinics, 4 to 7 nursing homes, and a variety of other services. With this organization came new goals of "population-based planning, decentralization, universal

---

[198] U.S. Department of Veterans Affairs. *Vet Center Program*. Retrieved June 20, 2018, from http://www.vetcenter.va.gov/
[199] Exceptions were made for veterans with service-connected disabilities or those discharged for disability or hardship near the end of their service obligation.

EXHIBIT 6.55. **Veterans Integrated Service Networks**

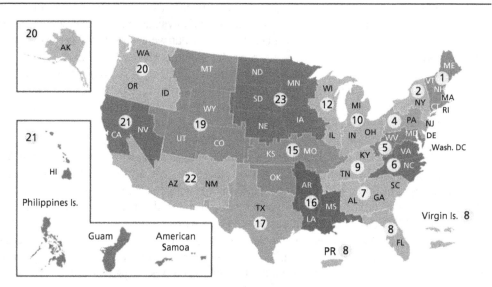

VISN 1: VA New England Healthcare System
VISN 2: New York/New Jersey VA Health Care Network
VISN 4: VA Healthcare - VISN 4
VISN 5: VA Capitol Health Care Network
VISN 6: VA Mid-Atlantic Health Care Network
VISN 7: VA Southeast Network
VISN 8: VA Sunshine Healthcare Network
VISN 9: VA MidSouth Healthcare Network
VISN 10: VA Healthcare System
VISN 12: VA Great Lakes Health Care System
VISN 15: VA Heartland Network
VISN 16: South Central VA Health Care Network
VISN 17: VA Heart of Texas Health Care Network
VISN 19: Rocky Mountain Network
VISN 20: Northwest Network
VISN 21: Sierra Pacific Network
VISN 22: Desert Pacific Healthcare Network
VISN 23: VA Midwest Health Care Network

Source: U.S. Department of Veterans Affairs. *Locations: Veterans Integrated Service Networks (VISN).* Retrieved June 20, 2018, from https://www.va.gov/directory/guide/division.asp?dnum=1

availability of primary care, a shift to outpatient care from inpatient care, and an emphasis on measuring health-care performance on the outcome of patient treatment." The transformation resulted in a change in the ratio of outpatient visits to inpatient admissions from 29:1 in 1995 to more than 100:1 in 2006[200] as well as a dramatic improvement in quality. VISNs can be compared to the "newer" concept of Accountable Care Organizations, described earlier.

Starting in the early 2000s, the VA system became increasingly stressed, in part due to aging Vietnam veterans and then those returning from Iraq and Afghanistan. For example,

> the United States Court of Appeals for the Ninth Circuit accused the Department of Veterans Affairs of 'unchecked incompetence' and unconscionable delays in caring for veterans with mental health problems ... [For example,] the agency had no suicide prevention officers at any of its outpatient clinics and that 70 percent of its health facilities had no systems to track potentially suicidal patients.[201]

Further, in January 2011, the

> OIG [Office of Inspector General] reported that VARO [VA Regional Office] staff inconsistently processed temporary 100 percent disability evaluations. OIG projected that VARO staff did not correctly process evaluations for approximately 27,500 Veterans and that, since January 1993, VBA [Veterans Benefits Administration] has paid Veterans a net $943 million without adequate medical evidence.[202]

Moreover, the OIG found that medical license monitoring was inconsistent and fragmented across its VA medical facilities.

By 2014, the VA was in full crisis, not only for long delays in care and lapses in quality but also for issuing false statements about wait times. To remedy this situation, Congress passed the Veterans Access, Choice, and Accountability Act of 2014, P.L. 113–146 (Choice Program).[203] The purpose of the act was to give beneficiaries the opportunity to access community providers if the required service was not provided by their VA facility, if they could not make an appointment for necessary care within 30 days, and/or if physical access barriers existed, such as living more than 40 driving miles from the nearest facility. This program did not solve the problems as intended, despite about one third of beneficiaries receiving care outside the VA system. With Choice Program funding running out, Congress

---

[200]Kessee, N. (2009). Overview of the Department of Veterans Affairs. In: P. F. Pasquina & R. A. Cooper (Eds.), *Care of the Combat Amputee* (Chapter 5). Washington, DC: Office of the Surgeon General, United States Army Falls Church, Virginia Borden Institute, Walter Reed Army Medical Center. Retrieved June 20, 2018, from http://ke.army .mil/bordeninstitute/published_volumes/amputee/CCAfrontmatter.pdf

[201]Editorial: "More excuses and delays from the V.A." (2011, August 22). *New York Times,* A18 (New York ed.).

[202]Opfer, G. J. (Inspector General, Department of Veterans Affairs). Major Management Challenges, FY 2012. Retrieved June 21, 2018, from https://www.va.gov/oig/pubs/VAOIG-2012-MMC.pdf

[203]U.S. Department of Veterans Affairs. VHA Office of Community Care. Veterans Choice Program. Retrieved June 18, 2018, from https://www.va.gov/COMMUNITYCARE/programs/veterans/VCP/index.asp#resources

passed the VA Maintaining Internal Systems and Strengthening Integrated Outside Networks (MISSION) Act of 2018.[204] Signed into law by the president on June 6, 2018, it appropriated $5.2 billion in mandatory funding to extend the Choice Program until a new, consolidated Veterans Community Care Program became operational. Under this Care Program, the eligibility standards for private options are far broader than the Choice Program's 40 miles and 30-day wait criteria. Further, it requires the VA to: coordinate veterans' coverage and care outside of the region where they reside; ensure the scheduling of medical appointments in a timely manner; ensure continuity of care and services; and ensure veterans do not experience a lapse in healthcare services. In addition to these requirements, the act also:

- Consolidates the agency's multiple private-care programs;
- Authorizes the VA to contract with an outside company to streamline billing;
- Expands the existing caregiver program by extending stipends and other benefits to veterans of all eras, not just families of injured post-9/11 veterans;
- Requires review of all underused hospitals, leading to possible closures;
- Expands a telehealth program;
- Provides new tools to recruit medical professionals to address thousands of vacancies; and
- Requires negotiating contracts with private walk-in clinics, starting with a demonstration program in Arizona with the drugstore chain CVS.

The CBO estimated that the MISSION Act will result in *an additional* 640,000 veterans each year going outside the VA system at a cost of $46.5 billion over a 5-year period.[205] Considering that the expansion budget is $5.2 billion, many veterans groups are worried about the financial solvency of this program.

Current Status. The current status of the VA and the benefits it provides can be summarized from the Department of Veterans Affairs 2019 budget.[206] The 2019 budget request for discretionary funding totals $88.9 billion, of which $76.5 billion (including medical care collections) is requested for VA Medical Care. The 2019 mandatory funding request totals $109.7 billion.

[204]VA Maintaining Internal Systems and Strengthening Integrated Outside Networks (MISSION) Act of 2018. Retrieved June 18, 2018, from https://www.congress.gov/bill/115th-congress/senate-bill/2372

[205]Congressional Budget Office. (2018, May 14). H.R. 5674. VA Maintaining Internal Systems and Strengthening Integrated Outside Networks Act of 2018. Retrieved June 20, 2018, from https://www.cbo.gov/system/files/115th-congress-2017-2018/costestimate/hr5674.pdf?wpisrc=nl_health202&wpmm=1

[206]U.S. Department of Veterans Affairs. (2019). *Annual budget submission: President's budget request fiscal year 2019.* Retrieved June 21, 2018, from https://www.va.gov/budget/products.asp Note: The VA is required to submit annual budget requests.

This money will support 366,358 full-time equivalent (FTE) employees and more than 9.3 million veterans who are enrolled for benefits. More specifically, this budget funds the following activities:

- Medical care for 7.0 million patients
- Modernization of VA's electronic health record system to improve quality of care. This initiative includes a system to be installed by Cerner to coordinate with the Department of Defense (DoD) and Coast Guard.
- Expansion of mental health services
- Disability compensation benefits for 4.9 million veterans and 432,000 survivors
- Pension benefits for 269,000 veterans and 200,000 survivors
- Hiring an additional 225 fiduciary employees to ensure protection for VA's most vulnerable veterans who are unable to manage their VA benefits
- Strengthening VA's infrastructure through $1.1 billion in major construction and $706.9 million in minor construction for priority infrastructure projects, and $1.4 billion in Non-Normal Recurring Maintenance (NMR) Education assistance programs serving nearly 1 million students
- Vocational rehabilitation and employment benefits for over 149,000 veterans
- A home mortgage program with a portfolio of nearly 3 million active loans
- The largest national cemetery system, projected to inter more than 134,000 veterans and eligible family members in 2019

Eligibility and priority status to receive healthcare (and other) benefits depends on a number of factors, including service record (where the veteran served and length of service),[207] service-connected illness and/or disability, and income.[208]

The actual spending for health services is a trade-off between how many persons the VA wants to cover and what it can afford based on final congressional approval. The terms of resource allocation were laid out in the Veterans' Health Care Eligibility Reform Act of 1996 (P.L. 104–262, 110 Stat. 3177), which mandated that the VA deliver healthcare services to veterans with service-connected disabilities; to those unable to pay for necessary medical care; and to specified groups of veterans, such as former prisoners of war and veterans of World War I. The remainder of available services could be provided on a resource- and funding-available basis. In 2008, an extension of the Veterans Programs Enhancement Act of 1998 (P.L. 105–368) gave eligible veterans access to this system for 5 years after honorable discharge, without having to demonstrate financial need or a service-connected disability (SCD). After that time, veterans are placed into certain standardized, prioritized categories that specify their ongoing needs. Given the annual budget, the Secretary of Veterans Affairs

[207] VA/Vets.gov. *Health care benefits eligibility.* Retrieved June 21, 2018, from https://www.vets.gov/health-care/eligibility/
[208] U.S. Department of Veterans Affairs. *Annual income limits—Health benefits.* Retrieved June 21, 2018, from http://nationalincomelimits.vaftl.us This site provides a calculator for financial eligibility.

decides which categories will receive funding. The priority groups, from highest to lowest (P1through P8), are as follows:[209]

P1   Veterans who have SCDs rated 50% or more disabling (or two or more SCDs that together are 50% or more disabling) veterans deemed to be unemployable because of service-connected conditions.

P2   Veterans with SCDs rated 30% or 40% disabling.

P3   Veterans who are former prisoners of war; were awarded the Purple Heart or Medal of Honor; were discharged because of SCDs; have SCDs rated 10% or 20% disabling; or were disabled as a result of treatment or vocational rehabilitation.

P4   Veterans who are receiving aid and attendance benefits or are housebound and veterans whom VA has determined to be catastrophically disabled as a result of a non-service-connected illness or injury.

P5   Veterans who do not have SCDs or who have noncompensable SCDs rated 0% disabling and whose annual income and net worth are below VA's national means-test thresholds; veterans who are receiving VA pension benefits; and veterans who are eligible for Medicaid benefits.

P6   Compensable 0% service-connected veterans; veterans exposed to ionizing radiation during atmospheric testing or during the occupation of Hiroshima and Nagasaki; Project 112/SHAD participants;[210] veterans of the Mexican border period or of World War I; veterans who served in the Republic of Vietnam between January 9, 1962, and May 7, 1975; veterans of the Persian Gulf War who served between August 2, 1990, and November 11, 1998; veterans who served on active duty at Camp Lejeune for at least 30 days between August 1, 1953 and December 31, 1987;[211] veterans who served in a theater of combat operations after November 11, 1998 as follows: Currently enrolled veterans and new enrollees who were discharged from active duty on or after January 28, 2003, are eligible for the enhanced benefits for 5 years postdischarge.

---

[209]U.S. Department of Veterans Affairs. *Volume II: Medical programs and information technology programs. Congressional submission FY 2019 funding and FY 2020 advance appropriations* (p. 51). Retrieved June 21, 2018, from https://www.va.gov/budget/docs/summary/fy2019VAbudgetVolumeIImedicalProgramsAndInformationTechnology.pdf

[210]From 1962 to 1973 the Department of Defense tested biological and chemical warfare vulnerability for land (Project 112) and sea (Shipboard Hazard and Defense-SHAD) active military. See U.S. Department of Veterans Affairs: About Project 112 and Project SHAD. Retrieved June 21, 2018, from https://www.publichealth.va.gov/exposures/shad/basics.asp

[211]This benefit is for those exposed to toxins in the drinking water at this base. See U.S. Department of Veterans Affairs. *Exposure to contaminated drinking water at Camp Lejeune*. Retrieved June 21, 2018, from https://www.benefits.va.gov/COMPENSATION/claims-postservice-exposures-camp-lejeune-water.asp

P7 Veterans with gross household income below the geographically adjusted VA income limit for their resident location, and who agree to pay copays; veterans with gross household income above the VA and the geographically adjusted income limit for their resident location, and who agree to pay copays; veterans with noncompensable 0% service-connected and: Subpriority a: Enrolled as of January 16, 2003, and who have remained enrolled since that date and/or placed in this subpriority due to changed eligibility status or Subpriority b: Enrolled on or after June 15, 2009 whose income exceeds the current VA or geographic income limits by 10% or less.

P8 Veterans with gross household incomes above the VA income limits and the geographically adjusted income limits for their resident location, and who agree to pay copays; veterans who have non-service-connected conditions and: Subpriority c: Enrolled as of January 16, 2003, and who have remained enrolled since that date and/or placed in this subpriority due to changed eligibility status or Subpriority d: Enrolled on or after June 15, 2009, whose income exceeds the current VA or geographic income limits by 10% or less.

Veterans not eligible for enrollment are those not meeting the criteria above; Subpriority e: Noncompensable 0% service-connected (eligible for care of their SC condition only); or Subpriority g: Non-service-connected.

If a veteran *is* eligible, the VA is required[212] to make available certain services, called the Medical Benefits Package. (Please see Exhibit 6.56.) The patient's personal VA physician determines the "need" for care, which is defined as care or service that will promote, preserve, and/or restore health.

In addition to the Medical Benefits Package, certain persons may be eligible for long-term care benefits (including nursing homes) through three types of institutions: VA-owned and operated Community Living Centers (CLC), state veterans' homes (owned and operated by the states but subsidized by VA payments), and the contract community nursing home program (privately owned homes under contract with the VA). Each program has its own admission and eligibility criteria that depend on: whether the reason for admission is a SCD and, if so, what percentage the veteran is disabled; financial need; and space availability. Unlike copays for medical benefits (which are determined by the priority category of the beneficiary), applicable long-term care copays are based on financial need.

Future Prospects. Despite the declining numbers of veterans (please see Exhibit 6.57), it is unknown if costs will also continue to proportionately decline. Expenses will depend not only on these projections but also on such factors as veterans of future conflicts, newly discovered illnesses and disabilities for existing and future veterans, and those who choose to be covered by other insurance (work, Medicare, or Medicaid). Further, despite best prices for items like pharmaceuticals, the VA is also subject to costs associated with advancing medical technology.

---

[212] 38 U.S.C. §§ 1710(a)(1), (2), 1701(5), (6).

EXHIBIT 6.56. VA Provided Care Under the Medical Benefits Package

Basic Care

- Outpatient medical, surgical, and mental healthcare, including care for substance abuse.
- Inpatient hospital, medical, surgical, and mental healthcare, including care for substance abuse.
- Prescription drugs, including OTC drugs and medical and surgical supplies available under the VA national formulary system.
- Emergency care in VA facilities. (Emergency care in non-VA facilities in certain conditions.)
- Bereavement counseling.
- Comprehensive rehabilitative services other than vocational services.
- Consultation, professional counseling, training, and mental health services for the members of the immediate family or legal guardian of the veteran.
- Durable medical equipment and prosthetic and orthotic devices, including eyeglasses and hearing aids.
- Home health services.
- Reconstructive (plastic) surgery required as a result of a disease or trauma but not including cosmetic surgery that is not medically necessary.
- Respite, hospice, and palliative care.
- Payment of travel and travel expenses for eligible veterans.
- Pregnancy and delivery service, to the extent authorized by law.
- Completion of forms.

Preventive Care

- Immunizations
- Periodic medical exams
- Healthcare assessments
- Health education, including nutrition education
- Screening tests

VA Cannot Provide the Following Services

- Abortions and abortion counseling
- Cosmetic surgery except where determined by VA to be medically necessary for reconstructive or psychiatric care

- Drugs, biologicals, and medical devices not approved by the FDA unless the treating medical facility is conducting formal clinical trials under an Investigational Device Exemption (IDE) or an Investigational New Drug (IND) application, or the drugs, biologicals, or medical devices are prescribed under a compassionate use exemption.

- Gender alteration

- Health club or spa membership

- *In vitro* fertilization

- Services not ordered and provided by licensed/accredited professional staff

- Special private duty nursing

- Hospital and outpatient care for a veteran who is either a patient or inmate in an institution of another government agency if that agency has a duty to give the care or services.

Source: Military.com. *Veterans medical benefits package*. Retrieved June 21, 2018, from https://www.military.com/benefits/veterans-health-care/veterans-medical-benefits-package.html

In addition to addressing concerns of cost and eligibility, the VA will be required to continue implementing and monitoring quality improvement programs. This expectation comes from specific quality initiatives underway and the VA's desire to enhance system transparency. However, much needs to be done to rebuild trust. For example:

> As of June 2017, the Department of Veterans Affairs (VA) publicly reported 35 health care quality measures on the *Hospital Compare* website ... [However], VA Central Office officials told GAO that they have not systematically assessed the completeness and accuracy of the clinical information across VAMCs [VA Medical Centers] and the extent to which this affects the accuracy of its quality measures because they have focused on other priorities ... As a

EXHIBIT 6.57. Veterans Population Projections 2017–2037

The total veteran population is predicted to decline from 20.0 million in 2017 to 13.6 million in 2037.

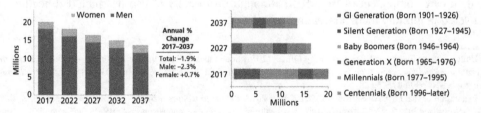

Source: U.S. Department of Veterans Affairs: Veterans Population Projections 2017–2037. Retrieved from https://www.va.gov/vetdata/docs/demographics/new_vetpop_model/vetpop_infographic_final31.pdf

result, VA does not have assurance that the quality measures it publicly reports on *Hospital Compare* and its own website accurately reflect the performance of its VAMCs and provide veterans with the information they need to make informed choices about their care.[213]

Active Military/Retirees and Dependents. Unlike most healthcare "systems" in the United States, the military health system (MHS) is guided by a mission statement, which it refers to as the MHS Quadruple Aim.[214] The Quadruple Aim's goals are:

- *Increased Readiness.* Ensuring that the total military force is medically ready to deploy and that the medical force is ready to deliver healthcare anytime, anywhere in support of the full range of military operations, including humanitarian aid missions.

- *Better Health.* Reducing the generators of ill health by encouraging healthy behaviors and decreasing the likelihood of illness through focused prevention and the development of increased resilience.

- *Better Care.* Providing a care experience that is patient and family centered, compassionate, convenient, equitable, safe, and always of the highest quality.

- *Lower Cost.* Creating value by focusing on quality, eliminating waste, and reducing unwarranted variation; considering the total cost of care over time, not just the cost of an individual healthcare activity.

To accomplish its mission, the MHS is composed of three parts. First, active military personnel (including commissioned corps of the PHS) can receive care on base. Second, veterans can receive care in VA facilities for qualified services. Finally, because these latter two facilities and some services are not always available, the Department of Defense (DoD)[215] provides health insurance for active and retired military personnel, reservists, and eligible dependents. Access to private services started only after passage of the Dependents Medical Care Act of 1956; before that time, the federal government did not provide off-base healthcare benefits to dependents of active military personnel. This assistance was formalized in 1966 with the Military Medical Benefits Amendments, forming what became known as the Civilian Health and Medical Program of the Uniformed Services (CHAMPUS). The 1994 Defense Authorization Act changed the program name to TRICARE. TRICARE is the civilian care component of the MHS, although historically it also has included healthcare delivered in military medical treatment facilities.

---

[213]United States Government Accountability Office. (2017, September). *VA healthcare quality: VA should improve the information it publicly reports on the quality of care at its medical facilities.* Retrieved June 21, 2018, from https://www .gao.gov/assets/690/687523.pdf

[214]Evaluation of the TRICARE Program. *Fiscal Year 2018. Report to Congress by the TRICARE Management Activity (TMA).* Retrieved June 21, 2018, from https://www.health.mil/Reference-Center/Reports/2018/05/09/Evaluation-of-the-TRICARE-Program-Fiscal-Year-2018-Report-to-Congress

[215]Managed by TRICARE Management Activity (TMA) under the authority of the Assistant Secretary of Defense (Health Affairs).

TRICARE services are delivered through Military Treatment Facilities (MTFs) or private sector providers. After October 1, 2018, administration and management of the 932 MTFs were transferred from their military departments (each under their respective service branch Surgeon General) to the centralized Defense Health Agency.[216] The facilities are generally on or near a U.S. military base and typically are staffed by military, civil service, and contract personnel.

To administer TRICARE and enable beneficiaries to access the private sector, the DoD has contracted with insurance companies to act as TPAs. In this role, they: establish and maintain provider networks; provide enrollee support, such as operating service call centers to field complaints and answering plan benefit/enrollment questions; and provide administrative services, such as enrollment, care authorization, and claims processing.

Pharmacy and dental benefits are handled separately through other contracts, such as through TRICARE retail network pharmacies, the TRICARE Pharmacy Home Delivery program, and the premium-based TRICARE Dental Program.

Starting in 2018, there were two administrative regions: Humana was awarded the contract for the East, and Health Net Federal Services (a division of Centene) received the Western region contract.

With the exception of active duty service members (who are assigned to the TRICARE Prime option and pay no out-of-pocket costs for TRICARE coverage), MHS beneficiaries may have a choice of TRICARE plan options[217] depending upon their status (e.g., active duty family member, retiree, reservist, child under age 26 ineligible for family coverage, Medicare-eligible, etc.) and geographic location. Each plan option has different beneficiary cost-sharing features. Pharmacy copayments are established separately and are the same for all beneficiaries under each option. Although some smaller TRICARE plans are available to select subgroups, most military users receive their healthcare through two major plans: TRICARE Prime, and TRICARE Select.[218] (In general and except for Medicaid, TRICARE is the secondary payer when the beneficiary has other insurance.)

TRICARE Prime is an HMO-style option in which beneficiaries typically get most care at a MTF. Certain retirees may be eligible to enroll in this option (for an annual enrollment fee) if they live within or near a designated Prime Service Area. Active duty family members must enroll annually (at no cost) if they wish to participate in the plan.

---

[216]"As a means of reducing duplication, DoD established the Defense Health Agency (DHA) in 2013 to administer the MHS and to combine shared services. The Congress gave DHA additional administrative responsibilities for the military treatment facilities in the National Defense Authorization Act for Fiscal Year 2017 (NDAA; Public Law 114-328)." Congressional Research Service (2018, April 20). *Defense primer: Military health system.* Retrieved June 22, 2018, from https://fas.org/sgp/crs/natsec/IF10530.pdf

[217]See MyTRICARE.com. *Plans and programs.* Retrieved June 22, 2018, from https://www.mytricare.com/internet/tric/tri/mtc_nprov.nsf/sectionmap/LrnAbtTRCR_PlnsandPrgrms and Tricare: Health Plans. Retrieved from https://www.tricare.mil/Plans/HealthPlans

[218]Starting January 1, 2018, TRICARE Extra and TRICARE Standard were merged to become TRICARE Select.

Under *TRICARE Select*, when beneficiaries choose an in-network provider for medical care, their cost sharing is lower than if they choose an out-of-network provider. In this respect, the structure is like a PPO (described more fully below in the Managed Care section). All beneficiaries need to enroll in TRICARE Select to receive coverage. Enrollment will be free until January 1, 2020. Beginning in 2020, current working-age retirees who wish to use Select must pay an enrollment fee of $150 for individual coverage or $300 for family coverage. (Please see Exhibit 6.58 for trends in the number of eligible TRICARE beneficiaries by beneficiary group and Exhibit 6.59 for TRICARE beneficiary plan choice by age group.)

Exhibit 6.60 highlights an example of the extent of government subsidies to lower costs for TRICARE members (retirees).

As far as quality, TRICARE monitors metrics and institutes improvement activities to fulfill elements of the MHS mission statement. For example, in addition to patient satisfaction surveys, TRICARE assesses metrics on Medical Readiness, Improving Clinical Outcomes, and Improving Safety.

Summary. The MHS, particularly TRICARE, is a unique system with a clear mission statement and well-defined goals. However, it faces the same cost/quality/access issues as does the corresponding civilian sector without demonstrating clear superiority or even parity. Recent evaluations have recommended changes in plan structures (including increase cost sharing) as well as improvements in access, quality, and safety.[219]

EXHIBIT 6.58. **Trends in the Number of Eligible TRICARE Beneficiaries by Beneficiary Group, Fiscal Years 2015–2017**

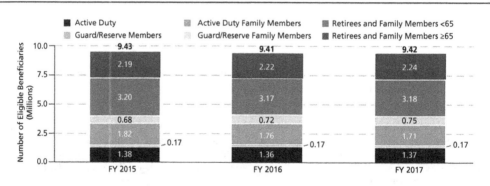

Source: Evaluation of the TRICARE Program: Fiscal Year 2018 Report to Congress by the TRICARE Management Activity (TMA).

---

[219] Congressional Budget Office. (2017, October). *Approaches to changing military health care.* Retrieved June 23, 2018, from https://www.cbo.gov/system/files/115th-congress-2017-2018/reports/53137-approachestochangingmilitaryhealth care.pdf

EXHIBIT 6.59. TRICARE Beneficiary Plan Choice by Age Group

Plan Type	0–17	18–24	25–44	45–64	≥65	Total[a]
Prime Enrolled	1,278,726	881,319	1,493,814	1,049,500	2,296	4,705,655
Prime	1,247,377	860,721	1,473,694	1,005,722	1,940	4,589,454
USFHP	31,349	7,698	15,910	43,778	356	99,091
TYA Prime	0	12,900	4,210	0	0	17,110
Non-Enrolled	673,324	265,287	515,557	832,418	19,428	2,306,014
Standard/Extra	516,442	207,503	327,833	772,410	4,268	1,828,456
TRS	148,466	32,831	171,992	32,471	16	335,776
Direct Care Only	31	3,997	7,529	5,971	14,144	31,672
Plus	6,278	1,671	3,425	16,902	995	29,271
TYA Standard	0	18,242	4,153	0	0	22,395
TRR	2,107	1,043	625	4,664	5	8,444
Medicare-Eligible	39	1,076	33,697	147,477	2,222,185	2,404,474
TFL	9	596	18,183	87,674	1,937,042	2,043,504
Plus[b]	0	4	120	1,204	181,096	182,424
Direct Care Only	1	12	315	6,695	57,342	64,365
Prime	24	404	14,022	48,781	369	63,600
USFHP	1	20	412	2,226	45,887	48,546
Other/Unknown	4	40	645	897	449	2,035
Total	1,952,089	1,147,682	2,043,068	2,029,395	2,243,909	9,416,143

[a] The totals in the right-hand columns of the tables may differ slightly from ones shown in other sections of this report. Reasons for differences may include different data pull dates, end-year vs. average populations, and different data sources.
[b] Among Medicare eligibles, 179,003 with TRICARE Plus also have TFL. These numbers are not included in the TFL row.
TRS = TRICARE Reserve Select; TRR = TRICARE Retired Reserve; TFL = TRICARE for LIFE; TYA = Tricare Young Adult; USFHP = Uniformed Services Family Health Plan. Standard/Extra is now TRICARE Select.

Source: Evaluation of the TRICARE Program: Fiscal Year 2018, Report to Congress by the TRICARE Management Activity (TMA), op. cit.

EXHIBIT 6.60. **TRICARE Retiree Coverage Costs with the National Average Employer-Provided Family Coverage**

2018	TRICARE Prime	TRICARE Select	Employer Provided[a]
Premium (annual)	$578	$0	$5,817
Deductible	$0	$300	$2,650
Catastrophic Cap	$3,000	$3,000	Variable
Min.-Max Out of Pocket	$578–$3,000	$300–$3,000	$5,817–$8,467

[a] Kaiser Family Foundation and Health Research & Educational Trust 2017 Annual Survey of Employer Health Benefits

Source: Frost, P. (2018, March 28). *One chart shows how military health care costs compare to civilians' fees.* Retrieved June 23, 2018, from https://www.military.com/paycheck-chronicles/2018/03/28/one-chart-shows-how-military-health-care-costs-compare-to-civilians-fees.html

Federal Employee Health Benefit Program. The Federal Employee Health Benefit Program (FEHBP) is not an insurance plan but rather is a nationwide arrangement by which the federal government, as an employer, subsidizes health insurance premiums for eligible federal workers and retirees, including postal employees. As of calendar year 2014 (when the ACA insurance provisions started), members of Congress and certain congressional staff are no longer eligible to enroll in plans offered under FEHB as employees but may be eligible to enroll in retirement. The reason this program is noteworthy is that over the past five decades, advocates of health reform have proposed this scheme for Medicare and universal coverage. Its background and features are, therefore, explained below.

Consistent with the post–World War II trend for employer-sponsored insurance, the Truman and Eisenhower administrations supported shared-cost coverage for federal employees. Several proposals by the Civil Service Commission (now the U.S. Office of Personnel Management [OPM]) failed to get congressional approval. By 1957, although 78% of government workers had private health insurance (including an employee group sponsored by postal workers), individuals paid for premiums on their own.[220] When, in the late 1950s, the federal government considered universal health insurance, its workers insisted that their health plan should preserve the freedom of choice they enjoyed when they purchased their own coverage. Congress bowed to this pressure on September 28, 1959, when it passed Public Law 86–382, establishing the FEHBP, which became operational on July 1, 1960.[221] The features of this law are noteworthy for a variety of reasons, not the least of which is that it pioneered concepts now common to health insurance products. (Please see Exhibit 6.61.)

---

[220] U.S. Congress Senate hearings before the Subcommittee on Insurance of the Committee on Post Office and Civil Service on S. 94 (86th Congress, 1st session). April 15, 1959.

[221] For this and other relevant laws concerning the FEHBP, see Blom, K. B., & Cornell, A. S. (Congressional Research Service) (2015, July 22). *Laws affecting the Federal Employees Health Benefits (FEHB) Program.* Retrieved June 23, 2018, from https://fas.org/sgp/crs/misc/R42741.pdf

EXHIBIT 6.61. **Pioneering Concepts in Public Law 86–382, Passed on September 28, 1959**

- The law is about 8½ pages of text that clearly explains congressional intent and leaves the details of implementation to the OPM. Compare this succinctness with the ACA of 2010, at 906 pages.

- Eligibility cannot be based on health status and coverage cannot be canceled except for reasons of fraud and nonpayment of premiums. Compare this provision to those in the ACA.

- The OPM was to contract with both service plans (including prepaid group practices—the forerunners of HMOs) and indemnity plans. Compare this requirement to the HMO Act (PL 93–222) of 1973.

- Health plans combined both basic benefits and "major medical" (catastrophic) coverage. This coverage also included a pharmaceutical plan. Such comprehensiveness was not universal in the private insurance arena till at least the 1980s. It still does not exist with respect to Medicare unless the beneficiary purchases supplemental coverage and a Part D plan.

- No premium differentials exist among beneficiaries based on age, health status, or geographic location. Especially pertinent is that retirees and their spouses pay the same as active workers. This mandate is contained in Chapter 89 Title 5 of the U.S. Code. Compare this provision to numerous initiatives for community rating (construed in many different ways, e.g., at the county or state level).

- If beneficiaries are no longer eligible, they can obtain "a temporary extension of coverage during which [they] may exercise the option to convert, without evidence of good health, to a non-group contract." Compare this provision to the enactment of the Consolidated Omnibus Budget Reconciliation Act of 1985.

- Since it is regulated by federal law, the FEHBP supersedes state insurance regulations. Compare this circumstance to the Employee Retirement Income Security Act of 1974, which enabled businesses to self-insure under terms not restricted by state health insurance laws.

- Beneficiaries can join national health plans in addition to locally sponsored ones. This possibility became a reality for self-insured company plans only after passage of ERISA in 1974. It is still not an option for employees whose employers purchase commercial policies, though Republican proposals may move the market in this direction.

Each year, OPM negotiates health benefits and premiums with private insurance plans to provide comprehensive benefits for eligible beneficiaries at a cost of more than $40 billion.[222] Funds for current employees come from congressional appropriations for salaries and benefits for each unit of government. Although premium prices vary greatly depending on plan benefits, cost sharing, and who is covered, by statute the government generally pays 72% of the weighted average premium of all health benefit plans participating in the FEHBP, but no more than 75% of any particular plan's premium; enrollees pay the difference.

---

[222] Blom, K. B., & Cornell, A. S. (Congressional Research Service) (2016, February 3). *Federal Employees Health Benefits (FEHB) program: An overview*. Retrieved June 24, 2018, from https://fas.org/sgp/crs/misc/R43922.pdf

Several features about the contracting are peculiar to the FEHBP:

- Most national PPO premiums are based on *experience rating* of the entire plan over the previous year. (It cannot be based on experience at the individual level.) Most HMO rates are calculated using *community rating*.

- OPM adds a charge to each plan's premium, limited by law to 1% of the premium, to cover its costs for program administration.

- The premium that OPM pays an experience-rated plan contains a "service charge" or profit, which is calculated according to detailed regulations. This profit is based on each year's assessment by OPM of the plan's performance on six factors:

  (1) contractor performance on accurate and timely claims processing, handling of claims disputes, and general beneficial innovations; (2) contract cost-risk factors, including group size (smaller enrollments receive credit for higher risk), certain enrollee demographics, and the plan's willingness to assume risk; (3) federal socioeconomic programs, such as programs to deter drug abuse, which are evaluated by considering the quality of the contractor's policies and procedures and the extent of unusual effort or achievement demonstrated; (4) capital investments (this is a general federal acquisition factor but seldom applicable under FEHB); (5) cost control, such as contractor-initiated efforts to improve benefit design, cost sharing, or innovative peer review procedures; and (6) independent development of administrative systems that improve cost efficiency and for which the contractor assumed the development costs. Each of these profit factors is scored with regard to the plan's performance in the previous year, and the sum of the scores determines the profit percentage.[223]

- OPM maintains in the U.S. Treasury contingency reserve funds for all FEHB plans. In general, contingency reserves are used to offset unexpected increases in spending or premium increases in later years...

  For FFS plans, OPM is authorized to charge plans up to 3% of their premium to establish and maintain contingency reserves... FFS plans can use their reserves to offset larger-than-anticipated claims, or, if the balance becomes larger than necessary, the reserves can be drawn down and used to offset a premium increase in the subsequent year. FFS plans can draw down these reserves as claims are paid.

  For HMO plans, OPM also charges plans up to 3% of their premium to establish and maintain contingency reserves. However, unlike those for FFS plans, the contingency reserves for HMO plans can be used only by OPM if OPM approves an adjustment during an annual reconciliation process that usually takes place in March.[224]

In addition to the above methodology, in 2016, the FEHB started a quality-based payment program called the Plan Performance Assessment (PPA). (Please see Exhibit 6.62.) In 2018, the first three performance areas were weighted at 65% while contract oversight counted for the remaining 35%.

---

[223] Ibid.
[224] Ibid.

EXHIBIT 6.62. Performance Areas and Domains of the FEHB Plan Performance Assessment

Performance Area	Domain
Clinical quality	Preventive care
	Chronic disease management
	Medication use
	Behavioral health
Customer service	Communication
	Access
	Claims
	Member experience/engagement
Resource use	Utilization management
Contract oversight	Contract performance
	Responsiveness to OPM
	Contract compliance
	Technology management and data security

Source: U.S. Office of Personnel Management Healthcare and Insurance (2017, December 14). *FEHB Program Carrier Letter No. 2017-15: Plan performance assessment—Consolidated methodology.* Retrieved June 24, 2018, from https://www.opm.gov/healthcare-insurance/healthcare/carriers/2017/2017-15.pdf

Currently, the FEHBP provides healthcare coverage through these plans to about 8.3 million federal employees, retirees, and their dependents.[225] While participation in FEHBP is voluntary, in 2017, about 84% of federal workers were enrolled in the program.[226] The types of products from which beneficiaries can choose are limited by statute and include: Consumer-Driven and High-Deductible plans; FFS plans; PPOs; and HMOs. In 2018, the OPM contracted with 83 insurers, which offered about 262 different plan options. Despite these many choices,

about two-thirds of FEHBP participants in 2015 were enrolled in one of the two options offered as part of the Blue Cross Blue Shield Association's (BCBSA) nationwide FFS

[225]OPM.gov: Open season briefing. October 2018. https://www.opm.gov/healthcare-insurance/healthcare/reference-materials/2018-openseason.pdf Retrieved April 13, 2019.
[226]US Office of Personnel Management: 2017 Federal Employee Benefits Survey Report. April 2018. Retrieved April 13, 2019 from https://www.opm.gov/policy-data-oversight/data-analysis-documentation/employee-surveys/2017-federal-employee-benefits-survey-results.pdf

plan... [B]y 2015 it was the largest in 98 percent of counties. Over this same time period, the median county market share held by BCBSA also increased—from 58 percent in 2000 to 72 percent in 2015.[227]

Of note is that enrollees in these plans are extremely satisfied, accounting for a plan change rate of 5% to 7% per year (compare to some private markets which can have a 25% turnover rate).

In the past few years, this program has been able to keep premium increases far below private sector rates; raises have declined from 6.4% in 2016 to 1.3% in 2019.[228] To address concerns about future price increases and maintain current satisfaction rates, the OPM requested[229] certain actions from health plans for fiscal year 2019:

- Modifying cost sharing for high-value and low-value benefits to help ensure members are getting the most value for their healthcare dollar

- Implementing high-performance tiered provider networks that offer reduced cost sharing for members who choose a provider(s) from such a network

- Reducing cost sharing when members take action to manage chronic conditions or obtain higher-quality or more efficient care through creative provider or vendor partnerships (e.g., patient-centered medical home [PCMH], cancer management)

- Improving enrollee engagement and decision support through online portals and other key communication methods

- Exploring innovative models that include other cost management techniques, such as new evidence-based utilization management (UM) in medical or specialty pharmacy

- Addressing the opioid abuse epidemic

- Taking action to improve medication adherence, drug UM, and the alignment of formularies to established clinical guidelines

- Requiring that members are charged the lesser of the prescription price or applicable copayment amount for prescription medications

- Promoting innovative HDHP plan design, where the premium pass-through amount to a member's HRA or HSA account is no longer limited to 50% of the plan deductible

- Clarifying coverage of genetic testing

- Continuing emphasis on population health

- Planning proposals to describe communication pathways to ensure members receive updated information about Tdap and HPV vaccinations

---

[227] Ibid.

[228] OPM.gov: Open season briefing, October 2018, op. cit.

[229] Spielman, AP (U.S. Office of Personnel Management Healthcare and Insurance): FEHB Program Carrier Letter No. 2018-01. January 23, 2018. Retrieved June 24, 2018 from https://www.opm.gov/healthcare-insurance/healthcare/carriers/2018/2018-01.pdf

While in recent years the ACA has been the model and vehicle for delivering the aim of universal healthcare, prior to that time, many policy analysts favored the FEHBP model to accomplish this goal. Proponents pointed to the high participation rate, low administrative costs, and high retention rate. They also claimed competition among commercial plans, as managed by the OPM, would lower costs and shift the risk to the insurer.[230]

Bovbjerg summarized the application of the FEHBP principles to health reforms in this way:

> First, selection issues can be severe and program altering. It seems very likely that stronger countermeasures will be needed for a new exchange than the FEHBP has as yet deployed. Second, it is challenging to maintain a wide spread of benefit packages for enrollees to choose among. Plausibly, better risk adjustment or other anti-selection mechanisms would assist in achieving this goal. Third, the FEHBP approach of negotiating with health plans and maintaining reserves that can be used to offset unexpected costs in a given year or temper year-to-year premium fluctuations is an alternative to direct public regulation of premiums.[231]

Opponents claim that, while such as system may work for small businesses, schemes to apply the model to Medicare would cause market distortions; sicker beneficiaries would choose either traditional Medicare, if still available, or plans with richer benefits. They also doubt the cost savings available. Further, seniors do not have enough information to make informed decisions about what plans to choose and tend to stay with current providers.

Because the marketplace is very different today, new analysis would need to be conducted to determine the feasibility of adopting the FEHBP or a like scheme to address the country's healthcare problems.

Managed Care

Background. Kaiser-Permanente has been previously cited as an example of the origins of managed care. Despite the attractiveness of such plans, by the early 1980s, they had only achieved commercial insurance market penetration of about 4%. Two factors subsequently catalyzed the rapid growth of health maintenance organizations (HMOs): passage of the TEFRA of 1982 and the deterioration of the economy. Recall that one portion of TEFRA mandated a phase-in of a DRG system to pay hospitals for inpatient services for Medicare recipients. In response, hospitals, fearing losses from this fixed reimbursement, increased their fees to private customers. At the same time, from 1979 to 1984, the United States experienced a recession, from which it recovered only slowly. The healthcare implication of these events was that companies spent more on premiums at a time when their revenues were shrinking. Employers often faced healthcare bills whose magnitude equaled or exceeded their net margins. Further, as mentioned previously, in December 1990 the Financial Accounting

---

[230] Pear, RA: Proposal for Medicare Is Unlike Federal Employee Plan. NY Times May 2, 2011, p. A18. Retrieved June 25, 3028 from http://www.nytimes.com/2011/05/02/health/policy/02medicare.html?_r=1&hpw

[231] Boybjerg, RR: Lessons for Health Reform from the Federal Employees Health Benefits Program: Timely Analysis of Immediate Health Policy Issues Urban Institute. August 12, 2009. Retrieved June 25, 2018 from http://www.urban.org/url.cfm?ID=411940

Standards Board (FASB) issued Statement 106, requiring publicly traded companies to recognize on their financial statements the full future obligation of healthcare benefits. In the case of some large companies, these obligations were in excess of $1 billion. (In 2005, a similar decision was made by the Government Accounting Standards Board, Rule No. 45, for state and local governments.)

In order to address this economic burden, employers demanded that insurance companies design products that would control these significant annual premium increases. Another feature the employers required was low employee out-of-pocket expenses. The reason for this latter request was that employee share of total health expenses had declined from about 55% in 1960 to about 20% in 1990. (According to the Office of the Actuary of CMS, this figure declined further to about 15% by 2000.) Because of this employee expectation, as well as results of collective bargaining, employers were locked into these out-of-pocket targets. As previously discussed, when the mandate is for low premiums and low out-of-pocket expenses, the only feasible insurance product will target provider-induced demand by limiting the provider network. The proliferation of HMOs thus resulted from these employer requirements; subsequently, other products such as Preferred Provider Organizations (PPOs) and Point of Service (POS) plans also emerged. By 1992, the majority of employer-sponsored plans were some type of managed care, with the traditional FFS plans declining to 8% of the market (from 96% in 1984). The change in payment method from uncontrolled FFS to discounted fee schedules (or capitation), implementation of extensive utilization review processes (to curb provider-induced demand), and the very rapid change in itself in the composition of the health insurance marketplace provoked strong hostility by many healthcare providers. Since employers and other payers controlled the funding, however, the plans continued to grow. (Please see Exhibit 6.63.) When the economy rebounded in the 1990s, employers were faced with a dilemma: They still wanted to hold down healthcare costs, but, in order to compete for and retain talented employees, they needed to offer more choice in health plans and other benefits. The plans themselves also needed to offer more freedom of choice of providers to their customers. PPOs and POS plans, therefore, replaced HMOs as the predominant managed care models.

In order to fully appreciate the subject of managed care, one must first understand the definition, delivery network structure, and operational features of these plans. Because the prototype managed care organization is the HMO, it will be considered first.

Definitions and Their Implications. Definitions of managed care are as varied as the types of plans and those who belong to and are affected by them. These differing definitions, as well as the subsequent establishment of hybrids that draw from diverse plan characteristics, have made evaluation research in this area very difficult to conduct and interpret. One must therefore be very careful in accepting findings without a close scrutiny of definitions and study methods.

Exhibit 6.64 provides several definitions of managed care that have been put forth by a variety of different organizations. With regard to the first four definitions, note the organizational bias in their formulation. The definition that captures the ideal and promise of managed care is, ironically, the last one, which has a non-American origin. The one part of the

EXHIBIT 6.63. Distribution of Health Plan Enrollment for Covered Workers, by Plan Type, 1988–2018

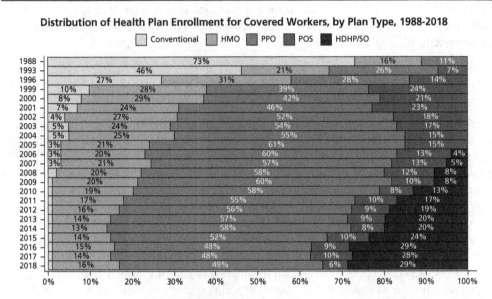

Distribution of Health Plan Enrollment for Covered Workers, by Plan Type, 1988-2018

Note: Information was not obtained for POS plans in 1988 or for HDHP/SO plans until 2006. A portion of the change in plan type enrollment for 2005 is likely attributable to incorporating more recent Census Bureau estimates of the number of state and local government workers and removing federal workers from the weights. See the Survey Design and Methods section from the 2005 Kaiser/HRET Survey of Employer-Sponsored Health Benefits for additional information.

Source: Kaiser Family Foundation: 2018 Employer Health Benefits Survey. Section 5: Market Shares of Health Plans. October 3, 2018 https://www.kff.org/reportsection/2018-employer-health-benefits-survey-section-5-market-shares-of-health-plans/ Retrieved April 13, 2019.

EXHIBIT 6.64. Definitions of Managed Care

Managed Care Is . . .

"a set of techniques used by or on behalf of purchasers of healthcare to manage healthcare costs by influencing patient care decision making through case-by-case assessment of the appropriateness of care prior to its provision." —Institute of Medicine

"a variety of interventions of healthcare delivery and financing intended to eliminate unnecessary and inappropriate care and to reduce cost." —Congressional Budget Office

"systems that integrate the financing and delivery of appropriate healthcare services to covered individuals." —Health Insurance Assn. of America (now America's Health Insurance Plans)

"systems or techniques generally used by third-party payers expressly to provide what they consider an appropriate mix of medical and social services at the lowest cost to payers and patients." —American Medical Association

"[a] process to maximize the health gain of a community within limited resources, by ensuring that an appropriate range and level of services are provided, and by monitoring on a case-by-case basis to ensure that they are continuously improved to meet national targets for health and individual health needs." —Roseleff and Lister, *European healthcare trends: Towards managed care in Europe*

definition that is not applicable to the U.S. experience is "within limited resources." Although cost containment is an important part of managed care, neither private nor governmental insurers in this country have explicit budgets beyond which they will not provide services. It is interesting that the United States turned to managed care as a solution to cost problems while in other countries these plans developed to address quality and access problems in the public system. We now focus on HMOs.

I define an HMO in this way:

> An HMO is a healthcare plan that delivers comprehensive, coordinated medical service to voluntarily enrolled members on a prepaid basis.

Several parts of this definition require a more detailed explanation. First is the key word "comprehensive." With regard to scope of services, many traditional non-HMO plans covered acute care but not routine preventive services.[232] A founding precept of an HMO is the provision of care that prevents illness and maintains health. In fact, for all the bad press these plans have received, the research indicates that HMOs *do* provide more preventive care than other forms of insurance coverage.[233] Another part of the comprehensiveness is financial coverage. For example, before enactment of the ACA, most insurance products had lifetime limits on health plan payments, ranging from $1 million to $5 million. HMOs never had such caps.

The next key concept is "coordinated medical service." This term implies that someone is directing the care to ensure it is delivered in a high-quality, cost-effective manner. While the term "gatekeeper" is often applied to this function, it is more appropriate to say that it is the responsibility of a *primary care physician*. Primary care is defined as:

> the provision of integrated, accessible healthcare services by clinicians who are accountable for addressing a large majority of personal healthcare needs, developing a sustained partnership with patients, and practicing in the context of family and community.

> The term *integrated* is used to denote the provision of comprehensive, coordinated, and continuous services that provide a seamless process of care.[234]

Note that essential features in this definition are that these physicians must be capable of caring for a majority of common conditions (such as diabetes, asthma, high blood pressure, and arthritis) and can treat patients on a long-term basis in whatever setting they need care. The specialties that fit this definition, therefore, are family medicine, internal medicine, and pediatrics. The HMO requires that patients coordinate care through their primary care physicians; except in emergency situations, the HMO generally will only pay for services[235] that the primary care physician authorizes. Because this process restricts freedom of patients

---

[232]This paucity of coverage and incomplete funding was one reason for inclusion in the ACA of the requirement for certain preventive coverage without out-of-pocket expenses.

[233]Miller, R. M., and Luft, H. S. (2002). HMO plan performance update: An analysis of the literature, 1997–2001. *Health Affairs*, 21: 63-86, 2002 This early article's findings have been replicated by subsequent research and monitoring of the quality of these plans.

[234]Vanselow, N. A., Donaldson, M. S., & Yordy, K. D. (1995). A new definition of primary care. *JAMA, 273,* 192.

[235]The word "services" will be used for medical care, but it also includes products such as pharmaceuticals and medical devices/equipment.

to self-direct access to specialists of their choice, it has become a source of dissatisfaction with HMO plans. Other healthcare arrangements (such as PPOs) may not require these referrals in all cases.

A "new" concept that draws on the principles of coordination of care by a primary care physician is the "medical home." (Please see Exhibit 6.65 for features agreed upon by all

EXHIBIT 6.65. **Patient-Centered Medical Home**

The PCMH is an approach to providing comprehensive primary care for children, youth and adults. The PCMH is a healthcare setting that facilitates partnerships between individual patients, and their personal physicians, and when appropriate, the patient's family . . .

Principles

Personal physician—each patient has an ongoing relationship with a personal physician trained to provide first contact, continuous and comprehensive care.

Physician directed medical practice—the personal physician leads a team of individuals at the practice level who collectively take responsibility for the ongoing care of patients.

Whole person orientation—the personal physician is responsible for providing for all the patient's healthcare needs or taking responsibility for appropriately arranging care with other qualified professionals. This responsibility includes care for all stages of life: acute care; chronic care; preventive services; and end-of-life care.

Care is coordinated and/or integrated across all elements of the complex healthcare system (e.g., subspecialty care, hospitals, home health agencies, nursing homes) and the patient's community (e.g., family, public and private community-based services).

Quality and Safety

- Practices advocate for their patients.

- Evidence-based medicine and clinical decision-support tools guide decision making.

- Physicians in the practice accept accountability for continuous quality improvement through voluntary engagement in performance measurement and improvement.

- Patients and families actively participate in decision-making, quality improvement, and feedback.

- Practices go through a voluntary recognition process by an appropriate non-governmental entity

- Payment: The payment structure should be based on the following framework:

- It should allow for separate fee-for-service payments for face-to-face visits. (Payments for care management services that fall outside of the face-to-face visit, as described above, should not result in a reduction in the payments for face-to-face visits.)

- It should recognize case mix differences in the patient population being treated within the practice.

- It should allow physicians to share in savings from reduced hospitalizations associated with physician-guided care management in the office setting.

- It should allow for additional payments for achieving measurable and continuous quality improvements.

Source: Excerpted from American Academy of Family Physicians, American Academy of Pediatrics, American College of Physicians, and American Osteopathic Association, Joint Principles of the Patient-Centered Medical Home, March 7, 2007. Retrieved June 26, 2018, from https://www.aafp.org/dam/AAFP/documents/practice_management/pcmh/initiatives/PCMHJoint.pdf

four major primary care organizations.)[236] Medical homes are seen as the essential core of Accountable Care Organizations. (Please see Chapter 4, "Hospitals and Healthcare Systems.") Note the similarity of this concept to that of the role of the primary care physician in an HMO setting. However, also note that while the payment recommendation mentions sharing savings, it stresses FFS payments rather than capitation.

The final essential feature of the HMO definition is the prepaid method of compensation: that is, capitation. Individual primary care providers (or the medical groups to which they belong) receive monthly payments from insurance companies based on the number of patients assigned to them. Adjustments are usually made by age and sex of individuals. The amount received on behalf of an individual patient is usually called the "per member per month" (PMPM) payment.

The reason HMOs can perform better than other types of plans in containing costs is that they are designed to change physician behavior. As Exhibit 6.66 illustrates, physician behavior accounts for about 75% of healthcare expenses. One reason health systems fail to achieve successful cost containment strategies is that they usually address only the amount of payment to providers and suppliers rather than the method of payment that will result in a

EXHIBIT 6.66. Physicians' Control of Healthcare Expenses

Sectors under Physician Control	Amount Spent in 1993 in Billions	Percentage of Total
Hospital care	$363	38.6%
Physicians	$176	18.7%
Drugs and devices	$ 87	9.2%
Nursing homes	$ 76	8.1%
Subtotal	$702	74.6%
Sections not controlled		
Other (such as alternate site care)	$ 93	9.9%
Dental	$ 92	9.8%
Administration	$ 54	5.7%
Subtotal	$239	25.4%
Total	$941	100.0%

Source: U.S. Departments of Health & Human Services and Commerce; Alex. Brown & Sons, Inc. (A division of Raymond James)—original document no longer available.

---

[236] For more information on how medical homes formed, see *Health Affairs* (May 2010), Special Edition: Reinventing primary care.

change in behavior. Capitation is a hallmark of HMOs. If a plan does not involve capitation, it is not truly an HMO, no matter what it calls itself.[237] Since in a capitated plan the services are prepaid, the physician does not increase revenue by doing more. Capitation, therefore, addresses the financial incentives of provider-induced demand that occurs in a FFS setting.

The concern with capitation, of course, is that the physician will be tempted to withhold services. In addressing this issue, however, Berwick noted: "If anything, the data suggest hazards and ethical problems in the overuse of services in fee-for-service settings, rather than its underuse in capitated care."[238] Since the capitated primary care physician is at financial risk for providing services, it is in his or her best interest to provide more preventive care and personally perform as many routine procedures as possible. For example, instead of referring patients, many internists are capable of providing routine gynecologic exams, performing diabetic foot exams, and removing simple skin lesions.

Applying the principles of insurance presented at the beginning of this chapter, physicians should realize that in a capitated scheme, for specified services, they now assume the same risk as an insurer. It is important, therefore, that they make sure the patients are of average risk for illness (a problem for some academic medical centers) and that the number of patients is sufficient to provide adequate cash flow to spread the risk of catastrophic cases. One of the biggest mistakes physicians can make is to "try out" capitation with a small number of patients.

To summarize, what differentiates HMOs from noncapitated schemes is financial and clinical accountability aided by enhanced coordination of care.

Types of Health Maintenance Organizations. In order to understand the types of plans in this sector, one must understand the different organizational structures of HMOs. An important point to remember is that *the type of HMO is defined by how the physicians are organized and their relationship to the insurance company (health plan).*

The first type of plan is a *staff model*. In this arrangement, physicians are employees of the plan and, therefore, only see patients who belong to that HMO. They receive salaries as well as performance bonuses based on such measures as number of patients seen, compliance with cost-control measures, and meeting quality goals. Although physicians are not capitated under this scheme, their employment status, supervision, and reward structure make this model a true HMO. Also, since these physicians are employees, their management decision-making abilities may be restricted. Companies often waste time and expense if they market their services and products to physicians in staff model HMOs. The true business decision makers are plan executives. Common examples of this arrangement are employer and

---

[237] The exception to this absolute statement is when physicians are salaried, such as in a staff-model HMO. In this case, the group is usually capitated. Still, the compensation system does not reward them for doing more.

[238] Berwick, D. M. (1996). Payment by capitation and the quality of care. *The New England Journal of Medicine 335*, 1227–1231. This classic paper's conclusions have been supported by subsequent research and independent evaluations of health plans and providers. For example, Timbie et al. found that: "Overall, MA [Medicare Advantage] outperformed FFS [fee-for-service] on all 16 clinical quality measures." Timbie, J. W., Bogart, A., Damberg, C. L., Elliott, M. N., Haas, A., Gaillot, S. J.... Paddock, S. M. (2017). Medicare advantage and fee-for-service performance on clinical quality and patient experience measures: Comparisons from three large states. *Health Services Research, 52*(6), 2038–2060.

union-sponsored plans, which hire full-time physicians to care for all employee and family healthcare needs.

The second type of plan is the *group model*. In this arrangement, physicians belong to a medical group that has a mutually exclusive relationship with a health insurance plan. In other words, the plan's patients only see the group's physicians, and the group only cares for those patients enrolled in the plan. The group is capitated, and physicians within the group determine the distribution of funds among themselves. The decision-making authority in this model is split between the plan and the group. For example, pharmaceutical companies may convince the plan (or its designated pharmaceutical benefit manager) to offer its products to members. These companies then need to convince the group's leadership, and often individual physicians, to use these medications. The prototype of a group model is the relationship between Kaiser and the Permanente Medical Group.

In order to be able to compete with organizations like Kaiser-Permanente, in the early 1970s, health plans were formed to give individual physicians access to capitated insurance contracts. These plans were often organized around county medical societies; the first was in the San Joaquin Valley in California. Since the physicians still retained their medical practices, this third model is called an "individual practice association" (IPA). In the first iteration of this arrangement, the health plan contracted with each individual physician. In the next version, physicians organized into virtual medical groups for purposes of contracting with health plans. Under this arrangement, the organizing entity can be a hospital (so-called hospital-based IPA), medical society, or freestanding company. The plan then contracts with and pays capitation to the IPA, which, in turn, pays member physicians on a fee or capitation basis. Unlike group and staff model physicians, those who belong to an IPA can see fee-for-service patients and contract with multiple plans, including other HMOs. The decision makers are even more decentralized in this setting. They consist of the plan executives, IPA administrators, and individual physicians.

The fourth type of plan is the *network model*, an organizational hybrid between the group and IPA models. This arrangement was started in 1971 by Mervin Shalowitz, MD, at CNA Insurance Company in Chicago and was aptly named "Intergroup." In network models, plans contract with established *medical groups* to provide care to enrolled members. It has thus been called an IPA of groups. Unlike IPAs, these groups are actual legal entities in which physicians share practice revenues and expenses. As is the case with IPAs, physicians in network models also see non-HMO patients and can contract with multiple plans. The decision makers here are the plan executives, group leadership, and individual physicians. Since physicians are organized in groups, reaching them is logistically easier than with the original IPA model.

As mentioned above, one of the public's most significant criticisms about HMOs has been their lack of freedom of choice; the plan will not pay for care outside the contracted network (except for emergencies). In order to grow market share in the 1990s, HMOs adopted four tactics. First, they shifted from the capital-intensive and smaller geographic network of staff and group models to IPA and network models. By 2004, IPA and network arrangements had close to 80% of the HMO market. Second, in order to respond to customer concerns about the rising price of premiums, the plans held down provider reimbursement levels. They implemented this tactic at a time when physicians and hospitals were adopting expensive new technologies (e.g., more childhood immunizations, better and more expensive chemotherapy options, new laboratory diagnostics, and additional invasive and diagnostic radiology procedures). In effect, plans shifted the financial risk of these higher-level services to the providers. Third, plans relaxed the referral requirements, allowing some patients to see specialists without first contacting their primary care physician. Finally, benefits were extended, often without adequate increases in premiums. The most significant benefit, and the one that caused the greatest financial impact, was prescription drug coverage, which will be discussed further below.

Distribution of HMO Premiums and Its Behavioral Implications. Understanding how managed care plans allocate their premiums will elucidate how they provide incentives for physicians to change their behavior. This behavioral change transitions them from a fragmented, fee-for-service environment to a more coordinated HMO setting. (Please see Exhibit 6.67 for a schematic of this distribution.) While this example is generally valid for most plans, there are numerous variations in both the amounts allocated to each category as well as what items are contained in each.

The first category describes physician or group financial responsibilities when they accept risk for paying all professional and diagnostic services—often called a *full professional risk contract*. Under this scheme, physicians receive capitation every month for all patients assigned to their care. Out of that sum, they must pay for nearly all professional services, diagnostic tests, and therapies (physical, speech and occupational). Also included are immunizations and medication administered in outpatient settings, such as chemotherapy. Whatever is left is used to pay themselves for *their* services and to cover practice expenses. In order to protect themselves against catastrophic financial losses from providing proper care to their patients, physicians must have reinsurance (stop-loss insurance). This protection is either provided by the health plan or purchased on the open market. One

EXHIBIT 6.67. Distributing Prepaid Premiums

40% Physician Capitation	40% Hospital Fund	20% Health Plan Expenses
Physician fees:	Inpatient charges	Operating expenses
Inpatient	Surgicenter (facility only)	Pharmaceuticals
Outpatient	Skilled nursing facility	*Reinsurance for special services*:
Referrals	Durable medical equipment	Transplants
Outpatient services:		Chronic hemodialysis
Laboratory		Psychiatry/chemical dependency
Radiology		
Therapies		
Stop-loss insurance	Stop-loss insurance	Stop-loss insurance

reason why many physicians and groups have been financially hurt by full professional risk contracts is they neglected to obtain such coverage. To highlight the risk of these arrangements, the California Medical Association estimates that from 1996 to 2004, 126 medical groups in that state closed or went bankrupt, affecting about 36,000 physicians and 3.8 million health plan enrollees. The American Medical Association reported that the majority of medical groups in California that participated in risk-capitated arrangements did not have reinsurance. Another reason for these bankruptcies is that groups assumed risk for services they could not fully control, such as pharmaceuticals.[239]

Health plans refer to the next fund by a variety of names, such as: hospital fund, medical incentive fund, shared risk fund, and Part A fund (corresponding to benefits covered by Medicare Part A). It always covers institutional expenses for hospital and skilled nursing home care, and usually home care and durable medical equipment (from wheelchairs to home hospital beds to intravenous pumps). Again, it is important to make sure that reinsurance exists for these services since some groups are also at risk for losses in this fund. In contrast to the capitation reinsurance, which is often specified in terms of dollars spent *per person per contract year* (at least $10,000), the reinsurance for institutional services may be in terms of dollars spent *per hospitalization* (about $50,000 or more) or *number of in-patient days,* after which the benefit will apply (e.g., after 30 days in the hospital the reinsurance will start to pay back this fund).

In contrast to Medicare's use of DRGs, managed care plans usually pay hospitals on the basis of pre-negotiated, per-diem fees. (Please see the Hospital Inpatient Payment Methods section of Chapter 4.) These fees are all-inclusive daily payments; the total is thus based on the patient's length of stay in the hospital, *regardless of the number, cost, or intensity of services*. The per diems vary only by level and by type of service used in the hospital (i.e., different charges apply for intensive care, general medical/surgical care, obstetrics, newborn nursery, and psychiatry). The magnitude of per diems across all services is in the order of thousands of dollars per day with significant local area variations. For reference, the cost of skilled nursing home care is typically about one third that of a general medical/ surgical day.

Before discussing the health plan expense category, please refer to Exhibit 6.68, which provides a brief survey of research over three decades for the reasons HMOs have lower costs than other types of insurance coverage. Rather than viewing these statements as conflicting, one should appreciate that they reflect an evolution of the marketplace. Recall that under a fee-for-service scheme, primary care physicians are paid on a daily basis; the longer the patient stays in the hospital, the greater the compensation. In a capitated plan, since these physicians receive one monthly fee, longer stays do not yield larger payments. Hospital length of stay reduction, however, is principally due to another feature of physician compensation in HMO arrangements: *Contracts between physicians and HMOs often contain*

---

[239]For more insights into these dynamics, see Robinson, J. C. (2001). Physician organization in California: Crisis and opportunity. *Health Affairs, 20*(4), 81–96 and Bodenheimer, T. (2000). California's beleaguered physician groups, Can they survive? *The New England Journal of Medicine, 342*, 1064–1068.

EXHIBIT 6.68. Reasons for HMO Cost Savings

- "Total costs (premium and out-of-pocket) for [HMO] enrollees are 10 to 40 per cent lower than those for comparable people with [indemnity] health insurance. Enrollees in health-maintenance organizations have about as many ambulatory visits as comparison groups. Most of the cost differences are attributable to hospitalization rates about 30 per cent lower than those of conventionally insured populations. These lower hospitalization rates, in turn, are due almost entirely to lower admission rates; the average length of stay shows little difference. There is no evidence that health-maintenance organizations reduce admissions in discretionary or 'unnecessary' categories; instead, the data suggest lower admission rates across the board."[a]

- "Health maintenance organizations (HMOs) achieve their cost savings through lower rates of hospital admissions... The rate of discretionary surgery was lower in the HMO, while the rate of nondiscretionary surgery was equivalent in the two systems. For medical admissions, rates of discretionary and nondiscretionary admissions were lower in the HMO. There were no observable adverse effects on health from the lower rates of nondiscretionary hospitalization, either because the net effect on health was small or because the HMO substituted appropriate ambulatory services. We conclude that HMO reductions in hospitalization rates do not occur 'across the board'; discretionary surgery is selectively avoided."[b]

- "Although research has indicated that HMOs have been effective in limiting medical costs, there is mixed evidence in the literature on how they achieve these savings... Our results indicate that HMOs tend to enroll a younger but not much healthier population than traditional fee-for-service plans, suggesting that self-selection is not a major contributor to HMO cost savings."[c]

- A study at a group model HMO, the Carle Clinic in Urbana, Illinois,

  yielded three important findings. First...HMO patients with the same disease as their FFS [fee-for-service] counterparts made more use of lower-cost providers (more midlevel providers and generalists), avoided higher-cost providers (fewer specialists and ER visits), and received arguably more cost-effective services (less expensive ancillary services and more selective use of specialists). Second...HMO care used fewer expenditures—expressed as total outpatient dollars and adjusted for...case mix...Our results suggest that most of the savings occurred for the patients with average health and that the healthiest and sickest patients tended to receive the same total outpatient resources regardless of insurance.

  Third, savings occurred because the HMO chose which physicians cared for their patients.[d]

- In a study comparing HMO with fee-for-service enrollees who were employees of the State of Massachusetts, after studying eight medical conditions, the authors found that HMO costs were lower because

  47% of differences in plan costs are attributable to differences in the likelihoods that patients in the two types of plans suffer from these conditions. On average, approximately 3% of the difference between plans in total costs for *all* conditions results from differing incidence rates. Price differences are the other major component, explaining 45% of cost differences in total. This provides strong evidence that price differentials are a key source of cost differences, although our results must be qualified by our inability to separate pure price effects from the effects of unobserved, within-age-and-sex-cohort selection. Finally, treatment-intensity differences explain only a small part of cost differences. The indemnity plan offers more intense treatment only for live births.

> The HMOs, in contrast, offer more intensive treatment for AMI [heart attacks] and possibly for colon cancer . . . we have the positive finding that cost savings by HMOs are not achieved through curtailing essential medical treatments.[e]

[a] Luft, H. (1978). How do health-maintenance organizations achieve their "savings"? *New England Journal of Medicine, 298,* 1336–1343.

[b] Siu, A.L., et al. (1988). Use of the hospital in a randomized trial of prepaid care. *JAMA, 259,* 1343–1346.

[c] Taylor, A. K., et al. (1995). Who belongs to HMOs: A comparison of fee-for-service versus HMO enrollees. *Medical Care Research Review,* 52, 389–408.

[d] Flood, A.B., et al. (1998). How do HMOs achieve savings? The effectiveness of one organization's strategies. *Health Services Research,* 33, 79–99.

[e] Altman, D., et al. (2002). Enrollee mix, treatment intensity, and cost in competing indemnity and HMO plans. *Journal of Health Economics,* 22, 23–45.

provisions whereby both parties share savings in the hospital fund; the split is usually about 50–50, but physicians can get as much as 65% of the surplus. Consider that even with a per diem of $1,000, with each day saved, physicians can earn at least $500. While some believe that this design encourages doctors to withhold hospital services, research does not support this contention. Further, physicians should realize that restricting appropriate care not only exposes them to potential litigation but can cost more in the long run. The important feature to appreciate is that *under this payment arrangement, total physician compensation depends on efficiently and effectively delivering and coordinating an appropriate mix of services.* Therefore, these physicians will highly value products or services that can help them achieve this mix.

The third column lists expenses that are, strictly speaking, solely the financial responsibility of the health plan. Of course, since the total premium is fixed, any amounts allocated to these expenses will cause less to be available for the other two funds. The operating costs (often called sales, general and administrative expenses [SG&A]) should be about 8% to 10% of premium in well-run plans. Many companies, however, allocate 15% or more to this category in order to build in a small up-front profit margin. (It should be noted that historical profit margins for these plans have been in the 3% to 5% range. This figure will change as more companies merge and diversify into other healthcare-related services.) As mentioned previously, the ACA mandates that nonmedical expenses cannot be greater than 15% for large employer plans and 20% for those covering small groups and individuals.

Pharmaceuticals have been one of the most rapidly rising components of health plan costs. Prior to the 1990s, with the exception of Medicaid, self-administered medications were not usually included in health insurance benefits. According to data from CMS on national health expenditures, in 1990, individuals paid 59% of prescription drug costs; by 2008, that figure declined to 21% and was 16% in 2016.[240] As far as actual expenditures,

---

[240] Kamal, R., & Cox, C. (Kaiser Family Foundation). (2012, December 20). What are the recent and forecasted trends in prescription drug spending? Out-*of-pocket costs for Rx drugs are expected to increase, but will likely represent a smaller portion of overall Rx spending.* Retrieved June 26, 2018, from https://www.healthsystemtracker.org/chart-collection/recent-forecasted-trends-prescription-drug-spending/?_sf_s=recent+trends#item-start

pharmaceuticals can account for about $120 PMPM.[241] The significance of this number is highlighted by the fact that it often exceeds the budgeted capitation for primary care physicians. In order to address these rapidly rising pharmaceutical costs, all health plans have adopted one or more of the strategies listed in Exhibit 6.69. (This topic will be addressed in more detail in Chapter 7, "Healthcare Technology.") The opportunities for managed care companies to reduce costs also present challenges to pharmaceutical companies and pharmacies seeking to maximize their revenues.

EXHIBIT 6.69. Strategies to Lower Pharmaceutical Costs

- Establishment of Formularies
- Drug utilization review programs
- Increase premiums
- Increase patient out-of-pocket expenses (usually copayments but now coinsurance is being more frequently used)
- Patient's ability to use HSAs and Consumer Driven Health Plans
- Tiered benefit structures (Usually in the form of copayments, patients pay the least for generics, more for branded drugs on formulary and most for non-formulary drugs.)
- Requiring generic substitution when available (This requirement is not legal in all states.)
- Prior authorization for certain high cost or commonly misused drugs
- Physician bonus incentives for achieving cost, formulary adherence, and/or generic prescription targets
- Use of wholesalers (if the plan manages its own pharmaceutical benefits)
- Contracting with PBM firms.
- In-house pharmacies
- Coverage of over-the-counter medication that can substitute for prescription drugs (e.g., ibuprofen [Motrin] and ranitidine [Zantac])
- Mail order arrangements that lower patient copayments and decrease dispensing and overhead costs (Usually these arrangements give patients 90-day supplies of medications; local pharmacies often provide this service at the same price.)
- Lowest price guarantees (particularly for government payers)
- Quantity targets for pricing (private payers rebates; government payers price reductions
- Comparative cost/benefit studies, not just placebo comparisons for efficacy (e.g., NICE in England)
- Expectations for value-added services (e.g., monitoring, education, and/or disease management programs)
- Performance payments (i.e., if the drug does not work, then there is no payment)

---

[241] Milliman Research Report. (2016). *Commercial specialty medication research: 2016 benchmark projections*. Retrieved June 26, 2018, from http://www.milliman.com/uploadedFiles/insight/2016/commercial-specialty-medication-research .pdf

One important term previously mentioned is "formulary." Managed care organizations, or companies that manage prescription drug benefits by contract for them (called pharmaceutical benefit management [PBM] companies), provide plan members with a list of medications for which the insurer will pay something toward their costs. This list, called a formulary, is usually published according to the therapeutic class of medication: for example, antihypertensives, antibiotics, birth control, and so on. The health plan or PBM negotiates discounts with pharmaceutical companies or wholesalers for certain medications. The drugs for which they are able to obtain the best prices will appear as "preferred" in the formulary. Most prescription drug benefits have at least three "tiers" of payments, with associated increasing copayments: generics, preferred formulary drugs, and nonpreferred formulary drugs. (Sometimes the formulary includes only preferred medications; in this case, the nonpreferred drugs are called nonformulary.) The larger PBM firms and their market shares are displayed in Exhibit 6.70.

The last item in Exhibit 6.67 is services for which the plan carves out the responsibility from capitation; the plan then either assumes the risk itself or contracts with a separate entity to manage these conditions. If an outside organization assumes the responsibility, it may be paid on a fee-for-service basis, bundled/packaged, capitated, and/or have a component

EXHIBIT 6.70. **Pharmacy Benefit Management Market Share, by Total Equivalent Prescription Claims Managed, 2017**

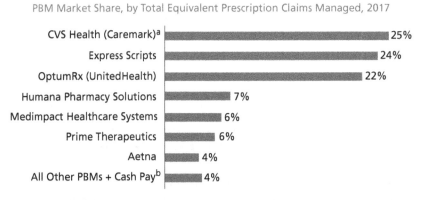

PBM Market Share, by Total Equivalent Prescription Claims Managed, 2017

CVS Health (Caremark)[a]	25%
Express Scripts	24%
OptumRx (UnitedHealth)	22%
Humana Pharmacy Solutions	7%
Medimpact Healthcare Systems	6%
Prime Therapeutics	6%
Aetna	4%
All Other PBMs + Cash Pay[b]	4%

[a] Excludes claims processed by Aetna. For 2017, CVS Health changed its publicly reported computation of equivalent prescription claims filled in network pharmacies.

[b] Figure excludes cash pay prescriptions that use a discount card processed by one of the 7 PBMs shown on the chart.

Note: Drug Channels Institute research and estimates. Total equivalent prescription claims includes claims at a PBM's network pharmacies plus prescriptions filled by a PBM's mail and specialty pharmacies. Includes discount card claimes. Note that figures may not be comparable with those of previous reports due to changes in publicly reported figures of equivalent prescription claims. Total may not sum due to rounding.

Source: Drug Channels Institute. (2018, February). *The 2018 Economic Report on U.S. Pharmacies and Pharmacy Benefit Managers*. Retrieved March 15, 2019 from http://drugch.nl/pharmacy

of cost/quality performance. Some managed care plans have diversified into businesses that provide these services to their members as well as to members of other plans. For example, UnitedHealth Group has a subsidiary called United Behavioral Health. The services that are most often carved out are chemical dependency/behavioral health and organ transplants.

Disease Management. Plans are increasingly also looking at carving out certain disease categories for special and often separate treatment. This process encompasses what has become known as disease management. (Please see Exhibit 6.71 for a definition by the trade group for these companies.) Such carve-outs often involve contracts for services with companies[242]

EXHIBIT 6.71. Definition of Disease Management

Disease management is a system of coordinated healthcare interventions and communications for populations with conditions in which patient self-care efforts are significant.

Disease management

- Supports the physician or practitioner/patient relationship and plan of care;
- Emphasizes prevention of exacerbations and complications utilizing evidence-based practice guidelines and patient empowerment strategies; and
- Evaluates clinical, humanistic, and economic outcomes on an ongoing basis with the goal of improving overall health.

Disease management components include[a]

- Population identification processes;
- Evidence-based practice guidelines;
- Collaborative practice models to include physician and support-service providers;
- Patient self-management education (may include primary prevention, behavior modification programs, and compliance/surveillance);
- Process and outcomes measurement, evaluation, and management;
- Routine reporting/feedback loop (may include communication with patient, physician, health plan and ancillary providers, and practice profiling).

[a] Full-service disease management programs must include all six components. Programs consisting of fewer components are disease management support services.

Source: Care Continuum Alliance (CCA). *Definition of Disease Management*. Retrieved June 28, 2018 from http://www.carecontinuum.org/dm_definition.asp

---

[242]For a list of accredited disease management organizations, please see NCQA. *Other healthcare organizations. Disease Management*. Retrieved June 28, 2018, from https://reportcards.ncqa.org/#/other-health-care-organizations/list?program=Disease%20Management

specializing in such conditions as congestive heart failure (CHF), chronic obstructive pulmonary disease (COPD), asthma, diabetes, and chemical dependency/behavioral health. In evaluating the success of these initiatives, one should ask what would happen to the overall coordination of care if many of the major diseases were handled on a subspecialty basis out of the purview of the patient's primary care physician.

Research shows that the effectiveness of these programs is extremely variable since they differ in their structures, scope, care models (such as who provides the care and how much they communicate with the patient's physician), and the disease entity being treated. For example, deBruin et al. reviewed 31 papers

> describing disease management programs for patients with diabetes (n = 14), depression (n = 4), heart failure (n = 8), and COPD (n = 5). Twenty-one studies reported incremental healthcare costs per patient per year, of which 13 showed cost-savings. Incremental costs ranged between −$16,996 and $3,305 per patient per year. Substantial variation was found between studies in terms of study design, number and combination of components of disease management programs, interventions within components, and characteristics of economic evaluations.[243]

Despite these cautions and, in numerous cases, lack of evidence, many companies still ask their insurance plans to provide disease management programs.

To summarize, HMOs offer the opportunity to coordinate care across a continuum of services and sites. Coordination is facilitated by aligning the financial incentives of the physicians with the best use of all services and products to achieve the most efficient and effective outcomes. This scheme provides a number of marketing opportunities, from enhancing physician efficiency to reducing hospital stays or admissions to developing more cost-effective pharmaceutical benefit plans. Knowledge of the incentives and reimbursement arrangements is the key to developing value-added products and services.

Preferred Provider Organizations. Preferred provider organizations (PPOs) emerged as an alternative to HMOs because they give patients more freedom of choice of providers. According to the original definition by the American Association of PPOs:[244] "PPOs, while difficult to define, have a number of common operational elements." These elements are:

- Insurer or third parties contract with a panel of providers. Often the provider network is larger than a comparable HMO network; however, in view of continuing cost escalations, many of these networks are becoming more select.

---

[243]de Bruin, S. R., Heijink, R., Lemmens, L. C., Struijs, J. N., & Baan, C. A. (2011). Impact of disease management programs on healthcare expenditures for patients with diabetes, depression, heart failure or chronic obstructive pulmonary disease: A systematic review of the literature. *Health Policy, 101*(2), 105–121.

[244]In 2012 the American Association of Preferred Provider Organizations (AAPPO) and the Third Party Administrators Association of America (TPAAA) merged to form The American Association of Payers, Administrators and Networks (AAPAN). Retrieved June 28, 2018, from http://aapan.org/Home.aspx

- They negotiate a fee schedule with these providers. Instead of capitation, these providers are paid on a discounted fee-for-service basis. The rates are usually based on a percentage (above or below) the local Medicare payment rates, usually ranging from 80% to 140% of RBRVS.
- The providers agree to abide by a utilization review process. Since the health plan is paying claims, the utilization review can be more administratively complex than in an HMO setting, where physicians are financially as well as clinically responsible for care and may tend more to self-monitoring.
- Patients are not locked in (i.e., if they obtain care outside the panel of contracted providers, they will retain some coverage, though not as comprehensive as if they had stayed within the network).

  In an HMO, except for emergencies, all care must be approved and referred by the patient's primary care physician. If a patient seeks such care without a referral, the patient will be fully responsible for the bill. In a PPO, if the patient sees a contracted doctor (with or without a referral), the plan pays that doctor according to the fee schedule, usually with some limited coinsurance. If the patient sees a noncontracted provider, the plan requires the patient to pay more of the bill, but still pays something.

Since these operational details can be quite different among plans, the validity of research about their operations is problematic.

While PPOs proliferated during the managed care backlash of the 1990s, rising health-care costs have forced these plans to increasingly behave more like HMOs: Provider networks are narrowing, fee schedules are more "aggressive," utilization review is stricter with more disease management, and financial penalties are increasing for going to noncontracted providers or using nonpreferred products. These changes, along with HMOs adopting several open features, have caused some convergence in the design of these two very different types of insurance.

An important caution is notable for providers and suppliers dealing with PPOs. Some of these companies contract with other plans that use their PPO rates and networks without the knowledge of the providers and suppliers; they are essentially selling their contractual relationships to a third party. These arrangements are called silent PPOs, because those delivering the services or providing products are unaware of these secondary contracts. When payments are due, it can be difficult to identify the responsible party. Contracts must, therefore, specify who is financially responsible or prohibit such behavior.

Point-of-Service Plans. Point-of-service (POS) plans are a hybrid between HMOs and PPOs and may incorporate any number of features of each. For example, some plans have HMO-like benefits if the patient stays with his or her assigned primary care physician but switch to PPO-like fees if the patient prefers to see another contracted physician. Other types of arrangements may include plan-set cost targets; if costs are less than a certain amount, the plan may share the difference with providers. Because of the extreme number of variations, no single definition or list of characteristics adequately defines this type of plan.

Stakeholder Requirements and Desires for Managed Care Success. In a managed care setting, relationships among the different stakeholders can create opportunities for conflict or productive relationships. The conditions for creating opportunities for mutual benefit are outlined below. (With regard to HMOs, the terms "primary care physicians" and "groups" refer to IPA and network models, respectively.) What hospitals and health plans require from each other for a workable business arrangement can be inferred from the explanations below. What patients desire from insurance was discussed earlier in this chapter.

Primary Care Physicians/Groups Want Health Plans to

- *Do benefit interpretations.* When an issue arises about benefits, plans often place the burden of explaining coverage on the physician; this circumstance often causes conflict between patient and physician. Although physicians must understand benefits, the plan should be the sole source of this information for the majority of patient inquiries.

- *Leave them alone to manage their business* (i.e., not micromanage). In PPOs, particularly, plans often require preauthorization that adds nothing to reducing unnecessary utilization or improving quality of care. For example, when asked to authorize a hospitalization for pneumonia, one plan's only question was which lung was affected.

- *Share profits as befits a partnership.* Physician incentives should be aligned with rewards for efficient and effective care across a continuum of services and be commensurate with the total workload. For example, PPOs require primary care physicians do much more nonclinical work compared to traditional fee-for-service or professional risk capitation plans; for example, they must obtain permission to refer for specialty care or medication treatments. The extra administrative burden is, most often, not compensated.

- *Give at-risk, capitated physicians enough patients to diffuse risk or develop creative payment schedules until those enrollment targets are met.* Recall that under these schemes, physicians become insurance companies and are subject to the conditions of insurance risk. One such condition is adequate numbers of enrollees to diffuse the risk. Physicians should have a panel of at least 350 non-Medicare members of average risk before starting to accept capitated risk arrangements.

- *Provide timely and accurate eligibility and payment data, preferably online.* This statement seems rather obvious in a world with rapid, electronic financial transactions; however, because much data still requires manual input, healthcare information systems frequently contain erroneous or untimely data. For example, HMO member eligibility lists often do not accurately correlate with the capitation the plans owe. Also, contracted provider lists are not always up-to-date, causing problems for both referring physicians and their patients.[245]

---

[245]This problem is so prevalent that laws have been passed addressing it. One of the first was in California, which requires weekly updating of provider lists. See Weintraub, D. (2015, October 15). New law will require state to keep provider directories updated. *California Health Report*. Retrieved June 30, 2018, from https://www.calhealthreport.org/2015/10/15/new-law-will-require-state-to-keep-provider-directories-updated/

- *Set capitation based on realistic risk, compensating for adverse selection.* Some physicians or groups, such as those at academic medical centers, attract sicker patients; capitation must account for this fact.

- *Provide appropriate stop-loss insurance for most conditions and first dollar reinsurance for high cost cases that primary care physicians cannot usually manage (e.g., transplantation).* As mentioned above, this provision protects physicians from unlimited downside financial risk.

- *Help physicians obtain favorable supplier contracts (in the case of HMO arrangements).* As previously explained, physicians in these arrangements are at financial risk for such services as specialty consultations and outpatient diagnostics such as laboratory and radiology services. Health plans have the contacts and market power to help these physicians negotiate and obtain better contracts than they could alone. Unfortunately, many plans do not help in this regard.

Primary Care Physicians/Groups Want Hospitals to

- *Be price competitive but also be able to profit on managed care contracts.* When fee-for-service was the prevalent mode of payment, hospitals negotiated managed care fees based on their marginal costs of filling a few more unused beds; now that managed care predominates, hospital revenue from these plans must also cover total costs.

- *Be competitive on quality and scope of services.* Physicians will not be able to attract sufficient numbers of patients unless the public perceives that the hospitals to which they admit are of high quality. Also, the range of quality services must be broad enough to allow physicians to coordinate as much as possible of their patients' care at or through these facilities.

- *Help negotiate reasonable fees for hospital-based physician services.* Again, recall that in capitated contracts, physicians are responsible for paying professional fees. Certain hospital-based physician specialists have a monopoly on providing services in that setting. These specialties include but are not limited to pathology, emergency medicine, anesthesia, radiology, and neonatology. Unless hospital administrators assist primary care physicians/groups with these negotiations, these capitated physicians may use a different hospital or be forced to refuse HMO contracts.

- *Offer packaged (bundled) services.* These packages involve combining services from a variety of functional areas to deliver a discrete episode of care for a fixed price. For example, consider the previously common thallium stress test (a nuclear medicine study to assess reduced blood flow in the heart causing chest pain or other related symptoms).[246] The patient exercises on a treadmill while the heartbeat is monitored for changes that would indicate abnormal stress. At peak exercise, thallium is injected,

---

[246]While this technology has been replaced by ultrasound imaging, it is used as more complex example to illustrate this issue.

and the patient's heart is scanned by a nuclear medicine camera. This scan is compared to one done later, after the patient has rested. The one piece of diagnostic information that this series of procedures yields is whether the patient is likely to have circulatory problems in the heart, requiring further diagnostic tests or interventions. Because of the different functional areas involved, at least four bills can be generated: the cardiologist who performs the stress test, the radiologist who reads the scans, and separate facility bills for both the stress test and radiology scans. Hospitals should understand that the managed care customers who pay for these services (health plans and physicians) want both predictability of cost and also ease of payment. By packaging this service into one bill and providing the referring physician with one report that contains all diagnostic information, the hospital can offer a value-added service to these customers. Other opportunities for packaging have included cardiac bypass surgery, cataract surgery, and prostate biopsies. In the latter two cases, specialist physicians have understood this packaging concept better than hospitals and have set up these services on their own in freestanding surgical centers.

Managed Care Plans Want Primary Care Physicians Who

- *Practice high-quality medicine.* Plans are subject to scrutiny from outside agencies and rely on physicians to provide a high level of care.

- *Practice efficiently.* PPOs, in particular, rely on physicians to use resources appropriately, since these plans are based on a discounted fee-for-service system. These resources should be used for medically necessary care and be provided in a timely fashion.

- *Provide care that is patient-friendly as well as easy to use and access.* One of the criteria employers use when selecting health plans is their ability to provide these features.

Hospitals Want Physicians Who

- *Practice medicine economically, by using services appropriately and delivering care efficiently.* As explained previously, hospital payments are usually fixed by day (per diem) or diagnosis (DRG). Physicians must, therefore, help hospitals live within these budgets. This feature is the way physicians can help hospitals profit from managed care contracts.

- *Deliver quality care.* This subject is related the physicians' desire for the hospital to provide a high level and scope of quality services.

- *Cooperate with them in contracting with other physicians and health plans as well as participate in packaging services.*

- *Are available to serve all segments of the hospital's patients.* Hospitals have missions to serve their communities; fulfillment of this mission requires participation of physicians on staff of these institutions.

Current Trends. Managed care is an evolving sector that has experienced significant changes over the past several decades. A few of these changes are highlighted below.

In the past, many states required health insurance plans to be nonprofit and to charge community-based rates. (Recall the origin of the Blue Cross plans.) When the laws changed and the Blue Cross/Blue Shield Association allowed member plans to be for-profit, many converted to this status. They then began to do more individual or company-specific underwriting. With this conversion also came consolidation of plans, mainly by acquisitions. The fastest period of consolidation was from 1994 to 2004, when the number of plans decreased from 556 to 465, while enrollment increased from about 55 to 79 million. Plans that started out as HMOs also learned that, in order to compete in the market, they needed to offer their customers more choice; as a result, the majority of HMO companies offer PPO and POS options. Many PPOs, however, chose not to enter the HMO sector.

With the emergence of different forms of managed care plans, local market conditions required flexibility in physician compensation. (Please see Exhibit 6.72 for examples of some of these payment methods.) In addition to using different payment methods to drive desired utilization patterns, plans also developed and began enforcing clinical practice standards. These standards decreased utilization in some instances (e.g., unnecessary day-before-surgery admissions) but also increased other services (e.g., preventive care such as immunizations). Also, as mentioned, over time, plans increased patient cost sharing to address consumer-induced demand. A result of these measures was that inpatient hospital utilization decreased.

As also mentioned, during the economic expansion of the mid- to late 1990s, health plans realized that customers were demanding more provider choice and expanded benefits. These customers, however, were also accustomed to the lower prices HMOs charged compared to other types of plans. Recalling the trade-off among premiums, out-of-pocket expenses, and freedom of choice of providers, the only way plans could deliver on all three of these dimensions *and* enhance benefits was to shift more financial risk to providers without paying them more. For example, the per diems or DRGs that they paid hospitals included ever more

EXHIBIT 6.72. Different Methods Managed Care Plans Use to Compensate Physicians

- Discount fee-for-service payments for all (mainly in PPOs)
- Full professional risk capitation for groups or primary care physicians
- Capitation for primary care physicians only for *their* services; specialists paid on a discount of fee for service
- Capitation for both primary care physicians and specialists
- Discount fee for service for primary care physicians and capitation for specialists (This method is rarely used but has been employed in areas with a primary care shortage and surplus of specialists.)
- Global payment to physicians as part of a defined service package (e.g., a global fee to a radiation oncologist for a course of radiation therapy as opposed to the usual per-visit fee)

sophisticated and costly technology; at the same time, the high-margin, less-ill patients who made up for lower-paying managed care contracts were not being admitted to the hospitals to the same extent as they were in the past. Also, hospitals found it difficult to demand higher rates because occupancies were lower and they needed to cover fixed costs. Fortunately, during better economic times, they could rely on investment returns to help cover their reduced operating margins.

As far as physicians and medical groups, many grew very dependent on managed care contracts for patient volume and could not afford to cancel them when they were asked to provide more services without commensurate compensation. Those who received capitation were particularly affected since they were also responsible for increased technological costs (diagnostics, immunizations, and treatments, such as chemotherapy). As mentioned previously, many groups that also assumed some financial risks for pharmacy benefits, particularly in California, went bankrupt. The legislative response in that state was prohibition against assumption of such contractual risk.

At the time of these changes, previously mentioned state mandates proliferated in response to voter demands to restrict managed care's cost controls. Among these mandates were requirements that plans remove restrictions on access to certain specialists by eliminating the requirement for primary care referrals (so-called open access provisions). A common example of the latter requirement is women's access to gynecologists. For instance, in Illinois, women are entitled to see an OB/GYN without referral from their internist or family physician; however, this legislation was not well thought out. After passage of the law, women started to see OB/GYNs not affiliated with their primary care physicians or groups. In many cases, when these women were hospitalized, it was at facilities where their primary care physicians were not on staff. The result was lack of coordination of care for the patients' other medical conditions. Further, the primary care physicians were expected to pay the bills for the services the OB/GYN ordered. Subsequently, the law was amended to allow the health plan to require women to see an OB/GYN affiliated with their primary care physician. The lesson here is that such provisions can destroy the advantages of coordinated care, with possible decrements in quality and increased costs.

Because the public believes that health plans achieve profitability by withholding care, legal actions of a variety of types have been instituted against these firms. One of the most famous was a 1993 award of $89 million against Health Net, a California HMO, which was found guilty of withholding payment for a bone marrow transplant for a woman who was diagnosed with metastatic breast cancer at age 38.[247] The irony is that the science did not subsequently support this intervention.[248]

The public's criticism of managed care (particularly HMOs) has been largely colored by the relative lack of freedom to choose providers. As a consequence of voter demand for freedom of choice of providers, some states passed laws often called "any willing provider provisions." Such laws require health plans to contract with any physician and/or pharmacy

---

[247]Eckholm, E. (1993, December 30). $89 million awarded family who sued H.M.O. *New York Times*.

[248]Welch, G. H., & Mogielnocki, J. (2002). Presumed benefit: Lessons from the American experience with marrow transplantation for breast cancer. *British Medical Journal, 324*, 1088–1092.

that meet their criteria and are willing to sign a standard agreement. Unfortunately, the legislators did not carefully consider the potential consequences of these regulations. The most obvious result is that having a greater number of providers increases administrative costs; these costs must, in turn, be passed along to the purchaser. Another consequence is that, while the providers are willing to meet the terms on signing the agreement, they may not be able to meet cost and quality performance targets in the short or long run. Subsequent contract cancellation is time consuming, potentially exposes the plan to litigation, and is disruptive to patients if they need to be transferred to other physicians. An additional important consideration is the change in market risk structure that these laws cause. Recall that in a capitated scheme, physicians are essentially small insurance companies and depend on sufficient numbers of people signed up with them. If these laws cause the capitated population to be spread among more physicians, any one of them will have fewer patients, thus increasing financial risk.

In addition to health plans shifting risk to providers, both the plans and employers have shifted more financial responsibility to patients. One method that was seriously considered before passage of the ACA was a *defined contribution* scheme: Employers set a fixed amount they were willing to contribute to purchase health insurance, leaving employees to shop for the plan that met their coverage needs at a price they wanted to spend (including such out-of-pocket payments as copayments, coinsurance, and deductibles). While few employers actually follow this strategy, health plans started to offer more flexibility to allow employees to design their own insurance coverage. However, with this flexibility came more responsibility for patients to pay out-of-pocket charges. This trend is demonstrated in Exhibit 6.73 with respect to deductibles. For employees who had a deductible, the amount also rose: from an average of $584 in 2006 to $1,505 in 2017. Other forms of out-of-pocket expenses have also risen for patients. (Please see Exhibit 6.74 for one example of copayment trends.)

EXHIBIT 6.73. **Percentage of Covered Workers in a Plan that Includes a General Annual Deductible for Single Coverage, by Plan Type, 2006–2017**

	2006	2007	2008	2009	2010	2011	2012	2013	2014	2015	2016	2017
HMO												
All Small Firms	17%	14%	25%	27%	34%	38%	33%	44%	59%	46%	44%	41%
All Large Firms	10%	20%[a]	18%	12%	25%[a]	27%	29%	40%	26%	40%	47%	37%
All Firms	12%	18%	20%	16%	28%	29%	30%	41%	37%	42%	46%	38%
PPO												
All Small Firms	69%	72%	73%	74%	80%	76%	76%	78%	83%	85%	85%	78%
All Large Firms	69%	71%	66%	74%	76%	83%	77%	82%	8S	84%	84%	86%
All Firms	69%	71%	68%	74%	77%	81%	77%	81%	85%	85%	84%	86%

					POS							
All Small Firms	35%	53%ª	59%	63%	64%	68%	58%	78%ª	69%	80%	81%	71%
All Large Firms	28%	41%	41%	58%	70%	71%	63%	49%	72%ª	61%	66%	58%
All Firms	32%	48%	50%	62%	66%	69%	60%	66%	70%	72%	76%	65%
					ALL PLANS							
All Small Firms	56%	60%	65%	67%	73%	75%	72%	77%	82%	82%	82%	77%
All Large Firms	54%	59%	56%	61%	68%ª	74%	73%	78%	80%	81%	83%	83%
ALL FIRMS	55%	59%ª	59%	63%	70%ª	74%	72%	78%ª	80%	81%	83%	81%

HDHP: High Deductible Health Plan; SOs: Savings Options
ª Estimate is statistically different from estimate for the previous year shown (*p* < .05).
Note: Small Firms have 3–199 workers; Large Firms have 200 or more workers. Average general annual health plan deductibles for PPOs, POS plans, and HDHP/SOs are for in-network services. By definition, all HDHP/SOs have a deductible.
Source: Kaiser Family Foundation (2007, September 19). *2017 employer health benefits survey section 7: Employee cost sharing.* Retrieved June 30, 2018, from https://www.kff.org/report-section/ehbs-2017-section-7-employee-cost-sharing/

EXHIBIT 6.74. **Among Covered Workers with a Copayment for a Primary Care Physician Office Visit, Distribution of Copayments, 2006–2018**

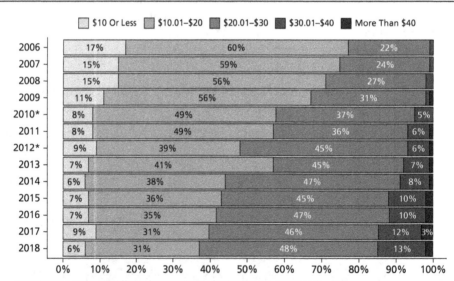

* Distribution is statistically different from distribution for the previous year shown (p < .05).

Source: Kaiser Family Foundation: 2018 Employer Health Benefits Survey. Section 7: Employee Cost Sharing. October 3, 2018. https://www.kff.org/report-section/2018-employer-health-benefits-survey-section-7-employee-cost-sharing/ Retrieved April 14, 2019.

SUMMARY

What are the next likely measures that will transform the health insurance market? Several factors will contribute to this answer. First, employers continue to be interested in expanding existing initiatives outside traditional insurance providers and narrowing the networks that are provided. (Please see Exhibit 6.75 for examples.)

Second, federal actions to undo the ACA will expand opportunities for purchasers of insurance. A prominent example is Association Health Plans (AHPs). On October 12, 2017, President Trump issued Executive Order 13813, "Promoting Healthcare Choice and Competition Across the United States," which stated: "It shall be the policy of the executive branch, to the extent consistent with law, to facilitate the purchase of insurance across State lines and the development and operation of a healthcare system that provides high-quality care at affordable prices for the American people."[249] As a result of that Executive Order, on June 21, 2018, the U.S. Department of Labor (DOL) published final regulations that expand the ERISA definition of who can form multi-employer health plans—another term for AHPs.

EXHIBIT 6.75. **Among Firms Offering Health Benefits, Percentage of Firms Whose Largest Plan Has Various Features, by Firm Size, 2017**

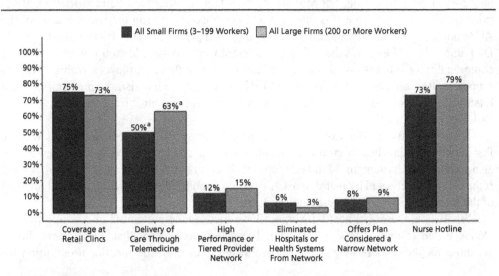

ª Estimate is statistically different from estimate for all other firms not in the indicated size category (p < .05)

Source: Kaiser Family Foundation (2017, September 19). *2017 employer health benefits survey, section 14: Employer practices and health plan networks.* Retrieved July 3, 2018, from https://www.kff.org/report-section/ehbs-2017-section-14-employer-practices-and-health-plan-networks/

---

[249]Executive Order 13813 of October 12, 2017: *Promoting healthcare choice and competition across the United States.* Retrieved July 3, 2018, from https://www.federalregister.gov/documents/2017/10/17/2017-22677/promoting-healthcare-choice-and-competition-across-the-united-states

The DOL stated that the purpose of this change is to allow "employees of small employers and working owners . . . to obtain coverage that is not subject to the regulatory complexity and burden that currently characterizes the market for individual and small group health coverage and, therefore, can enjoy flexibility with respect to benefit package design comparable to that enjoyed by large employers."[250] As Keith noted, the advantage of this change is that "[a]s a single multi-employer plan under ERISA, AHPs do not have to comply with many of the Affordable Care Act's . . . most significant consumer protections, such as the law's rating rules and the essential health benefits."[251] AHPs will still need to accept enrollees without regard to health status but can adjust premiums based on gender, age, geography, and industry. Implementation of some terms of this rule started August 20, 2018; others became effective after April 1, 2019. However, in April, 2019 court decisions held that AHPs were not valid because, among other issues, they did not meet ERISA definitions for an employer. Appeals are expected. The impact on insurance exchange plans is not yet known, but the fear is that healthier people will opt for the AHPs, leaving the exchange membership comparatively sicker. The result will be even higher exchange premiums, leading to the need for more federal subsidies. Higher exchange premiums will also cause even more nonsubsidized people to drop their coverage. Facing these potential problems, the State of NY, along with 10 other states and the District of Columbia, sued the Department of Labor (DoL) over the above-mentioned final rule. On March 28, 2019 U.S. District Court Judge John D. Bates ruled that: "The Final Rule was intended and designed to end run the requirements of the ACA, but it does so only by ignoring the language and purpose of both ERISA and the ACA. DOL unreasonably expands the definition of "employers" to include groups without any real commonality of interest and to bring working owners without employees within ERISA's scope despite Congress's clear intent that ERISA cover benefits arising out of employment relationships. Accordingly, these provisions are unlawful and must be set aside . . ."[252] The DoL has yet to appeal.

An additional consideration may come from the states. In 2006, Massachusetts was the first state to mandate health insurance enrollment for its residents. In May 2018, New Jersey also added that requirement. Mandate proposals in other states are being considered as well. If these laws are enacted by many states, they could counter the effects of the federal removal of the mandate that was effective January 1, 2019.

Finally, purchasers of health insurance have focused their attention on a concept called "Value-Based Insurance Design" (VBID). The general concept is that stakeholders should get more for the amount they spend on healthcare. However, the functional definition for

---

[250]Definition of "Employer" under Section 3(5) of ERISA-Association Health Plans A Rule by the Employee Benefits Security Administration on 06/21/2018. Retrieved July 3, 2018, from https://www.federalregister.gov/documents/2018/06/21/2018-12992/definition-of-employer-under-section-35-of-erisa-association-health-plans#footnote-1-p28912

[251]Keith, K. (2018, June 21). Final rule rapidly eases restrictions on non-ACA-compliant association health plans. *Health Affairs Blog*. Retrieved July 3, 2018, from https://www.healthaffairs.org/do/10.1377/hblog20180621.671483/full/

[252]State of New York, et al. Plaintiffs v. United States Department of Labor, et al. Defendants: Civil Action No. 18-1747 (JDB). United States District Court for the District of Columbia Filed 03/28/19 Retrieved May 23, 2019, from https://affordablecareactlitigation.files.wordpress.com/2019/03/5940153-0-12659.pdf

VBID varies widely. For example, in June 2018, the House Committee on Ways and Means and the Joint Economic Committee held meetings on VBID that focused on expanding allowable benefits to be paid from HSAs.[253] CMS has focused its VBID activities on Medicare Advantage plans:

> The Medicare Advantage Value-Based Insurance Design (VBID) Model is an opportunity for Medicare Advantage plans to offer supplemental benefits or reduced cost sharing to enrollees with Centers for Medicare & Medicaid Services (CMS)-specified chronic conditions, focused on the services that are of highest clinical value to them. The model tests whether this can improve health outcomes and lower expenditures for Medicare Advantage enrollees.[254]

The private sector has used VBID to mean both use of evidence-based medical practice and guarantees by providers and suppliers of results. For example, if a drug does not work as intended, the payer will not have to reimburse the supplier. More will be discussed about the concept of value at the end of Chapter 9.

In conclusion, this chapter first presented the basic principles of health insurance and what makes a condition insurable. It then discussed the evolution of the health insurance industry in the United States, with explanations of the current status of employer-sponsored plans. Next, it considered government-sponsored programs, particularly their source and use of funds, as well as their suitability for single national models. The managed care presentation that followed showed how customers and business partners must understand each other's needs for the system to work effectively. Finally, some insights were presented for recent and future trends for this sector. While this chapter should bring you up to date on all these topics, you should be aware that this sector is rapidly changing; constant environmental assessment is therefore essential.

---

[253] University of Michigan Center for Value-Based Insurance Design: Press Release: V-BID Highlighted at Two Congressional Hearings June 6, 2018. Retrieved July 3, 2018 from http://vbidcenter.org/press-release-v-bid-highlighted-at-two-congressional-hearings-last-week/

[254] CMS.gov. *Medicare Advantage value-based insurance design model*. Retrieved July 3, 2018, from https://innovation.cms.gov/initiatives/vbid/

CHAPTER

7

HEALTHCARE TECHNOLOGY

SECOND WITCH.

> Fillet of a fenny snake,
> In the cauldron boil and bake;
> Eye of newt and toe of frog,
> Wool of bat and tongue of dog,
> Adder's fork and blind-worm's sting,
> Lizard's leg and owlet's wing,
> For a charm of powerful trouble,
> Like a hell-broth boil and bubble.

ALL.

> Double, double toil and trouble;
> Fire burn and cauldron bubble.

—William Shakespeare, *Macbeth*, Act 4, Scene 1

Any sufficiently advanced technology is indistinguishable from magic.

—Arthur C. Clarke, *Profiles of the Future: An Inquiry Into the Limits of the Possible*

DEFINITION AND FRAMEWORKS FOR STUDY

Medical technology is defined as "[t]he drugs, devices, and medical and surgical procedures used in medical care, and the organizational and supportive systems within which such care is provided."[1] Since this definition is quite broad, one must look for a meaningful framework to approach this topic. The U.S. National Library of Medicine proposes two methods: analysis based on the *physical nature* of the technology (e.g., drugs, therapeutic devices, and diagnostics) and consideration based on *how the technology is used* (e.g., screening, diagnosis, and treatment). These methods are outlined in Exhibit 7.1. This chapter will combine elements of both frameworks. The first part of this chapter will discuss some major trends and key issues in healthcare technology. The second part will consider issues concerning healthcare technology's contribution to cost (raising and lowering) as these costs relate to prevention, screening, diagnosis, and treatment. The goal of this chapter is to raise questions

---

[1] Office of Technology Assessment (1978). *Assessing the efficacy and safety of medical technologies* (p. xii). Retrieved July 3, 2018, from http://ota.fas.org/reports/7805.pdf The Office of Technology Assessment (OTA) was created when Congress passed Public Law 92-484 in 1972. Its task was to furnish Congress (and the American people) with unbiased evaluations of technology, including those applied to healthcare. While the law that created the OTA was not repealed, it closed on September 29, 1995 because the Republican Congress withheld its funding.

that should be constantly asked as we evaluate new technology and reevaluate existing technology. The significant issues discussed below are not in order of importance but follow a logical flow of topics that relate to one another. While illustrative examples in each section come from selected types of technology, the reader should infer that principles apply to the entire spectrum of the definition.

EXHIBIT 7.1. Frameworks for Studying Healthcare Technology

1. Physical Nature

   For many people, the term "technology" connotes mechanical devices or instrumentation; to others, it is a short form of "information technology," such as computers, networking, software, and other equipment and processes to manage information. However, the practical application of knowledge in healthcare is quite broad. Main categories of health technology include the following.

   - *Drugs*: e.g., aspirin, beta-blockers, antibiotics, cancer chemotherapy

   - *Biologics*: e.g., vaccines, blood products, cellular and gene therapies

   - *Devices, equipment and supplies*: e.g., cardiac pacemaker, magnetic resonance imaging (MRI) scanner, surgical gloves, diagnostic test kits, mosquito netting

   - *Medical and surgical procedures*: e.g., acupuncture, nutrition counseling, psychotherapy, coronary angiography, gall bladder removal, bariatric surgery, cesarean section

   - *Public health programs*: e.g., water purification system, immunization program, smoking prevention program

   - *Support systems*: e.g., clinical laboratory, blood bank, electronic health record system, telemedicine systems, drug formulary

   - *Organizational and managerial systems*: e.g., medication adherence program, prospective payment using diagnosis-related groups, alternative healthcare delivery configurations

   Certainly, these categories are interdependent; for example, vaccines are biologics that are used in immunization programs, and screening tests for pathogens in donated blood are used by blood banks.

2. Purpose or Application

   Technologies can also be grouped according to their healthcare purpose, i.e.:

   - *Prevention*: protect against disease by preventing it from occurring, reducing the risk of its occurrence, or limiting its extent or sequelae (e.g., immunization, hospital infection control program, fluoridated water supply)

   - *Screening*: detect a disease, abnormality, or associated risk factors in asymptomatic people (e.g., Pap smear, tuberculin test, screening mammography, serum cholesterol testing)

   - *Diagnosis*: identify the cause and nature or extent of disease in a person with clinical signs or symptoms (e.g., electrocardiogram, serological test for typhoid, x-ray for possible broken bone)

   - *Treatment*: intended to improve or maintain health status or avoid further deterioration (e.g., antiviral therapy, coronary artery bypass graft surgery, psychotherapy)

   - *Rehabilitation*: restore, maintain or improve a physically or mentally disabled person's function and well-being (e.g., exercise program for post-stroke patients, assistive device for severe speech impairment, incontinence aid)

■   *Palliation*: improve the quality of life of patients, particularly for relief of pain, symptoms, discomfort, and stress of serious illness, as well as psychological, social, and spiritual problems. (Although often provided for progressive, incurable disease, palliation can be provided at any point in illness and with treatment, e.g., patient-controlled analgesia, medication for depression or insomnia, caregiver support.)

Source: U.S National Library of Medicine, National Information Center on Health Services Research and Health Care Technology (NICHSR). *HTA [health technology assessment] 101: II. Fundamental concepts.* Retrieved July 3, 2018, from https://www.nlm.nih .gov/nichsr/hta101/ta10104.html#Heading7

Of further note is that not all technologies fall neatly into single categories: Many tests and other technologies used for diagnosis also are used for screening. Some technologies are used for diagnosis as well as treatment (e.g., coronary angiography to diagnose heart disease and to guide percutaneous coronary interventions). Implantable cardioverter defibrillators detect potentially life-threatening heart arrhythmias and deliver electrical pulses to restore normal heart rhythm. Electronic health record systems can support all these technological purposes or applications. Information technology (IT) will be discussed in detail in Chapter 8, "Information Technology."

MAJOR TRENDS IN HEALTHCARE TECHNOLOGY

Safety

The first important issue in healthcare technology is safety. According to the World Health Organization (WHO): "Patient safety is the absence of preventable harm to a patient during the process of health care. The discipline of patient safety is the coordinated efforts to prevent harm, caused by the process of health care itself, from occurring to patients."[2]

A conceptual framework for studying this subject is outlined in Exhibits 7.2 and 7.3.

EXHIBIT 7.2.   **10 High-Level Classes for Studying Patient Safety**

1.   Incident type

2.   Patient outcomes

3.   Patient characteristics

4.   Incident characteristics

5.   Contributing factors/hazards

6.   Organizational outcomes

7.   Detection

8.   Mitigating factors

9.   Ameliorating actions

10.   Actions taken to reduce risk

---

[2]Retrieved July 6, 2016, from http://www.who.int/patientsafety/about/en

EXHIBIT 7.3. **Conceptual Framework for the International Classification for Patient Safety**

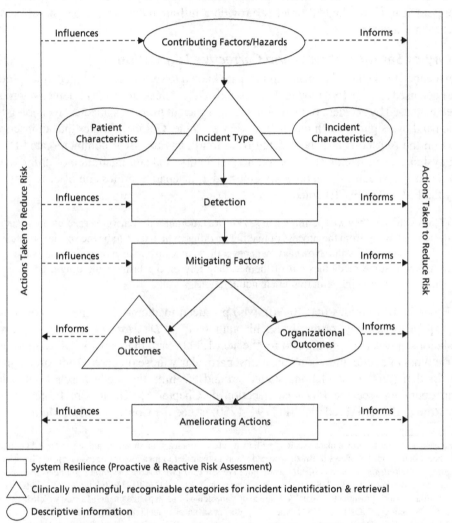

System Resilience (Proactive & Reactive Risk Assessment)

Clinically meaningful, recognizable categories for incident identification & retrieval

Descriptive information

The solid lines represent the semantic relationships between the classes. The dotted lines represent the flow of information.

Source: WHO. (2009, January). *Conceptual framework for the international classification for patient safety, version 1.1. Final technical report.* Retrieved July 3, 2018, from http://www.who.int/patientsafety/taxonomy/icps_full_report.pdf

Exploring the special issues of safety is best accomplished by first reviewing the background of its relevant history. The focus here will be on the regulations that govern U.S. healthcare technology and how they evolved to address problems this technology created. While not all these laws are, strictly speaking, related to safety issues, major legislation will be presented in chronological order to provide a full appreciation of how these measures relate to one another.

History of Safety Problems and Corrective Legislation

As evidenced by the fact that many animals are known to self-medicate,[3] medicinal products have been used since before modern humans existed. While adulterated or defective products (whether caused by accident or intention) are also ancient problems, medical technology regulation and oversight is much more recent. For example, Goldberg[4] notes that an inscription found on the Acropolis at Athens dated from fourth century BCE commemorated Evanor, the Physician, as inspector of drugs. While preparation and administration of drugs was the province of physicians, the apothecary emerged as a separate profession of drug preparers. Pliny the Elder (23–79 CE) noted:

> [T]he doctors, if they will permit me to say so, are ignorant—they are governed by names: so detached they are from the process of making up drugs, which used to be the special business of the medical profession. Nowadays whenever they come on books of prescriptions, wanting to make up some medicines out of them ... they rely on the fashionable druggists' shops which spoil everything with fraudulent adulterations.[5]

Pedanius Dioscorides (ca. 40–90), who practiced medicine in Rome, is known as the father of pharmacology, primarily for his authorship of *De Materia Medica*; in its many translations, it was the standard text for the next 1,500 years. In this work, Dioscorides notes diverse types of adulteration of medications, particularly those prepared from foreign plants. The "modern" era of regulations started around the time the medical school at Salerno began operating (see the Physicians section of Chapter 5, "Healthcare Professionals"). Holy Roman Emperor Frederick II (1194–1250) issued the Constitutions of Melfi in 1231,[6]

---

[3]Examples include red and green macaws, along with many other animals, who eat clay to aid digestion and kill bacteria, and female woolly spider monkeys in Brazil who add plants to their diet to increase or decrease their fertility. (Shurkin, J. *Animals that self-medicate: Many animal species have created their own pharmacies from ingredients that commonly occur in nature.* Retrieved July 3, 2018, from http://www.pnas.org/content/111/49/17339.full.pdf). These findings contradict Sir William Osler's proclamation that: "A desire to take medicine is, perhaps, the greatest feature which distinguishes man from other animals." (Osler, W. [1891, March 27]. Recent advances in medicine. *Science*, 170–171.)

[4]Goldberg, A. (1986). Development of drug regulating authorities. *British Journal of Clinical Pharmacology, 22,* 67S–70S.

[5]*Pliny's Natural History*, Book XXV (1949–54). From the 10-volume edition. Trans. H. Rackham (vols. 1–5, 9) W.H.S. Jones (vols. 6–8), and D. E. Eichholz (vol. 10). Cambridge, MA: Harvard University Press.

[6]For a full English translation, see Powell, J. M. (trans.). (1971). *The Liber Augustalis or Constitutions of Melfi promulgated by the Emperor Frederick II for the Kingdom of Sicily in 1231.* Syracuse, NY: Syracuse University Press.

in which, among other provisions, he addressed the handling of medications. The laws in this document (as well as additional ones in the *Novae Constitutiones Regni* Siciliae of 1241) stipulated that: medicine and pharmacy be separate professions (especially, physicians could not make drugs); apothecaries[7] were to make drugs "under control" of physicians; physicians and apothecaries were prohibited from collusion; the drug-making process was to be conducted "faithfully according to the arts and the conditions of men in the presence of sworn witnesses"; certain medications could not be sold after 1 year; and a fee schedule for medications was set. Those who violated the statutes were dealt with thusly: "[I]f those appointed ... are proved to have committed frauds in the office granted to them, we order that they should be put to death."

From Salerno, these regulatory practices spread rapidly to other countries on the continent and then to England. "The earliest code of quality control in Britain appears to be that of the Ordinances of the Guild of Pepperers in Soper Lane in 1316. In the 12th century the pepperers were responsible for the distribution of imported drugs and spicery (which included spices, sugar, confectionary and fruit)."[8]

The combination of trade in spices and drugs was not unusual, since many spices were used in medicinal preparations.[9] Although the Pepperers were supposed to monitor guild members for product adulteration, by 1423, the city authorities of London (through the Commonalty of Physicians and Surgeons) appointed two independent drug inspectors who had the power to bring offenders before the mayor and alderman of the city. In 1428, the Pepperers were incorporated as the Worshipful Company of Grocers, to which apothecaries belonged.[10] In 1540, Henry VIII empowered the Royal College of Physicians of London (which he chartered in 1518) to appoint four of its fellows as inspectors of the London apothecaries: "[T]he representatives of the Faculty were empowered to examine apothecaries' wares for defective, corrupt, etc., wares, drugs and stuff. Here we have the prototype of the pure food and drug acts of the present day, save that it was the Faculty of Physic, and not the town prosecutor, who acted as inspector."[11]

---

[7]The term used in the Latin was actually *Confectionarii* (confectioners).

[8]Griffen, J. P. (2013). A history of drug regulation in the UK. In J. P. Griffin, J. Posner, & G. R. Barker (Eds.), *The textbook of pharmaceutical medicine* (7th ed.) (pp. 319–346). Belfast: Blackwell.

[9]"It was not just life-threatening illnesses that nutmeg was said to cure. A growing interest in the medicinal value of plants had led to an explosion in the number of dietary books and herbals, all of which claimed that nutmeg and other spices for beneficial in combating a host of minor ailments. For chesty coughs, Doctors recommended mulled wine suffused with nutmeg. Cloves were said to cure earache, peppers stifled colds, while those embarrassed with trapped wind were recommended to take an extraordinary pot-pourri of 15 spices including cardamom, cinnamon and nutmeg ..." From: Milton, G. (1999). *Nathaniel's nutmeg or, the true and incredible adventures of the spice trader who changed the course of history* (p. 18). New York: Penguin Books.

[10]According to the Oxford English Dictionary (OED), the name "grocer" refers to "One who buys and sells in the gross, i.e. in large quantities."

[11]Boston, C. A. (1916, April). Medical legislation in the United States 1. *Medical Times*, 113–116.

By the mid-16th century, apothecaries had become what we would today call community pharmacists. Given their independent practice, for many years they petitioned to separate from the grocers. Finally, on December 6, 1617, King James I granted a royal charter for incorporation of the Worshipful Society of Apothecaries[12] of London.

> In 1704 the Society won a key legal suit (known as the Rose Case) against the Royal College of Physicians in the House of Lords, which ruled that apothecaries could both prescribe and dispense medicines. This case led directly to the evolution of the apothecary into today's general practitioner of medicine. Just over a century later, because of the Apothecaries' Act of 1815, the Society was given the statutory right to conduct examinations and to grant licences to practise Medicine throughout England and Wales, as well as the duty of regulating such practice.[13]

It was only with passage of the English Food and Drugs Act of 1875 that the right of physicians to inspect pharmacies was withdrawn.

American medical product regulation[14] is even more recent and is characterized by legislation that largely *reacted* to problems; rarely, if ever was it proactive. In 1800, following Dr. Benjamin Waterhouse's demonstration in this country that smallpox vaccine was effective,[15] fake versions were widely marketed. To ensure a pure, effective source for this vaccine, Congress passed the Vaccine Act of 1813, authorizing Baltimore physician John Smith to be the sole agent to "preserve the genuine vaccine matter and to furnish the same to any citizen." Following an outbreak of smallpox in North Carolina in 1821, thought to be caused by a contaminated lot of vaccine, a U.S. House of Representatives committee recommended that responsibility for vaccine regulation should go back to state and local governments; the Vaccine Act was repealed in 1822.

With respect to medication regulation, in 1820, representatives from all 22 state medical societies were invited to Washington, DC, to establish the U.S. Pharmacopeia, the first compendium of standard drugs for the United States. The 11 representatives who attended created a list containing 217 drugs, which was to be used to identify medications as well as

---

[12]The word "apothecary" came into use in Britain in the 13th century. According to the OED it came from the late Latin *apothēcārius*, meaning storekeeper. Thus, the term originally referred to: "One who kept a store or shop of nonperishable commodities, spices, drugs, comfits, preserves, etc."

[13]*History of the worshipful society of apothecaries of London*. Retrieved July 3, 2018, from http://www.apothecaries.org/history

[14]This section will focus laws concerning medical products used within the United States, that is, manufactured in or imported into this country, but not exported abroad.

[15]Smallpox inoculation (what we now generically call vaccination) was practiced sporadically in the United States in the late 17th century. Of particular note was George Washington's letter to Dr. William Shippen Jr. of February 6th 1777: "Finding the Small pox to be spreading much and fearing that no precaution can prevent it from running through the whole of our Army, I have determined that the troops shall be inoculated. This Expedient may be attended with some inconveniences and some disadvantages, but yet I trust in its consequences will have the most happy effects. Necessity not only authorizes but seems to require the measure, for should the disorder infect the Army in the natural way and rage with its usual virulence we should have more to dread from it than from the Sword of the Enemy." The full letter is available at https://founders.archives.gov/documents/Washington/03-08-02-0281 Retrieved July 3, 2018.

ensure they met strength, quality, purity, and consistency standards.[16] It is important to note that prior to this time, quality had to be observed as the drugs were compounded; advances in chemistry in the late 18th and early 19th centuries allowed testing of medications *after* their manufacture.[17]

The chemical testing methods and new pharmacopeia were put to good use when problems arose regarding adulterated medication administered to soldiers during the Mexican-American War (1846–1848). Federal investigators found that most of this medication was imported from Europe. In response, Congress passed the Drug Importation Act of 1848, which required appointment of special customs inspectors at six major ports of entry[18]—New York, Boston, Philadelphia, Baltimore, Charleston, and New Orleans—who were tasked with checking the "quality, purity, and fitness for medical purposes" of imported drugs. Further, the Act required that all imported drugs be labeled with the name of the manufacturer and the place of preparation. As a standard for inspection for each drug, the special agents were to employ not just the U.S. Pharmacopeia, but those of Edinburgh, London, France, and Germany. According to a history of the U.S. Customs and Border Patrol: "The law was initially successful, but after 2 years its effectiveness was soon undercut by political cronyism[19] that filled the special examiner posts with unqualified personnel. A lack of proper enforcement at some ports also arose from ineffective standards and methods of analysis."[20]

The law remained until its repeal in 1922.

The next major crisis occurred in late 1901. In this pre-antibiotic era, treatment of some conditions was accomplished with antiserums (i.e., antibodies derived from animal blood

---

[16] Subsequently, the decision makers included representatives from the pharmacy community. Currently, governance is conducted by a Board comprising officers and trustees representing: the medical sciences (2); the pharmaceutical sciences (2); an at-large capacity (3); and the public interest (1). Today, the " ... U.S. Pharmacopeial Convention (USP) is a scientific nonprofit organization that sets standards for the identity, strength, quality, and purity of medicines, food ingredients, and dietary supplements manufactured, distributed and consumed worldwide. USP's drug standards are enforceable in the United States by the Food and Drug Administration, and these standards are used in more than 140 countries." Retrieved July 3, 2018, from http://www.usp.org/about-usp

[17] A prominent reference used in this process was: Beck, L. C. (1846). *Adulterations of various substances used in medicine and the arts, with the means of detecting them: Intended as a manual for the physician, the Apothecary and the artisan.* New York: Samuel S. and William Wood.

[18] Collectors at other ports were authorized to secure the services of "some reasonable person" to test the purity of drugs. It was not until 1856 that Congress authorized the first special examiner on the West Coast at the port of San Francisco.

[19] The best contemporaneous description of the political nature of these appointments is by Nathaniel Hawthorne, who was appointed Surveyor for the District of Salem and Beverly and Inspector of the Revenue for the Port of Salem in April 1846. In the opening section of *The Scarlett Letter* (The Custom-House), he starts his description of the appointees thusly: " ... I found few but aged men. They were ancient sea-captains, for the most part, who, after being tossed on every sea, and standing up sturdily against life's tempestuous blast, had finally drifted into this quiet nook, where, with little to disturb them, except the periodical terrors of a Presidential election, they one and all acquired a new lease of existence ... " [Hawthorne, N. (1850). *The scarlett letter*. Boston: Ticknor and Fields]. Hawthorne, a Democrat, lost his job in 1848 after Whig candidate Zachary Taylor won the presidency.

[20] The U.S. Customs Department was originally part of the Treasury Department, since its main task was to collect import taxes (customs). Today it is part of the Department of Homeland Security. See https://www.cbp.gov/sites/default/files/documents/mexicanamericanwar.pdf (accessed July 3, 2018).

[often horses]), which were injected into the sick patients. One of these treatments was horse serum for diphtheria, a particularly lethal disease in children. Since there were no federal laws to control biologics, each state was responsible for its own quality control. In 1901, 13 children in St. Louis died from tetanus that was caused by anti-diphtheria serum contaminated with bacterial spores. In response to this tragedy, Congress passed the Biological Products Act of 1902, often referred to as the Biologics Act. This law, which became effective August 21, 1903, pioneered the premarket approval (PMA) of pharmaceuticals by mandating that both producer and facility obtain licenses. Further, all products were required to have a label with the product name, expiration date, and address and license number of the manufacturer.

Implementation of this law was also responsible for the emergence of two important U.S. agencies. The Marine Hospital Service (MHS) was started in 1798 to provide medical care to merchant seamen. "In the 1880s, the MHS had been charged by Congress with examining passengers on arriving ships for clinical signs of infectious diseases, especially for the dreaded diseases cholera and yellow fever, in order to prevent epidemics."[21] In 1887, the MHS set up a facility on Staten Island that came to be called the Hygienic Laboratory; it moved to Washington, DC, 4 years later. In addition to testing the purity of air and water, the lab was to investigate "infectious and contagious diseases and matters pertaining to the public health." In 1889, Congress established the U.S. Public Health Service (USPHS), Commissioned Corp as the uniformed body of the MHS. In 1902, the MHS was renamed the Public Health and Marine Hospital Service. (In 1912, the name was shortened to the Public Health Service.)[22] When the Biologics Act of 1902 became operational, the USPHS was given responsibility for its enforcement, and the Hygienic Lab was tasked with evaluation of specimens. These actions gave birth to the modern Public Health Service (PHS), and the Hygienic Lab evolved into the National Institutes of Health (NIH). Today, the NIH is comprised of 27 different institutes and centers.[23] Each has its own research agenda, which can focus on, for example, a particular part of the body (National Eye Institute), a disease category (National Cancer Institute), an organ system (National Heart, Lung and Blood Institute), a disease process (National Institute of Allergy and Infectious Diseases), or a general area of support (National Library of Medicine and the Centers). The institutes and centers administer their own budgets, and all but three receive their funding directly from Congress. Although the Food and Drug Administration (FDA) became responsible for regulating biologics in 1972, laws affecting biologics (such as biogenerics; see below) are still regulated by amendments to the Public Health Service Act.

---

[21] *A Short History of the National Institutes of Health*. Retrieved July 3, 2018, from https://history.nih.gov/exhibits/history/index.html

[22] The USPHS became part of the Department of Health, Education and Welfare (DHEW) when the latter was established in 1953. After the independent Department of Education was founded in 1980, DHEW became known as the Department of Health and Human Services. See the chapter on Medicare for the HHS organization chart.

[23] For a complete list and descriptions, see *List of NIH Institutes, Centers, and Offices*. Retrieved July 3, 2018, from https://www.nih.gov/institutes-nih/list-nih-institutes-centers-offices

Not long after the Biologics Act was passed, American journalists[24] began to uncover a host of social ills that prompted federal legislative action. On June 30, 1906, President Theodore Roosevelt signed the Federal Food and Drugs Act of 1906 (called the Pure Food and Drug Act) "[f]or preventing the manufacture, sale, or transportation [through interstate commerce] of adulterated or misbranded or poisonous or deleterious foods, drugs, medicines, and liquors, and for regulating traffic therein, and for other purposes." This legislation, more than any previous law, significantly changed how pharmaceuticals are regulated in the United States. The major drug provisions of the Act are outlined below:

1. The Secretaries of the Treasury, Agriculture, and Commerce and Labor were to set uniform rules and regulations for "carrying out the provisions of this Act, including the collection and examination of specimens of foods and drugs manufactured or offered for sale." The actual examinations of specimens of foods and drugs (including those that were imported) were tasked to the Bureau of Chemistry in the Department of Agriculture (the forerunner of the FDA).[25]

2. The term "drug," was defined as "all medicines and preparations recognized in the United States Pharmacopeia or National Formulary for internal or external use, and any substance or mixture of substances intended to be used for the cure, mitigation, or prevention of disease of either man or other animals."

3. A drug was considered "adulterated" if it "differed from the standard of strength, quality, or purity, as determined by the test laid down in the United States Pharmacopeia or National Formulary official at the time of investigation." If the drug varied from those standards, it could still be legally sold if its label clearly stated its actual strength, quality, and purity. In either case, a drug is considered adulterated if "its strength or purity fall below the professed standard or quality under which it is sold."

4. A drug was considered "misbranded" if its package or label contained "any statement, design, or device regarding such article, or the ingredients or substances contained

---

[24]Upton Sinclair's *The Jungle* is the most famous of these exposés and was responsible for food purity laws. Samuel Hopkins Adams was the reporter credited with exposing the "patent medicine" industry in his series of articles in *Collier's Magazine* starting on October 7, 1905. He started the series, collectively called "The Great American Fraud," by stating: "This is the introductory article to a series which will contain a full explanation and exposure of patent-medicine methods, and the harm done to the public by this industry, founded mainly on fraud and poison." The term "patent medicine" usually meant over-the-counter medication that was trademarked ("branded") but not necessarily patented.

[25]Starting in 1867, the Division of Chemistry of the Department of Agriculture began investigating the contamination of agricultural produce and subsequently reviewed misbranding and use of dangerous chemical preservatives. In 1901 its name was changed to the Bureau of Chemistry and then, in 1927, to the Food, Drug, and Insecticide Administration. In 1930 the name was shortened to the Food and Drug Administration (FDA). In 1940, the FDA was transferred (along with the Public Health Service) to the Federal Security Agency (started in 1939). President Eisenhower's "Reorganization Plan No. 1 of 1953," abolished the Federal Security Agency and created the Department of Health, Education, and Welfare (HEW), to which the FDA was transferred. In 1969, the FDA became part of the Public Health Service within HEW, along with such other organizations such as the NIH and Centers for Disease Control (CDC—now called the Centers for Disease Control and Prevention). With the creation of an independent Department of Education in 1980, HEW became the Department of Health and Human Services (HHS), where the FDA is still organizationally located.

therein which shall be false or misleading in any particular." Drugs were also considered misbranded if their origin was mislabeled, if they were an "imitation of or offered for sale under the name of another article," or if the contents of the package were removed and replaced in whole or in part with other contents. In order to specifically address a widespread problem with medicines that surreptitiously contained narcotics and other substances, a drug was considered to be misbranded if its package failed to have a statement on the label regarding "the quantity or proportion of any alcohol, morphine, opium, cocaine, heroin, alpha or beta eucaine, chloroform, *cannabis indica*, chloral hydrate, or acetanilide, or any derivative or preparation of any such substances contained therein."

Unlike the Biological Products Act of 1902, however, the Pure Food and Drugs Act of 1906 did not include provisions for premarket testing or approval. A further serious gap in this legislation became apparent several years later. In 1911, the Supreme Court ruled that the 1906 law applied only to false labeling, not to false claims about the drug's performance.[26] To fix the problem, in 1912, Congress passed the Sherley Amendment (named after Congressman Joseph Swagar Sherley, D-KY) which added to the definition of mislabeling: "If its package or label shall bear or contain any statement, design, or device regarding the curative or therapeutic effect of such article or any of the ingredients or substances contained therein, which is false and fraudulent." The Supreme Court upheld this provision on subsequent challenge.[27]

Despite this fix, three additional problems remained. First, the 1906 law with its 1912 amendment prohibited false labeling but not false advertising. Second, before a case could be successfully prosecuted, the burden of proof was *on the government* to show that the claims were false and fraudulent.

Third, while the contents of the drug needed to be labeled correctly, individuals could still use them indiscriminately and physicians could recommend or dispense them at will—sometimes to great profit. This abuse particularly applied to narcotics (a forerunner by a century of the current opioid abuse problem). Because of the perceived high and growing rates of addiction, some states passed laws limiting importation and use of narcotics. However, it was easy to circumvent these laws by obtaining the drugs from states with fewer restrictions. Further, states resisted federal government intervention in what they considered an internal regulatory prerogative. In order to address this problem at the national level, Congress enacted the Harrison Narcotics Act of 1914 (named after Congressman Francis Burton Harrison, D-NY). The law was passed as a revenue measure, and its enforcement thus fell under the Division of Internal Revenue of the Treasury Department. Physicians

---

[26] See U.S. Supreme Court: U.S. v. Johnson (1911) No. 433. Argued: April 13, 1911Decided: May 29, 1911. Writing for the majority, Justice Holmes wrote: "… we are of opinion that the phrase is aimed not at all possible false statements, but only at such as determine the identity of the article, possibly including its strength, quality, and purity …"

[27] See U.S. Supreme Court: Seven Cases of Eckman's Alternative v. United States of America and Six cases of Eckman's Alternative v. United States of America. Nos. 50, 51. Argued December 2, 1915. Decided January 10, 1916. Justice Holmes again wrote the majority opinion.

(or dentists or veterinarians) who wished to prescribe such substances were required to register with the local Internal Revenue Collector and pay $1.00 per year, in return for which the professionals received a tax stamp with their name and a unique, permanent registration number. This tax stamp (certificate) was to be displayed in a "conspicuous place." If physicians wanted to prescribe one of the controlled substances, they had to write a prescription containing not only the drug information but also the date; their name, address, and registration number; and the patient's name and address. If physicians wanted to keep such medications in their office or medical bag (for home visits), they needed to order duplicate forms from the government and keep records of their individual dispensing.[28] The registration processes also applied to importers and distributers. These measures were the foundation of the requirements for physicians (and nurse practitioners and physician assistants) to supply certain written information for controlled substances and to obtain a unique Drug Enforcement Administration (DEA) identification number. But problems arose with the Act's enforcement. The law permitted "dispensing or distribution of any of the aforesaid drugs to a patient by a physician, dentist or veterinary surgeon registered under this Act *in the course of his professional practice* [emphasis added]"; however, it did not define the limits of this highlighted term. The result, as Sacco[29] points out, was:

> The Treasury viewed patient drug maintenance using these substances as beyond medical scope, and many physicians were arrested, prosecuted, and jailed. Under authority of the Harrison Act, the Narcotic Division of the Internal Revenue Bureau closed down state and city narcotic clinics and sent drug violators to federal penitentiaries … Ultimately, physicians stopped prescribing drugs covered under the Harrison Act, thereby sending users to the black market to seek out these substances.

Passage of the next major law was, again, the result of a tragedy. By the early 1930s, the FDA was collecting many examples of great harm to patients caused by deficiencies in the Pure Food and Drug Act of 1906; although contents needed to be accurately represented, there was no formal government approval required to market new drugs. The press was also pushing for reforms (as was the case in 1906). Examples of injurious medications

> included Banbar, a worthless "cure" for diabetes that the old law protected; Lash-Lure, an eyelash dye in which a number of women suffered injuries to their eyes, including one con-firmed case of permanent blindness … ; Radithor, a radium-containing tonic that sentenced users to a slow and painful death; and the Wilhide Exhaler, which falsely promised to cure tuberculosis and other pulmonary diseases.[30]

---

[28] For an excellent contemporaneous description of the process, see Lengfeld, F. (1915). The Harrison Anti-Narcotic Act. *California State Journal of Medicine, XIII*, 182–183.

[29] Sacco, L. N. *Drug enforcement in the United States: History, policy, and trends* (Congressional Research Service R43749). Retrieved July 3, 2018, from https://www.fas.org/sgp/crs/misc/R43749.pdf

[30] FDA. *Part II: 1938, Food, Drug, Cosmetic Act*. Retrieved July 3, 2018, from https://www.fda.gov/AboutFDA/History/FOrgsHistory/EvolvingPowers/ucm054826.htm

Congress had been debating how to fix these problems for 5 years when, in October 1937, a drug disaster occurred. In 1932, Polish-born bacteriologist and pathologist Gerhard Domagk found that the red dye Prontosil cured streptococcal infections in mice.[31] Subsequently it was shown that Prontosil was converted to sulfanilamide (its active ingredient) in the body. After this discovery, sulfanilamide became the world's first effective antibacterial drug—a true "wonder drug," as many called it. Pharmaceutical companies rushed to produce it in powder and pill forms, and it was mass marketed. In this setting, the S.E. Massengill Company of Bristol, Tennessee, thought that a liquid form of the medication would sell well, particularly in the pediatric market. As Akst points out:[32]

> Massengill's chief chemist concocted a solution of 10 percent sulfanilamide, 72 percent diethylene glycol [DEG is a highly toxic analog of ethylene glycol, the active ingredient in antifreeze], and 16 percent water. The company's internal control lab approved the solution's appearance, taste, and fragrance—it was flavored with raspberry extract, saccharin, and caramel, among other ingredients—and by September 1937, Massengill had distributed 240 gallons of the liquid, called Elixir Sulfanilamide, across the country. Soon after the drug was distributed, several patients in Tulsa, Oklahoma became severely ill, some dying of kidney failure. (Most of the medication had been distributed to Tulsa and across Mississippi.) Tulsa physicians notified the Chicago-based American Medical Association about the deaths and analysis of the liquid at the University of Chicago revealed the cause to be DEG.[33]

By the time the medication was recalled, 107 people had died, most of them children.

Prosecution of the company's owner, Sam Massengill, highlighted the problem with the Pure Food and Drug Act. The medication's label contained exactly what was in it; so, with respect to accurate content, no law was violated. However, successful charges of mislabeling were brought on a technicality: An "elixir" was supposed to be an alcoholic solution, and the medication contained DEG instead of alcohol. The maximum fine for such mislabeling was assessed—$26,000.[34]

Congress was finally spurred into passing new comprehensive legislation to close the regulatory loopholes of the previous law. The result was the Federal Food, Drug, and Cosmetics Act (FD&C Act) of 1938, which is the backbone of modern medical technology legislation. (Many subsequent laws are amendments to this Act and refer to its provisions.) The FD&C Act had several significant new provisions with respect to the medical field. Specifically, it:

1. Brought medical devices under FDA regulation. Prior to that time, enforcement of regulations for medical devices was under jurisdiction of the Post Office Department and the Federal Trade Commission (FTC), since many of them were sold through the mails

---

[31] For this achievement, he received the Nobel Prize in Physiology or Medicine in 1939.

[32] Akst, J. (2013, June 1). The Elixir Tragedy, 1937. *The Scientist*. Retrieved July 3, 2018, from http://www.the-scientist.com/?articles.view/articleNo/35714/title/The-Elixir-Tragedy1937

[33] It is noteworthy that pharmacologist Frances Oldham Kelsey participated in the analysis. She was subsequently credited with holding up importation of thalidomide in the United States after she joined the FDA in 1960.

[34] For more details on this story, see Ballentine, C. (1981, June). Taste of raspberries, taste of death: The 1937 Elixir Sulfanilamide incident. *FDA Consumer Magazine*. Retrieved July 3, 2018, from https://www.fda.gov/downloads/AboutFDA/WhatWeDo/History/Origin/ucm125604.doc

and subject to interstate commerce laws. For purposes of regulation, the Act treated devices like drugs except for an exemption from PMA. The law defined a device as

> an instrument, apparatus, implement, machine, contrivance, implant, *in vitro* reagent, or other similar or related article, including any component, part, or accessory, which is—
>
> i.   recognized in the official National Formulary, or the United States Pharmacopeia, or any supplement to them,
>
> ii. intended for use in the diagnosis of disease or other conditions, or in the cure, mitigation, treatment, or prevention of disease, in man or other animals, or
>
> iii. intended to affect the structure or any function of the body of man or other animals, and which does not achieve its primary intended purposes through chemical action within or on the body of man or other animals and which is not dependent upon being metabolized for the achievement of its primary intended purposes.

2. Created the category of "new drugs" which were subject to heightened reviews under the new law. The term "new drug" was defined as any human drug:

> the composition of which is such that such drug is not generally recognized, among experts qualified by scientific training and experience to evaluate the safety and effectiveness of drugs, as safe and effective for use under the conditions prescribed, recommended, or suggested in the labeling thereof, except that such a drug not so recognized shall not be deemed to be a "new drug" if at any time prior to June 25, 1938, it was subject to the Food and Drugs Act of June 30, 1906, as amended, and if at such time its labeling contained the same representations concerning the conditions of its use [or] the composition of which is such that such drug, as a result of investigations to determine its safety and effectiveness for use under such conditions, has become so recognized, but which has not, otherwise than in such investigations, been used to a material extent or for a material time under such conditions.

The primary example of an excluded drug was aspirin.

3. Required that if a drug met the definition of "new," it had to be tested in humans and proven safe. In this respect, compared to the 1906 law, *the burden of proof was shifted to the pharmaceutical company*.

4. Required that drug labels contain instructions so that patients could use medications safely.

5. Repealed the Sherley Amendment requirement to prove intent to defraud in drug misbranding cases.

6. Authorized factory inspections.

Despite this legislation, the laws governing pharmaceuticals still had some major problems. One social issue that arose was whether the public should have free access to medication without a physician's prescription. Another issue was that, as a result of the FD&C

Act, drugs dispensed by a physician's written prescription were exempt from some labeling requirements (name and place of business of manufacturer, distributor or packer, quantity of contents, common or usual name, and, under some circumstances, narcotics labeling).[35] Because no law existed that specified which medications required prescriptions (other than narcotics), the designations were left to manufacturers, who found it less restrictive and more profitable to require a physician's order to obtain their products. The result, as a history of the FDA notes,[36] is that:

> Licensed doctors ... became deputies and spoilsmen in the growing system of controls. Consumers had to pay for the drug and a visit to the doctor. These new privileges for doctors were the bounty of the government's regimentation of the drug industry and assault on consumers' freedom to self-medicate. Dependence on doctors was further institutionalized and legitimated by making it difficult for consumers to gain information, in particular by the labeling and advertising controls that prohibited information or mandated unintelligibility.

In order to remedy these problems, in 1944 the FDA defined a prescription-only drug as one that,

> because of its toxicity or other potentiality for harmful effect or the method of its use or the collateral measures necessary to its use, is not generally recognized among experts qualified by scientific training and experience to evaluate its safety and efficacy, as safe and efficacious for use except by or under the supervision of a physician, dentist, or veterinarian.[37]

But the choice of over-the-counter (OTC) or prescription designation was still up to the drug company; some chose to market the *same drug* OTC while others decided it could be sold only with a prescription. With the intent to standardize how drugs were offered and make OTC drugs safer and more available to the public, Congress passed the Durham-Humphry[38] Amendment to the FD&C Act in 1951. The law gave the FDA the authority to designate which drugs can be sold OTC and which must be dispensed only by prescription. The relevant section that amended the FD&C Act stated that drugs which were to be dispensed only by prescription were those

> intended for use by man which ... because of its toxicity or other potentiality for harmful effect, or the method of its use, or the collateral measures necessary to its use, is not safe for use except under the supervision of a practitioner licensed by law to administer such drug; or is limited by an approved application ... to use under the professional supervision of a practitioner licensed by law to administer such drug.

---

[35] Federal Food, Drug, and Cosmetic Act of June 25, 1938, Pub. L. No. 75-717 (1938), reprinted in: Dunn, C. W. *Federal Food, Drug, and Cosmetic Act: A Statement of Its Legislative Record* 14 (1938) (current version at 21 U.S.C. § 353(b) (2004)) This labeling exemption also came from a 1939 FDA regulation mandating that any drug for which adequate directions for lay use could not be prepared must be sold only by prescription.

[36] FDA Review. History of Federal Regulation: 1902–Present. Retrieved July 3, 2018, from http://www.fdareview.org/ 01_history.php#p06

[37] 9 Fed. Reg. 12,255, 12,255–56 (Oct. 10, 1944).

[38] It is noteworthy both Carl Thomas Durham (D-NC) and Hubert H. Humphry (D-MN), who was to become Lyndon Johnson's Vice President, both started their careers as pharmacists.

Further, the medications that the FDA mandated for prescription status were required to carry the label: "Caution: Federal law prohibits dispensing without prescription."[39] The law permitted the FDA to exempt drugs from prescription designation if it was "not necessary for the protection of the public health." This amendment, however, was weaker than the FDA regulations because it merely mandated prescription-only status for drugs that were unsafe without professional supervision; the regulations had restrictions for drugs that were also ineffective.

In the next decade, rapid scientific developments allowed many new medications to get to market quickly because regulations allowed their approval if the FDA did not act on a New Drug Application (NDA) in a timely fashion. In this permissive climate, yet another tragedy caused passage of legislation that led to more controls. In 1957, the West German pharmaceutical company Chemie Grünenthal GmbH (now Grünenthal GmbH) released a medication originally intended as a sedative but that subsequently was prescribed for pregnant women to ease the symptoms of morning sickness. In the next 5 years, the drug, thalidomide, was successfully marketed in 46 countries. On September 12, 1960, the William S. Merrell Company of Cincinnati (an American licensee for the drug) submitted an NDA to the FDA. However, Dr. Frances Kelsey, who was in charge of its review, was concerned about its safety documentation, since some medical reports in late 1960 suggested that thalidomide might cause neuropathy (nerve damage) in some users.[40] In November 1961, Chemie Grünenthal removed the drug from the market because of strong global evidence that thalidomide caused severe birth defects, a problem widely publicized in the press with photos of the malformed children.[41] Because of the fortuitous withholding of thalidomide, Congress finally passed a version of legislation that had been proposed as early as 1959. The result was the Kefauver-Harris Amendments of 1962 (named after Senator Carey Estes Kefauver, D-TN, and Rep. Oren Harris, D-AK), which made major changes to pharmaceutical regulation, including these six:

1. The burden of proof for safety formally shifted from the FDA to the pharmaceutical company. Now the FDA was required to *act* on an NDA rather than letting the drug come to market through inaction. This change from *premarket notification* to *premarket approval* moved the regulations in line with the Biological Products Act of 1902.

---

[39]The Food and Drug Administration Modernization Act of 1997 allowed a change in this language "removing the requirement that prescription drugs be labeled with 'Caution: Federal law prohibits dispensing without prescription' and adding in its place a requirement that prescription drugs be labeled with 'Rx only' or 'only,'" See FDA Backgrounder on FDAMA. Retrieved July 3, 2018, from https://www.fda.gov/RegulatoryInformation/LawsEnforcedbyFDA/Significant AmendmentstotheFDCAct/FDAMA/ucm089179.htm

[40]Harris, S. B. (1992). The right lesson to learn from thalidomide. Retrieved July 3, 2018, from http://yarchive.net/med/fda.html

[41]A little-known fact was that "Though the drug was never approved in this country, [the William S. Merrell Company] distributed [thalidomide] to over 1,000 physicians under the guise of investigational use. Over 20,000 Americans received thalidomide in this 'study', including 624 pregnant patients, and about 17 known newborns who suffered the effects of the drug." *The History of Drug Regulation in the United States* Drug Efficacy (p. 6). Retrieved July 3, 2018, from http://www.fda.gov/downloads/aboutfda/whatwedo/history/productregulation/promotingsafeandeffectivedrugsfor100years/ucm114468.pdf

2. In order to be approved, the drug had to demonstrate efficacy as well as safety. The FDA was also required to review all NDAs that had been marketed from 1938 to 1962 to determine whether these drugs were also efficacious and safe.

3. The FDA was empowered to access company production and control records in order to evaluated compliance with Good Manufacturing Practice (GMP).

4. The control of prescription drug advertising was transferred to the FDA from the FTC.

5. The FDA became responsible for preclearing all human trials. Of particular importance in this obligation was a requirement that patients involved in the studies must give their informed consent.

6. The FDA was to preclear product labeling rather than enforce its accuracy retrospectively.

While these measures were a big step toward safer and more efficacious medicines, they produced an unwanted effect. Ward points out that "[a]s clinical tests became more complicated and required more trials, the time from the granting of the patent to market approval rose from five to seven years in 1960 to nine to twelve years in 1975. That reduced the average time that a marketed drug enjoyed patent protection by half."[42]

As a result, there was a substantial decline in drug innovation.[43] Thus, from this law emerged the current problem facing any technology regulatory body: weighing the benefit to society of quick introductions against the potential harm from unknown problems.

When the Kefauver-Harris Amendments were passed in 1962, Congress also considered similar legislation applying to medical devices; while the FDA had to determine whether a device was safe and efficacious, there was no requirement for premarket testing, review, or approval. However, as was the case with medications, it was only after a crisis that a law was passed regulating devices.

In 1968, Dr. Hugh Davis introduced the Dalkon shield intrauterine device (IUD) through a company he co-owned. By 1970, over 600,000 units were on the U.S. market when A. H. Robbins bought the company and made some modifications to the product design. By June 1974, A. H. Robbins had sold about 2.2 million devices in the United States when it suspended sales because of reports of 4 to 6 related deaths as well as thousands of injuries (particularly uterine perforation and pelvic infections) and unwanted pregnancies.[44]

As a result of the Dalkon shield problem (as well as reports of pacemaker malfunctions), Congress finally passed the medical device regulation law it had debated for so long. The Medical Device Amendments of 1976 categorized products *already on the market* into three

---

[42]Ward, M. R. (1992, October 31). Drug approval overregulation. *The Cato Institute*. Retrieved July 3, 2018, from http://www.cato.org/sites/cato.org/files/serials/files/regulation/1992/10/reg15n4e.html

[43]Peltzman, S. (1973). An evaluation of consumer protection legislation: The 1962 drug amendments. *Journal of Political Economy*, 81(5), 1049–1091.

[44]Litigation related to these deaths and complications dragged on for more than two decades. By March, 1985, the company declared bankruptcy to protect itself from further suits. In order to settle legal claims, A. H. Robbins set up the first fixed-asset trust ($2.48 billion), which started making payment offers in March 1990. The trust was terminated in April 2000 and the records were transferred to the University of Virginia Law Library (retrieved July 3, 2018, from http://ead.lib.virginia.edu/vivaxtf/view?docId=uva-law/viul00041.xml) In December, 1989, American Home Products bought A. H. Robbins.

categories for purposes of regulation—Class I, Class II, and Class III—based on the risk they posed to patients (low, moderate, and high, respectively).[45] While each class has its own regulatory requirements, all must comply with five general requirements:

1. Registration of establishments involved in bringing the product to market, e.g., manufacturers, distributors, repackagers and relabelers, and foreign firms.

2. Listing with the FDA all devices to be marketed.

3. Adherence to GMPs, which, according to the FDA, "are a set of procedures to ensure that devices are manufactured to be safe and effective through quality design, manufacture, labeling, testing, storage, and distribution."[46]

4. Labeling devices or *in vitro* diagnostic products.

5. Premarket notification submission to the FDA via 510(k) process (see below).

Regulatory specifics of each class are as follows:[47]

Class I. The above general requirements "are sufficient to provide reasonable assurance of the safety and effectiveness of the device." Many Class I devices are exempt from premarket notification. Examples include elastic bandages, examination gloves, and hand-held surgical instruments.

Class II. These devices "cannot be classified as Class I because the general controls by themselves are insufficient to provide reasonable assurance of safety and effectiveness." They may include new devices for which information or special controls are available to reduce or mitigate risk. Particular controls may include special labeling requirements, mandatory performance standards, and postmarket surveillance. Currently "15% of all device types classified in Class II are subject to special controls." Although most Class II devices require premarket notification via the 510(k) process (see Exhibit 7.4), a few are exempt by regulation. It is estimated that 90% of medical devices have been authorized to be marketed in the United States through the 510(k) process.[48] Examples of Class II devices include powered wheelchairs, infusion pumps, and surgical drapes.

---

[45]For details on these classifications see *Classify your medical device* at: http://www.fda.gov/MedicalDevices/DeviceRegulationandGuidance/Overview/ClassifyYourDevice/default.htm Also see *General controls for medical devices* at: http://www.fda.gov/medicaldevices/deviceregulationandguidance/overview/generalandspecialcontrols/ucm055910.htm (accessed July 3, 2018)

[46]As part of the GMP oversight authority, the Amendments also empowered the FDA "to deal with the notification, repair, replacement, and refund of defective devices, and to ban any device that presents a substantial deception or substantial unreasonable risk of injury or illness." See Rados, C. (2006). Medical device and radiological health regulations come of age. *FDA Consumer Magazine* (The Centennial Edition/January–February 2006). Retrieved July 3, 2018, from https://www.fda.gov/downloads/AboutFDA/WhatWeDo/History/ProductRegulation/UCM593521.pdf

[47]Johnson, J. A. (2012, June 25). FDA regulation of medical devices. Congressional Research Service 7–570. Retrieved July 3, 2018, from https://fas.org/sgp/crs/misc/R42130.pdf

[48]See Underwriters Lab (UL). *U.S. medical device clearance: Navigating the FDA 510(k) premarket approval process for medical devices*. Retrieved July 3, 2018, from https://library.ul.com/wp-content/uploads/sites/40/2015/02/UL_WP_Final_U.S.-Medical-Device-Clearance-Navigating-the-FDA-Premarket-Approval-Process-for-Medical-Devices_v5_HR.pdf; and FDA. *510(k) submission process*. Retrieved July 3, 2018, from https://www.fda.gov/MedicalDevices/DeviceRegulationandGuidance/HowtoMarketYourDevice/PremarketSubmissions/PremarketNotification510k/ucm070201.htm

EXHIBIT 7.4. Explanation of the 510(k) Process

Each person who wants to market in the U.S., a Class I, II, and III device intended for human use, for which a Premarket Approval application (PMA) is not required, must submit a 510(k) to FDA unless the device is exempt from 510(k) requirements of the Federal Food, Drug, and Cosmetic Act ... A 510(k) is a premarket submission made to FDA to demonstrate that the device to be marketed is at least as safe and effective, that is, substantially equivalent (SE), to a legally marketed device ... that is not subject to PMA. Submitters must compare their device to one or more similar legally marketed devices and make and support their substantial equivalency claims. A legally marketed device ... is a device that was legally marketed prior to May 28, 1976 ... for which a PMA is not required, or a device which has been reclassified from Class III to Class II or I, or a device which has been found SE through the 510(k) process. The legally marketed device(s) to which equivalence is drawn is commonly known as the "predicate."

What Is Substantial Equivalence

A 510(k) requires demonstration of substantial equivalence to another legally U.S. marketed device. Substantial equivalence means that the new device is at least as safe and effective as the predicate.

A device is substantially equivalent if, in comparison to a predicate, it:

- has the same intended use as the predicate; *and*
- has the same technological characteristics as the predicate; *or*
- has the same intended use as the predicate; *and*
- has different technological characteristics and the information submitted to the FDA does not raise different questions of safety and effectiveness; *and*
- demonstrates that the device is at least as safe and effective as the legally marketed device.

A claim of substantial equivalence does not mean the new and predicate devices must be identical. Substantial equivalence is established with respect to intended use, design, energy used or delivered, materials, chemical composition, manufacturing process, performance, safety, effectiveness, labeling, biocompatibility, standards, and other characteristics, as applicable ....

When a 510(k) Is Required

A 510(k) is required when:

- Introducing a device into commercial distribution (marketing) for the first time. After May 28, 1976 (effective date of the Medical Device Amendments to the Act), anyone who wants to sell a device in the U.S. is required to make a 510(k) submission at least 90 days prior to offering the device for sale ...
- You propose a different intended use for a device which you already have in commercial distribution ... Note that prescription use to over the counter use is a major change in intended use and requires the submission of a new 510(k).
- There is a change or modification of a legally marketed device and that change could significantly affect its safety or effectiveness. The burden is on the 510(k) holder to decide whether or not a modification could significantly affect safety or effectiveness of the device.

Source: FDA. *Premarket notification 510(k)*. Retrieved July 3, 2018, from http://www.fda.gov/MedicalDevices/DeviceRegulation andGuidance/HowtoMarketYourDevice/PremarketSubmissions/PremarketNotification510k/

Class III. These devices "cannot be classified as a Class I device because insufficient information exists to determine that the application of general controls are sufficient to provide reasonable assurance of the safety and effectiveness of the device"; "cannot be classified as a Class II device because insufficient information exists to determine that the special controls ... would provide reasonable assurance of [their] safety and effectiveness"; and are "purported or represented to be for a use in supporting or sustaining human life or for a use which is of substantial importance in preventing impairment of human health [or present] a potential unreasonable risk of illness or injury." These devices must, therefore, undergo extensive clinical trials to prove they are safe and effective and pass an FDA PMA process. Examples include heart valves, silicone gel–filled breast implants, implanted cerebellum stimulators, metal-on-metal hip joints, and certain dental implants.

One category of devices that did not exist in 1976 was electronic media (e.g., electronic medical records and mobile applications.) Since such devices became available the FDA has slowly rolled out selective regulations. For example, the FDA issued a guidance statement that it would not examine low-risk general wellness devices, defined as "products that meet the following two factors: (1) are intended for only general wellness use ... and (2) present a low risk to the safety of users and other persons." Examples "may include exercise equipment, audio recordings, video games, software programs and other products that are commonly, though not exclusively, available from retail establishments (including online retailers and distributors that offer software to be directly downloaded)."[49] More will be said about this topic in Chapter 8.

For about 20 years after the passage of the Kefauver-Harris Amendments in 1962, there remained a class of pharmaceuticals that were available only on a trial basis under Investigational New Drug (IND) approval. The reason for this status was that their potential market for sales did not warrant the cost of clinical trials to prove safety and efficacy to allow them to obtain approval under an NDA. Since they were neither reviewed (as the 1962 amendments required) nor withdrawn, they were called *orphan drugs*; the diseases treated by these medications were thus called orphan diseases. By the 1970s, products in this category included "drugs for single usage, drugs for chronic diseases, drugs with anticipated legal liability, drugs for use in diseases endemic to third world countries, and unpatentable drugs."[50]

At that time, the prevailing business model for pharmaceutical companies was to develop "blockbuster drugs," often defined as those with more than $1 billion in annual sales. The strategy for producing these drugs required coming up with products that could be sold to large numbers of patients with common conditions, such as hypertension, diabetes, common infections, and the like.

---

[49] FDA. *Digital health*. Retrieved July 3, 2018, from https://www.fda.gov/MedicalDevices/DigitalHealth/default.htm
[50] Huyard, C. (2009). How did uncommon disorders become "rare diseases"? History of a boundary object. *Sociology of Health & Illness, 31*(4), 463–477.

In order to encourage development of potentially unprofitable drugs and respond to lobbying by organizations representing patients with rare conditions,[51] Congress passed the Orphan Drug Act in 1983. The Act provided pharmaceutical companies with:

1. Federal funding of grants and contracts to perform clinical trials of orphan products.

2. A tax credit of 50% of clinical testing costs.

3. An exclusive right to market the orphan drug for 7 years from the date of marketing approval.

4. Enhanced coordination with the FDA throughout the drug's development.

5. Priority FDA review.

6. A waiver of drug application fees.[52]

Initially, the Act was aimed at drugs for which there was "no reasonable expectation" that U.S. sales would support their development. The vagueness of that description and lack of resultant company interest caused passage of a 1984 amendment changing the definition of the targeted products to those used for "rare diseases," defined as any disease or condition that "(A) affects less than 200,000 persons in the United States, or (B) affects more than 200,000 in the United States and for which there is no reasonable expectation that the cost of developing and making available in the United States a drug for such disease or condition will recovered from sales in the United States of such drug."[53]

Of note is that the Orphan Drug Act does not allow deviation from regulatory requirements applied to nonorphan drugs and does not extend product patent life. (It only extends marketing exclusivity.) A 1988 amendment to the Act requires sponsors to apply for orphan drug designation *before* submitting an NDA or a product license application to the FDA. The regulatory administration of this Act is carried out by the Office of Orphan Product Development.[54]

The success of this Act can be measured by the number of medications brought to market as the result of its enactment. Because of the high cost of development and lengthy approval process (about 90 months in 1982–1983, two thirds of which was taken up with

---

[51] See *National Organization for Rare Disorders*. Retrieved from http://rarediseases.org/about/what-we-do/history-leadership

[52] Institute of Medicine (US) Committee on Accelerating Rare Diseases Research and Orphan Product Development; M. J. Field, & T. F. Boat (Eds.) (2010). *Rare diseases and orphan products: accelerating research and development*. Washington, DC: National Academies Press (US). Retrieved from http://www.ncbi.nlm.nih.gov/books/NBK56187

[53] FDA: Orphan Drug Act. Relevant Excerpts (Public Law 97-414, as amended). Last updated August 2013. Retrieved from http://www.fda.gov/ForIndustry/DevelopingProductsforRareDiseasesConditions/HowtoapplyforOrphanProductDesignation/ucm364750.htm

[54] "The Board shall be comprised of the Assistant Secretary for Health of the Department of Health and Human Services and representatives, selected by the Secretary, of the Food and Drug Administration, the National Institutes Health, the Centers for Disease Control, and any other Federal department or agency which the Secretary determines has activities relating to drugs and devices for rare diseases or conditions. The Assistant Secretary for Health shall chair the Board." SEC. 227 of the Public Health Service Act [42 USC 236].

clinical trials[55]), pharmaceutical companies brought to market fewer than 10 drugs for rare conditions between 1973 and 1983.[56] Today, the Orphan Drug Product designation database[57] contains about 3,800 entries. Further, the FDA says its Orphan Grants Program has been used to bring more than 45 products to marketing approval.

As explained below in the Specialty Pharmaceuticals section, the effect of this law has tremendous implications for increasing costs of medical care. The regulatory reasons for this problem include these six loopholes in the Orphan Drug Act.

1. *Orphan status requires prevalence data from the United States.* Tax benefits and market exclusivity do not take into account foreign product sales, which, for example, in the case of some infectious diseases (such as tropical parasites), may be considerable.

2. *Market exclusivity is much broader protection than a patent.* The former grants a treatment monopoly to prevent entrance of competitors whose products have similar effects on the disease; the latter merely protects the chemical entity. The only way a new medication can challenge the market protection of the established orphan drug is if the company "provides a reasonable hypothesis that their product is 'clinically superior' to the approved product by means of greater effectiveness, greater safety, or that it provides a major contribution to patient care (MC-to-PC)."[58] The FDA emphasizes that a claim of clinical superiority will be "evaluated on a case-by-case basis for each drug product"; that is, there is no prescription for making this determination when comparing it to the existing orphan drug.[59] However, *clinical superiority cannot be claimed based on lower cost, greater patient compliance, or increased quality of life.* The Act specifies that the only circumstance that allows the FDA to categorically grant permission to another company to offer another drug in this category is when the market exclusivity holder "cannot assure the availability of sufficient quantities of the drug to meet the needs of persons with the disease or condition for which the drug was designated."

---

[55]Reichert, J. M. (2003). Trends in development and approval times for new therapeutics in the United States. *Nature Reviews: Drug Discovery*, 2(9), 695–702.

[56]Office of Orphan Products Development, FDA. Retrieved July 3, 2018, from http://www.fda.gov/AboutFDA/CentersOffices/OfficeofMedicalProductsandTobacco/OfficeofScienceandHealthCoordination/ucm2018190.htm

[57]FDA. *Search orphan drug designations and approvals.* Retrieved July 3, 2018, from https://www.accessdata.fda.gov/scripts/opdlisting/oopd/listResult.cfm

[58]FDA. *Frequently asked questions (FAQ)—designating an orphan product.* Retrieved July 3, 2018, from http://www.fda.gov/ForIndustry/DevelopingProductsforRareDiseasesConditions/HowtoapplyforOrphanProductDesignation/ucm240819.htm

[59]Guidance from the FDA provides additional clarification of the MC to PC issue: "The following factors, when applicable to severe or life-threatening diseases, _may in appropriate cases, be taken into consideration_ [emphases added] when determining whether a drug makes a major contribution to patient care: convenient treatment location; duration of treatment; patient comfort; reduced treatment burden; advances in ease and comfort of drug administration; longer periods between doses; and potential for self-administration." Department of Health and Human Services. Food and Drug Administration. 21 CFR Part 316 [Docket No. FDA–2011–N–0583] RIN 0910–AG72 Orphan Drug Regulations: Final rule. Federal Register Vol. 78, No. 113 Wednesday, June 12, 2013. Rules and Regulations (pp. 35117–35135). Retrieved July 3, 2018, from https://www.gpo.gov/fdsys/pkg/FR-2013-06-12/pdf/2013-13930.pdf

3. *A drug can obtain orphan status for more than one indication if each condition affects fewer than 200,000 people.* This loophole encourages companies to separate disease categories as much as possible, even if the drug treats a broad group. It is difficult, therefore, to classify *overall* drug use by disease or category. As examples, medications used to treat one autoimmune disease may also be used to treat a different autoimmune condition. Further, it may also be used to treat a different class of disease, such as cancers.

4. *A pharmaceutical company can obtain orphan drug designation if one of the indications is a rare disease and other indications are for much more prevalent conditions.* Another variant on this theme is that a company can obtain orphan status for a rare condition and physicians can prescribe the drug for "off-label" (nonapproved) indications. In either case, the pharmaceutical company charges orphan drug (i.e., high) prices for all uses. As an example of these practices, Daniel et al. state that

> rituximab, which was initially FDA approved for use in the treatment of follicular non-Hodgkin's lymphoma, is the number 1 selling medication approved as an orphan drug. It is currently used to treat a wide variety of conditions, ranks as the 12th all-time bestselling medication in the United States, and generated over $3.7 billion in US sales in 2014.[60]

The overall significance of this issue was highlighted in a report by AHIP:[61] Of 46 orphan drugs available between 2012 and 2014, 22 were used for nonorphan diseases; prices for orphan drugs used primarily for nonorphan diseases increased by 37%, while those used primarily for orphan indications rose by 12%; and almost half of all drugs approved by the FDA in 2015 were orphan drugs.

5. *Orphan status is granted based on disease prevalence at the time of approval.* Regulations do not take into account growth of the affected population over the life of the market exclusivity. This problem was highlighted when azidothymidine (AZT) was approved as a drug for AIDS.

6. *Orphan drug status can be granted to a company that does not develop the drug and also for a drug that is not new.* In other words, if new research shows an older, generic drug can be used to treat a rare condition in the United States, a company other than the one that developed it can obtain orphan designation and market exclusivity. For example, by 1990, thalidomide (see above) received orphan drug status for treatment of leprosy and a complication of bone marrow transplants.[62] In 1998, Celgene received orphan drug designation for thalidomide for treatment of the blood disease multiple myeloma.[63]

---

[60]Daniel, M.G., Pawlik, T. M., Fader, A. N., Esnaola, N. F., & Makary, M. A. (2016). The Orphan Drug Act: Restoring the mission to rare diseases. *American Journal of Clinical Oncology, 39*(2), 210–213.

[61]AHIP [originally called America's Health Insurance Plans]. (2016, October). Orphan drug utilization and price changes (2012–2014) (Data Brief). Retrieved July 3, 2018, from https://www.ahip.org/wp-content/uploads/2016/10/OrphanDrug_DataBrief_10.21.16.pdf

[62]Blakeslee, S. (1990, April 10). Scorned thalidomide raises new hopes. *New York Times*, C3.

[63]FDA. *Drug approval package: Thalomid (thalidomide) capsules approval date: July 16, 1998.* Retrieved July 3, 2018, from https://www.accessdata.fda.gov/drugsatfda_docs/nda/98/020785s000_ThalidomideTOC.cfm

The next safety initiative was once more due to a tragedy. In 1982, 7 people died in the Chicago area when they took Tylenol to which a tamperer (who was never found) had added cyanide.[64] The rapid and complete product recall, as well as redesign of the packaging to prevent tampering, have been used in many business schools as a case study about Johnson & Johnson's effective and ethical corporate crisis response.

Likewise, the swift FDA response was unprecedented. On November 5, 1982, the agency published regulations for "tamper-resistant packaging" covering most OTC products. The regulatory authority and specifications subsequently became part of amendments to the FD&C Act, and the term "tamper-resistant" was replaced with "tamper-evident." Briefly, if the packaging is not compliant with tamper-evident specifications and/or labeling requirements, the FDA is empowered to charge the manufacturer with "misbranding."[65]

The next major piece of legislation (the Hatch-Waxman Act) was unusual in its liberal-conservative joint sponsorship as well as its compromise between competing business factions.[66] The situation at the time of its passage was the following: To prevent competitors from copying their drugs, brand name manufacturers patented their chemical discoveries *before* they knew the drugs would be marketable. The patent life for these new entities (called pioneer drugs) was 17 years.[67] However, by 1984, mean FDA approval times had jumped to 37.2 months (more than 15 months longer than in the previous decade), and clinical trial times had ballooned to 71.7 months,[68] thus shortening effective patent protection lives, on average, to less than half their previous times.

Prior to 1984, generic companies had two problems that impeded their product development. First, "all information in an IND and NDA was regarded as confidential proprietary business information that could not be revealed by the FDA to the public or any competitor, and could not be used as the basis for any subsequent approval of a generic version of the pioneer new drug."[69] Second, the generic companies had to duplicate all the animal and human trials in order to get an NDA. Thus, to help their respective businesses, branded manufacturers wanted patent extension (which generic drug companies opposed) and generic manufacturers wanted an easier application process once patent life expired (which branded

---

[64]For a contemporary account, see McFadden, R. D. (1982, October 2). Poison deaths bring U.S. warning on Tylenol use. *New York Times*, A1.

[65]"A tamper-evident package is one having one or more indicators or barriers to entry which, if breached or missing, can reasonably be expected to provide visible evidence to consumers that tampering has occurred." Title 21: Food and Drugs Chapter C Part 211—Current Good Manufacturing Practice for Finished Pharmaceuticals. §211.132 Tamper-evident packaging requirements for over-the-counter (OTC) human drug products. Last amended, Nov. 4, 1998. Retrieved July 3, 2018, from http://www.ecfr.gov/cgi-bin/retrieveECFR?gp=1&SID=9637de728e02c1d070d9196bdee28347&ty=HTML&h=L&mc=true&n=pt21.4.211&r=PART#se21.4.211_1132

[66]For an interesting narrative on the origins of this law, See Richert, L. (2014). *Conservatism, consumer choice and the Food and Drug Administration during the Reagan era: A prescription for scandal* (pp. 133–140). New York: Lexington Books.

[67]As a result of the Uruguay Round Agreements Act of 1994, after June 8, 1995, the patent life of drugs was extended from 17 to 20 years from the date of the first filing of the patent application. The Act was part of U.S. compliance with the Uruguay Round of international negotiations that created the World Trade Organization from its predecessor, the General Agreement on Tariffs and Trade.

[68]Reichert, J. M., op. cit.

[69]Hutt, P. B. (2013). The regulation of drug products by the U.S. Food and Drug Administration. In J. P. Griffin, J. Posner, & G. R. Barker (Eds.), *The textbook of pharmaceutical medicine* (7th ed.). Belfast: Blackwell.

drug companies opposed). The compromise achieved by Utah Senator Orrin Hatch, a conservative Republican, and California Representative Henry Waxman, a liberal Democrat, was officially named the Drug Price Competition and Patent Term Restoration Act of 1984; however, it is commonly called the Hatch-Waxman Act. The following are its essential features:

1. Instead of submitting a time-consuming and costly NDA, the process was streamlined for generic manufacturers so they could submit an Abbreviated New Drug Application (ANDA). In making this submission, the application

    must state one of the following:

    I.   that the required patent information relating to such patent has not been filed;

    II.   that such patent has expired;[70]

    III. that the patent will expire on a particular date; or

    IV.   that such patent is invalid or will not be infringed by the drug, for which approval is being sought.

    A certification under paragraph I or II permits the ANDA to be approved immediately, if it is otherwise eligible. A certification under paragraph III indicates that the ANDA may be approved on the patent expiration date.[71]

    If challenged by the branded drug manufacturer, a Paragraph IV certification is risky, for reasons detailed below.

2. Rather than having to conduct original research, generic drug companies need only demonstrate bioequivalence[72] to the branded drug if the generic is essentially a duplicate.

3. Some generics have the same active ingredient as the branded drug but vary because they have a different route of administration, dosage form, strength or frequency of administration, or are manufactured with a different chemical than the original (such as a salt). For these drugs, the company must submit information according to

---

[70]Generic drugmakers can find a list of approved, safe, and effective drugs as well as patent and exclusivity information in the FDA publication: Approved Drug Products with Therapeutic Equivalence Evaluations (Orange Book). https://www.fda.gov/Drugs/InformationOnDrugs/ucm129662.htm Retrieved April 18, 2019. Once a generic has been approved as equivalent, it will also be listed.

[71]FDA. *Small business assistance: 180-day generic drug exclusivity*. Retrieved August 16, 2016, from http://www.fda.gov/Drugs/DevelopmentApprovalProcess/SmallBusinessAssistance/ucm069964.htm

[72]Bioequivalence is determined by pharmacokinetic studies that look at what happens to active drug levels in the blood over time after the medication is administered. Two measures are important: the peak concentration (the highest level the medication achieves) and "area under the curve" (the total amount of medicine measured in the blood from when it is first given to when it is no longer detectable). To be considered bioequivalent, these measures must be between 80 and 125% of the branded reference drug, with a confidence level of testing of 90%. For a much more extensive explanation, see Guidance for Industry. Bioequivalence Studies with Pharmacokinetic Endpoints for Drugs Submitted Under an ANDA. Draft Guidance. U.S. Department of Health and Human Services Food and Drug Administration Center for Drug Evaluation and Research (CDER). December 2013. Retrieved July 3, 2018, from http://www.fda.gov/downloads/drugs/guidancecomplianceregulatoryinformation/guidances/ucm377465.pdf

Section 505(b)(2) of the Act, sometimes called a paper NDA. This application requires less information than a full NDA but more than an ANDA.

4. To compensate the branded drug company for its development and increased times for regulatory approval (which use up patent exclusivity life), the patent can be extended by a maximum of 5 years or a total of 14 years of effective patent life, whichever is less.

The results of these measures on drug development were dramatic. By 2012 (8 years after passage of the Hatch-Waxman Act), ANDAs and NDAs went from about 50 each to about 500 and 100, respectively.[73]

Despite these provisions to aid generic drug companies, branded drug manufacturers still have legal methods to help them extend their holds on product exclusivity. Some of these techniques are explained below.

1. *When a generic drug company files an ANDA, it must notify the NDA sponsor or patent holder.* However, the NDA sponsor or patent holder usually has several patents on the same product, not all of which run concurrently; therefore, within 45 days of receipt of a paragraph IV notice (see above), the patent holders can file a patent infringement suit against the ANDA applicant. Unless the courts reach an earlier decision, the FDA may not give final approval to the ANDA for at least 30 months from the date of the notice. Companies have used this tactic to slow the ANDA approval, sometimes claiming the last patent on the drug has not expired (even if that particular patent is not material to generic production of the chemical entity).[74]

2. *Improved formulations of a drug are often planned in a company's product pipeline.* By introducing this improvement before the old drug's patent expiration (a process called *next-generation preempt*), the branded pharmaceutical company can make generic production of its initial drug less desirable. An example of this practice was Forest Laboratory's (now part of Actavis) drug citalopram (Celexa). Several years before this antidepressant lost patent protection, the company launched its L-isomer escitalopram (Lexapro), which was at least as effective as Celexa but had fewer side effects.

3. *When a company's drug goes off patent, it can obtain another patent on a modified form, which has its own patent life.* This strategy is called *product extension*. A classic example was the Marion Merrell Dow (now part of Sanofi) drug Cardizem (diltiazem), used for hypertension and heart rhythm problems. The drug was originally administered 3 or 4 times a day; when the patent life expired, the company introduced a twice-daily product (Cardizem SR). When this latter formulation was due to go off patent, Cardizem CD, a once-daily product, was brought to market.

---

[73] Thayer, A. M. (2014). 30 years of generics. The door that legislation unlocked for generic drugs three decades ago has blown wide open. *Chemical & Engineering News, 92*, 8–16.

[74] See Carey, T. (2009, December 24). Generic manufacturers gain another advantage in disputing drug patents. Retrieved July 3, 2018, from http://pharmaceuticalcommerce.com/legal-regulatory/generic-manufacturers-gain-another-advantage-in-disputing-drug-patents/—a revealing, but unsuccessful, example of this tactic.

4. *When a company's brand is very strong and its drug is about to go off patent, the firm may want to introduce its own generic product,* called a *branded generic.* For example, for many years the McNeil Consumer Healthcare Division of Johnson & Johnson marketed the Motrin brand of ibuprofen. When the drug became a generic, the company still marketed it under the Motrin brand and preserved some sales.

5. *If a branded drug company faces patent expiration, it can manufacture the medication in partnership with a generic drug company.* The advantage derives from cooperation in not challenging a paragraph IV filing. If the partnering generic drug company is the first applicant to file a substantially complete ANDA requesting a paragraph IV certification and the patent holder does not challenge it, the generic product will be eligible for a 180-day period of exclusivity beginning from the date it begins commercial marketing. Since only one generic drug company is marketing the product, this time period affords significant profitability potential for the branded company because it can continue its manufacturing and maintain some of its pricing power. The generic drug maker saves money in litigation and manufacturing costs while sharing in the pricing benefit of the period of exclusivity. This "first-mover" exclusivity is the Act's incentive for generic drug firms to cooperate with branded manufacturers, since, if the challenge fails, the patent holder can prevent market entry by up to 30 months. (See item 1.) This strategy is sometimes called *producing an authorized generic.* In a variation of this process, the patent holder may partner with a generic drug company once another company has its generic product approved. This process is called *flanking.* GSK employed this strategy in 2003 when Apotek launched a generic version of the antidepressant Paxil; GSK then partnered with generic drug company Par Pharmaceutical to supply it with generic Paxil in return for royalties on U.S. sales.

6. *If a generic drug maker achieves the 180-day period of exclusivity, the branded drug manufacturer can pay that firm to withhold its product introduction.* This process is called *pay for delay.* According to a FTC study, these anticompetitive deals cost consumers and taxpayers $3.5 billion in higher drug costs every year.[75] For many years, the FTC has been suing companies that engage in the practice, claiming illegal anti-competitive behavior. In a June 2013 Supreme Court ruling, the Court stated "that the deals could potentially be a violation of antitrust law" but refused the FTC's request to declare them to be presumed to be illegal.[76] Despite the lack of definitive guidance, the FTC noted that there were fewer pay-for-delay deals in fiscal year 2014 (21) compared to 2012 (40).[77]

---

[75] Federal Trade Commission. *Pay-for-delay: When drug companies agree not to compete.* Retrieved July 3, 2018, from https://www.ftc.gov/news-events/media-resources/mergers-competition/pay-delay

[76] Bartz, D. (2016, January 13). Controversial "pay-for-delay" deals drop after FTC's win in top court. *Reuters Business News.* Retrieved July 3, 2018, from http://www.reuters.com/article/us-pharmaceuticals-patent-ftc-idUSKCN0UR2JA20160113

[77] *Agreements filed with the Federal Trade Commission under the Medicare Prescription Drug, Improvement, and Modernization Act of 2003. Overview of agreements filed in FY 2014—A report by the Bureau of Competition.* Retrieved July 3, 2018, from https://www.ftc.gov/system/files/documents/reports/agreements-filled-federal-trade-commission-under-medicare-prescription-drug-improvement/160113mmafy14rpt.pdf

In a potentially more far-reaching decision, in November 2016, the Supreme Court declined to hear an appeal by Glaxo of a ruling concerning a delay deal that did not involve an explicit cash payment.

> Teva sought to make a generic version of Lamictal, a drug used to treat epilepsy and bipolar disorder, which prompted Glaxo to file a patent infringement lawsuit. The drug makers later reached a deal, but Glaxo did not make a cash payment to Teva. Instead, Glaxo agreed to allow Teva to sell generic chewable and tablet forms of Lamictal before its patent expired. Moreover, Glaxo also agreed not to sell its own so-called authorized generic version of Lamictal, which would have competed with a version sold by Teva. This was the central issue, because payers that filed their own lawsuit [in addition to the FTC's] against the drug makers charged the settlement was unfair. How so? They maintained the deal paved the way for higher prices than if Teva had proceeded to sell a lower-cost generic.[78]

Despite these rulings, the FTC is still pursuing individual actions.

7. *When all other periods of exclusivity have lapsed on an approved and marketed product, if a branded drug maker can show it has studied the product's safety and efficacy for use in children, then it can receive an additional 6 months of exclusivity.* This extension is obtained through the FDA's Written Request (WR) process. Although this tactic was not part of Hatch-Waxman but originated in 1997 with the FDA Modernization Act (FDAMA), it is included here with other examples of how drug makers can extend the lives of their branded products.

8. *In order to avoid generic competition, a branded drug can go from prescription to OTC status.* The original drug maker can then keep its brand identity as a sales advantage, be a first mover in marketing its OTC version, and have a cost advantage because it is already manufacturing the drug. Examples of this approach include such companies as Astra Zeneca, which moved its branded gastrointestinal product Prilosec to OTC status.

Several years after the Hatch-Waxman Act was in place, the number of branded drugs going off patent decreased and generic drug makers were becoming much more desperate for new products. In 1987, Mylan experienced unusual difficulty getting ANDA approvals and hired a private investigator when the FDA did not address its complaints. Rummaging in the garbage of chemist Charles Chang, the FDA official in charge of the generic drug division, the investigator found evidence of payoffs that explained Mylan's troubles and other companies' success.[79] Mylan presented this evidence to the House Energy and Commerce Subcommittee on Oversight and Investigations, setting off a 6-year-long investigation. As Reid[80] explains, the result was that

---

[78]Silverman, E. (2016, November 7). Supreme Court lets pay-to-delay ruling against pharma stand. *STAT*. Retrieved July 3, 2018, from https://www.statnews.com/pharmalot/2016/11/07/supreme-court-pay-delay-glaxo-teva

[79]Freudenheim, M. (1989, September 10). Exposing the FDA. *New York Times*, Section 3 (Business) 1, 14.

[80]Reid, J. P. (1999). A generic drug price scandal: Too bitter a pill for the Drug Price Competition and Patent Term Restoration Act to swallow? *Notre Dame Law Revue, 75*(1), 309.

[i]nvestigators from the Departments of Justice and Health and Human Services discovered that not only had drug companies used cash and gifts to sway FDA officials, but some had also submitted fraudulent data with their ANDAs. Most shockingly, some generic companies had taken name brand drugs, repackaged them as samples of their own products, and submitted them for bioequivalency tests … As a result of the scandal, thirty individuals and nine drug companies were found guilty or admitted their role in FDA corruption.

Consequently, Congress passed the Generic Drug Enforcement Act of 1992, greatly enhancing penalties for illegal activities such as the ones that caused the scandal.

While the generic drug investigation was at its height, Congress also addressed weaknesses in the device regulations and passed the Safe Medical Device Act (SMDA) of 1990.[81] This law added the following requirements for medical devices:

1. In addition to the manufacturer, a "device user facility" (hospital, ambulatory surgical facility, nursing home, or outpatient treatment facility, but not a physician's office) is required to report events where there is a "probability that a device has caused or contributed to the death of a patient of the facility." This requirement added a new class of reporting organizations.

2. The 510(k) submission was changed from a notification procedure to a premarket approval process.

3. For purposes of a 510(k) submission, the Act clarified the definition of a new device as substantially equivalent

    > if it is at least as safe and effective as the predicate … has the same intended use as the predicate and has the same technological characteristics as the predicate; or has the same intended use as the predicate and has different technological characteristics and the information submitted to FDA does not raise new questions of safety and effectiveness and demonstrates that the device is at least as safe and effective as the legally marketed device

4. Manufacturers are required to adopt methods of tracking the devices, "the failure of which would be reasonably likely to have serious adverse health consequences and which is a permanently implantable device, or a life sustaining or life supporting device used outside a device user facility." (It would take another law, the Food and Drug Administration Amendments Act of 2007, for implementation of a unique device identifier requirement.)

5. The FDA[82] was granted power to "include performance standards for a class II device if the Secretary determines that a performance standard is necessary to provide reasonable assurance of the safety and effectiveness of the device."

---

[81] For a full transcript of the law see https://www.govtrack.us/congress/bills/101/hr3095/text Retrieved July 3, 2018.
[82] This law and others give the enumerated powers and responsibilities to the Secretary of HHS. For clarity, since it is the unit of HHS responsible for carrying out these laws, "the FDA" will be used in these descriptions instead of "the Secretary."

6. The FDA was given recall authority if "there is a reasonable probability that a device intended for human use would cause serious, adverse health consequences or death."

7. Manufacturers are required to conduct postmarket surveillance

> for any device of the manufacturer first introduced or delivered for introduction into interstate commerce after January 1, 1991, that is a permanent implant the failure of which may cause serious, adverse health consequences or death, is intended for a use in supporting or sustaining human life, or potentially presents a serious risk to human health.

8. The FDA may also "require a manufacturer to conduct postmarket surveillance for a device ... if [it] determines that postmarket surveillance of the device is necessary to protect the public health or to provide safety or effectiveness data for the device."

9. Recognizing that some devices were combinations of "a drug, device, or biological product," the Act empowers the FDA to designate the main function of the compound device and assign its regulation to the appropriate authority within the agency.[83] (See the discussion about the 21st Century Cures Act below for an update on this provision.)

10. The Act also set up the Humanitarian Use Device (HUD) program, creating an alternative pathway for getting market approval for medical devices that may help people with rare diseases or conditions. A HUD is defined as a "medical device intended to benefit patients in the treatment or diagnosis of a disease or condition that affects or is manifested in fewer than 4,000 individuals in the United States per year."[84]

Between enactment of the Hatch-Waxman Act and the SMDA, another safety issue arose: Companies (not the original manufacturer) were reimporting U.S.-made drugs originally sold abroad and selling them at discounted prices. This practice caused the following problems:

- Since the drugs were not under FDA supervision, they may have become "subpotent or adulterated" while out of the country.

- The practice was providing cover for importation of counterfeit medications.

- Reimported drugs were sold at deeply discounted prices to healthcare entities, which in turn sold them at below-wholesale prices to retail outlets. As the Act (see below) states, this practice "helps fuel the diversion market and is an unfair form of competition to wholesalers and retailers that must pay otherwise prevailing market prices."

---

[83] The FDA is still trying to streamline the process of sorting out these devices for regulatory review. See, for example: Nguyen, T., & Sherman, R. E. (2016, August 11). *Making continuous improvements in the Combination Products Program: The pre-RFD process.* (FDA Voice). Retrieved July 3, 2018, from https://blogs.fda.gov/fdavoice/index.php/2016/08/making-continuous-improvements-in-the-combination-products-program-the-pre-rfd-process

[84] See Guidance for Industry and Food and Drug Administration Staff: Humanitarian Use Device (HUD) Designations (2013, January 24). Retrieved July 3, 2018, from http://www.fda.gov/downloads/RegulatoryInformation/Guidances/UCM336515.pdf

An additional problem noted by regulators was that manufacturers' representatives were giving samples to physicians who, in turn, were selling them to patients without controls on monitoring expiration dates or adulteration.

To correct these practices, Congress passed the Prescription Drug Marketing Act of 1987. Signed by President Reagan in April 1988, the Act made illegal the reimportation of U.S. drugs by anyone other than the manufacturer; prohibited the sale of drug samples and the resale of drug products initially sold to healthcare institutions; and required state licensure of wholesale distributors of prescription drugs (the latter process was clarified by the Prescription Drug Amendments of 1992). The history of this Act is illustrative not only of how laws are passed to correct harmful practices but how the implementation process can take years (if ever) to implement.

A controversial part of the law required wholesalers to keep a detailed record of what happened to the drug through its chain of distribution ("pedigree"); however, that provision was not the only one that delayed its execution. Briefly, here is what happened:

1. The provisions of the law concerning drug samples became effective on October 20, 1988; the FDA's Proposed Rule on requirements of their distribution was issued on March 14, 1994; the Final Rule was issued on December 3, 1999.

2. The portion of the law that dealt with wholesalers was never totally resolved. It was last addressed in the Drug Supply Chain Security Act (DSCSA) [Title II of the Drug Quality and Security Act (DQSA)], which was signed into law on November 27, 2013. This law "removed the drug pedigree language and replaced it with new language in section 503(e) of the FD&C Act, which pertains to new licensing requirements and uniform national standards for wholesale distribution of prescription drugs [and] added product tracing requirements."[85]

3. The rules about importation of drugs have been modified over the years in response to the public's desire to obtain medication that is not available in the United States or is cheaper elsewhere. The issues concern drugs that are and are not FDA approved. For unapproved drugs, the FDA has issued guidance recommendations since the 1950s. It was only in 2007 that amendments to the FD&C Act[86] specified a waiver for individual importation: The FDA "may grant to individuals, by regulation or on a case-by-case basis, a waiver of the prohibition of importation of a prescription drug or device or class of prescription drugs or devices, under such conditions as the Secretary determines to be appropriate." Subsequently, language was added to address Canadian imports.[87] However, the language is broad and, hence, vague. This provision

---

[85] FDA. (2017, June 30). *Drug supply chain security act product tracing requirements frequently asked questions*. Retrieved July 3, 2018, from https://www.fda.gov/Drugs/DrugSafety/DrugIntegrityandSupplyChainSecurity/DrugSupply ChainSecurityAct/ucm487301.htm

[86] Amendments to Section 804 of the FD&C Act: Waiver authority [21 USC 384]: Congressional Record, V. 153, Pt. 8, April 30, 2007, to May 9 2007 (p. 10769).

[87] Federal Food, Drug and Cosmetic Act [As Amended through P.L. 113–5, Enacted March 13, 2013] Section 804 (p. 613). Retrieved July 3, 2018, from http://legcounsel.house.gov/Comps/FDA_CMD.pdf

is not enforced by law or regulation, but only through guidance statements that the FDA periodically issues.[88]

By 1992, backlogs at the FDA caused by lack of resources in personnel and equipment resulted in waits of over 30 months for drug approvals. Because companies were losing valuable patent life and patients were denied useful medications, Congress looked into ways to speed the process. Since it was unwilling to allocate more money for regulation, Congress passed the Prescription Drug User Fee Act (PDUFA) of 1992, authorizing the FDA to set up a fee schedule to charge applicants for review of their products.[89] By 1996–1997, the evaluation time declined by more than a year. Further, analysis of the economic and social benefits revealed that between extra producer profits ($7–$11 billion) and consumer welfare benefits ($7–$20 billion), the combined social surplus was between $14 and $31 billion. Moreover, the health benefits of the more rapid availability of drugs saved the equivalent of an estimated 140,000 to 310,000 life-years.[90]

New actions came with a change in presidential administrations. In March 1993, President Clinton created the National Performance Review (NPR), naming Vice President Gore as its leader. Tasked with "restoring Americans' trust in government," this program targeted 32 federal agencies that had 90% of the federal government's contact with the public (High Impact Agencies); among them was the FDA. The NPR was to work "in partnership with these agencies to help them focus on the three balanced measures of success: customers, employees, and getting results that matter to Americans."[91]

One result of this ongoing activity was the Food and Drug Administration Modernization Act of 1997.[92] This long and complex law puts into statute some processes with which the FDA was previously empowered and extended and clarified other procedures. For example, some of the application and approval processes were streamlined. Unfortunately, many of these provisions are still being implemented and modified. The following list is a very brief summary of some of them.

- If a drug maker obtains "information relating to the use of a new drug in the pediatric population [that] may produce health benefits in that population," the company can be

---

[88] See FDA. (2018, March 1). *Imported drugs raise safety concerns*. Retrieved July 3, 2018, from http://www.fda.gov/Drugs/ResourcesForYou/Consumers/ucm143561.htm; and Is it legal for me to personally import drugs? Retrieved from http://www.fda.gov/AboutFDA/Transparency/Basics/ucm194904.htm

[89] For current information on rates, see Prescription Drug User Fee Act (PDUFA). Retrieved July 3, 2018, from http://www.fda.gov/ForIndustry/UserFees/PrescriptionDrugUserFee Subsequent reauthorizations added FDA authority to use funds for postmarketing surveillance The law must be reauthorized every 5 years; on August 18, 2017, the president signed into law the Food and Drug Administration Reauthorization Act (FDARA), which includes the reauthorization of PDUFA through September 2022.

[90] Philipson, T., Berndt, E. R., Gottschalk, A. H. B., & Sun, E. (2008). Cost-benefit analysis of the FDA: The case of the prescription drug user fee acts. *Journal of Public Economics*, *92*, 1306–1325.

[91] Kemensky, J. (1999, January). *National Partnership for Reinventing Government (formerly the National Performance Review): A brief history*. Retrieved July 3, 2018, from http://govinfo.library.unt.edu/npr/whoweare/history2.html

[92] FDA. Backgrounder on FDAMA (The FDA Modernization Act of 1997). (1997, November 21). Retrieved July 3, 2018, from https://www.fda.gov/RegulatoryInformation/LawsEnforcedbyFDA/SignificantAmendmentstotheFDCAct/FDAMA/ucm089179.htm

awarded an additional 6 months of market exclusivity.[93] A subsequent law, the Best Pharmaceuticals for Children Act in 2002, which required mandatory pediatric testing of new drugs, was found to be illegal under the FD&C Act. This court decision led Congress to pass the Pediatric Research Equity Act of 2003, correcting language that accomplished the purpose of its predecessor.

- At the request of the sponsor of a new drug, the FDA shall "facilitate the development and expedite the review of [a] ... drug if it is intended for the treatment of a serious or life-threatening condition and it demonstrates the potential to address unmet medical needs for such a condition." These drugs are called "fast track products."

- The FDA is required to establish a data bank in the NIH, for use by the general public, to provide information on research relating to new drugs for serious or life-threatening diseases.

- The Act allowed drug makers

   to provide economic information about their products to formulary committees, managed care organizations, and similar large-scale buyers of health-care products. The provision is intended to provide such entities with dependable facts about the economic consequences of their procurement decisions. *The law, however, does not permit the dissemination of economic information that could affect prescribing choices to individual medical practitioners.* [Emphasis added].[94]

This last provision operates under the Affordable Care Act (ACA) prohibition on using economic considerations for recommending therapies.

- The FDA shall, "in consultation with the Director of the National Institutes of Health and with representatives of the drug manufacturing industry, review and develop guidance, as appropriate, on the inclusion of women and minorities in clinical trials." Appropriate inclusion of these populations is unfortunately still lacking.[95]

- The Act amends the Public Health Service Act to require the FDA to "take measures to minimize differences in the review and approval" of new biological products[96] and drugs.

- Previous law required the statement: "Caution: Federal Law prohibits dispensing without a prescription" to avoid misbranding violations. The Act changes the statement requirement to, at minimum, "Rx Only."

---

[93]FDA. (2016, November 30). Qualifying for Pediatric Exclusivity under Section 505A of the Federal Food, Drug, and Cosmetic Act: Frequently asked questions on Pediatric Exclusivity (505A). Retrieved July 3, 2018, from http://www.fda .gov/Drugs/DevelopmentApprovalProcess/DevelopmentResources/ucm077915.htm

[94]FDA Backgrounder on FDAMA, op. cit.

[95]For a deeper discussion of this issue, see Califf, R. M. (2016, January 27). 2016: The year of diversity in clinical trials (FDA Voice). Retrieved July 5, 2018, from http://blogs.fda.gov/fdavoice/index.php/2016/01/2016-the-year-of-diversity-in-clinical-trials

[96]" ... the term *biological product* means a virus, therapeutic serum, toxin, antitoxin, vaccine, blood, blood component or derivative, allergenic product, or analogous product, or arsphenamine or derivative of arsphenamine (or any other trivalent organic arsenic compound), applicable to the prevention, treatment, or cure of a disease or condition of human beings."

▪ The Act created an exemption for pharmacies that prepare drugs on-site (compounding pharmacies) "if the drug product is compounded for an identified individual patient based on the unsolicited receipt of a valid prescription order or a notation, approved by the prescribing practitioner, on the prescription order that a compounded product is necessary for the identified patient."

This clause was meant to preserve individualized drug treatments. Unfortunately, the exemption led to weak enforcement of preparation standards and a healthcare tragedy. Many physicians ordered steroid solutions from the New England Compounding Center in Framingham, Massachusetts; the drugs were for treatment of back pain (despite equivocal evidence of their effectiveness).

> In September 2012, the Centers for Disease Control and Prevention (CDC), in collaboration with state and local health departments and the Food and Drug Administration (FDA), began investigating a multistate outbreak of fungal meningitis and other infections among patients who received contaminated preservative-free MPA [medroxyprogesterone acetate] steroid injections from that pharmacy.[97]

This crisis led to passage of Title I of the Drug Quality and Security Act of 2013 that contains important provisions relating to the oversight of compounding of human drugs.[98]

▪ The Act requires that a pharmaceutical company that is the sole manufacturer of a drug that is "life-supporting, life-sustaining or intended for use in the prevention of a debilitating disease or condition" (and is not a product that was originally derived from human tissue and was replaced by a recombinant product) shall give the FDA 6 months' notice before its discontinuance."

▪ The Act eliminated local control of nonprescription drugs and subjected them to nationally uniform regulations. Further, these OTC medications are required to display on their labels the quantity and proportion of all active ingredients as well as an alphabetical listing of inactive ingredients.

▪ For the first time, manufacturers were allowed, under certain circumstances, to provide information about off-label use of their products. In the case of drugs, "off-label" means it is being prescribed under circumstances not approved by the FDA, that is, for a different disease or symptom, in a population that has not been included in the label, or with a different dosage level or formulation. For example, a drug may be approved to treat a certain kind of cancer but not another kind. This portion of the Act opened a debate about

---

[97]CDC. (2015, October 15). Multistate outbreak of fungal meningitis and other infections (updated). Retrieved July 5, 2018, from https://www.cdc.gov/hai/outbreaks/meningitis.html; see also Eichenwald, K. (2015, April 16). Killer pharmacy inside a medical mass murder case. *Newsweek*. Retrieved July 5, 2018, from http://www.newsweek.com/2015/04/24/inside-one-most-murderous-corporate-crimes-us-history-322665.html

[98]FDA. *Human drug compounding*. Retrieved July 5, 2018, from http://www.fda.gov/drugs/GuidanceCompliance RegulatoryInformation/PharmacyCompounding; and FDA. *Text of Compounding Quality Act*. Retrieved July 5, 2018, from http://www.fda.gov/Drugs/GuidanceComplianceRegulatoryInformation/PharmacyCompounding/ucm376732.htm

what information companies were allowed to disseminate. The conflict pits a company's constitutional right to free speech against the FDA's mandate to protect the health of the U.S. population through its regulatory authority over drug promotion and approval. (See the FDA mission statement below.)

These concerns about off-label use are well founded. Research has shown that off-label use:

- Is frequent and differs in different settings: from 21% in office-based practices[99] to 78.9% of children discharged from pediatric hospitals.[100]

- Has a significant lack of evidence-based indications. For example, in the office setting, 73% of off label use "had little or no scientific support,"[101] while in the intensive care unit, 48.3% of the off-label medication orders had grade C ["at least moderate certainty that the net benefit is small"][102] or no evidence."[103]

- Can lead to a much higher incidence of adverse drug reactions compared to approved drugs with good scientific evidence for their use.[104]

The result of this conflict has been a number of court cases addressing these competing interests. The first one of significance was *Washington Legal Foundation v. Michael Friedman and Donna Shalala*.[105] In granting summary judgment for the plaintiff, the court found that the FDA documents providing guidance on the information companies could disseminate "are contrary to rights secured by the United States Constitution and therefore must be set aside." More specifically, among other provisions, the court ordered that:

1. Defendants SHALL NOT [emphasis in original] in any way prohibit, restrict, sanction or otherwise seek to limit any pharmaceutical or medical device manufacturer or any other person:

    a) from disseminating or redistributing to physicians or other medical professionals any article concerning prescription drugs or medical devices previous published in a bona fide peer-reviewed professional journal, regardless of whether such article

---

[99]Radley, D. C., Finkelstein, S. N., & Stafford, R. S. (2006). Off-label prescribing among office-based physicians. *Archives of Internal Medicine* [Now called *JAMA Internal Medicine*], *166*(9), 1021–1026.

[100]Shah, S. S., Hall, M., Goodman, D. M., Feuer, P., Sharma, V., Fargason, C. Jr., ... Slonim, A. D. (2007). Off-label drug use in hospitalized children. *Archives of Pediatrics & Adolescent Medicine*, *161*(3), 282–290. [Published correction appears in *Arch Pediatr Adolesc Med., 161*(7): 655].

[101]Radley, D. C., et al., op. cit.

[102]*Grade* definitions. U.S. Preventive Services Task Force. (2018, June). *What the grades mean and suggestions for practice*. Retrieved July 5, 2018, from http://www.uspreventiveservicestaskforce.org/Page/Name/grade-definitions

[103]Lat, I., Micek, S., Janzen, J., Cohen, H., Olsen, K., & Haas, C. (2011). Off-label medication use in adult critical care patients. *Journal of Critical Care*, *26*(1), 89–94.

[104]Eguale, T., Buckeridge, D. L., Verma, A., Winslade, N. E., Benedetti, A., Hanley, J. A., & Tamblyn, R. (2015). Association of off-label drug use and adverse drug events in an adult population. *JAMA Internal Medicine*, *176*(1), 55–63. The only exception to this finding is when off-label medications have strong scientific evidence for their use.

[105]Washington Legal Foundation v. Michael Friedman [Acting Commissioner, FDA] and Donna Shalala [Secretary, Department of Health and Human Services]. U.S. District Court for the District of Columbia—36 F. Supp. 2d 418 (D.D.C. 1999), February 16, 1999.

includes a significant or exclusive focus on *unapproved uses for* drugs or medical devices *that are* approved by FDA *for other uses* and regardless of whether such article reports the original study on which FDA approval of the drug or device in question was based. [Emphasis in original.]

These types of court cases have continued to the present time, resulting in expansion of free speech rights for the manufacturers and causing the FDA to issue multiple revisions of permissible activities.[106]

- The Act sets conditions for the FDA to grant expanded use for drugs and devices that are still undergoing investigation

> for the diagnosis, monitoring, or treatment of a serious disease or condition in emergency situations ... [when] the licensed physician determines that the person has no comparable or satisfactory alternative therapy available to diagnose, monitor, or treat the disease or condition involved, and that the probable risk to the person from the investigational drug or investigational device is not greater than the probable risk from the disease or condition.

One caveat is that the "provision of the investigational drug or investigational device will not interfere with the initiation, conduct, or completion of clinical investigations to support marketing approval." This stipulation has had a major positive influence on the willingness of manufacturers to provide products for "compassionate use." Without it, if the product caused injury or death, it may not only taint the company in the eyes of the investor community, but also reduce subsequent FDA willingness to approve it.

- The Act formally sets the *mission of the FDA*, directing it to

> promote the public health by promptly and efficiently reviewing clinical research and taking appropriate action on the marketing of regulated products in a timely manner ... by ensuring that—

(A)   foods are safe, wholesome, sanitary, and properly labeled;

(B)   human and veterinary drugs are safe and effective;

(C)   there is reasonable assurance of the safety and effectiveness of devices intended for human use;

(D)   cosmetics are safe and properly labeled; and

(E)   public health and safety are protected from electronic product radiation.

It is curious that this provision occurs in the latter part of the document rather than at the beginning.

---

[106]For two excellent articles explaining off-label use as well as the current legal situation (respectively), see Wittich, C. M., Burle, C. M., & Lanier, W. L. (2012). Ten common questions (and their answers) about off-label drug use. *Mayo Clinic Proceedings, 87*(10), 982–990; and Richardson, E. (2016). Off-label drug promotion. *Health Affairs Health Policy Brief*. Retrieved July 5, 2018, from http://healthaffairs.org/healthpolicybriefs/brief_pdfs/healthpolicybrief_159.pdf

■ The Act sets outsourcing terms by which the FDA "may enter into a contract with any organization or any individual (who is not an employee of the Department) with relevant expertise, to review and evaluate" applications or submissions.

■ The Act requires registration of any "establishment within any foreign country engaged in the manufacture, preparation, propagation, compounding, or processing of a drug or a device that is imported or offered for import into the United States."

Significant major legislation was next passed to further speed drug approval: the Food and Drug Administration Amendments Act of 2007. Most of this Act concerned reauthorization or enhancement of previous legislation. The truly innovative part of this law was introduction of priority review vouchers for companies that developed drugs for FDA-specified "neglected tropical diseases." These companies could use this voucher for other drugs it developed or sell it to another company.[107] In 2012, the Food and Drug Administration Safety and Innovation Act (FDASIA) expanded the voucher system to cover rare pediatric diseases.

The subsequent important law came from the necessity to address technological progress. Biologic drugs had not only become a key addition to treatment regimens but were notably contributing to increasing healthcare costs. (See the Specialty Pharmaceuticals section below.) In anticipation of these drugs reaching their patent expirations, new legislation was needed to address generic versions (sometimes called biogenerics or biosimilars). While the Hatch-Waxman Act addressed the regulation of *chemical*-based generic medications, it did not cover those of *biologic* origin. Congress therefore approved the Biologics Price Competition and Innovation Act of 2009.[108] For a biologic to be an approved generic, this Act requires "that there are no clinically meaningful differences in safety, purity, and potency between a biosimilar product and the brand or product." After the FDA approves a Biological License Application (BLA) for the pioneer (original) drug, the company is awarded a 12-year market exclusive. The first approved biosimilar receives 1 year of exclusivity, but the company must give the pioneer drug firm 6 months' advance notice of its introduction. While a patent holder is free to exercise its legal rights if the patent life is still running, once the 12 years of market exclusivity are over, the FDA may approve a biosimilar BLA. (Contrast this process to the one in the Hatch-Waxman Act, described earlier.)

As mentioned briefly above, sometimes legislation is required to reauthorize previous provisions that have or are about to expire. The FDASIA[109] contains a number of such provisions. For example, it reauthorized user fees for drugs, devices, and generics (including biologics) and made permanent the Best Pharmaceuticals for Children Act and the Pediatric

---

[107] For an excellent review of vouchers, see Gaffney, A., & Mezher, M. (2018, April 30). *Regulatory explainer: Everything you need to know about FDA's priority review vouchers*. Retrieved July 5, 2018, from https://www.raps.org/regulatory-focus/news-articles/2017/12/regulatory-explainer-everything-you-need-to-know-about-fdas-priority-review-vouchers

[108] Title VII—Improving Access to Innovative Medical Therapies. Subtitle A—Biologics Price Competition and Innovation ("Biologics Price Competition and Innovation Act of 2009"). Retrieved July 5, 2018 from http://www.fda.gov/downloads/Drugs/GuidanceComplianceRegulatoryInformation/ucm216146.pdf The law was actually passed in 2010 as part of the Patient Protection and Affordable Care Act of 2010.

[109] Retrieved September 7, 2016, from https://www.congress.gov/bill/112th-congress/senate-bill/3187/text?overview=closed

Research Equity Act of 2003. Among the new features contained in that law are the following items:

- The FDA was mandated (in consultation with the National Coordinator for Health Information Technology and the chairman of the Federal Communications Commission) to produce "a report that contains a proposed strategy and recommendations on an appropriate, risk-based regulatory framework pertaining to health information technology, including mobile medical applications, that promotes innovation, protects patient safety, and avoids regulatory duplication." As mentioned above, the question is ongoing regarding whether the FDA should have regulatory authority over information technology; the basis for such power would be if such technology is classified a medical device.

- Many parts of the Act deal with enhanced registration and monitoring of both foreign and domestic facilities and importers. The law gives the FDA authority to designate a foreign entity to monitor plants in its respective country and set schedules for inspections based on risk of problems occurring. It also requires the FDA to accept foreign clinical trials if they are adequate under FDA approval standards (or explain in writing why the trial is not adequate). Of particular additional importance was the extension of the requirement for GMPs to raw materials used in drug production. To enforce these provisions, the law grants jurisdiction to the FDA for any violation occurring outside the United States if the product was intended for import into this country. See the Baxter heparin example in the Regulatory Inadequacy section below as an illustration of the importance of enforcing these provisions.

- Recognizing the emergence of drug-resistant bacteria, the Act specifies terms for priority review of certain antibiotics and an additional 5-year marketing exclusivity for drugs intended to treat a "qualifying pathogen" (i.e., one "that has the potential to pose a serious threat to public health"). Examples include methicillin-resistant *Staphylococcus aureus*, vancomycin-resistant *Staphylococcus aureus* and enterococcus, multidrug-resistant tuberculosis, and *Clostridium difficile*.

- In this Act, for the first time, a law addresses the science of nanotechnology. The FDA is directed to

  > intensify and expand activities related to enhancing scientific knowledge regarding nanomaterials included or intended for inclusion in products regulated under … statutes administered by the Food and Drug Administration, to address issues relevant to the regulation of those products, including the potential toxicology of such nanomaterials, the potential benefit of new therapies derived from nanotechnology, the effects of such nanomaterials on biological systems, and the interaction of such nanomaterials with biological systems.

- Another new subject contained in the legislation involves patient participation in product development discussions. Specifically, the FDA was directed to

  > develop and implement strategies to solicit the views of patients during the medical product development process and consider the perspectives of patients during regulatory discussions, including by fostering participation of a patient representative who may

serve as a special government employee in appropriate agency meetings with medical product sponsors and investigators.

- The Act enhances scrutiny of diverse patient populations to be included in clinical studies. It requires the FDA to submit a report to Congress explaining "the extent to which clinical trial participation and the inclusion of safety and effectiveness data by demographic subgroups including sex, age, race, and ethnicity, is included in applications."

- The Act contains provisions to anticipate and respond to drug shortages. It requires the sole manufacturer of a critical drug to give the FDA at least 6 months' notice of its discontinuance; authorizes the FDA to expedite drug application reviews or inspections in order to prevent a drug shortage; requires the FDA to submit an annual report to Congress on drug shortages and implement a strategic plan to address such shortages; requires the FDA to maintain a current list of drugs experiencing a shortage; and requires the Comptroller General of the United States to study the causes of drug shortages and to develop recommendations to prevent or mitigate them.

As of this writing, the most recent major legislation concerning healthcare technology is the 21st Century Cures Act (P.L. 114-255): An Act to accelerate the discovery, development, and delivery of 21st-century cures, and for other purposes, which was signed into law by President Barack Obama on December 13, 2016. This law was the result of major lobbying by the stakeholders who benefited from its passage. For example, "58 pharmaceutical companies, 24 device companies and 26 'biotech products and research' companies ... reported more than $192 million in lobbying expenses on the Cures Act and other legislative priorities."[110] Some technology-related portions of the law are highlighted below:

- The FDA is allowed to review drugs and devices based on "data summaries" from such sources as observational studies. Since randomized clinical trials (the "gold standard" for approval) are significantly more expensive and time consuming than the experiential sources, the fear is that rigorous scientific evaluations may be significantly weakened.

- Drug companies are allowed to promote off-label uses to insurance companies. Recall from the previous discussion that they were already allowed to discuss such uses with physicians.

- Combination products that have device and drug components can be evaluated through the faster device review process.

- Three research programs are identified for special funding: The Cancer Moonshot, the BRAIN Initiative, and the Precision Medicine Initiative. While the law designates $4.8 billion over 10 years (earmarked for the NIH), these funds are subject to annual appropriations.

- The FDA will receive an additional $500 million through 2026 to carry out the terms of the Act. However, critics say the FDA will still lack adequate resources to police food safety and monitor post marketing problems.

---

[110]Findlay, S., & Lupkin, S. (2016, December 7). Grab bag of goodies in 21st Century Cures Act. *Kaiser Health News.* Retrieved July 5, 2018, from http://khn.org/news/grab-bag-of-goodies-in-21st-century-cures-act

- The Act renews the voucher program that incentivizes companies to develop drugs to treat rare pediatric diseases.[111]

- As mentioned previously, for many years, regulators and industry representatives have considered regulating various software products as medical devices.

  Section 3060 of the Act exempts five categories of software from regulation as a medical device, including software used for administrative support, maintaining or encouraging a healthy lifestyle, electronic patient records, processing or displaying clinical data or related findings by a healthcare professional, and supporting or providing treatment recommendations.[112]

Given this legislative history, it is evident that the FDA is responsible for a significant scope of regulation and surveillance. Exhibit 7.5 summarizes its regulatory activities.

EXHIBIT 7.5. What Does FDA Regulate?

The scope of FDA's regulatory authority is very broad and its responsibilities are closely related to those of several other government agencies. Consumers are therefore often frustrated when trying to determine the appropriate regulatory agency to contact. The following is a representative list of product categories that fall under FDA's regulatory jurisdiction.

In general, FDA regulates:

Foods
Included under foods are:

- Dietary supplements

- Bottled water

- Food additives

- Infant formulas

- Other food products (although the U.S. Department of Agriculture [USDA] plays a lead role in regulating aspects of some meat, poultry, and egg products)

Drugs
Included under drugs are:

- Prescription drugs (both brand name and generic)

- Nonprescription (OTC) drugs

---

[111] Despite the voucher, tax law changes in 2017 decreased the incentive by reducing the tax credit for clinical-testing costs from 50% to 25%.

[112] FDA News. (2017, January 20). Software exclusions, breakthrough devices featured in 21st Century Cures Act. Retrieved July 5, 2018, from http://www.fdanews.com/articles/180147-software-exclusions-breakthrough-devices-featured-in-21st-century-cures-act?class=url

Biologics

Included under biologics are:

- Vaccines
- Blood and blood products
- Cellular and gene therapy products
- Tissue and tissue products
- Allergenics

Medical Devices

Included under medical devices are:

- Simple items like tongue depressors and bedpans
- Complex technologies such as heart pacemakers
- Dental devices
- Surgical implants and prosthetics

Electronic Products that Give Off Radiation

Included in this category are:

- Microwave ovens
- X-ray equipment
- Laser products
- Ultrasonic therapy equipment
- Mercury vapor lamps
- Sunlamps

Cosmetics

Included under cosmetics are:

- Color additives found in makeup and other personal care products
- Skin moisturizers and cleansers
- Nail polish and perfume

Veterinary Products

Included in this category are:

- Livestock feeds
- Pet foods
- Veterinary drugs and devices

Tobacco Products

Included under tobacco products are:

- Cigarettes
- Cigarette tobacco
- Roll-your-own tobacco
- Smokeless tobacco

Further, the FDA works with other government agencies that deal with the following issues:

Advertising

The FTC is a federal agency that regulates many types of advertising and protects consumers by stopping unfair, deceptive or fraudulent practices in the marketplace.

Alcohol

The Department of Treasury's Alcohol and Tobacco Tax and Trade Bureau (TTB) regulates aspects of alcohol production, importation, wholesale distribution, labeling, and advertising.

Consumer Products

The Consumer Product Safety Commission (CPSC) works to ensure the safety of consumer products such as toys, cribs, power tools, cigarette lighters, household chemicals, and other products that pose a fire, electrical, chemical, or mechanical hazard.

Drugs of Abuse

The Department of Justice's DEA works to enforce the controlled substances laws and regulations of the United States, including as they pertain to the manufacture, distribution, and dispensing of legally produced controlled substances.

Meat and Poultry

The USDA's Food and Safety Inspection Service regulates aspects of the safety and labeling of traditional (nongame) meats, poultry, and certain egg products.

Pesticides

The Environmental Protection Agency (EPA) regulates many aspects of pesticides. EPA sets limits on how much of a pesticide may be used on food during growing and processing and how much can remain on the food sold to consumers.

Vaccines for Animal Diseases

The USDA's Animal and Plant Health Inspection Service (APHIS), Center for Veterinary Biologics, regulates aspects of veterinary vaccines and other types of veterinary biologics.

Water

EPA regulates aspects of drinking water. EPA develops national standards for drinking water from municipal water supplies (tap water) to limit the levels of impurities.

Source: FDA 101. *An overview of FDA's regulatory review and research activities.* Retrieved July 5, 2018, from http://www.fda.gov/AboutFDA/WhatWeDo/ucm407684.htm

Special Safety Issues. Even with all the above regulations concerning healthcare technology, safety concerns remain. A brief discussion of current important problems follows.

Counterfeits. The U.S. FDA refers to the counterfeit problem using the abbreviation SSFFC, signifying Substandard, Spurious, Falsely labeled, Falsified, and Counterfeit medical products.[113]

While the United States has a relatively small percentage of products that fit into this category, increasing costs of prescription medication have boosted ordering from online pharmacies, some of which are located outside the country. In attempting to remedy this problem, the National Association of Boards of Pharmacy issues the Verified Internet Pharmacy Practice Sites (VIPPS) certificate, an accreditation that requires an internet pharmacy to comply with the licensing and survey requirements of its home state and each state to which it dispenses pharmaceuticals.[114]

Still, patients persist in using uncertified sites. The potential scope and complexity of the problem, when it does occur, can be staggering. For example, the largest counterfeit drug recall occurred in 2003, when 18 million Lipitor tablets were pulled off the market. The counterfeit process started with ingredients that were shipped from the Hong Kong office of a Swiss company to a manufacturer in Costa Rica; the drug was then repackaged in Nebraska and distributed primarily by still another company in Missouri.[115]

The FDA has developed a cooperative plan with other nations to try to combat SSFFC Medical Products. The framework for this effort is displayed in Exhibit 7.6.

Design flaws. Despite rigorous review processes for medical devices, sometimes only time and actual use will reveal unanticipated flaws. Two examples illustrate this problem.

In October 2007, Medtronic suspended worldwide distribution of its Sprint Fidelis family of defibrillation leads after 268,000 had been implanted worldwide.[116] The leads were thinner than previous versions to reduce clots in the blood vessels into which they were inserted and to make the insertion easier for the cardiologist. The problem was that the thinness also made them more susceptible to fracture, especially in younger, more active patients.[117]

As computerized physician order entry (CPOE) systems started being used in hospitals in the early 2000s, they were touted as reducing medical errors, thus enhancing patient safety. In most respects, these systems did accomplish their aims. However, after many systems were

---

[113]The terminology is the same as that used by the World Health Organization: Substandard, spurious, falsely labeled, falsified, and counterfeit (SSFFC) medical products. Fact sheet January 31, 2018. Retrieved July 5, 2018, from http://www.who.int/mediacentre/factsheets/fs275/en

[114]National Association of Boards of Pharmacy. Retrieved from http://www.nabp.net/programs/accreditation/vipps

[115]Case Study: Lipitor U.S. Recall 12/3/07. Retrieved July 5, 2018, from https://www.pfizer.com/files/products/LipitorUSRecall.pdf

[116]Defibrillators deliver a shock to the heart when a life-threatening rhythm occurs. This "lead" connects the electrical power source implanted under the skin of the chest with the tip in the heart where the shock is delivered.

[117]For more information on this recall, see *Medtronic recalls Sprint Fidelis cardiac leads: Questions and answers for consumers.* Retrieved July 5, 2018, from http://rifflawfirm.com/wp-content/uploads/2015/05/Medtronic-Recalls-Sprint-Fidelis-Cardiac-Leads_-Questions-and-Answers-for-Consumers.pdf; and FDA. *Class 1 device recall Medtronic Sprint Fidelis lead.* Retrieved from https://www.accessdata.fda.gov/scripts/cdrh/cfdocs/cfres/res.cfm?id=65383

EXHIBIT 7.6. FDA Global Strategic Framework for SSFFC Medical Products

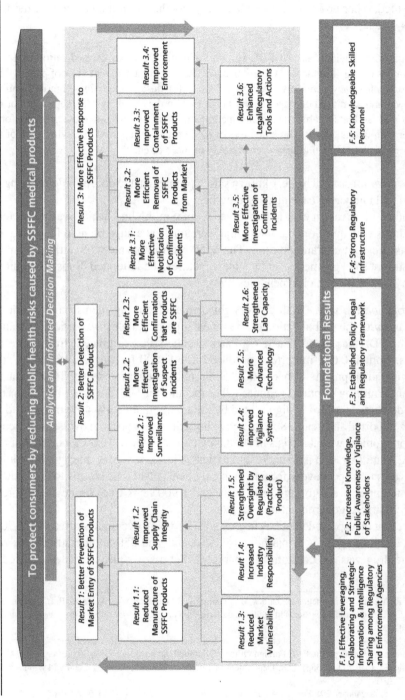

Source: FDA. *FDA global strategic framework for SSFFC medical products*. Retrieved July 5, 2018, from https://www.fda.gov/downloads/Drugs/ResourcesForYou/Consumers/BuyingUsingMedicineSafely/CounterfeitMedicine/UCM451841.pdf

implemented, other problems arose. One study, conducted at the Hospital of the University of Pennsylvania,

> [F]ound that a widely used CPOE system facilitated 22 types of medication error risks. Examples include fragmented CPOE displays that prevent a coherent view of patients' medications, pharmacy inventory displays mistaken for dosage guidelines, ignored antibiotic renewal notices placed on paper charts rather than in the CPOE system, separation of functions that facilitate double dosing and incompatible orders, and inflexible ordering formats generating wrong orders. Three quarters of the house staff reported observing each of these error risks, indicating that they occur weekly or more often.[118]

Deception/Tampering. The best-known safety problem in the deception/tampering category is the Tylenol tampering case discussed earlier.

Another, more recent example involved GlaxoSmithKline, which was convicted of selling "20 drugs with questionable safety that were made at a huge plant in Puerto Rico that for years was rife with contamination ... The $150 million payment to settle criminal charges was the largest such payment ever by a manufacturer of adulterated drugs. The outcome also provides $600 million in civil penalties."[119]

Regulatory inadequacy. Quality oversight of manufacturing plants has become a monumental task with the globalization of the medical product industry, particularly pharmaceuticals. The FDA has noted that it regulates products that originated from more than 150 countries, from 130,000 importers, produced in 300,000 foreign facilities. The number of FDA-regulated shipments at over 300 U.S. ports has quadrupled over 10 years and is now more than 24 million shipments annually. The fact that the U.S. drug supply chain is no longer solely a domestic concern is highlighted by the reality that nearly 40% of finished products are being imported and nearly 80% of active ingredients come from overseas sources.[120] The inspection problem was at a crisis in 2008, when the *New York Times* reported that "the Food and Drug Administration is so understaffed that, at its current pace, the agency would need at least 27 years to inspect every foreign medical device plant that exports to the United States, 13 years to check every foreign drug plant and 1,900 years to examine every foreign food plant, according to government investigators."[121]

The event that spurred the FDA to enhance its foreign oversight started in late 2007 when Baxter's anticlotting drug, heparin, caused 4 deaths and 350 additional adverse reactions. When the drug was pulled from the market in February 2008, it was discovered that the

---

[118] Koppel, R., Metlay, J. P., Cohen, A., Abaluck, B., Localio, A. R., Kimmel, S. E., & Strom, B. L. (2005). Role of computerized physician order entry systems in facilitating medication errors. *Journal of the American Medical Association*, *293*, 1197–1203.

[119] Harris, G., & Wilson, D. (2010, October 27). $750 million fine for drug maker of tainted goods. *New York Times*, A1.

[120] See Report to Congress on the FDA Foreign Offices. Submitted pursuant to Section 308 (c) of the FDA Food Safety Modernization Act (P. L. 111–353). U.S. Department of Health and Human Services, Food and Drug Administration. February 12, 2012.

[121] Harris, G. (2008, January 29). For F.D.A., a major backlog overseas. *New York Times*, A15.

Chinese plant where it was manufactured had no drug certification—neither China nor the FDA had inspected it. In this lapse, the FDA admitted that it had violated its own policy by allowing the supplier to become a major source of the medication for the United States.[122] The full investigation of this incident took 4 years and revealed that 22 Chinese companies may have been involved in producing contaminated heparin, which was linked to 81 possible deaths worldwide.

As previously mentioned, one result of this crisis was enactment of the FDASIA, signed into law on July 9, 2012 (P.L. 112-144). Title VII of the law expanded the FDA's examination authority and enhanced penalties.[123] The law, however, did not address the lack of ability to inspect products. Recognizing the need to work with other governments, in 2011, the FDA formulated the "Pathway to Global Product Safety and Quality."[124] The Pathway's Pillars require the agency to:

- Partner with foreign counterparts to create global coalitions of regulators to ensure and improve global product safety

- Build global data information systems and networks and proactively share data with peers

- Expand intelligence gathering, with an increased focus on risk analytics and thoroughly modernized information technology capabilities

- Effectively allocate agency resources based on risk, leveraging combined efforts of government, industry, and public and private third parties

By increasing the number of inspectors in India and China and partnering with European governments, inspections of domestic and foreign facilities (particularly the latter) for both drugs and devices have increased.[125] In 2017, the United States and the European Union agreed to mutual recognition of national inspection agencies to review manufacturing processes in their respective jurisdictions.[126]

Misuse of technology. Misuse of established and well-vetted technologies can have adverse outcomes with the risks of using some being greater than others. The ECRI[127] conducts research and reviews the danger of these technologies. The scope of this problem is illustrated in a recent list of technology hazards. (Please see Exhibit 7.7.)

---

[122]Bogdanich, W., & Hooker, J. (2008, February 16). China didn't check drug supplier, files show. *New York Times*, A1.

[123]The Food and Drug Administration Safety and Innovation Act (FDASIA). (2018). Retrieved July 5, 2018, from https://www.fda.gov/RegulatoryInformation/LawsEnforcedbyFDA/SignificantAmendmentstotheFDCAct/FDASIA/default.htm

[124]FDA. (2011, July 7). *Pathway to global product safety and quality.* Retrieved July 5, 2018 from https://www.hsdl.org/?view&did=4123 Of note is that this document is located on the Homeland Security website.

[125]FDA. 2017 Annual report on inspections of establishments in FY 2016. Retrieved July 5, 2018 from https://www.fda.gov/downloads/regulatoryinformation/lawsenforcedbyfda/significantamendmentstothefdcact/fdasia/ucm539110.pdf

[126]FDA News. (2017, March 9). U.S., E.U. agree on mutual recognition of drug manufacturing inspections. Retrieved July 5, 2018 from http://www.fdanews.com/articles/180801-us-eu-agree-on-mutual-recognition-of-drug-manufacturing-inspections

[127]Founded in 1968, ECRI (originally known as the Emergency Care Research Institute) started its focus in emergency medicine, resuscitation, and related biomedical engineering. Shortly thereafter it expanded its scope across all aspects of care involving medical products. See www.ecri.org

EXHIBIT 7.7. **2019 Top 10 Patient Safety Concerns**

1. Diagnostic Stewardship and Test Result Manage ment Using EHRs
2. Antimicrobial Stewardship in Physician Practices and Aging Services
3. Burnout and Its Impact on Patient Safety
4. Patient Safety Concerns Involving Mobile Health
5. Reducing Discomfort with Behavioral Health
6. Detecting Changes in a Patient's Condition
7. Developing and Maintaining Skills
8. Early Recognition of Sepsis across the Continuum
9. Infections from Peripherally Inserted IV Lines
10. Standardizing Safety Efforts across Large Health Systems

Source: ECRI: 2019 Top 10 Patient Safety Concerns Executive Brief. https://assets.ecri.org/PDF/White-Papers-and-Reports/2019-Top10-Patient-Safety-Concerns-Exec-Summary.pdf Retrieved April 17, 2019.

An important consideration in this category is problems that arise from technology which is used simply because it exists: the so-called *technological imperative*. As Fuchs described it: "[T]he physician's approach to medical care and health is dominated by what may be called a technologic imperative. In other words, medical tradition emphasizes giving the best care that is technically possible; the only legitimate and explicitly recognized constraint is the state of the art."[128]

The impetus to use technology in this fashion comes not only from a physician's desire to do everything possible for the patient; often it is incentivized by financial rewards and the fear of a malpractice lawsuit if the diagnosis is missed (no matter how remote the chance). The use of technology in this latter case is termed "defensive medicine." (See the discussion about costs of malpractice in the Malpractice and Defensive Medicine section below.)

The harm of the technological imperative is illustrated by the following example:

To the shock of many cancer experts, the most common cancer in South Korea is not lung or breast or colon or prostate. It is now thyroid cancer, whose incidence has increased fifteen-fold in the past two decades ... The thyroid cancer rate in the United States has more than doubled since 1994. Cancer experts agree that the reason for the situation in South Korea and elsewhere is not a real increase in the disease. Instead, it is down to screening, which is finding tiny and harmless tumors that are better left undisturbed, but that are being treated aggressively.[129]

---

[128]Fuchs, V. R. (1968). The growing demand for medical care. *New England Journal of Medicine, 279,* 190–195.
[129]Kolata, G. (2014, November 4). Study points to overdiagnosis of thyroid cancer. *New York Times,* sA4.

This increased use (and spurious cancer detection) followed the addition of coverage for thyroid ultrasound to screening exams.

Laboratory testing. An exception to the safety crisis-reaction sequence of laws was passage of the "Clinical Laboratories Improvement Act of 1967," or CLIA'67 (Section 5 of Public Law 90-174). The purpose of the Act was to regulate licensing of clinical labs engaged in interstate commerce. Because of advances in laboratory diagnostics and changes in business models in the mid-1980s, the DHHS commissioned a study to modify CLIA'67. The result was the *Final report on assessment of clinical laboratory regulations*, submitted in April, 1986.[130] Among its recommendations were federal standardization of regulations and a focus on measurement of objective outcomes to assess compliance. These recommendations found their way into Public Law 100-578, the *Clinical Laboratory Improvement Amendments of 1988.*[131] Final regulations were published in 1992, phased in through 1994, and amended in 1993, 1995, and 2003. Despite these changes, the law is still cited as CLIA '88. "In general terms, the CLIA regulations establish quality standards for laboratory testing performed on specimens from humans, such as blood, body fluid and tissue, for the purpose of diagnosis, prevention, or treatment of disease, or assessment of health."[132]

CLIA mandates that the FDA categorize laboratory tests according to seven dimensions:

1. Knowledge
2. Training and experience
3. Reagents and materials preparation
4. Characteristics of operational steps
5. Calibration, quality control, and proficiency testing materials
6. Test system troubleshooting and equipment maintenance
7. Interpretation and judgment

The FDA then ranks these items in complexity from 1 (lowest) to 3 (highest) to determine a test's overall complexity. "For commercially available FDA-cleared or approved tests, FDA scores the tests using these criteria during the pre-market approval process. The final score determines whether the test system is categorized as moderate or high complexity. Tests

---

[130]Kenney ML, Greenberg DP. Final report on assessment of clinical laboratory regulations. Submitted to the Office of the Assistant Secretary for Planning and Evaluation, DHHS, by Macro Systems, Inc., Silver Spring, MD, April 8, 1986. A more accessible form of the report is: Kenney, ML: Quality Assurance in Changing Times: Proposals for Reform and Research in the Clinical Laboratory Field. *Clin. Chem.* (1987) 33 (2): 328–336.

[131]Available at: https://www.govinfo.gov/content/pkg/STATUTE-102/pdf/STATUTE-102-Pg2903.pdf Retrieved May 31, 2019.

[132]CDC: Division of Laboratory Systems. https://www.cdc.gov/csels/dls/ Retrieved May 31, 2019.

developed by the laboratory or that have been modified from the approved manufacturer's instructions default to high complexity according to the CLIA regulations."[133]

CMS has the primary responsibility for the operation of the CLIA program through its Center for Medicaid and State Operations, Survey and Certification Group, and Division of Laboratory Services.

The CDC also plays an import role in the CLIA by:

▪ Providing analysis, research, and technical assistance

▪ Developing technical standards and laboratory practice guidelines, including standards and guidelines for cytology

▪ Conducting laboratory quality improvement studies

▪ Monitoring proficiency testing practices

▪ Developing and distributing professional information and educational resources

▪ Managing the Clinical Laboratory Improvement Advisory Committee (CLIAC)

For tests classified as moderate to high complexity, the laboratories or sites that perform these tests need to have a CLIA certificate, be inspected, and must meet the CLIA quality standards. The complexity standards also include qualification of personnel.

In addition to the tests classified as moderate to high complexity, CLIA also has a category whereby a test can be "waived" of certain requirements if it demonstrates low risk if an incorrect result is obtained.[134] Falling into this category are certain tests listed in the CLIA regulations; tests cleared by the FDA for home use; and tests that the manufacturer applies to the FDA for waived status by providing scientific data that verifies that the CLIA waiver criteria have been met. The sites that perform these tests must still have a CLIA certificate and be able to demonstrate they are following the manufacturer's instructions.

CLIA is funded by user fees and penalties[135] that CMS assesses for violators (listed in an annual report).[136]

In summary, the topic of safe healthcare technology can be characterized by reactive governmental measures in response to often predictable crises. Unfortunately, political considerations and special interests have prevented timely preemptive measures. Hope

---

[133]CDC: Test complexities. Available at: https://www.cdc.gov/clia/test-complexities.html Retrieved May 31, 2019.

[134]FDA: CLIA - Tests waived by FDA from January 2000 to present. https://www.accessdata.fda.gov/scripts/cdrh/cfdocs/cfClia/testswaived.cfm Retrieved May 31, 2019.

[135]Sanctions can include suspension from the program or monetary penalties that vary by type of infraction. See: CMS.gov: Civil Monetary Penalties (Annual Adjustments) https://www.cms.gov/Medicare/Provider-Enrollment-and-Certification/SurveyCertificationGenInfo/Civil-Monetary-Penalties-Annual-Adjustments.html Retrieved May 31, 2019

[136]CMS.gov: Laboratory Registry. https://www.cms.gov/Regulations-and-Guidance/Legislation/CLIA/Laboratory_Registry.html Retrieved May 31, 2019.

for improvement lies at the institutional levels and devotion to system-wide quality improvement. (Please see Chapter 9, "Quality.")

Bringing Healthcare Technology to Market

Before looking at restructuring trends, it is necessary to understand the current functions that are needed to bring a technology to market. In this section, the focus will be on the pharmaceutical industry, though, as mentioned previously, similar principles apply to medical devices and diagnostics. Exhibits 7.8 and 7.9 outline the new drug development process; highlights are explained in the next list.

- *Basic research/discovery.* Companies have traditionally carried out this function themselves in-house or by contracts with university partners. Recognizing the financial potential of such deals, universities have established technology transfer offices to handle such relationships. For example, in 2007, "Northwestern sold the rights to about half of its Lyrica royalties for $700 million ... Total royalties amounted to about $1.4 billion, including annual payments plus the value of the rights the university sold. ... Lyrica is now responsible for as much as 18% of the $10 billion Northwestern endowment."[137]

- *Clinical trials.*

   Clinical trials are conducted in a series of steps, called phases—each phase is designed to answer a separate research question.

   Phase I. Researchers first test a new drug or treatment in a small group of people for the first time to evaluate its overall safety, determine a safe dosage range, and identify side effects.

   Phase II. The drug or treatment is given to a larger group of people to see if it is effective and to further evaluate its safety.

   Phase III. The drug or treatment is given to large groups of people to confirm its effectiveness, monitor side effects, compare it to commonly used treatments, and collect information that will allow the drug or treatment to be used safely.[138]

- *Patent application.* Depending on when the developer realizes the potential success of the product, it applies for patent protection. As previously mentioned, this protection is separate from the market exclusivity the FDA can grant in certain cases.

---

[137]Lorin, J. (2016, August 18). The pill that made Northwestern rich. *Bloomberg BusinessWeek*. Retrieved July 5, 2018, from http://www.bloomberg.com/news/articles/2016-08-18/the-pill-that-made-northwestern-rich
[138]U.S. National Library of Medicine. Retrieved July 5, 2018, from http://ClinicalTrials.gov—Clinical Trial Phases. www.clinicaltrials.gov

EXHIBIT 7.8. Stages in the Typical Brand-Name Drug Development Process

New Drug Development Process: Steps from Test Tube to NDA Review

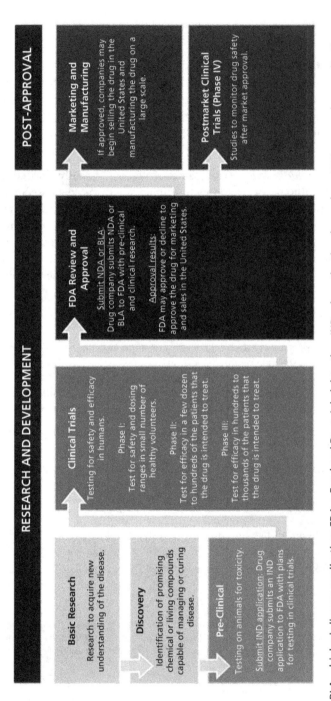

BLA = biologic license application; FDA = Food and Drug Administration; IND = investigational new drug; NDA = new drug application

Source: GAO. (2017, November). *Report to congressional requesters: Drug industry, profits, research and development spending, and merger and acquisition deals.* Retrieved July 5, 2018, from https://www.gao.gov/assets/690/688472.pdf

EXHIBIT 7.9. **Drug Discovery and Development**

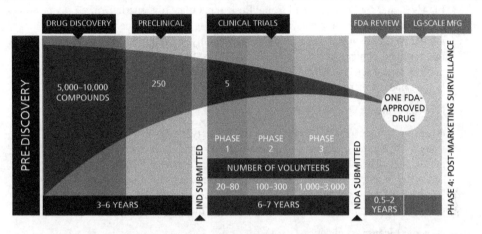

Source: PhRMA. *New medicines in development for diabetes, 2012*. Retrieved July 5, 2018, from http:// phrma-docs.phrma.org/sites/default/files/pdf/12-535phrmaoverviewdiabetes1109.pdf Also see PhRMA (2017, Spring). Biopharmaceuticals in Perspective. Retrieved July 4, 2018, from http://phrma-docs.phrma .org/files/dmfile/Biopharmaceuticals-in-Perspective-2017.pdf

■ *Regulatory application.* The common types of drug applications to the FDA[139] are:

Investigational New Drug (IND)

Current federal law requires that a drug be the subject of an approved marketing application before it is transported or distributed across state lines. Because a sponsor (the manufacturer or licensee or company) will probably need to ship the investigational drug to clinical investigators in many states, it must seek an exemption from that legal requirement. The IND is the means through which the sponsor technically obtains this exemption from the FDA.

New Drug Application (NDA)

When the sponsor of a new drug believes that enough evidence on the drug's safety and effectiveness has been obtained to meet FDA's requirements for marketing approval, the sponsor submits to FDA a new drug application (NDA). The application must contain specific technical data for review, including chemistry, pharmacology, medical, biopharmaceutics, and [statistical evaluation of the clinical trials]. If the NDA is approved, the product may be marketed in the United States. For internal tracking purposes, all NDA's are assigned an NDA number.

---

[139]Retrieved July 5, 2018, from http://www.fda.gov/Drugs/DevelopmentApprovalProcess/HowDrugsareDevelopedand Approved/ApprovalApplications

Abbreviated New Drug Application (ANDA)

An Abbreviated New Drug Application (ANDA) contains data that, when submitted to FDA's Center for Drug Evaluation and Research, Office of Generic Drugs, provides for the review and ultimate approval of a generic drug product. Generic drug applications are called "abbreviated" because they are generally not required to include preclinical (animal) and clinical (human) data to establish safety and efficacy. Instead, a generic applicant must scientifically demonstrate that its product is bioequivalent (i.e., performs in the same manner as the innovator drug)...

Over the Counter Drugs (OTC)

Over-the-counter (OTC) drugs play an increasingly vital role in America's health care system. OTC drug products are those drugs that are available to consumers without a prescription. There are more than 80 therapeutic categories of OTC drugs, ranging from acne drug products to weight control drug products. As with prescription drugs, CDER [Center for Drug Evaluation and Research] oversees OTC drugs to ensure that they are properly labeled and that their benefits outweigh their risks.

Biologic License Application (BLA)

Biological products are approved for marketing under the provisions of the Public Health Service (PHS) Act. The act requires a firm who manufactures a biologic for sale in interstate commerce to hold a license for the product. A biologics license application is a submission that contains specific information on the manufacturing processes, chemistry, pharmacology, clinical pharmacology and the medical effects of the biologic product. If the information provided meets FDA requirements, the application is approved and a license is issued allowing the firm to market the product.

- *Manufacturing.* This process ranges from sourcing of raw materials (including biologic substrates) to finished product production to packaging.
- *Marketing/Sales.* These functions range from internal company planning, to managing a sales force, to price negotiations with public and private entities, to ultimate product sales.
- *Postmarket surveillance (Phase IV study).* After the technology reaches the marketplace, it is constantly monitored for adverse reactions ranging from mild side effects to death.

Evolving Industry Structure

All of the functions above had traditionally been performed by the company itself in an integrated, single-entity business model. However, the structure of the healthcare technology industry has been changing in at least two major ways.

First, there has been a great deal of merger, acquisition, and alliance activity over the past 20 years, particularly in the pharmaceutical sector. (Please see Exhibit 7.10 for many prominent examples.)

A principal, though not exclusive, reason for these combinations is the desire of companies to fill their pipelines with new products as the older ones go off patent. The effectiveness

EXHIBIT 7.10. Pharma Industry Merger and Acquisition Analysis, 1995 to 2015

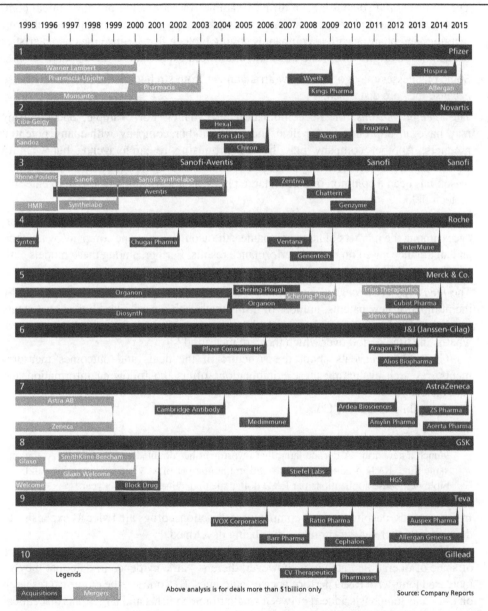

Source: Vij, R. (2016, February 17). *Pharma industry merger and acquisition analysis, 1995 to 2015*. Retrieved July 5, 2018, from http://revenuesandprofits.com/pharma-industry-merger-and-acquisition-analysis-1995-2015

of these strategies has been questioned for more than a decade, and the research results do not provide clear-cut answers. Some of the problems that confound evaluation include:

- The *nature of the companies* can differ. Examples include: large pharmaceutical company mergers, large pharmaceutical companies acquiring small ones, small biotech firms merging, and pharmaceutical companies buying biotech firms. Since the characteristics of each of the original firms are different, one would expect the results to vary.

- Some businesses may go into a new arrangement from strength while others may do so because they are distressed.

- The *specific reasons* for the combination also matter. For example, one company may have an unpromising pipeline and seek another company with many potential products. Another company may have a promising research agenda but want to diversify into a new class of products it has not investigated previously. This latter reason has been a common one when large pharmaceutical companies wish to enter the biotech field.

- The *operational nature* of the deals also varies. For example, there can be great differences among the mergers of large companies, the acquisition of one company by another, and an alliance based on mutual performance results. Further, among these models, cultural compatibilities can have varying degrees of importance.

- The *measures of success* across studies varies. For example, is success measured by the number of new patents, number of drugs that reach a particular clinical trial stage, number of NDAs, or product revenue? Also, when one or more of these metrics are used, what is the time period over which they are measured?

    Given these caveats about the structure of the deals and outcomes measurements, research evaluating these combinations offers the following information and conclusions:

    According to Bain & Co.:

    > [I]in the late 1990s, pharma companies spent an average of $1.1 billion to develop and launch a new drug. A decade later, that investment has doubled to $2.2 billion. At the same time, R&D productivity, measured in the number of new molecular entities and biologic license applications per R&D dollar spent, declined by 21% a year.[140]

In other words, despite growing company combinations, drugs are twice as expensive to develop, and there are fewer new drugs being developed.

    Large company mergers have achieved short-term cost savings through economies of scale of operational activities; however, there is "little evidence to date that they've increased long-term R&D performance or outcomes. By contrast, the empirical research on *alliances* [emphasis added] between smaller biotech firms and larger pharmaceutical

---

[140]Farcas, C., & van Biesen, T. (2009, June 26). The real reason Big Pharma mergers are wise. *Forbes*. Retrieved July 5, 2018, from http://www.forbes.com/2009/06/26/big-pharma-mergers-leadership-governance-acquisitions.html

entities is more encouraging in nature."[141] Further, "products developed in an alliance have a higher probability of success in the more complex late stage trials, particularly if the licensee is a large firm."[142] The reason for this latter finding may be that large-scale trials and regulatory expertise at a *global level* are required to ensure the critical factor of speed to market for these products.

The second trend in the industry restructuring has occurred as companies discovered benefits of outsourcing specialized functions; large companies then act as the coordinators of these activities. The important questions here are: What functions should companies outsource, and which should they keep in-house? A diversity of opinions and actual company actions highlight attempts to answer these questions. Using the above categories of product development, we can address the industry's current status.[143]

- *Basic research/discovery.* The Bain & Co. study mentioned above explains why this task should be moved, to a large degree, outside the company:

    > Innovation is one area where scale doesn't work ... Innovation can't be manufactured; it must be nurtured in a highly entrepreneurial environment. That argues for acquiring new compounds from a large global pool of smaller, independent, innovation-focused companies. In fact, the big pharma deals have better odds of success if the companies involved move quickly to reduce the scale of their internal research. They should shift 40% to 50% of their current innovation budgets to outside their newly merged companies.

    Indeed, there has been a trend toward larger companies using smaller ones as sources of new products. The financial deals usually take the form of some combination of up-front payments, milestone payments, and royalties. Another trend in this area is for larger companies to spin off parts of research and development functions into smaller companies. For example, in 2010, GSK spun off a biotech research group Convergence Pharmaceuticals in which it took an 18% stake.[144]

- *Clinical trials.* As companies seek to predict research costs and avoid staffing up for one-off clinical trials, they are increasingly hiring outside firms to manage these studies. The outside organizations that they employ are called contract research organizations (CROs). Companies may also hire outside firms (called functional service

---

[141] Grabowski, H., & Kyle, M. (2008). Mergers and alliances in pharmaceuticals: Effects on innovation and R&D productivity. In K. Klaus Gugler, B. Burcin, & B. B. Yurtoglu (Eds.), *Economics of corporate governance and mergers* (pp. 262–287). Northampton, MA: Edward Elgar.

[142] Danzon, P. M. (2016, Fall). Economics of the pharmaceutical industry. *NBER Reporter*. Retrieved July 5, 2018, from http://www.nber.org/reporter/fall06/danzon.html

[143] See, for example: Bounds, A. (2017, April 9). Pharma investors put less skin in the game as risk appetite wanes: Focus is on leaving marketing, manufacturing and global distribution to others. *Financial Times*. Retrieved July 5, 2018, from https://www.ft.com/content/f07ee806-1adf-11e7-bcac-6d03d067f81f?desktop=true

[144] Ward, A. (2014, June 15). GSK spin-off gears up for possible listing. *Financial Times*. Retrieved July 5, 2018, from https://www.ft.com/content/9bdf9b4a-f46a-11e3-a143-00144feabdc0

providers[FSPs]) for *portions* of these trials. This outsourcing activity was estimated at $36.27 billion in 2017 and expected to grow to $56.34 billion by 2023.[145]

Some observers of this trend disagree with its logic as a business strategy. For example, Christiansen et al.[146] believe a

> far better strategy would be to focus on the place in the value chain that is becoming decommoditized: the management of clinical trials, which are now an integral part of the drug research process and so a critical capability for pharmaceutical companies. Despite this, most drug makers have been outsourcing their clinical trials to contract research organizations such as Covance and Quintiles, better positioning those companies in the value chain. Acquiring those organizations, or a disruptive drug maker like Dr. Reddy's Laboratories, would help reinvent big pharma's collapsing business model.

In addition to outsourcing the performance of trials, large companies are increasingly also taking on investment partners to pay for the trials to mitigate their riskiness. Examples include NovaQuest Capital Management, LLC and Avillion, LLC.[147]

- *Regulatory filing and compliance.* Outsourcing regulatory affairs is particularly useful for small companies that do not have experience dealing with the FDA. This function is a core competency of larger firms. For both types of businesses, however, it is often helpful to hire an outside company to help with part of the process if they are filing outside the United States.

  External expertise with such tasks as language translation, application formatting, and identification of appropriate governmental agencies can be very helpful.

- *Sales and marketing.* This function has been the traditional province of large, well-established companies. Smaller firms, however, can incur large fixed costs by staffing up to promote just one product. Consequently, these firms often hire companies that can detail their products to potential purchasers or prescribers. Sometimes these outside firms are larger companies in the same sector that have a business arrangement to copromote a product.

- *Manufacturing.* Given the global nature of the sources or components of healthcare products, it is difficult for companies to directly own and control the manufacturing process from start to finish. Consider, for example, a pill. The raw ingredients, often coming from India or China, are transformed into a therapeutic chemical entity, after which it is crafted into a form (tablet, capsule, etc.) that can be swallowed. The final product must then be bottled, labeled, and shipped. All of these processes may be done at different sites by different companies.

---

[145] IGEA HUB. (2018). Top 10 CROs, 2018. Retrieved July 5, 2018, from https://www.igeahub.com/2018/03/15/top-10-global-cros-2018

[146] Christiansen, C. (2011, March 1). The big idea: The new M&A playbook. *HBR*, 49–57.

[147] See, for example: Roland D. (2017, May 1). Drug firms learn from Hollywood. *The Wall Street Journal*, B3.

With these restructuring trends comes an increase in system complexity. Even after the product has come to market, the relationships can be equally complex. (Please see Exhibit 7.11 for an example using relationships in the pharmaceutical industry.) Coordination of activities has become much more important to decrease the likelihood that errors will occur—perhaps leading to more and more costly regulation.

EXHIBIT 7.11. **Flow of Goods and Financial Transactions among Players in the U.S. Commercial Pharmaceutical Supply Chain**

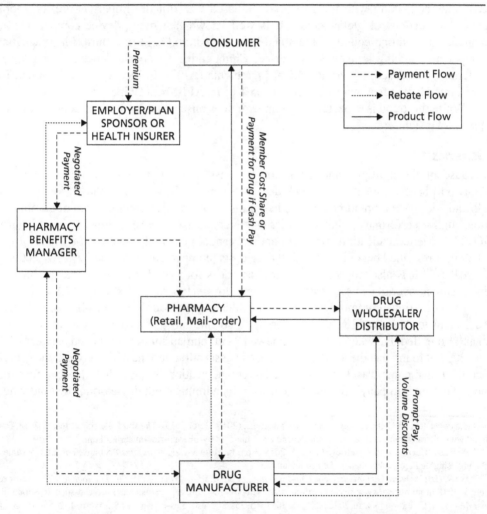

Source: Kaiser Family Foundation. (2005, February 28). *Follow the pill: Understanding the U.S. commercial pharmaceutical supply chain*. Retrieved July 5, 2018, from http://kff.org/other/report/follow-the-pill-understanding-the-u-s

Globalization

Globalization of healthcare technology is also characterized by mergers/acquisitions/ alliances and supply chain activity. The former group is highlighted in the pharmaceutical sector by the activity displayed in Exhibit 7.10. This globalization also involves the medical device industry. One example is the Shenzhen-based imaging company Mindray. The company entered the United States in 2004 and by 2006 was listed on the New York Stock Exchange. In 2008, it bought Datascope Patient Monitoring (a New Jersey–based company) for $200 million. Its strategy is to provide diagnostic imaging equipment at lower cost, thus competing with the likes of U.S.-based GE. Equally important are the supply chain implications of globalization. It is well known that many device components are manufactured in one country, assembled in a second, and sold in a third. Pharmaceutical component sourcing is likewise dispersed. China and India are the largest source of raw materials, called active pharmaceutical ingredients (APIs). In fact, China's dominance is highlighted by the fact that India imports 65% of *its* APIs from China.[148]

While this trend is expected to continue, it does raise concerns about accountability and quality oversight.

Generics

Because of the multiple, and often complex, issues around generics, this section will focus on pharmaceuticals. The FDA defines a generic drug as one that "is identical—or bioequivalent—to a brand name drug in dosage form, safety, strength, route of administration, quality, performance characteristics and intended use."[149] According to consulting firm IQVIA, generic medications (branded and unbranded) currently account for about 89% of all drugs prescribed but only 23% of all drug costs (compared to 86% and 29%, respectively, in 2013).[150] It is also important to note that prices for *branded* generics are significantly increasing as overall generic costs are trending down. (Please see Exhibit 7.12.)

Two questions commonly arise when evaluating generic drug use. First, are generics equivalent to their brand name counterparts? For the most part, the answer is yes. Davit et al.[151] reported that when the FDA reviewed 2,070 human studies conducted between 1996 and 2007, it found that the average difference in absorption into the body between the generic and the brand name was 3.5%. However, a few medications require that the same formulation (the same company's product) is consistently administered; the reason is that individual

---

[148]India dependent on China for key pharma raw materials. (2016, October 19). *The Week*. Retrieved July 5, 2018, from http://www.theweek.in/news/biz-tech/india-dependent-china-for-key-pharma-raw-materials.html

[149]U.S. FDA. *Generic drugs*. Retrieved July 5, 2018, from https://www.fda.gov/Drugs/ResourcesForYou/Consumers/BuyingUsingMedicineSafely/GenericDrugs/default.htm

[150]IQVIA. (2017, December). *Medicine use and spending in the U.S.: A review of 2017 and outlook to 2022*. Retrieved July 5, 2018, from https://www.iqvia.com/-/media/iqvia/pdfs/institute-reports/medicine-use-and-spending-in-the-us-a-review-of-2017-and-outlook-to-2022.pdf?_=1530817469251 See also, Kesselheim, A. S., Avorn, J. & Sarpatwari, A. (2016). The high cost of prescription drugs in the United States, origins and prospects for reform. *JAMA*, 316(8), 858–871.

[151]Davit, B. M., Nwakama, P. E., Buehier, G. J., Conner, D. P., Haidar, S. H., Patel, D. T., … Woodstock, J. (2009). Comparing generic and innovator drugs: A review of 12 years of bioequivalence data from the United States Food and Drug Administration. *Annals of Pharmacotherapy*, 43(10), 1583–1597.

EXHIBIT 7.12. **Express Scripts Prescription Price Index**

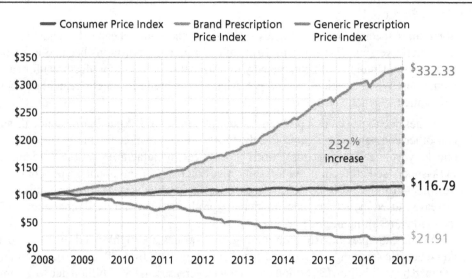

Source: Express Scripts. *2017 drug trend report*. Retrieved July 5, 2018, from http://lab.express-scripts .com/lab/drug-trend-report/~/media/2b56ec26c9a04ec2bcca0e9bf1ea8ff1.ashx

absorption and metabolism can sometimes vary dramatically. Examples of such products include warfarin (Coumadin), thyroxine (Synthroid), digoxin (Lanoxin), and diphenylhydantoin (Dilantin).

The second question that is commonly asked is: Are generics always cheaper? The answer is, increasingly, no. A 2015 survey commissioned by Bloomberg News found that of more than 21,000 generic drugs reviewed, in excess of 3,500 have at least doubled their prices since late 2007; the drugs were not in any particular class but ranged from basic chemotherapy medicines to older antibiotics.[152] The reason for these price increases include:

1. As is the case with orphan drugs, the potential market for some generic drugs is so small that it cannot support multiple producers. Example: Pyrimethamine (Daraprim) is a very old drug for treating the parasite toxoplasmosis. After Turing Pharmaceuticals bought the rights from GlaxoSmithKline (its sole manufacturer) in 2015, it raised the price by 5,000%, from $13.50 to $750 per pill.

2. Market consolidation can reduce the number of manufacturers, leading to higher prices. Example: Colchicine, a gout remedy known to the ancient Greeks, was manufactured

[152]Langreth, R., & Koons, C. (2015, October 6). 2,000% drug price surge is a side effect of FDA safety program. *Bloomberg News*. Retrieved July 5, 2018, from http://www.bloomberg.com/news/articles/2015-10-06/2-000-drug-price-surge-is-a-side-effect-of-fda-safety-program

in the United States by URL Pharma. In 2012, Takeda purchased the company and branded the drug (Colcrys). In doing so, it raised the price from about 25 cents to almost $6 per pill.

3. Sometimes special contractual deals make the brand name cheaper for patients than the generic version. Example: In 2011, after Lipitor (atorvastatin) became available as a generic, UnitedHealth contracted with Pfizer (the brand's manufacturer) for steep reductions. When a patient filled a prescription, the brand had a copayment of about $30 while the generic cost $50.

4. Shortages due to production problems. Example: In 2013, Hikma Pharmaceuticals and two other companies accounted for about 90% of the market for the generic antibiotic doxycycline. That year, these firms experienced manufacturing problems requiring FDA-supervised correction. As a result, prices increased from about $5 per course of treatment to about $100. By 2015, once the quality problems were corrected, this price increase caused these companies to increase production and attracted other entrants in the market, resulting in price declines.

While examples of extremely high generic prices are highlighted in the popular press, generic spending has declined each year from 2014; from 2016 to 2017, spending declined by $5.5 billion ($5 billion due to price decreases and $0.5 billion due to volume decreases).[153]

In the near future, the FDA's Office of Generic Drugs says it will focus on "postmarket evaluation of generics; equivalence standards for complex drug products and locally acting products, therapeutic equivalence evaluation ... computational tools ... research on evaluating modified release formulations, identifying the role replica design studies can play in determining bioequivalence and piloting surveillance methods for generics using the Sentinel program."[154]

Specialty Pharmaceuticals

These products need to be considered separately because they are growing in number and expense and account for the greatest part of increases in pharmaceutical costs. The following facts[155] highlight this trend:

- Specialty share of net spending across institutional and retail settings rose from 24.7% in 2008 to 46.5% in 2017.

- The largest proportion of new medicines launched in the last 5 years have been specialty drugs, and specialty share of spending has risen, while traditional net medicine spending has declined by more than $133 per person over the past decade.

---

[153]IQVIA. *Medicine use and spending in the U.S.: A review of 2017 and outlook to 2022*, op. cit.
[154]OGD aims to finish up work on scientific priorities from prior years. *FDANews Drug Daily Bulletin, 3* (2016, November). Retrieved July 5, 2018, from http://www.fdanews.com/articles/179108-ogd-aims-to-finish-up-work-on-scientific-priorities-from-prior-years
[155]IQVIA. *Medicine use and spending in the U.S.: A review of 2017 and outlook to 2022*, op. cit.

- In terms of prescription volume, specialty represents just 1.9% of prescriptions and 37.4% of spending in the same retail and mail-order distribution channels.

- In nonretail settings, specialty drugs represent 60% of invoice spending and 2.3% of standard unit volumes.

There is no uniform definition for these drugs, but they tend to share some or all the following characteristics:

1. Very expensive on a per-patient basis.

2. Indicated for treatment of chronic conditions.

3. Treat diseases that are often rare with few alternative therapies, such as orphan drugs.

4. Injectable but usually not self-administered. Exceptions include drugs for multiple sclerosis.

5. Often biological in origin. To repeat the definition,

> [t]he term "biological product" means a virus, therapeutic serum, toxin, antitoxin, vaccine, blood, blood component or derivative, allergenic product, protein (except any chemically synthesized polypeptide), or analogous product, or arsphenamine or derivative of arsphenamine (or any other trivalent organic arsenic compound), applicable to the prevention, treatment, or cure of a disease or condition of human beings.[156]

   The explosion in the biologics sector was aided by these factors: understanding of the genetic basis for diseases, the ability to rapidly and (relatively) cheaply sequence genetic material, passage of the Orphan Drug Act, and development of the biotechnology industry.

6. Frequently administered on an outpatient basis, particularly a physician's office. This aspect has profound reimbursement implications, since physicians can greatly profit from choosing more expensive medications rather than cheaper and equally effective alternatives.

7. Require special handling in their distribution channels (e.g., controlled temperature, reformulation before administration, patient education).

The five top categories of these drugs, in declining order of annual sales, are: (1) analgesics—anti-inflammatories; (2) multiple sclerosis; (3) anticancer agents; (4) antivirals (including hepatitis C and HIV treatments); and (5) endocrine and metabolic agents. These medications account for about 80% of spending in this class.[157]

---

[156]United States Code, 2011 Edition: Title 42—The Public Health and Welfare, Chapter 6A: Public Health Service Subchapter II—General Powers and Duties. Part F —Licensing of Biological Products and Clinical Laboratories subpart 1—biological products, Sec. 262—Regulation of biological products. Retrieved July 5, 2018, from https://www.gpo.gov/fdsys/pkg/USCODE-2011-title42/html/USCODE-2011-title42-chap6A-subchapII-partF-subpart1-sec262.htm

[157]Navitus Health Solutions. *2017 drug trend*. Retrieved July 5, 2018, from https://www.navitus.com/getdoc/1d79601c-59a6-47cf-bb81-a1c3bfea402c/Drug-Trend-Report_2017.aspx

Because these medicines are very expensive, payers have adopted a variety of strategies to control costs. These methods apply to all expensive technologies, not just specialty drugs.

1. *Employing disease management* (please see the Managed Care section in Chapter 6, "Payers"). Payers have internal units or hire outside companies to attend to patients with rare, high-cost diseases or conditions that are very common (such as diabetes and heart failure). The hope is that this special attention will result in more appropriate use of high-cost medications.

2. *Contracting with a specialty pharmacy/pharmaceutical benefit manager (PBM)*. Payers either have subsidiaries or contract with independent companies that manage pharmacy benefits on their behalf. Certain firms specialize in tracking and managing specialty pharmaceuticals. Prominent examples include: BriovaRX, which is a subsidiary of OptumRX, owned by UnitedHealth Group; CVS Caremark Specialty Pharmacy, owned by CVS Health; and Accredo, a division of Express Scripts. Contracts usually include management fees as well as incentives to control costs. Providers (such as physicians) must order the drugs from one of these companies.

3. *Requiring prior authorization*. When a drug is expensive, and often when it is first launched, payers want the option to review its necessity by using predetermined protocols. For example, a physician may need to call a special phone number (frequently staffed by a PBM) to get authorization to prescribe a medication. Obtaining this permission often does not prevent the drug's use but does determine whether the payer will cover its expense.

4. *Restricting off-label use*. When an FDA-approved medication can be used for nonapproved indications, payers will often check to make sure the patient's disease is one of the *approved* indications to ensure payment.[158]

5. *Implementing physician-developed guidelines*. When a treatment is very new and appears to effectively treat a disease, national guidelines may not be available. Payers will, therefore, often convene local experts to decide on appropriate use. This process may be ad hoc or as part of an ongoing review by the payer's Pharmacy and Therapeutics (P&T) Committee, which makes formulary decisions.

6. *Changing the benefit design*. On average, specialty pharmaceuticals are paid 60% from pharmacy benefits and 40% medical benefits.[159] (Variations from these figures can occur by insurer [e.g., Medicare, Medicaid, private payer] as well as by site of care [e.g., hospital, physician's office, home, etc.].) For example, a patient may be responsible only for a physician's office copayment while receiving a medication billed to the insurer at tens of thousands of dollars. Some plans have moved the basis for payment to the pharmacy benefit at a level that requires the patient to pay a coinsurance—often

---

[158] Japan provides an interesting international example with respect to off-label prescribing. If, for example, an oncologist uses one nonapproved medication in the treatment regimen, the insurer will not pay for *any* of the drugs used.

[159] *EMD Serono Specialty Digest* (14th ed.) (2018). Retrieved July 5, 2018, from https://specialtydigestemdserono.com/?id=jklyHFlrXSCnRIblnaAzxNDRDA7t5GHAcXSLNxHXjojAQqBtjUXQ4JOTLM+uUJ+9k1FMhevkooeEqryQ8cklM7hIijMoiBtzUx3PSsGJNzU=

thousands of dollars. Other strategies for shifting the benefit design include increasing deductibles or copayments for these medications. (Patient responsibility is, of course, subject to annual out-of-pocket limits.) This cost-control method is, however, flawed in the long run. Making patients responsible for any costs for goods or services works only if they can make choices about their care. Since these medications are often used for chronic and, frequently, life-threatening indications, there is no discretionary component. In fact, creating a financial barrier to their use may result in greater expenses for the payer if the patient does not take the medications. One way pharmaceutical companies are responding to these increased out-of-pocket expenses is by a method called *couponing*. These companies raise their charges for medications but provide patients with coupons to cover their increased out-of-pocket expenses. Some insurance plans have responded by banning use of the coupons or making their use less appealing for patients. For example, in 2018, PBM "Express Scripts and others introduced a new 'copay accumulator' approach for its corporate customers. The programs prevent copay card funds from counting toward a patient's required out-of-pocket spending before insurance kicks in on expensive specialty drugs, such as arthritis and HIV treatments."[160] The Centers for Medicare & Medicaid Services (CMS) has taken retaliation a step further by suing offenders. For example, when Pfizer contributed to a charity that helped patients pay for the company's drugs, CMS won a $23.85 million judgment. As U.S. Attorney Andrew Lelling said in a statement: "Pfizer knew that the third-party foundation was using Pfizer's money to cover the co-pays of patients taking Pfizer drugs, thus generating more revenue for Pfizer and masking the effect of Pfizer's price increases."[161]

7. *Selective contracting with infusion centers.* Since some providers charge more than others, insurance companies look to selective contracting to provide volume in return for lower prices for care.

8. *Bundling with service payment.* Instead of paying separately for the service component and medication, payers are contracting with providers to bundle the entire episode of care into one fee. For example, recall from Chapter 6 that Medicare's End Stage Renal Dialysis program requires injectable medications (such as erythropoietin) be billed with the global episode of dialysis. Other such initiatives include courses of treatment for cancers.

   It should be noted that part of this bundling process assumes payment is made for services that occur over a period of time, not just one encounter. Consider another example: treatment of high blood pressure. Instead of paying by episode, bundling would take into account such treatment components as additional medications required

---

[160]Erman, M., & Humer, C. (2018, July 5). Drugmakers try evasion, tougher negotiations to fight new U.S. insurer tactic. *Reuters*. Retrieved July 6, 2018, from https://www.reuters.com/article/us-usa-healthcare/drugmakers-try-evasion-tougher-negotiations-to-fight-new-u-s-insurer-tactic-idUSKBN1JV1AX

[161]Kaiser Health News. (2018, May 25). Pfizer settles with U.S. over practice of using charity to pay kickbacks to Medicare patients. Retrieved July 6, 2018, from https://khn.org/morning-breakout/pfizer-settles-with-u-s-over-practice-of-using-charity-to-pay-kickbacks-to-medicare-patients

to achieve the target pressure, laboratory tests needed to monitor the medication (e.g., to prevent side effects), and handling adverse reactions.

9. *Removing "buy and bill" incentives.* Physicians typically buy specialty pharmaceuticals from a specialty PBM or directly from the manufacturer. They then bill the insurance company at rates that are often significantly higher than acquisition cost. (The exception is Medicare Part B, which allows only a 6% markup over national average sales price. Please see Chapter 6 for more details.) Some insurers have instituted a process by which the physician orders the drugs and the company pays the PBM the acquisition cost. Obviously, this change has caused much resentment from physicians (e.g., oncologists) whose revenue largely depends on those markups.

10. *Establishing pay-for-performance metrics.* Insurance companies pay not only for the medications that work but also for those that do not. To mitigate this problem, insurers have contracted with pharmaceutical companies to pay only for the treatment courses that achieve a predetermined goal. For example, Merck "agreed to peg what the insurer Cigna pays for the diabetes drugs Januvia and Janumet to how well Type 2 diabetes patients are able to control their blood sugar."[162] Similar deals have been applied to more expensive medications, such as those that treat multiple sclerosis.[163]

11. *Sequencing multiple therapeutically equivalent medications.* Some treatment classes contain medications with similar efficacy and rates of side effects. However, the costs for each of these medications can vary significantly. For example, in 2014, the wholesaler acquisition cost (WAC) of a 30-day course of maintenance treatment for rheumatoid arthritis ranged from about $702 (Orencia, BMS) to $14,100 (Rituxan, Genentech). Other drugs in this class are priced at about $2,800.[164] Having physicians choose the lowest-cost effective drug in a class, and then the next most expensive if the first fails, can achieve significant savings.

12. *Incentivizing prescription of generic medications.* Many terms have been applied to generic forms of specialty medications. Differences among these terms are important because their approval and usage indications can vary. With respect to the "reference product" (original branded medication), *biosimilars*: (a) are very similar in structure; (b) do not have any clinically meaningful differences in safety and effectiveness; (c) are allowed to have only minor differences in clinically inactive components; and (d) cannot be automatically substituted. Biosimilars are sometimes called *follow-on biologics*. *Bioequivalent* or *interchangeable* medications are biosimilar but also meet other standards that allow pharmacists to substitute them for the reference product

---

[162]Pollack, A. (2009, April 22). Drug deals tie prices to how well patients do. *New York Times*, B1.

[163]See also Rubenfire, A. (2016, December 10). Pay-for-performance drug pricing: Drugmakers asked to eat costs when products don't deliver. *Modern Healthcare*. Retrieved July 6, 2018, from http://www.modernhealthcare.com/article/20161210/MAGAZINE/312109949?utm_source=modernhealthcare&utm_medium=email&utm_content=20161210-MAGAZINE-312109949&utm_campaign=dose

[164]Drugs for rheumatoid arthritis (2014). *The Medical Letter on Drugs and Therapeutics, 56*(1458), 127–132.

without the order of the prescriber. *Biobetter* medications are based on the reference product but claim to offer improvements.

Savings from these medications will be determined by their development and production costs, which are substantially more than nonbiologic medications. As a result, while generic nonbiologics are typically discounted by about 80%, biosimilars and bioequivalents may be discounted only by 15% to 30%.[165] However, because the reference drugs are so expensive, even this smaller reduction can be significant. "Cumulative potential savings to health systems in the European Union … and the U.S., as a result of the use of biosimilars, could exceed EUR50 billion in aggregate over the next five years and reach as much as EUR100 billion."[166] Some major specialty drugs losing patent protection in the near future include Herceptin (trastuzumab), June 2019; Avastin (bevacizumab), July 2019; Aranesp (darbepoetin alfa), May 2024; and Enbrel (etanercept), November 2028.

13. *Enabling pharmacists to substitute generics.* Once interchangeable medications are available, allowing pharmacists to substitute them for the reference products can save payers and patients money. Enabling laws to allow this substitution are the province of individual states and will be subject to much lobbying by pharmaceutical companies and others whose profits are lowered by this action.

14. *Using pharmacogenomics.* With advances in understanding how genes determine the effectiveness of therapies, physicians can better predict who will benefit from certain treatments, particularly very expensive ones. For example, the HER2-neu receptor protein predicts the response to Herceptin in breast cancer patients. Both clinicians and payers now require genetic profiles where drug choices depend on their results.

15. *Requiring step therapy.* For many conditions, successful treatment is often not achieved with a single dose of one medication. Instead, these diseases are treated with a series of medications in a stepwise fashion—escalating doses and/or use of more medications that may be more expensive and have more adverse effects. Payers often insist that practitioners follow guidelines for adjusting therapy before the most expensive medication is prescribed. For example, a patient with chronic asthma might be sequentially treated with an inhaled corticosteroid, long-acting beta agonist, and leukotriene receptor antagonist before omalizumab (Xolair) is administered.[167]

---

[165] Singh, S. (2016, May 3). Basics about biosimilars: The savings potential and the challenges. *CVSHealth Insights, 6.* Retrieved July 6, 2018, from https://payorsolutions.cvshealth.com/insights/basics-about-biosimilars

[166] IMS Institute for Healthcare Informatics [now part of IQVIA]. (2016, March). Delivering on the potential of biosimilar medicines: The role of functioning competitive markets. Retrieved July 6, 2018, from https://www .iqvia.com/-/media/iqvia/pdfs/institute-reports/delivering-on-the-potential-of-biosimilar-medicines.pdf?la=en& hash=03018A6A86DED8F901DDF305BAA536FF0E86F9B4&_=1530986176970

[167] National Asthma Education and Prevention Program, Third Expert Panel on the Diagnosis and Management of Asthma. (2007, August). *Guidelines for the diagnosis and management of asthma: Section 4, stepwise approach for managing asthma in youths ≥12 years of age and adults.* Bethesda, MD: National Heart, Lung, and Blood Institute. Retrieved July 6, 2018, from https://www.ncbi.nlm.nih.gov/books/NBK7222/figure/A2212/?report=objectonly See also *Global initiative for asthma: 2018 pocket guide for asthma management and prevention.* Retrieved from https://ginasthma.org/download/ 836

16. *Mandating specialist evaluation/use.* For some specialty medications, payers will authorize use only by practitioners with certain expertise and experience. Using the asthma example above, some companies will pay for omalizumab only if it is prescribed and administered by an allergist or pulmonologist.

17. *Reducing waste.* Ordering just the right dose for individual patients can save costs. For example, if a practitioner orders a multidose vial for more than one course of treatment, often extra medication is left over. Payment for more than a patient needs is costly. However, this extra medication can be used in other patients at no additional cost to the specialist. Strictly speaking, this practice is illegal when treating Medicare patients; however, enforcement is often lax.

18. *Payment using reference products or indexes.* Since many of these products are new, and sometimes unique, a manufacturer's pricing can be arbitrarily extremely high. By using a variety of reference and indexing techniques, payers can get closer to a true market rate. These techniques are commonly used by countries outside the United States that can mandate fee schedules for their national health plans. (Please see Exhibit 7.13 for a list of these methods.)

EXHIBIT 7.13. Reference/Index Pricing Methods and Example Countries

- *Lowest-priced identical chemical entity—active ingredient formulation, such as generics* (generic referencing)

    Examples: United States, Canada (some provinces), Sweden, Spain, Denmark

- *Lowest price in therapeutic class* (therapeutic referencing)

    Examples: Germany, the Netherlands, New Zealand, British Columbia

- Representative drug in class as benchmark for payment

    Examples: Most European countries

- *Market basket of prices from different countries*

    Example: Canada (Patented Medicine Prices Review Board)

- Maximum price lowest of list of comparison countries

    Example: Brazil

- Total cost per time period comparisons

    Examples:

    Weighted average monthly treatment cost in therapeutic categories (Australia, e.g., for ACE inhibitors, statins, calcium channel blockers, proton pump inhibitors, and selective serotonin reuptake inhibitors)

    Defined daily dose (DDD) cost of therapy, average cost within a category (Germany)

■ Additional opportunity for pharmacist ability/mandate to substitute: generic and/or therapeutic class

   Examples:

   Notify patient of generic equivalent, patient decides (Finland, South Africa, and Slovakia)

   Mandatory substitution of lowest-cost generic alternative (Sweden)

   A variation on this method for lowering costs applies exclusively for the patient's benefit. Many U.S. insurance companies forbid pharmacists to tell patients when their drugs are cheaper when they pay out of pocket than they are if patients are using their insurance and paying a copayment (or coinsurance). This prohibition is called a "gag clause." Legislators are currently looking into such arrangements and considering making the practice illegal.[168]

19. *Gathering data*. Finally, payers must have timely and accurate access to data to ensure compliance with whichever of the above methods it chooses to employ.

Patents

While the issue of U.S. patents is discussed above, an international issue has affected American companies. World Trade Organization (WTO) agreements allow governments to issue *compulsory licenses* that permit, without approval of the patent holder, the manufacture, import, and sale of cheaper generic versions of drugs. This permission is granted in special cases, such as a national public health emergency.[169] Some African countries as well as Brazil and Thailand have used compulsory licenses to circumvent the high costs of medications to treat HIV infection and cancers.

Genomics and Precision Medicine

The WHO defines genomics as

the study of genes and their functions, and related techniques.

The main difference between genomics and genetics is that genetics scrutinizes the functioning and composition of the single gene whereas genomics addresses all genes and their interrelationships in order to identify their combined influence on the growth and development of the organism.[170]

The introduction of genomics into healthcare technology marks a departure from traditional medical practice that is built around diagnosis and treatment of the "average"

---

[168]Firozi, P. (2018, July 5). The Health 202: "Gag clauses" mean you might be paying more for prescription drugs than you need to. *Washington Post*. Retrieved July 5, 2018, from https://www.washingtonpost.com/news/powerpost/paloma/the-health-202/2018/07/05/the-health-202-gag-clauses-mean-you-might-be-paying-more-for-prescription-drugs-than-you-need-to/5b3a36ca1b326b3348addc4a/?noredirect=on&utm_term=.714601c14174

[169]World Trade Organization. (2018, March). Compulsory licensing of pharmaceuticals and TRIPS. Retrieved July 6, 2018, from https://www.wto.org/english/tratop_e/trips_e/public_health_faq_e.htm

[170]WHO. *Human genomics in global health*. Retrieved from http://www.who.int/genomics/geneticsVSgenomics/en/

patient. With the emergence of genomics, the focus has shifted to customizing treatments for individual patients, a process often called *personalized medicine*. However, this method of care is extremely time-consuming and expensive. The approach has therefore shifted to surveying many characteristics of individuals across large populations. Researchers gather disease-specific information as well as genetic, environmental, and lifestyle differences so that customized individual therapies can be informed by these large data sets. This new approach is called *precision medicine*. As explained by the National Academy of Sciences:

> "[P]recision medicine" refers to the tailoring of medical treatment to the individual characteristics of each patient. It does not literally mean the creation of drugs or medical devices that are unique to a patient, but rather the ability to classify individuals into subpopulations that differ in their susceptibility to a particular disease, in the biology and/or prognosis of those diseases they may develop, or in their response to a specific treatment. Preventive or therapeutic interventions can then be concentrated on those who will benefit, sparing expense and side effects for those who will not.[171]

Though the genetic part of precision medicine started with Gregor Mendel's presentation of his plant hybridization research in 1865, accelerated scientific discoveries began in 1953 when Watson and Crick "discovered" the double helix structure of DNA.[172] The promise of clinical utility for DNA sequencing got a boost in 2003 when the federally financed Human Genome Project announced completion of its work in sequencing the human genome. At the start of this project, its director, Dr. Francis Collins, stated that knowledge from the research

> will dramatically accelerate the development of new strategies for the diagnosis, prevention, and treatment of disease, not just for single-gene disorders but for the host of more common complex diseases (e.g., diabetes, heart disease, schizophrenia, and cancer) for which genetic differences may contribute to the risk of contracting the disease and the response to particular therapies.[173]

However, in 2010, 10 years after the first, preliminary, human genome results were announced, the prospects for its utility were more guarded. As Khoury et al. wrote:

> Never before has the gap between the quantity of information and our ability to interpret it been so great. Whole-genome sequencing will produce abnormal results in all who are tested: everyone will have positive results, false positives and false negatives. Some results may prove harmful; some will be useless. Preserving the health benefits of genomics while minimizing the harms will be an important research goal.[174]

---

[171]Committee on A Framework for Developing a New Taxonomy of Disease, National Research Council, National Academy of Sciences. (2011). *Toward precision medicine, building a knowledge network for biomedical research nd a new taxonomy of disease*. Washington, DC: The National Academies Press.

[172]See National Human Genome Research Institute. All about the Human Genome Project (HGP). Retrieved July 6, 2018, from https://www.genome.gov/10001772

[173]Collins, F. S. (1999). Consequences of the Human Genome Project. *The New England Journal of Medicine, 341*, 28–37.

[174]Khoury, M. J., Evans, J., & Burke, W. (2010). A reality check for personalized medicine. *Nature, 464*, 680.

The problem with realization of the benefits of genomic research are twofold. First, although there are many examples of single mutations strongly identified with diseases (e.g., HER2 and BRCA 1 and 2), many conditions are associated with numerous mutations at differing sites. These multiple variations make it difficult to pin down the causes of diseases and, hence, cures. A related problem is that the presence of some of these mutations does not necessarily imply that the associated disease is inevitable.

The second problem concerns important gene modifications not typically detected by routine sequencing. These modifications are called *epigenetic* changes. The word "epigenetic" literally means "on top of the gene" and is most frequently characterized by addition of a methyl group on a gene:[175] this change disrupts the cell's ability to "read" the affected sequence, thus turning a function on or off. The effects of these changes vary from cell to cell and in which organ they occur. They can be functional, causing normal cell differentiation, or dysfunctional, leading to unrestrained tumor growth if a suppressor gene is silenced. Like basic genetic codes, epigenetic changes can also be passed to offspring. Therefore, until epigenetic changes can be routinely sequenced and are fully understood, mere genetic mapping will not give an unambiguous picture of disease mechanisms.

Despite these caveats, several business models have been developed that rely on population-based genetic data. Some of these models are described below.

1. *Collection of genetic data from large groups can potentially elucidate disease mechanisms to guide the design of gene-based cures.* An early company example is deCode Genetics (now owned by Amgen). Founded in 1996 in Reykjavik, the company's idea was to gather genetic data from the homogenous and relatively inbred Icelandic population, looking for small coding differences (single nucleotide polymorphisms called SNPs, pronounced "snips")[176] that could cause diseases. The revenue model was sale of this information to other companies that would use it to develop diagnostic and therapeutic products. Two years later, Dr. J. Craig Venter founded Celera (now part of Quest Diagnostics), a private company that directly competed with the federally sponsored Human Genome Project in speed and cost to complete mapping of the human genome.[177] Venter's business model was also to gather genetic code differences and make them available commercially.

    As sequencing equipment has become faster and cheaper, more individual genomes can be sequenced and compared. (Please see Exhibit 7.14 for the progress of this technology.) In addition to entry of other business-to-business companies in this sequencing sector, this lower cost has also led to formation of business-to-consumer companies, like

---

[175] Another epigenetic modification can involve histones—the proteins around which DNA wraps itself. Changes in histones can cause DNA to be wound tightly or loosely, thus giving cellular replication mechanisms harder or easier access to genetic transcription.

[176] U.S. National Library of Medicine. (2018, July 3). *What are single nucleotide polymorphisms (SNPs)?* Retrieved July 3, 2018, from https://ghr.nlm.nih.gov/primer/genomicresearch/snp

[177] For a detailed accounting of the very contentious race to finish coding the human genome, see Shreeve, J. (2004). *The genome war: How Craig Venter tried to capture the code of life and save the world.* New York: Knopf.

EXHIBIT 7.14. **Cost of Sequencing One Genome**

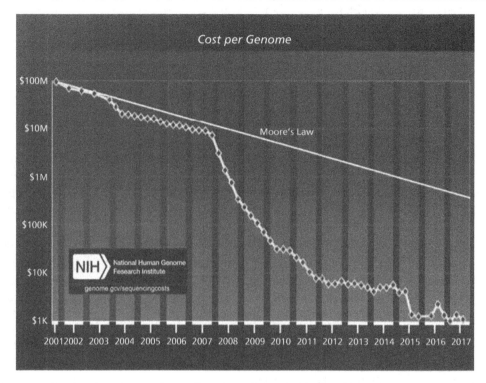

Source: National Human Genome Research Institute. (2018, April 25). *DNA sequencing costs: Data from the NHGRI Genome Sequencing Program (GSP)*. Retrieved July 6, 2018, from https://www.genome.gov/sequencingcostsdata

23 and Me. From a sputum sample submitted by mail, for about $100 the company will sequence certain "high-risk" genes rather than the entire genetic sequence. Concerns have arisen about the predictive value of these findings and what individuals can and will do with the information. The recommendations the company provided to customers with their results were so worrisome that, after November 22, 2013, the FDA prohibited the company from furnishing interpretations of the findings; it was then directed to supply only ancestral information and basic genetic data. In response, 23andMe subsequently resubmitted an application under the regulatory pathway for low-to-moderate risk devices. On April 6, 2017, the FDA allowed the company to directly market to the

public its screening for the likelihood to develop 10 diseases, including Parkinson's, Alzheimer's, and celiac disease.[178]

2. *Pharmacogenomics uses gene sequencing data to help physicians predict the effectiveness of certain drugs for specific diseases as well as the likelihood of side effects.* This tool was described in the earlier Specialty Pharmaceuticals section for drugs used for oncology. It has also been proven useful for such conditions as schizophrenia.[179]

3. *Techniques are being developed to diagnose cancers from small amounts of DNA circulating in the blood: so-called liquid biopsies.* However, other methods of detection may be more useful at earlier stages of the disease when tumor cells have not entered the bloodstream.

4. *Methods for targeted gene insertions or deletions have recently become available.* Using research on adaptive mechanisms of bacteria, these techniques are based on CRISPR (clustered regularly interspaced short palindromic repeats) and CRISPR-associated (Cas) genes.[180] While this therapy has enormous potential to treat such genetic conditions as hemophilia and sickle cell disease, ethical issues still need to be fully considered, since this technology can also be used to "improve" individuals, not just cure known diseases. For example, consider the implications of using this knowledge to manipulate fetal genes. Also, information about unintended complications from this technology continues to emerge.[181]

5. Another medical application of this technology is insertion of genes in plants and yeast to cause them to "manufacture" drugs.

6. *Nontargeted introduction of genes to correct defects is also being developed.* The first such treatment was Glybera (alipogene tiparvovec), each dose containing trillions of viruses that carry functioning copies of the lipoprotein lipase gene. Patients who lack the enzyme the gene produces cannot properly process fats in the blood. The problem is not effectiveness but cost—the therapy's price is $1 million.[182]

---

[178]See FDA allows marketing of first direct-to-consumer tests that provide genetic risk information for certain conditions. (2017, April 6). Retrieved July 6, 2018, from https://www.fda.gov/NewsEvents/Newsroom/PressAnnouncements/ucm551185.htm

[179]Foster, A., Miller, D. D., & Buckley, P. (2007). Pharmacogenetics and schizophrenia. *Psychiatric Clinics of North America, 30*(3), 417–435.

[180]Sander, J. D., & Joung, J. K. (2014). CRISPR—Cas systems for editing, regulating and targeting genomes. *Nature Biotechnology, 32,* 347–355.

[181]See, for example: Charlesworth, C. T., Deshpande, P. S., Dever, D. P., Dejene, B., Gomez-Ospina, N., Mantri, S., ... Porteus, M. H. (2018, January 5). *Identification of pre-existing adaptive immunity to Cas9 proteins in humans: bioRxiv* (Cold Spring Harbor Laboratory). Retrieved July 6, 2018, from https://www.biorxiv.org/content/early/2018/01/05/243345.article-info

[182]Regalado, A. (2016, May 4). The world's most expensive medicine is a bust. The first gene therapy approved in the Western world costs $1 million and has been used just once. The doctor who tried it says the price is "absolutely too high." *MIT Technology Review.* Retrieved July 7, 2018, from https://www.technologyreview.com/s/601165/the-worlds-most-expensive-medicine-is-a-bust

As more information becomes available, genetic behavior will have more useful roles in individualizing treatments. At present, there are many worries about use of this knowledge, including usefulness to predict disease, ability to institute effective treatments, and concern about ethical issues of genetic manipulation.

Disruptive Innovation

The term "disruptive innovation" was originally defined and explained in 1995 by Clay Christensen and colleagues.[183] Ten years later, Professor Christensen reviewed this concept and how the term has been misapplied. He defines disruption as:

> a process whereby a smaller company with fewer resources is able to successfully challenge established incumbent businesses. Specifically, as incumbents focus on improving their products and services for their most demanding (and usually most profitable) customers, they exceed the needs of some segments and ignore the needs of others. Entrants that prove disruptive begin by successfully targeting those overlooked segments, gaining a foothold by delivering more suitable functionality—frequently at a lower price. Incumbents, chasing higher profitability in more-demanding segments, tend not to respond vigorously. Entrants then move upmarket, delivering the performance that incumbents' mainstream customers require, while preserving the advantages that drove their early success. When mainstream customers start adopting the entrants' offerings in volume, disruption has occurred.[184]

The example Christensen most frequently cites is in the computer industry. Originally, computers were large and expensive machines used for complex tasks, such as research calculations and military applications. Disruptive companies, like Apple, introduced products that were much lower cost and served an overlooked segment—individual users. Companies such as IBM ignored these entrants as they improved products for their traditional customers. We know the outcome—personal computers replaced the original equipment in all but a few applications, such as supercomputers.

Disruptive innovation as defined by Christensen does not, however, describe all innovative technologies that significantly change the way medicine is practiced or delivered. Disruptive innovations can come into common practice without altering the relationship among cost, quality, and access, or it may force a trade-off decision among these health system dimensions. By contrast, a truly "disruptive technology" will add value to the healthcare system by improving one or more dimensions without a required trade-off. The result is a new Pareto optimal state.

Consider the following example to illustrate this point. Prior to 1970, when diabetic patients needed blood sugar tests, they went either to their doctors' offices or a local hospital to have blood drawn. The sample was then processed by a hospital or commercial

---

[183]Bower, J. L., & Christensen, C. M. (1995, January–February). Disruptive technologies: Catching the wave. *HBR*, 43–53.

[184]Christensen, C. M., Raynor, M., & McDonald, R. (2015, December). What is disruptive innovation? *HBR*, 44–53. For application of this concept to healthcare, see Hwang, J., & Christensen, C. M. (2008). Disruptive innovation in healthcare delivery: A framework for business-model innovation. *Health Affairs, 27*(5), 1329–1335.

laboratory. The results typically took a day, after which physicians called the patients back with results and further instructions on management. In 1970, the Ames Company launched its Reflectance Meter,[185] which gave physicians and emergency rooms a tool with which to perform point-of-care blood sugars, thus increasing access and timeliness of care. Further, the test was cheaper than assays performed in large laboratories. Over time, the "glucometer" machines became cheaper and portable, allowing patients to perform testing at home or elsewhere. Portability gave patients the ability to perform more tests and thus better control their blood sugars. Thus, this technology lowered cost per test, improved access, and enhanced quality by allowing patients to better regulate their blood sugars. This example also points out another exception to the disruptive innovation story: an expensive, institutionally based technology becomes cheaper and easier to use and moves to the point of care. This trajectory is far more common than that of "disruptive innovations."

Another example of a disruptive technology is the introduction of newer oral anticoagulants (medications that slow blood clotting). These medications have a variety of uses, such as preventing stoke in patients with atrial fibrillation and treating those with existing blood clots. Introduced into clinical use in 1954, warfarin[186] (dicoumerol) was the first oral medication for this indication. While effective, its daily dosing is very individual and often requires frequent blood testing to maintain a therapeutic blood level. Further, there are many drugs with which it interacts, and patients must adhere to some dietary restrictions. Since the main side effect is bleeding, it is often underdosed. On the positive side, if bleeding occurs, the medication can be easily reversed.

Because of those problems, the need arose for oral medications with standard dosing that did not require frequent tests, had fewer drug interactions and food restrictions, and performed as well or better than warfarin. The first such drug was dabigatran (Pradaxa), originally introduced in Europe in 2008 and approved by the FDA for stroke prevention in 2010. Rivaroxaban (Xarelto), which acted by a different mechanism,[187] followed shortly thereafter. Subsequent research showed that these medications performed at least as well as warfarin and had fewer bleeding episodes. The results looked so good that, in 2011, one industry report[188] predicted that by the end of 2013, as much as 50% of warfarin use could

---

[185] Between 1965 and 1970, Ames Company and Boehringer Mannheim produced chemical strips that turned colors depending on the glucose content of the blood place on it. However, the results were "semi-quantitative." On April 22, 1968, Anton Hubert Clemens of Ames Company filed a patent for a "Reflectance Meter." When blood was placed on the chemically treated strip and the strip was then inserted into this machine, it displayed an actual number—the patient's blood glucose. Ames Company (then a division of Miles Laboratories, which Bayer subsequently purchased) commercially launched the Reflectance Meter in 1970, though the patent (3604815) was not granted until September 14, 1971. Since then, many companies have produced their own glucometers, and by competition, lowered the cost even further.

[186] This drug was discovered by Dr. Karl Paul Link in 1941 at the Wisconsin Alumni Research Fund, hence the name WARFarin. It was isolated from spoiled sweet clover that was causing some cows to bleed and have spontaneous abortions. Since the 1940s it has been used as a rat poison. Human use as an anticoagulant became more widespread after it was used to treat President Eisenhower when he had a heart attack in 1955.

[187] Dabigatran is a thrombin inhibitor, while rivaroxaban is a Factor Xa inhibitor.

[188] *Medco 2011 drug trend report*. (2012, April). Retrieved July 7, 2018, from http://lab.express-scripts.com/lab/insights/industry-updates/the-new-drug-trend-report-is-available Medco is now part of Express Scripts.

be replaced by these new oral anticoagulants. However, two concerns slowed adoption. First, while bleeding was less frequent with the newer drugs, when it did occur, it was not reversible. Further, the medication is long-lasting; for example, in the elderly (the greatest users of these drugs), it can take 11 to 13 hours for half of rivaroxaban, the shortest-acting medication in this class, to be eliminated from the body. Second, while these newer drugs are more convenient for the patient, physicians who switched to them lost revenue from the frequent blood tests that were needed to monitor warfarin use. Still, market share increased from 6% in 2011 to about 48% by 2014.[189] Market share now appears to be increasing more rapidly due to two developments. First, many physicians who were reluctant to use the new medicines became more familiar with their performance. Second, and perhaps more importantly, in October 2015, the FDA approved the monoclonal antibody idarucizumab (Praxbind) for the reversal of the anticoagulant effects of dabigatran. While this medication should mitigate some concerns about uncontrolled bleeding, it works only with dabigatran and carries a wholesale cost of $3,500.

HEALTHCARE TECHNOLOGY'S CONTRIBUTION TO COSTS BY STAGE OF CARE

Overview

As explained in the chapter's introduction, this section will analyze how healthcare technology contributes to costs, as we consider its application to prevention, screening, diagnosis, and treatment.

First, we need to define two terms that frame how costs of technology are evaluated. The first term is *cost-benefit*. For our purposes, this term means that at the cost of a given technology, a certain benefit is derived. The benefit can be expressed by such metrics as lives saved, improved pain control, or reduced recurrence of an illness. This term is often incorrectly confused with *cost-effective*, which refers to the subjective *value of the benefit* of the technology at its stated cost. For example, consider a drug with a given condition that will prevent 1 death per 1,000 affected people. The cost of preventing 1 death is $1 million. The cost-benefit statement is a simple fact: Saving 1 life per 1,000 patients costs $1 million. The cost-effective evaluation, however, considers whether that 1 saved life per 1,000 patients is *worth* an expenditure of $1 million or if that sum can be used to better effect on another intervention for the same or a different condition.

Quality-Adjusted Life Years

One way that policy makers measure cost-effectiveness is by calculating the expense of a technology associated with *gains over time in the quality of life* of its recipients. This idea

---

[189]Barnes, G. D., Lucas, E., Alexander, G. C., & Goldberger, Z. D. (2015). National trends in ambulatory oral anticoagulant use. *The American Journal of Medicine, 128*(12), 1300–1305. e2.

led to the conceptualization of a quality-adjusted life year (QALY).[190] QALY calculations involve measuring the length of life extended by the technology, weighted by the quality of that extension:

$$QALY = \text{Length of Life Extended by the Technology} \times \text{Quality}$$

where quality is measured on a scale ranging from zero for death to 1 for perfect health.

The basic assumptions for calculating QALYs include:[191]

1. A resource-allocation decision must be made.
2. The outcomes of the alternatives can be specified in terms of health states, changes, and durations.
3. Resources are limited, and each alternative has resource implications (costs).
4. A major objective of the decision maker is to maximize health of the population, subject to resource constraints.
5. Health is defined as value-weighted time (QALYs) over the relevant time horizon.
6. Value is measured in terms of preference (desirability).
7. Each individual is risk neutral with respect to longevity and has utility that is additive across time.
8. Value scores (preferences) measured across individuals can be aggregated and used for the group.
9. QALYs can be aggregated across individuals; that is, "a QALY is a QALY" regardless of who gains/loses it.

One of the shortcomings of using QALYs to evaluate alternatives is that all of these assumptions may not be met. For example, in the United States, there is no explicit budget for healthcare; hence, the concept of saving resources on one technology so it can be used elsewhere may be meaningless in practice. (See assumption 3 above.)

In addition to problems with these assumptions, there are many methodologic issues to consider in using QALYs to evaluate the benefit of technology. Among these concerns are:

- What benefit do we choose to measure the effect on the quality of life? Is it simply an extension of longevity, or factors such as pain relief, increased independence, less medication, and so on?
- Extension of life is a linear measure whereas quality of life is not measured on a linear scale.

---

[190] Although the concept was formulated about 1970 as a measure of quality of life, this term was first used in Zeckhauser, R., & Shephard, D. S. (1976). Where now for saving lives? *Law and Contemporary Problems, 40,* 5–45. A related concept, developed in the early 1990s, is the disability-adjusted life year (DALY). For a discussion of the differences, see: Sassi, F. (2006). Calculating QALYs, comparing QALY and DALY calculations. *Health Policy and Planning, 21,* 402–440.

[191] Weinstein, M. C., Torrance, G., & McGuire, A. (2009). QALYs: The basics. *Value in Health, 12,* S5–S9.

- Since QALYs are measured over the length of the technology's benefit, the calculation strongly favors interventions in the young.

- The method of quality assessment can produce different results. For example, do we ask individuals hypothetical questions about their preferences for their own health and then aggregate the results? Or do we ask policy makers what they believe the best decisions are for populations? Do we ask individuals who would currently benefit (or be harmed) by a technology what *their* risk preferences are? Or do we ask individuals what they would do *if* they needed the technology at a future time?

- The scales used to measure quality are varied and include: EQ-5D (EuroQol); Health Utilities Index (HUI II and HUI III); Quality of Well-Being Scale (QWB); 15D; and SF-6D (derived from SF-36). Results are not consistent across the scales.

Despite all these caveats, policy makers in many countries often decide whether they will allow (and pay for) a new technology by calculating its associated QALYs and comparing that figure to a predetermined cutoff or with the QALYs for existing technology for the same condition. For example, the National Institute for Health and Care Excellence (NICE) in the United Kingdom uses QALY cutoff calculations to set benefits depending on the nature of the condition: £20,000 to £30,000 per QALY for standard treatments and £100,000 to £300,000 per QALY for rare diseases.[192] However, since technology rationing is not determined by cost in the United States, QALYs are often calculated but not used in policy decisions.

Core Cost Issues

In addition to the cost-benefit determination, another consideration about the costs of technology is its fundamental role as a driver of total healthcare costs. Indeed, it can be argued that if all waste in the healthcare system were eliminated and prices were frozen, technology would be the clear cause of future cost increases.[193] New medications for chronic conditions have highlighted this issue. For example, prices of for Sovaldi ($1,000 per pill, or $84,000 per course) and Harvoni ($1,125 per pill, or $94,500 per course) as treatments for hepatitis C infections have called attention to the problem of high-cost pharmaceuticals. (Please see the Specialty Pharmaceuticals section above for a discussion of this issue.)

The core issue of technology costs was explained by Weisbrod[194] more than 25 years ago in his classic article, "The Health Care Quadrilemma." In it, he explained the reasons for the rising costs of technology and the interplay with healthcare coverage:

[I]t is clear that much of the growth in health care expenditures during the post–World War II period has resulted not from increased prices for existing technologies, but from the price

---

[192]Paulden, M. (2017). Recent amendments to NICE's value-based assessment of health technologies: implicitly inequitable? *Expert Review of Pharmacoeconomics & Outcomes Research*, *17*(3), 239–242.

[193]While other factors, such as the aging population, might also be said to contribute to rising costs, the application of technology to this population might be argued as the root cause.

[194]Weisbrod, B. (1991). The health care qyuadrilemma: An essay on technological change, insurance, quality of care, and cost containment. *Journal of Economic Literature*, *29*(2), 523–552.

for new technologies. Newly developed technologies have driven up both costs of care and the demand for insurance, while also expanding the range of services for which consumers demand insurance. At the same time, expanding insurance coverage, which includes more people as well as a growing array of health care inputs, has provided an increased incentive to the R & D sector to develop new technologies, and a growing incentive for subsets of consumers who could benefit from particular new technologies to seek a wider definition of what would be covered by insurance.

Weisbrod presciently concluded that this relationship is dynamic and will continue to change as the reimbursement models for care evolve, particularly with a shift to having provider organizations bear more financial responsibility for patient care.

Given the above considerations, we now turn to evaluating the costs of technology by type of application. In doing so, recall Chapter 1, "Understanding and Managing Complex Healthcare Systems," where cost was explained as comprising the interplay among price, volume, and intensity. Here, technology is considered part of the intensity component. The intensity can be lower (as with generic medications) or higher (as with newer biologic pharmaceuticals).

Prevention

We first consider the well-known instances where certain preventive technologies have reduced costs for targeted populations. For example, the use of appropriate preventive, maintenance medications and immunizations have markedly reduced emergency room visits, hospitalizations, and mortality for patients with asthma. Further, it has long been known that immunizations, in general, can be cost-saving. A few long-established examples are listed below.

- "A routine, universal rotavirus immunization program would prevent 1.08 million cases of diarrhea, avoiding 34,000 hospitalizations, 95,000 emergency department visits, and 227,000 physician visits in the first five years of life ... The program would provide a net savings of $296 million to society."[195]

- "The model was used to compare costs and benefits of a combined vaccination programme (CVP) including tetanus, diphtheria, and acellular pertussis (dTap) administered at age 12, compared to current practice ... From the societal perspective, the CVP would be cost saving [Canadian] $858,106 at 10 years for the cohort." [196]

- If hepatitis A prevalence is 53% in patients with chronic liver disease, then immunizing this select group against this infection will save over $11,000 per 100 patients.[197]

---

[195]Tucker, A. W., Haddix, A. C., Bresee, J. S., Holman, R. C., Parashar, U. D., & Glass, R. I. (1998). Cost-effectiveness analysis of a rotavirus immunization program for the United States. *Journal of the American Medical Association, 279,* 1371–1376.

[196]Iskedjian, M., Walker, J. H., & Hemels, M. E. (2004) Economic evaluation of an extended acellular pertussis vaccine programme for adolescents in Ontario, Canada. *Vaccine, 22,* 4215–4227.

[197]Duncan, M., Hiroa, W. K., & Tsuchida, A. (2002). Prescreening versus empirical immunization for hepatitis A in patients with chronic liver disease: a prospective cost analysis. *American Journal of Gastroenterology, 97,* 1792–1795.

The cost-savings from prevention are not always so straightforward. For example:

A cost-effectiveness analysis was performed before initiation of the varicella vaccination program [to prevent chickenpox in children] in the United States. The results of the study indicated a savings of $5.40 for each dollar spent on routine vaccination of preschool-aged children when direct and indirect costs were considered. When only direct medical costs were considered, the benefit-cost ratio was 0.9:1.0.[198]

In other words, this vaccine saved money only when such expenses as parents' lost work time were considered.

Screening

For screening tests to have a positive cost-benefit for a particular condition, they must meet three criteria: (1) asymptomatic people can have the disease; (2) periodic screening can detect the disease; and (3) early detection and treatment can lead to a favorable outcome. Very often, tests meet only two of the three criteria. For example, since ovarian cancer tests have very high rates of false positive results, screening for this disease meets the first and third criteria but not second one. Before population-targeted chest computerized tomography (CT) scanning, screening for lung cancer met the first two criteria but not the third.[199] Even if screening shows a positive cost benefit, it may not be cost-effective. For instance, when the recommendations for lung cancer screening were changed in 2014, policy makers were balking at the $9.3 billion cost.[200]

Diagnosis

While the diagnostic process seems to be straightforward, several associated practices and beliefs needlessly increase costs.

The first belief is an overestimation in the need for technology to ensure diagnostic correctness.

---

[198]Marin, M., Güris, D., Chaves, S. S., Schmid, S., & Seward, J. F. (2007, June 22). Prevention of varicella, recommendations of the Advisory Committee on Immunization Practices (ACIP). *MMWR Recommendations and Reports*. Retrieved July 7, 2018, from https://www.cdc.gov/mmwr/preview/mmwrhtml/rr5604a1.htm

[199]U.S. Preventive Services Task Force. (2005). Lung cancer screening: Recommendation statement. *American Family Physician, 71*(6), 1165–1168.

[200]Steenhuysen, J. (2014, May 14). New lung cancer screening guidelines could cost Medicare $9.3 billion. *Reuters Health News*. Retrieved January 25, 2015, from http://www.reuters.com/article/us-health-cancer-lung-idUSKBN0DU20420140514. The recommendations for lung cancer screening are still not clear. For example, Redberg and O'Malley, commenting about a large VA study, wrote: "The findings are fascinating: a low take-up of LCS (58%), a high rate of incidental findings (41%), a low rate of detection of lung cancer [1.5%], and all for a highly resource-intensive program. From the data reported, we calculate that for every 1,000 people screened, 10 will be diagnosed with early-stage lung cancer (potentially curable), and 5 with advanced-stage lung cancer (incurable); 20 will undergo unnecessary invasive procedures (bronchoscopy and thoracotomy) directly related to the screening; and 550 will experience unnecessary alarm and repeated CT scanning (with its associated irradiation). Whether the benefits from this program outweigh the harms, and whether LCS is a wise investment of considerable resources required for screening and training, remains to be adequately evaluated with robust economic and utility analyses." Redberg, R. F., & O'Malley, P. G. (2017). Important questions about lung cancer screening programs when incidental findings exceed lung cancer nodules by 40 to 1. *JAMA Internal Medicine, 177*, 311–312.

EXHIBIT 7.15. **Patient Confidence with Physician Evaluation**

Evaluation Type	Confidence Level[a]			
	Median Visual Analog Scale Score	Interquartile Range	95% CI	No. (%) Who Had This Completed[b]
History and physical examination only	20	1, 72	16–25	77 (7)
History and physical examination and blood work	84	50, 100	80–85	271 (23)
History and physical examination, blood work, and ultrasonographic examination	85	55, 100	84–87	22 (2)
History and physical examination, blood work, and CT	90	60, 100	88–91	436 (37)

[a] Confidence levels with respect to medical evaluations were obtained from all participants.

[b] This column indicates the number of subjects who underwent the stated diagnostic evaluation. The total for this column does not equal the entire sample (n = l,168) because some patients may have undergone alternative evaluations. For example, participants who had a medical history and physical examination, a urinalysis, and a CT (for a nephrolithiasis diagnostic evaluation) would not be included in this column.

Source: Baumann, B. M., Chen, E. H., Mills, A. M., Glaspey, L., Thompson, N. M., Jones, M. K., & Farner, M. C. (2011). Patient perceptions of computed tomographic imaging and their understanding of radiation risk and exposure. *Annals of Emergency Medicine. 58*(1), 1–7.

For example, Baumann et al.[201] documented markedly increased patient satisfaction when "blood work" and CT scans were added to a physical exam in the emergency room. (See Exhibit 7.15.)

A related problem is that many patients do not understand that some diagnoses are made by history and physical exam alone, so they often demand unnecessary tests. An example is Parkinson's disease.

Not all blame should be placed on patients. Diagnostic tests are often paid at a relatively higher rate than cognitive services, creating a financial incentive to perform more tests. For example, Medicare pays $18.35 for a medical office electrocardiogram, which requires not more than a minute of a physician's time to interpret (and a few minutes of a technician's time to obtain); a 15–20-minute office visit is paid $78.02.[202] A related issue is that

---

[201] Baumann, B. M., Chen, E. H., Mills, A. M., Glaspey, L., Thompson, N. M., Jones, M. K., & Farner, M. C. (2011). Patient perceptions of computed tomographic imaging and their understanding of radiation risk and exposure. *Annals of Emergency Medicine, 58*(1), 1–7.

[202] The rates are 2018 nonfacility Medicare rates for CPT codes 93000 ("ECG with at least 12 leads; interpretation and report") and 99213 (intermediate office visit) for locality 0610216. See CMS.gov *Physician fee schedule search.* Retrieved July 7, 2018, from https://www.cms.gov/apps/physician-fee-schedule/search/search-results.aspx?Y=0&T=0& HT=0&CT=2&H1=99213&C=67&M=1

more testing leads to more findings, but not all findings are related to the purpose of the investigation or even warrant intervention.

Treatment

In this section, we first need to distinguish between two terms that are often misused interchangeably: efficacy and effectiveness. If a technology is *efficacious*, it has been shown to produce the expected result under ideal conditions. These ideal conditions usually involve a carefully selected population and highly trained and experienced researchers whose work is guided by rigorous protocols. *Effective* technologies, in contrast, are those that work in "real-world" settings.[203]

A number of treatments that have been proved efficacious in clinical trials fail to achieve their desired benefits in everyday practice. For example, medication inhalers are highly efficacious for people with asthma and chronic lung disease (chronic obstructive pulmonary disease, COPD); however, many misuse these devices and do not get their full benefits, leading to disease exacerbations.[204]

A major issue in considering costs of treatment is: On whom are we using the technology? Great progress has been made in evidence-based medicine that guides decisions about which patients will benefit most from which interventions. Further, genomic research has provided guidance about which patients will be helped by certain medications. These aids lower the costs of furnishing technology to those who will not benefit. However, despite this evidence, the recommendations are not always followed. For example, although guidelines are clear, prescription of inappropriate antibiotics is still widespread. The unwanted effects of such prescribing can add costs due to such complications as *Clostridium difficile* infection, allergic reactions, and fungal infections. Treating these problems can double the actual costs of prescribing[205] and add to global issues of mortality from drug-resistant bacteria.

One method of lowering treatment costs has been employing the least-costly effective medications, particularly generic drugs. For example, 2012 was a watershed year for patent expirations, notably for Lipitor (for hyperlipidemia), Plavix (for several conditions as an antiplatelet agent), Seroquel (for psychosis), Singulair (for asthma), Actos (for diabetes), and Lexapro (for depression). According to the IMS Institute for Healthcare Informatics, in that year, the loss of exclusivity cost drug companies $28.9 billion and reduced real per-capita spending on pharmaceuticals by 3.5%.[206] However, the cheapest medication is not always

---

[203]See (1) Gartlehner, G., Hansen, R. A., Nissman, D., Lohr, K. N., & Carey, T. S. (2006). *Criteria for distinguishing effectiveness from efficacy trials in systematic reviews* (p. 3). Rockville, MD: Agency for Healthcare Research and Quality (US); (Technical Reviews, No. 12.). Retrieved July 7, 2018, from https://www.ncbi.nlm.nih.gov/books/NBK44029/pdf/Bookshelf_NBK44029.pdf and (2) Singal A. G., Higgins, P. D., & Waljee, A. K. (2014). A primer on effectiveness and efficacy trials. *Clinical and Translational Gastroenterology, 5*, e45.

[204]Press, V. G., Arora, V. M., Shah, L. M., Lewis, S. L., Ivy, K., Charbeneau, J., … Krishnan, J. A. (2011). Misuse of respiratory inhalers in hospitalized patients with asthma or COPD. *Journal of General Internal Medicine, 26*(6), 635–642.

[205]M. Kulvick, MD, MBA, based on research at ETLA, The Research Institute of the Finnish Economy, Personal communication, January 2017.

[206]IMS Health. (2013, May 9). *Total real per capita spending on medicines fell 3.5 percent; fewer doctor office visits, and non-emergency hospital admissions; prescription use down 0.1 percent.* Note: In 2016 IMS and Quintiles merged to become QuintilesIMS. In November, 2017 the company was renamed IQVIA (www.iqvia.com).

the least costly overall choice. For example, some diseases (like hypertension) need multiple medications to achieve appropriate results, require laboratory tests to monitor side effects, entail multiple office visits for monitoring, and have additional costs due to unanticipated adverse reactions. The same logic applies to devices. For example, the cost of an implantable device is important, but one must also add the cost of hospitalization, recovery time (in and out of the hospital), need for ancillary services (like rehabilitation), and long-term monitoring (like pacemaker function checks). Thus, the *total* cost of treatment must be calculated, not just attention to the cheapest technology component.

One further consideration about generic medications is the potential problem of interchangeability among manufacturers' products. As explained above, a generic medication can have bioequivalence between 80% and 125% of the reference medication. For most generics (such as antibiotics), the clinical difference among different forms is not meaningful. However, as mentioned above, there are some medications for which very small difference in dosage can make a large clinical difference. Such medications are said to have a narrow "therapeutic index." One important example of such a drug is levothyroxine, used in treatment of hypothyroidism (underfunctioning thyroid gland). "Given the multiple sources of variation in the effects of a dose of the drug, there is no good reason to introduce another one by substituting a generic that could be switched without the prescriber's knowledge from one refill to the next."[207]

The only way to ensure effectiveness and cost containment is to make sure the patient receives the same manufacturer's generic medication throughout the entire course of treatment.

Yet another way technology has lowered costs is by introducing truly new innovations. For example, prior to the introduction of the gastric acid–lowering medications cimetidine and ranitidine in the 1970s, many patients with peptic ulcer disease (ulcers affecting the stomach and duodenum) needed surgical treatment that, in many cases, resulted in life-long morbidity. When these histamine-blocking medications (and subsequently proton pump inhibitors) were introduced, the number of surgeries for peptic ulcer disease dropped to insignificant numbers. With discovery of the bacterium *H. pylori* as the cause of this problem and development of diagnostic testing and treatment regimens for it, the disease has been substantively controlled at a much-reduced cost.

An additional cost consideration of treatment needs to be addressed: the expense of handling the side effects or complications of technologies. These events can be classified as *expected* (such as those following chemotherapy), *possible* (i.e., known but idiosyncratic, like allergies) or *unexpected* (unanticipated reactions). Adverse events can be further classified by *when* they occur. The following are some noteworthy examples. (Please see Exhibit 7.16 for others.)

Some Examples of Side Effects of Technology

Immediate

Drugs. Allergies or side effects, e.g., from antibiotics or chemotherapy

---

[207] Generic Levothyroxine. (2004, September 20). *The Medical Letter on Drugs and Therapeutics, 46*, 77–78.

Devices. "The Medtronic Sprint Fidelis (Fidelis) implantable cardioverter-defibrillator (ICD) transvenous high-voltage lead began to fracture soon after it was introduced in 2004. The manufacturer voluntarily removed Fidelis leads from the market in 2007 after 268,000 were implanted worldwide."[208]

Procedures. Morbidity/mortality (e.g., infections, bleeding, or death).

Delayed

Drugs. Use of dethylstilbestrol (DES) from 1938 to 1971 to reduce miscarriages was found to cause a rare vaginal cancer (clear cell carcinoma) in the daughters exposed to the drug in utero.[209] Taking the diet drugs fenfluramine or dexfenfluramine (Redux) caused heart valve problems.[210]

Devices. X-ray treatment for facial acne (first proposed in 1938) was found to increase the incidence of thyroid cancer 25 to 40 years later.[211]

One final consideration with respect to treatments is the review of clinical trials at the institutional level. This process includes evaluation of drugs, devices, and procedures (which the FDA does not review). The organization-specific group that is responsible for approving and reviewing research is usually called an institutional review board (IRB). According to the FDA:

an IRB is an appropriately constituted group that has been formally designated to review and monitor biomedical research involving human subjects. In accordance with FDA regulations, an IRB has the authority to approve, require modifications in (to secure approval), or disapprove research. This group review serves an important role in the protection of the rights and welfare of human research subjects.[212]

The IRB must register with the FDA, and an institution can choose a registered, external IRB if it does not wish to organize one itself. A single, external IRB is often beneficial when multisite clinical trials are being conducted.

---

[208]Hauser, R. G., Maisel, W. H., Friedman, P. A., Kallinen, L. M., Mugglin, A. S., … Hayes, D. L. (2011). Longevity of sprint fidelis implantable cardioverter-defibrillator leads and risk factors for failure: Implications for patient management. *Circulation, 123,* 358–363.

[209]CDC. (2018, July 7). *DEC history.* Retrieved July 7, 2018, from https://www.cdc.gov/des/consumers/about/history.html

[210]Centers for Disease Control and Prevention (CDC). (1997, November 14). Cardiac valvulopathy associated with exposure to Fenfluramine or Dexfenfluramine: U.S. Department of Health and Human Services Interim Public Health Recommendations. *Morbidity and Mortality Weekly Report, 46*(45), 1061–1066. Retrieved July 7, 2018, from https://www.cdc.gov/mmwr/preview/mmwrhtml/00049815.htm

[211]Kotulak, R. (1978, March 6). Acne X-ray linked to thyroid cancer. *Chicago Tribune,* 1.

[212]FDA. *Institutional review boards frequently asked questions—information sheet guidance for institutional review boards and clinical investigators.* Retrieved July 7, 2018, from https://www.fda.gov/RegulatoryInformation/Guidances/ucm126420.htm

EXHIBIT 7.16. Other Technologies Found to Be Ineffective or Harmful for Some or All Indications

- Autologous bone marrow transplantation with high-dose chemotherapy for advanced breast cancer
- Antiarrhythmic drugs
- Bevacizumab for metastatic breast cancer
- Colectomy to treat epilepsy
- Electronic fetal monitoring during labor without access to fetal scalp sampling
- Episiotomy (routine or liberal) for birth
- Extracranial-intracranial bypass to reduce risk of ischemic stroke
- Gastric bubble for morbid obesity
- Gastric freezing for peptic ulcer disease
- Hormone replacement therapy for preventing heart disease in healthy menopausal women
- Hydralazine for chronic heart failure
- Intermittent positive pressure breathing
- Mammary artery ligation for coronary artery disease
- MRI (routine) for low back pain in first 6 weeks
- Optic nerve decompression surgery for nonarteritic anterior ischemic optic neuropathy
- Oxygen supplementation for premature infants
- Prefrontal lobotomy for mental disturbances
- Prostate-specific antigen (PSA) screening for prostate cancer
- Quinidine for suppressing recurrences of atrial fibrillation
- Rofecoxib (COX-2 inhibitor) for anti-inflammation
- Sleeping facedown for healthy babies
- Supplemental oxygen for healthy premature babies
- Thalidomide for sedation in pregnant women
- Thymic irradiation in healthy children
- Triparanol (MER-29) for cholesterol reduction

Source: Fundamental concepts and issues—Health Care Technology Assessment by the National Information Center on Health Services Research & Health Care Technology. Retrieved July 7, 2018, from https://www.nlm.nih.gov/nichsr/hta101/ta10104.html

OTHER CONSIDERATIONS

Many other considerations about healthcare technology have prompted discussions among scientists, politicians, religious leaders, ethicists, lawyers, and others. Some of these issues are considered briefly below.

Religious Issues

A consistent debate throughout history has been whether the application of technology to human health is consistent with religious teachings. Perhaps the historically best-known instance is the use of anesthesia to lessen the pain of childbirth. In the mid-19th century, ether and chloroform anesthesia were coming into use with surgical procedures. When the subject of using anesthesia in deliveries was raised, physicians were unsure whether it was safe for mother and child and whether it did not impede normal labor. However, a major objection to its use was that lessening this pain was a contravention of divine punishment for "Eve's sin," viz. "In pain shall you bear children" (Gen. 3:16). Even the father of American obstetrics, Dr. Charles Meigs, pondered the religious implications: "The question is often propounded as to the Beneficence that ordained woman to the sorrow and pain of them that travail in childbirth."[213] It wasn't until Dr. John Snow administered chloroform anesthesia to Queen Victoria during the birth of Prince Leopold (her eighth of nine children) in 1853 that the practice started to be more accepted from a scientific and religious viewpoint;[214] the queen, after all, was head of the Church of England. A more recent and persistent religious objection by some to medical technology concerns its use for birth control drugs (oral contraceptives), devices (IUDs), and procedures (tubal ligations and vasectomies).

Ethical Issues

In addition to religious considerations, ethical issues abound with respect to medical technology. One reason for these problems is that our capacity to understand ethical implications lags considerably behind our ability to innovate. A detailed discussion of medical ethics is beyond this book,[215] but two issues offer examples on this topic.

1. *Fair allocation of limited resources.* Who gets the resources? What metrics should we use: Years of life left? Contributions to society? Ability to afford care? Do we want the

---

[213]Meigs, C. D. (1849). *Obstetrics: The Science and the Art* (p. 318). Philadelphia: Wood.

[214]An editorial in *The Lancet* on May 14, 1853 expressed incredulity that the Queen had received anesthesia: "In no case could it be justifiable to administer chloroform in perfectly ordinary labor; but the responsibility of advocating such a proceeding in the case of the Sovereign of these realms would, indeed, be tremendous." This concern was balanced by the following anecdote: During a visit to the Queen after Prince Leopold's birth, Prime Minister Gladstone asked her how she liked Dr. Snow's chloroform. The Queen replied "Very well, Mr. Gladstone." To which he noted: "The bishops are not pleased." "Then let the bishops have the babies, Mr. Gladstone," she responded.

[215]For more in-depth consideration of medical ethics, see, for example: Callahan, D. (1987). *Setting limits, medical goals in an aging society.* New York: Touchstone; and Daniels, N. (2008). *Just health, meeting health needs fairly.* New York: Cambridge University Press.

rich to be able to get resources if *they* can afford to do so, or will the rule be that if everyone cannot have access, none will get it?

One example of this problem was in the early days of hemodialysis. Scarce resources caused rationing on an emergency basis only when the kidney failure was considered reversible.[216] A second problem that has occurred is determining who gets influenza vaccine when shortages occur because of distribution delay or manufacturing problems.[217] A third ongoing issue is allocation of scarce human organs for transplantation.

2. *Genetic manipulation.* Insertion, deletion, or modification of genetic coding has posed ethical issues from their inception.[218] A further controversy has concerned use of embryonic stem[219] cells to treat such conditions as Parkinson's disease.

End-of-Life Costs

This issue was discussed in Chapter 2, "Determinants of Utilization of Healthcare Services and Products," but will be expanded here. Newer technology has contributed to increasing the cost of dying as well as the cost of living. Modern attention to this issue can perhaps be dated to 1980, when noted health services researcher and economist Eli Ginzberg wrote "The High Cost of Dying."[220] Since then, many policy makers have pointed to this issue as a major cause of rising healthcare costs and advocated programs to address it. However, the evidence across several decades does not support the premise of this argument or its remedies. One reason is that it is often difficult to tell when an illness will be the terminal event in a someone's life. Still, it is important to distinguish between aggressive, life-saving care and futile, end-of-life care. The following research over the past several decades demonstrates the general lack of effectiveness of measures to reduce end-of-life costs:

■ "None of the individual studies of cost savings at the end of life associated with advance directives, hospice care, or the elimination of futile care are definitive. Yet they all point in the same direction: cost savings due to changes in practice at the end of life are not likely to be substantial."[221]

---

[216]Ross, W. (2012). God panels and the history of hemodialysis in America: A cautionary tale. *Journal of Ethics, 14*(11), 890–896.

[217]See, for example: Fukuda, K., O'Mara, D., & Singleton, J. A. (2002). How the delayed distribution of influenza vaccine created shortages in 2000 and 2001. *P&T, 27*(5), 235–242.

[218]An excellent and easily read introduction to this topic is: U.S. National Library of Medicine: What are the ethical issues surrounding gene therapy? [See references on this site] Retrieved July 3, 2018, from https://ghr.nlm.nih.gov/primer/therapy/ethics

[219]Lo, B., & Parham, L. (2009). Ethical issues in stem cell research. *Endocrine Reviews, 30*(3), 204–213. This article provides a good discussion of the topic, including an explanation of the different types of stem cells.

[220]Ginzberg, E. (1980). The high costs of dying. *Inquiry, 17*(4), 293–295. The article is not a research piece, but about the last year of his mother's life (she died at 94). It concerns his actions to restrain hospitalizations and testing that would not have improved her quality of life but increased costs significantly.

[221]Emanuel, E. J., & Emanuel, L. L. (1994). The economics of dying—The illusion of cost savings at the end of life. *New England Journal of Medicine, 330*, 540–544.

■ "[T]he data available at present—and they are admittedly meager—do not support the frequently voiced or at least implied assumption that the high medical expenses at the end of life are due largely to aggressive, intensive treatment of patients who are moribund. For one thing, the data show that the number of decedents with very high medical expenses which suggest the use of expensive, high-technology interventions is quite small. For another, we do not know how many of the patients who died were clearly terminal patients ... What the data suggest, although they do not prove it, is that today, as in previous periods, most sick people who die are given the kind of medical care generally given the sick—and such care is expensive, especially for patients who are sicker than the average. Thus, the data from the studies conducted to date do not provide a basis for a policy of singling out one group of patients for cost-containment strategies."[222]

■ "Unfortunately, when studied in randomized trials, most conceptually promising end-of-life interventions have failed. The few trials that have documented improvements in one or more patient-centered outcomes were small- scale tests, typically conducted in academic settings."[223]

■ ["W]e estimate that only 11% of individuals in the highest cost group are in their last year of life. Efforts to improve the quality of care for this group are clearly warranted; however, expecting such interventions, if limited to those at the end of life, to have a meaningful impact on overall health care costs is misguided. Not only is this group small, but the window of time for a significant impact on costs is limited by the patients' life expectancy. Furthermore, our findings confirm the need to focus on those with chronic serious illnesses, functional debility, and persistently high costs."[224]

Media's Role in Increasing Technology Costs

It is well known that the popular media publishes very early-stage experimental findings that can have long-term benefits. Such announcements have been particularly frequent concerning treatments for such prevalent and serious conditions as Alzheimer's disease and certain cancers. These articles, however, are usually quick to point out that the findings in animal studies or in cell cultures are many years away from human application. Of far more harm, however, have been publications in peer-reviewed journals that skew findings to positive outcomes over negative findings.[225] The conclusions can raise public expectations and demand for newer, but not necessarily more effective, technology.

[222]Scitovsky, A. A. (2005). "The high cost of dying": What do the data show? *Milbank Quarterly, 83*(4), 825–841.

[223]Halpern, S. D. (2015). Toward evidence-based end-of-life care. *New England Journal of Medicine, 373*(21), 2001–2003.

[224]Aldridge, M. D., & Kelley, A. S. (2015). The myth regarding the high cost of end-of-life care. *American Journal of Public Health, 105*(12), 2411–2415.

[225]Chou, R., Aronson, N., Atkins, D., Ismaila, A. S., Santaguida, P., Smith, D. H., ... Moher, D. (2008, November 18). Assessing harms when comparing medical interventions. In *Methods guide for effectiveness and comparative effectiveness reviews*. Rockville, MD: Agency for Healthcare Research and Quality. Retrieved July 7, 2018, from https://www.ncbi.nlm.nih.gov/books/NBK47098

One of the best-known studies exposing this problem was by Turner et al.,[226] who studied publication of antidepressant trials. They found that:

> According to the published literature, it appeared that 94% of the trials conducted were positive. By contrast, the FDA analysis showed that 51% were positive. Separate meta-analyses of the FDA and journal data sets showed that the increase in effect size ranged from 11 to 69% for individual drugs and was 32% overall … We cannot determine whether the bias observed resulted from a failure to submit manuscripts on the part of authors and sponsors, from decisions by journal editors and reviewers not to publish, or both.

Malpractice and Defensive Medicine

One could argue that medical malpractice results from an inappropriate use of technology—either too little (failure to diagnose or treat) or too much (performance of needless or unnecessary procedures or treatments). The questions here are: Do malpractice costs significantly add to the overall cost of care? If so, what can be done about this problem?

Many scholarly articles have produced conflicting results about the significance of malpractice and the cost of care. The reasons are at least twofold. First, accurate data is hard to obtain from private sources, such as insurance companies and self-insured hospitals (which may settle cases privately). Many of the conclusions, therefore, are from analyzing Medicare data, which is easier to get. Second, authors evaluate data sources from different time spans. The problem with this latter sourcing was highlighted by Shaffer et al.: "Between 1992 and 2014, the rate of malpractice claims paid on behalf of physicians in the United States declined substantially. Mean compensation amounts and the percentage of paid claims exceeding $1 million increased, with wide differences in rates and characteristics across specialties."[227]

Therefore, analysis based on different partial time periods can yield different conclusions.

Even given the partial availability of data and differences in their sources, the figure for the cost of malpractice most quoted is $55.64 billion (in 2008 dollars), or 2.4% of healthcare spending.[228] Of that amount, $45.59 billion is due to the practice of "defensive medicine" (i.e., practitioners overtreating patients to avoid malpractice suits). The defensive medicine costs are mostly due to additional hospitalizations rather than excesses in the outpatient setting. The authors do note, however, that the quality of data to support the defensive medicine figure is "low." More recently, research by Reschovsky and Saiontz-Martinez[229] (who studied costs among Medicare patients) confirm the findings that most defensive

[226] Turner, E. H., & Tell, R. A. (2008). Selective publication of antidepressant trials and its influence on apparent efficacy. *New England Journal of Medicine, 358*(3), 252–260.

[227] Schaffer, A. C., Jena, A. B., Seabury, S. A., Singh, H., Chalasani, V., & Kachalia, A. (2017). Rates and characteristics of paid malpractice claims among U.S. physicians by specialty, 1992–2014. *JAMA Internal Medicine, 177*(5), 710–718.

[228] Mello, M. M., Chandra, A., Gawande, A. A., & Studdert, D. M. (2010). National costs of the medical liability system. *Health Affairs, 29*(9), 1569–1577.

[229] Reschovsky, J. D., & Saiontz-Martinez, C. B. (2018). Malpractice claim fears and the costs of treating medicare patients: A new approach to estimating the costs of defensive medicine. *Health Services Research, 53*(3), 1498–1516.

medicine costs are due to hospitalizations and postacute care utilization, and that the practice varies widely by specialty. The authors further note:

> While we conclude that defensive medicine likely contributes substantially to health care costs among Medicare beneficiaries, it is important to reiterate that these results do not support the positions of those arguing for or against tort reforms, per se. Previous research shows that malpractice liability tort reforms that make filing malpractice claims more difficult or place limits on potential awards have very little association with physicians' malpractice liability fears and subsequently on defensive medicine costs. Moreover, not all defensive medicine is necessarily bad; it can be quality-enhancing. We found that, in some instances, greater concern about malpractice liability is associated with lower costs, although we cannot assess whether this is a reflection of better quality care, avoidance behaviors, or methodological or data limitations.

Even the Congressional Budget Office (CBO) has weighed in on this issue with respect to reducing deficits.[230] Its recommendations would reduce mandatory spending by about $55 billion and increase revenue by about $7 billion between 2017 and 2026. Still, in line with many previous estimates, the CBO says its proposals would reduce total healthcare spending only by about 0.5%.

The conclusions of the above research, as well as of other older studies, indicate that, although there are opportunities for improvement, malpractice expenses and defensive medicine add little to overall healthcare costs.

SUMMARY

Healthcare technology has brought us the benefit of longer life and the ability to cope with physical and emotional problems. However, with those benefits come great costs—not always monetary in nature. In order to gain the most from healthcare technology, we must constantly reassess what exists as well as develop novel innovations that provide better value. Further, we must always evaluate the place of these technologies in our culture with respect to religious, ethical, and moral beliefs. As Arthur M. Schlesinger noted: "Science and technology revolutionize our lives, but memory, tradition and myth frame our response."[231]

---

[230]Congressional Budget Office: Options for Reducing the Deficit: 2017 to 2026. Chapter 5, Mandatory Spending Health Option 13, Limit Medical Malpractice Claims. Pp. 259–261. December 8, 2016. Retrieved July 7, 2018 from https://www.cbo.gov/sites/default/files/114th-congress-2015-2016/reports/52142-breakout-chapter5.pdf The recommended changes would: (1) cap awards for noneconomic damages at $250,000; (2) cap awards for punitive damages either at $500,000 or at twice the value of awards for economic damages (such as for lost income and medical costs), whichever is greater; (3) shorten the statute of limitations to 1 year from the date of discovery of an injury for adults and to three years for children; (4) establish a fair-share rule (under which a defendant in a lawsuit is liable only for the percentage of a final award that is equal to his or her share of responsibility for the injury) to replace the current rule of joint-and-several liability (under which each defendant is individually responsible for the entire amount of an award); (5) allow evidence of claimants' income from collateral sources (such as life insurance payouts and health insurance reimbursements, which can reduce the costs to claimants of being harmed) to be introduced at trial; and (6) cap attorneys' fees. (Typically, attorneys charge fees equal to one third of total awards and waive their fees if no award is made; the cap would reduce that percentage for larger awards.)

[231]Schlesinger, A. M. (1999). *The cycles of American history*. First Mariner Books Edition (p. xii). New York: Houghton Mifflin Harcourt.

CHAPTER

8

INFORMATION TECHNOLOGY

FALSTAFF.

> ... An old lord of the council rated me the other day in the street
> about you, sir, but I marked him not, and yet he talked very wisely, but
> I regarded him not, and yet he talked wisely, and in the street, too.

PRINCE HENRY.

> Thou didst well, for wisdom cries out in the streets and no man
> regards it.

—Shakespeare, *Henry IV, Part I,* Act 1, Scene 2

> Our inventions are wont to be pretty toys, which distract our attention
> from serious things. They are but improved means to an unimproved
> end. We are in great haste to construct a magnetic telegraph from
> Maine to Texas; but Maine and Texas, it may be, have nothing
> important to communicate.

—Henry David Thoreau, *Walden*

> Where is the wisdom we have lost in knowledge?
> Where is the knowledge we have lost in information?

—T. S. Eliot, Choruses from "The Rock"

INTRODUCTION

Gathering and using information for the healthcare system is a vast and rapidly evolving subject. Books and articles on this subject have ranged from the technical aspects of computer science to managing networks of integrated systems.[1] This chapter is intended for nontechnical healthcare professionals who work with information specialists. Such collaboration is essential for designing systems to improve the healthcare of those they serve as well as the financial health of the organizations in which they work. Unlike other chapters in this book, the nature of this topic requires explanations with many more organizational names, acronyms, and abbreviations. Further, many of these terms have changed over a short period of time as technology evolves and organizational responsibilities have been transformed. Histories of the evolution of this sector are included because the reader who wishes a deeper understanding of the topics will need guidance to sort out this massive and often confusing

---

[1]For a good general text on the subject, see Wager, K. A., Lee, F. W., & Glaser, J. P. (2017). *Health information systems: A practical approach for health care management* (4th ed.). San Francisco: Jossey-Bass.

terminology. Further, if a particular term or topic comes up, this chapter provides a good reference for its understanding. For those who wish only an overview of these subjects, skipping over the detailed sections will still yield a good overall understanding.

DEFINITIONS

Because of legislated requirements and financial penalties, governmental definitions will be presented for two key terms.

> *Health information* "means any information, whether oral or recorded in any form or medium, that—(A) is created or received by a health care provider, health plan, public health authority, employer, life insurer, school or university, or health care clearinghouse; and (B) relates to the past, present, or future physical or mental health or condition of an individual, the provision of health care to an individual, or the past, present, or future payment for the provision of health care to an individual."[2]

> *Health information technology* "means hardware, software, integrated technologies or related licenses, intellectual property, upgrades, or packaged solutions sold as services that are designed for or support the use by health care entities or patients for the electronic creation, maintenance, access, or exchange of health information."[3]

The term "information technology" is often abbreviated "IT" or "HIT" for *health information technology*; however, in many other countries, the term that is used is "information and communication technology," or ICT.

Three additional and related terms also require definitions because they are often used incorrectly and interchangeably.

> An *electronic medical record* (EMR) is "[a]n electronic record of health-related information on an individual that can be created, gathered, managed, and consulted by authorized clinicians and staff within one health care organization."

> An *electronic health record* (EHR) is "an electronic record of health-related information on an individual that conforms to nationally recognized interoperability standards and that can be created, managed, and consulted by authorized clinicians and staff across more than one health care organization."

> A *personal health record* is "[a]n electronic record of health-related information on an individual that conforms to nationally recognized interoperability standards and that can be drawn from multiple sources while being managed, shared, and controlled by the individual."[4]

---

[2] Social Security Act Sec. 1171. [42 U.S.C. 1320d].

[3] Public Law 111–5—February 17, 2009: American Recovery and Reinvestment Act. Title XIII—Health Information Technology: The "Health Information Technology for Economic and Clinical Health Act" or the "HITECH Act." Section 3000.

[4] These latter three definitions are from: The National Alliance for Health Information Technology: Report to the Office of the National Coordinator for Health Information Technology on Defining Key Health Information Technology Terms, April 28, 2008. Retrieved July 11, 2018, from http://www.hitechanswers.net/wp-content/uploads/2013/05/NAHIT-Definitions2008.pdf

A few more terms are also important and concern HIT "functionality." The Food and Drug Administration (FDA) categorizes functionality into three groups for purposes of regulation (which will be discussed later):

1. *Administrative functionalities* [include but are not limited to] admissions, billing and claims processing, practice and inventory management, scheduling, general purpose communications, analysis of historical claims data to predict future utilization or cost-effectiveness, determination of health benefit eligibility, population health management, reporting of communicable diseases to public health agencies and reporting on quality measures pose limited or no risk to patient safety.

2. *Health management functionalities* include but are not limited to health information and data exchange, data capture and encounter documentation, electronic access to clinical results, some clinical decision support, medication management, electronic communication and coordination, provider order entry, knowledge management, and patient identification and matching.

3. *Medical device functionality* [comprises such functions] as computer-aided detection software and remote display or notification of real-time alarms from bedside monitors.[5]

The interrelationship of these three elements is displayed in Exhibit 8.1.

Consider also a fourth category overlying the three displayed in the table: *decision-support functionality*, which draws on one or more of the three underlying categories to help the user make administrative and/or clinical decisions.

EXHIBIT 8.1.   **Three Categories of Health IT Functionality**

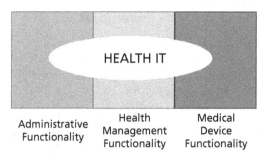

Administrative Functionality | Health Management Functionality | Medical Device Functionality

Source: FDASIA Health IT Report (2014, April). *Proposed Strategy and Recommendations for a Risk-Based Framework*. Retrieved July 11, 2018 from https://www.fda.gov/downloads/AboutFDA/CentersOffices/OfficeofMedicalProductsandTobacco/CDRH/CDRHReports/UCM391521.pdf

---

[5]FDASIA Health IT Report. (2014, April). *Proposed Strategy and Recommendations for a Risk-Based Framework*. Retrieved July 11, 2018, from https://www.fda.gov/downloads/AboutFDA/CentersOffices/OfficeofMedicalProductsandTobacco/CDRH/CDRHReports/UCM391521.pdf

Finally, a few common terms require clarification. For purposes of this chapter, I propose the following simple usages:

Data: Facts

Information: How you interpret the facts

Knowledge: How you use information to make decisions

Wisdom: How you use knowledge of your experience to make better decisions

BACKGROUND AND KEY ISSUES IN HEALTH INFORMATION TECHNOLOGY

Collection, Classification, and Ordering of Data

In order to start making sense of data, a standardized method of collection, classification, and ordering must be in place. This issue is critically important to health services research as well as cost accounting for healthcare products and services.

The history of healthcare information systems starts with recording the stories of patient illnesses and treatments for them. It should be noted that most of the early records show what their authors believed were successful interventions rather than failures. Further, what was recorded was information thought to be important in the context of the existing science. For example, in the 18th century, a treatise might be published on *how* to bleed a patient but not on *whether* bleeding was effective. Further, the type of information collected has always reflected demands of such elements as social and economic factors. For example, with respect to social issues, concerns about domestic abuse have led to routine questioning about feeling safe at home. With regard to economics, the demands for documentation for reimbursement for services have led to the need to record such clinically irrelevant information as how much time was spent with a patient and the measurement of the complexity of the problem being treated. Given this continuing need to collect, name, and classify medical information, it is useful to begin with a historical accounting.

The ancient Egyptians, Hippocrates, and Galen were among the early notable recorders of patient cases and treatments. The purpose of these records was to teach students and provide physicians with a guide for treating future patients. In that sense, they were used for deductive reasoning. The written "facts," however, were based on a single physician's experience. There were at least three problems with that method. First, there was no standard nomenclature for classifying findings into categories so they could be compared. What the physician recorded were collections of signs (objective findings) and symptoms (the patient's subjective experience of the illness, such as pain) without any organizing principles. Current scientists face the same problem with the emergence of new diseases and reclassification of existing ones, such as those now based on genetic information. Second, the treatments were not analyzed objectively to understand what worked and what did not work. Although Roger Bacon (1214–1284) is usually credited[6] with originating what we now consider the "scientific method" for analyzing problems, those techniques were not used in medicine until centuries later. Finally, the data were not organized in a systematic way that took into account patient variables.

The resolution to these problems in the English-speaking world[7] started with John Graunt (1620–1674), the father of epidemiology and demographics, who published analyses of the English Bills of Mortality starting in 1662.[8] These Bills of Mortality were often-inaccurate, local collections of causes of death by year. Graunt corrected and collated the data and paired them with other material, like birth records and environmental factors, to compile such useful information as life tables (predicting the percentage of persons who will live to each successive age and their life expectancy year by year) and displays of time trends for certain diseases (especially the plague).[9]

The most notable early call for classification of diseases can be dated to 1676, when the English physician Thomas Sydenham (1624–1689) published *Medical Observations Concerning the History and the Cure of Acute Diseases*.[10] In its preface, Sydenham espoused the concept that illnesses be classified into disease categories:

> [I]t is necessary that all diseases be reduced to definite and certain species, and that, with the same care which we see exhibited by botanists in their phytologies; since it happens, at present, that many diseases, although included in the same genus, mentioned with a common nomenclature, and resembling one another in several symptoms, are, notwithstanding, different in their natures, and require a different medical treatment.

Sydenham was influential not only in England but on the continent as well. Following his call for classification of diseases, Montpelier professor François Boissier de Sauvages de Lacroix (1706–1777), better known as Sauvages, published *Nosologia methodica sistens*

---

[6]Bacon adopted his ideas from the Arabian scientist Abu Ali Hasan Ibn al-Haitham (965–1040 CE), known in the West as Alhazan. Alhazan, in turn, adopted ideas about inductive reasoning from Aristotle.

[7]Death registries date from mid 15th Century Italy, mainly to track cases of plague. See Byrne, J. P. (2012). *Encyclopedia of the black death*, Vol. 1, ABC-CLIO (p. 113). Santa Barbara.

[8]Graunt, J. (1662). *Natural and political observations mentioned in a following index, and made upon the bills of mortality. With reference to the government, religion, trade, growth, ayre, diseases, and the several changes of the said city*. Thomas Roycroft for John Martin, and so on. Printed for the Royal Society, London. The publication was for the Royal Society, of which Graunt was a charter member (fellow).

[9]For a good article on Graunt's accomplishments, see Rothman, K. J. (1996). Lessons from John Graunt. *Lancet*, *347*(8993), 37–39.

[10]It is not known whether Sydenham was influenced by the work of Graunt. Of note is that, despite his prominence, Sydenham was not a fellow of either the Royal Society or the Royal College of Physicians. If he were a fellow of the former society, he might have had occasion to hear Graunt present his findings. Sydenham, T. (1843). *Medical observations concerning the history and the cure of acute diseases* [Observationes Medicae Circa Morborum Acutorum Historiam et Curationem] (Preface to the 3rd ed., p. 13). In R. G. Latham, *The works of Thomas Sydenham, M.D. translated from the Latin edition of Dr. Greenhill*, Vol. 1. Printed for the Sydenham Society, London. Retrieved July 11, 2018, from https://ia801408.us.archive.org/29/items/worksofthomassyd01sydeuoft/worksofthomassyd01sydeuoft.pdf

morborum classes juxtà Sydenhami mentem & botanicorum ordinem [Nosological method for the classification of diseases after the ideas of Sydenham and botanical organization] in 1763.[11] Sauvages took the idea of botanical organization from his friend Carl von Linné (Linnaeus) (1707–1778), to whom he sent botanical specimens. In his text, Sauvages classified diseases by class, order, and specific condition.

Sauvages's system, in turn, was adopted by the eminent Edinburgh physician and teacher William Cullen (1710–1790) when he published *Synopsis Nosologiae Methodicae*[12] in 1769. Cullen's classification of diseases became the standard in the latter part of the 18th and early 19th centuries and framed the way English-speaking physicians thought about and practiced medicine. The importance of this fact is that many American physicians trained in Britain, particularly in Edinburgh, and brought those ideas to the United States. Notable among Edinburgh's medical students were Benjamin Rush (1746–1813), signer of the Declaration of Independence and Surgeon General in the Continental Army, and John Morgan (1735–1789) and William Shippen, Jr. (1736–1808), cofounders of America's first medical school in Philadelphia (now the University of Pennsylvania Medical School).

When England enacted a law establishing a *national* registration of births and deaths in 1837, Cullen's classification was used to gather the data. (Of importance for the United States

---

[11]Boissier de Sauvages de Lacroix, F: *Nosologia methodica sistens morborum classes juxtà Sydenhami mentem & botanicorum ordinem* Amstelodami: sumptibus Fratrum de Tournes, 1768. Many sources give 1763 as the first date of publication; however, the frontispiece of available editions list the date as 1768. Retrieved July 11, 2018, from https://ia800504.us.archive.org/20/items/nosologiamethodi01bois/nosologiamethodi01bois.pdf

[12]Cullen, W. (1769). *Synopsis nosologiæ methodicæ, exhibens clariss virorum Sauvagesii, Linnæi, Vogelii, Sagari, et Macbridii, systemata nosologicaedidit suumque proprium systema nosologicum adjecit Guliemus Cullen.* Edinburgh, first published in 1769. As the Latin title explains, this book is a *synopsis* of nosological methods of other physicians to which Cullen's own system is added. In the first edition, he cites only the systems of Sauvages, Linné, and Vogel. A subsequent edition was published in 1785. The first edition is available at https://ia800604.us.archive .org/5/items/SynopsisNosologiaeMethodicae/Cullen_SynopsisNosologiaeMethodicae_1769.pdf. An 1827 English translation is available at https://ia801309.us.archive.org/32/items/b22020846/b22020846.pdf Both retrieved July 11, 2018. *Linnæi* is Carl von Linné (1707–1778), who is known for his botanical classification, but was trained as a physician and authored the medical text: *Genera Morborum In Auditorum Usum* [Disease classification with attention to use] Crist. ErH. Steinert Uppsala, 1763 Available at https://books.google.com/books/about/Genera_morborum.html?id=B5o_AAAAcAAJ Retrieved July 7, 2018. *Vogelii* is Rudolph Augustin Vogel (1724–1774), professor of surgery and then first professor of the medical faculty in Göttingen. The book to which Cullen referred is *Definitiones generum morborum praeside Rudolpho August, Vogel* [Description of the classification of disease supervised by Rudolph Augustin Vogel.] Göttingen, 1764. Although attributed to Vogel, in the historical literature, the book was actually the doctoral thesis of his student Gottfried Christoph Stender. *Sagari* is Johann Baptist Michael Edler von Sagar (1702–1778), an epidemiographer from the Austro-Hungarian empire (in what is now Slovenia) who published a nosological system modeled on Sauvages: *Systema morborum symptomaticum secundum classes, ordines, genera et species, cum characteribus, differentiis et therapejis.* [Organization of disease symptoms according to classes, orders, genera and species.] Vienna, 1776. *Macbridii* is David MacBride (1726–1778), a well-known Irish physician and surgeon who published a popular text: *A Methodological Introduction to the Theory and Practice of Physic.* London, 1772 (In Book III Section II of this work, he discusses "Diseases arranged according to the Systemic Method, into Classes Orders, Genera and Species.") Unlike the other works mentioned in this section, this one was first published in English. The Latin version was published in Utrecht in 1778.

is that this law was used as a model for the first state registry in Massachusetts in 1842.)[13] William Farr, one of the early key figures in the field of modern epidemiology, was appointed the first Compiler of Abstracts at the General Register Office. In presenting the results of the collected data, Farr firstly recognized the problems of single-observer findings:

> Only a limited number of facts fall under the notice of a single observer. His opinions, when they are the results of his own experience, are stated in general terms, and are often adopted by others in entirely different circumstances. Notwithstanding the constancy of nature, this leads to serious practical errors ... Diseases are more easily prevented than cured, and the first step to their prevention is the discovery of their exciting causes. The registry will show the agency of these causes by numerical facts and measure the intensity of their influence.[14]

Farr then acknowledged the need to standardize nomenclature so that sense could be made of the collated national data:

> The advantages of a uniform statistical nomenclature, however imperfect, are so obvious, that it is surprising no attention has been paid to its enforcement in Bills of Mortality. Each disease has, in many instances, been denoted by three or four terms, and each term has been applied to as many different diseases: vague, inconvenient names have been employed, or complications have been registered instead of primary diseases. The nomenclature is of as much importance in this department of inquiry as weights and measures in the physical sciences, and should be settled without delay.[15]

Farr's studies in this and subsequent annual reports were the "first to make extensive use of the standardized mortality rate to adjust for differences in age distribution in different sub-groups."[16] Using census data, he also developed methods for analyzing occupational mortality. Further, in 1864, he "was the first to publish work containing material calculated

---

[13]"The English Registration Act of 1837 served as the prototype of the first state registration law in the United States, enacted by Massachusetts in 1842. In the years following, births and deaths were registered in a few of the largest cities and several states. In 1855, the American Medical Association (AMA) adopted a resolution urging its members to take immediate and concerted action in petitioning legislative bodies to establish offices for the registration of vital events. By 1900, 10 states and the District of Columbia had met the requirements of the U.S. Bureau of the Census for admission to the U.S. Death Registration Area. The compilation of annual mortality statistics for the United States began with these states in 1900. Nationwide coverage was achieved in 1933 ... " Moriyama, I. M., Loy, R. M., & Robb-Smith, A. H. T. (2011). *History of the statistical classification of diseases and causes of death* (p. 2). Washington, DC: U.S. Government Printing Office. (DHHS publication; no. (PHS) 2011–1125). Retrieved July 11, 2018, from https://www.cdc.gov/nchs/data/misc/classification_diseases2011.pdf

[14]Farr, W. (1839). Appendix P: Letter to the Registrar-General from William Farr, Esq., respecting Abstracts of the recorded Causes of Deaths registered during the Half-year ending December 31, 1837, with numerous Tables. In First Annual Report of the Registrar-General of Births, Deaths and Marriages in England (pp. 88–89). London. Printed by W. Clowes and Sons, Stamford Street for Her Majesty's Stationery Office. Retrieved July 11, 2018, from https://babel.hathitrust.org/cgi/pt?id=nyp.33433087546358;view=1up;seq=8

[15]Ibid., p. 99.

[16]Whitehead, M. (2000). William Farr's legacy to the study of inequalities in health. *Bulletin of the World Health Organization, 78*(1), 86–87. Retrieved July 11, 2018, from http://www.who.int/bulletin/archives/78(1)86.pdf

and printed by a machine;"[17] that is, he was the first to use a computer to analyze medical data.

Initial attempts at developing an *international standardization* for disease classification occurred in 1853 with the Statistical Congress in Brussels. The many nations present (including the United States) considered standardization of statistics for topics ranging from meteorology, to emigration, to agriculture. The reasons for the congress and the case for healthcare were stated thusly:

> Statistics ... are the instruments by which the truth or fallacy of principles is unanswerably tested; and by them comparisons may be instituted. But there can be no comparison without a common point and a common channel. This is wanting in statistics. They are collected in all countries, but without unity of purpose they reveal no phenomena, and illustrate no universal law; without uniformity in the forms and language of statistical documents they afford no basis for comparison ...—The law of population is the most important subject of statistics ... Considering the extreme importance of a uniform nomenclature of diseases equally applicable to all countries, the attention of learned men is to be called to the question for further consideration at some future congress.[18]

Farr was named a vice president of the congress and, with Marc d'Espine of Geneva, was charged with crafting a classification that would be acceptable to all nations.

After much debate at a second meeting of the International Statistical Congress, held in Paris in 1855, no international adoption was forthcoming. "However, the general arrangement and structure of the list originally proposed by Farr, including the principle of classifying diseases by etiology (cause) followed by anatomic site, survives in the present classification."[19] By the 1857 meeting, a resolution was passed requiring that countries only use physician-reported causes of death (which were not always the case) using the nomenclature the congress endorsed. Unfortunately, many localities (much less countries) continued to record statistics using their own methods and terms. Many, however, did pattern their systems after Farr's anatomic classification.

Attempts at standardization continued for many years thereafter. One of the most significant advances was a nomenclature first published by the Royal College of Physicians of London in 1869.[20] The same year, the Surgeon General of the U.S. Army suggested that the

---

[17] He used a "Difference Engine" originally invented in 1837 by the Swede Per Georg Scheutz (1785–1873). The machine (based on Charles Babbage's design of 1815) was further refined and was exhibited at the Paris Exposition in 1855. After Farr saw it at the Exhibition, he "persuaded Bryan Donkin & Co to build one in England. It cost £1,200, comprised 4,320 parts, and weighed nearly 10 cwt. Farr used it to calculate life tables based on 6,470,720 deaths in England between 1841 and 1851." Dunn, P. M. (2002). Dr. William Farr of Shropshire (1807–1883): Obstetric mortality and training. *Archives of Disease in Childhood—Fetal and Neonatal Edition, 86*, F67–F69.

[18] Levi, L. (1854, March). Resume of the statistical congress, held at Brussels, September 11th, 1853, for the purpose of introducing unity in the statistical documents of all Countries. *Journal of the Statistical Society of London, 17*(1), 1–14. Retrieved July 11, 2018, from https://www.jstor.org/stable/pdf/2338350.pdf

[19] Moriyama, I. M., et al., op. cit., p. 11.

[20] *The nomenclature of diseases drawn up by the joint committee appointed by the Royal College of Physicians of London* (1869). Printed for the Royal College of Physicians by W. J. & S. Golbourn, London. Retrieved July 11, 2018, from https://ia600301.us.archive.org/26/items/nomenclaturedis00londgoog/nomenclaturedis00londgoog.pdf

American Medical Association (AMA) adopt this scheme for American physicians. After turning down the request, the AMA published its own *Nomenclature of Diseases* in 1872. Unlike the Royal College of Surgeons, which continued to update its nomenclature, the AMA abandoned its project after the first edition.

The next significant step toward a uniform classification was in 1891 at the International Statistical Institute (ISI; the successor to the International Statistical Congress) in Vienna in 1891. Jacques Bertillon[21] (1851–1922), chief of Statistical Services of the City of Paris, was appointed chair of a committee to standardize a list of causes of death. What became known as the Bertillon classification was adopted at the ISI's 1893 meeting in Chicago as the basis for subsequent publications entitled *International List of Causes of Death*. It "was based on the classification of causes of death used by the City of Paris, which, since its revision in 1885, represented a synthesis of English, German, and Swiss classifications. The classification was based on the principle, adopted by Farr, of distinguishing between general diseases and those localized to a particular organ or anatomical site."[22] Acceptance of this taxonomy received another boost at the American Public Health Association (APHA) meeting in Ottawa in October 1897, where it was recommended for use by all registrars of vital statistics in Canada, the United States, and Mexico. The following year, the APHA recommended the classification be revised every 10 years in order to keep up with the progress of science.

At the 1899 ISI meeting in Kristiania,[23] the classification was further endorsed for widespread use, and the APHA recommendation for decennial revisions was adopted. Following the latter action, the first International Conference for the Revision of the *International List of Causes of Death* was held in Paris in August 1900. That conference led to the First Revision (*International List of Causes of Death* [*ICD–1*]), which was recommended for adoption starting in 1901. The next conferences were held about every 9 to 10 years thereafter, until the 1990s.

When the World Health Organization (WHO) was created in 1948, it became responsible for the *ICD*. In that year, the revisions incorporated into *ICD*-6 also included categories for morbidity; hence, the meaning of *ICD* was changed to International Classification of Diseases.

The *ICD* has been altered by many countries for their individual needs. For example, in the United States in 1962, no procedure codes were available.[24] To fill that need, an *ICD* version was developed and called *ICDA* (the added "A" meant Adapted). In 1966, *ICDA*-8 was modified to include additional detail for coding hospital and morbidity data.

---

[21] Jacques Bertillon was grandson of Achille Guillard, who introduced the resolution requesting Farr and d'Espine to prepare a uniform classification at the first International Statistical Congress in 1853. Jacques was also the older brother of Alphonse (1853–1914) who was the first to advocate "mug shots" for criminals. Infamously, Alphonse supplied the flawed handwriting analysis used to convict Alfred Dreyfus.

[22] World Health Organization. *History of the development of the ICD*. Retrieved July 11, 2018, from http://www.who.int/classifications/icd/en/HistoryOfICD.pdf

[23] The name for Oslo from 1877 until 1925.

[24] Around this time the AMA's *Standard Nomenclature of Diseases and Operations* was replaced by *Current Medical Terminology*, which in turn became *Current Procedural Terminology*. See further on for an explanation of these works.

By 1979, healthcare providers were using the ICD's, Ninth Revision, Clinical Modification (*ICD*-9-CM),[25] which classified diagnoses (Volumes 1 and 2) and procedures (Volume 3). More recently, the *ICD* codes used in the United States are *ICD*-10-CM and *ICD*-10-PCS (Procedural Coding System), the latter employed for inpatient hospital procedures. The former codes are maintained by the National Center for Health Statistics (part of the Centers for Disease Control and Prevention [CDC]), while the Centers for Medicare and Medicaid Services (CMS) is responsible for the latter codes. These codes are important for both research purposes (their original intent) as well as to determine insurance coverage and diagnosis-based payments, such as diagnosis related groups (DRGs).

Although the latest revision, *ICD*-10, has been in *international* use since 1995, the United States used *ICD*-9 from 1979 to October 1, 2015. This delay was caused by several factors: the anticipated problems computers would face in 2000 (so-called Y2K issues); not wanting a code change to interfere with the Medicare requirements that EMRs be in place by 2014; and the complexity of the different format (i.e., *ICD*-9 was mostly numeric and had about 5,000 categories while *ICD*-10 is alphanumeric and has about 8,000 categories). As an example of format change, the *ICD*-9-CM code for high blood pressure of unknown cause was 401.0; the *ICD*-10-CM code is I10. Consider the impact this change had on software programs that needed to capture this new system. Proponents of the change claimed the new format would make for easier handling by computerized systems. *ICD*-11 was published in 2018 with subsequent conferences planned to discuss changes.[26] It is not known when the United States will adopt this new version; however, impediments to its implementation will not be as great as the change to its current form.

***

Once the data has been collected and classified, it needs to be presented in a logically useful format. The two most frequently used medical formats are the hospital chart and physician's office record.

The patient's hospital record has been traditionally organized according to functions, for example, physician orders, patient progress notes (sometimes combined and sometimes separate among all practitioners caring for the patient, viz. physicians, nurses, therapists, etc.), laboratory tests, imaging exams, and such documents as consultations and operative reports. Even with computerized records, these divisions still comprise the retrievable sections. For most of medical history, physician *outpatient* notes have been either nonexistent or cursory. When they were present, they represented a simple record of each visit in chronological order. In addition to clinical encounter information, however, hospital and physician outpatient records are also needed for quality improvement, clinical research, and billing; however, their formats did not often lend themselves to any of those activities.

---

[25] The term *adapted* was replaced by *clinical modification*, or CM.
[26] WHO. ICD-11 for Mortality and Morbidity Statistics (ICD-11 MMS), 2018 version. Retrieved July 11, 2018, from https://icd.who.int/browse11/l-m/en

The organization of clinical records underwent a major change in the 1960s with the efforts of physician Lawrence Leonard ("Larry") Weed (1923–2017). He noted that, while scientists focus on one problem and carry out investigations to resolution, physicians deal with many people, each of whom may have multiple problems that need to be addressed at irregular intervals. Further, some problems resolve, while others are chronic. The solution, in his words, "is to orient data around each problem. Each medical record should have a complete list of all the patient's problems, including both clearly established diagnoses and all other unexplained findings that are not yet clear manifestations of a specific diagnosis, such as abnormal physical findings or symptoms."[27]

His system is called the Problem Oriented Medical Record (POMR), and it has become the standard format for medical record keeping in the United States. The POMR has two components. The first, as mentioned above, is an ongoing list of patient conditions: diagnoses, symptoms, clinical findings (such as isolated laboratory abnormalities), medications, and allergies. The second part of the system is the format of each in-person patient encounter, for which Weed coined the acronym SOAP. The first part of the note, Subjective, records the patient's description of and experience with the problem (e.g., its duration, severity, and exacerbating or ameliorating factors). The second portion, Objective, reports such facts as vital signs (blood pressure, pulse, temperature, weight, height); observations about the patient (such as "anxious," "in no apparent pain," or "appears older than stated age"); findings of the physical exam, even if normal; and test results, such as laboratory and imaging exams. The third part, Assessment, is the clinician's thoughts about the cause of the problem (diagnosis) based on the previous two steps. Finally, given the assessment, a Plan is formulated to address each problem (i.e., treatments, further tests, and/or watchful waiting).

Of special importance is that the POMR has been easily adapted to EMRs because, in the 1960s, Weed and colleagues anticipated use of such computerized systems. In fact, he and Jan Schultz pioneered one of the first EMRs in 1976: the Problem Oriented Medical Information System (PROMIS).[28] Using touch-screen technology, it used the POMR to track problems and link clinical findings to diagnoses.

Terminology/Coding

Just as it is necessary to have a standardized data collection *framework*, it is also essential to be able to use a *common language* for the data being gathered. Further, that language must be encoded so it can be easily and clearly transmitted among stakeholders.

---

[27] Weed, L. L. (1968). Medical records that guide and teach. *The New England Journal of Medicine, 278*(11), 593–600.

A second part of the article was published as: Weed, L. L. (1968). Medical records that guide and teach. *The New England Journal of Medicine, 278*(12), 652–657. For a personal history and further rationale behind the POMR, see Wright, A., Sittig, D. F., McGowan, J., Ash, J. S., & Weed, L. L. (2014). Bringing science to medicine: An interview with Larry Weed, inventor of the problem-oriented medical record. *Journal of the American Medical Informatics Association, 21*(6), 964–968. Retrieved July 11, 2018, from https://academic.oup.com/jamia/article/21/6/964/788963

[28] Schultz, J. R. *A history of the PROMIS technology: An effective human interface.* Retrieved July 7, 2018, from http://www.campwoodsw.com/mentorwizard/PROMISHistory.pdf

Despite earlier efforts to adopt the Royal College of Physicians terms (see above), in the United States this task really began with a Bureau of the Census publication in 1920. The book explained its purpose thusly:

> To make possible medical discussion and to facilitate the interchange of ideas, therefore, it is necessary that we all speak the same medical language, that we all call the same diseases by the same names that we all call, for example, the febrile condition resulting from infection with the bacillus typhosus, either typhoid fever, or else enteric fever. It makes no difference which we call it so long as we all call it by the same term and understand what the term means.[29]

Notwithstanding this publication, some large hospitals (e.g., Bellevue in New York City, Massachusetts General Hospital in Boston, and Johns Hopkins University Hospital in Baltimore) still used their own terminology.

At the suggestion of Dr. George Baehr[30] (1887–1978), on March 22, 1928, the New York Academy of Medicine invited medical societies, hospitals, public health organizations, and other significant organizations to a national conference on disease nomenclature. At the second meeting of the National Conference on Nomenclature of Disease in 1930, the attendees achieved consensus,[31] and the results were first published in 1932.[32] At the time of the third revision in 1937, the AMA assumed responsibility for its preparation and publication. The 1942 revision added a standard nomenclature of surgical operations and was renamed *Standard Nomenclature of Diseases and Operations* (SNDO). (This action laid the groundwork for the standard naming of procedures and publication of the *Current Procedural Terminology* [CPT], explained below.)

At the time the last edition of SNDO was published in 1961, users realized that because it was designed for clinical rather than epidemiological use, the nomenclature was not very useful for retrieval of records for research study. Further, as prospects for computerized coding emerged,[33] the system did not appear to be useful for that purpose. As a result of these problems, the AMA published a new book called *Current Medical Terminology 1963*,[34] which contained "information about symptoms, signs, diagnostic testing, pathology, and treatment for listed diseases."[35] In this transition, however, procedure terms were dropped. The name

---

[29]Rogers, S. L. (1920). *Standard nomenclature of diseases and pathological conditions, injuries and poisonings for the United States Department of Commerce Bureau of the Census* (p. 5). Washington, DC: Government Printing Office. Retrieved July 11, 2018, from https://ia902306.us.archive.org/19/items/standardnomencla00unitiala/standardnomencla00unitiala.pdf

[30]Trained in pathology, Baehr was familiar with European classifications from his studies on the continent. In addition to his practice of pathology at Mt. Sinai Hospital in New York City, he was well connected through his other professional activities. He established the Health Insurance Plan (HIP) in New York and was on the board of New York City Board of Hospitals and the State Public Health Council. In 1945, the Surgeon General of the United States appointed him to the first NIH Scientific Advisory Board. Retrieved July 11, 2018, from http://icahn.mssm.edu/about/ait/archives/collection/george-baehr

[31]Standard classified nomenclature of disease. *JAMA, 110*(7), 509–511, 1938 [No author listed].

[32]Logie, H. B. (1932). *National conference on nomenclature of disease*. New York: The Commonwealth Fund.

[33]Bruce, R. A. (1962). Current medical terminology. *JAMA, 181*(11), 1015.

[34]*Current medical terminology*. Chicago: American Medical Association. 1962.

[35]Borman, K. R. (2017). Medical coding in the United States: Introduction and historical overview. In M. Savarise & C. Senkowski (Eds.), *Principles of coding and reimbursement for surgeons* (p. 4). Switzerland: Springer International.

was changed in later editions to *Current Medical Information and Terminology* (CMIT). The final version was published in 1981.

With cessation of CMIT, two requirements were again lacking: a standard description for procedures and a common language (terminology). These needs were filled by two separate initiatives.

To address medical *procedure descriptions*, starting in 1966, the AMA issued *Current Procedural Terminology* (CPT). The current edition is CPT-4, and it is used by physicians and other providers to bill payers for their services.

The recent efforts to *standardize language* started in 1965 when the College of American Pathologists (CAP) published *Systematized Nomenclature of Pathology* (SNOP) for use in their profession. In 1975, this book was modified and extended for use in other parts of medicine and became the *Systematized Nomenclature of Medicine* (SNOMED). After subsequent revisions,[36] in 2002, SNOMED terminology was officially merged with the National Health Service's Clinical Terms Version 3 (CTV3) to become SNOMED CT (Clinical Terms). Also at that time, the term "SNOMED" became its official name rather than an acronym for its original meaning. In 2007, a consortium of nine countries[37] formed the International Health Terminology Standards Development Organization (IHTSDO) and acquired the intellectual property rights to all versions of SNOMED from the CAP. As of December 31, 2016, the organization moved its offices to London, where IHTSDO was adopted as the incorporated name in England and SNOMED International became its global trading name. The organization now has 29 members and over 5,000 individual and organizational affiliates.

According to its website:[38]

> SNOMED CT is a terminology that can cross-map to other international terminologies, classifications and code systems. Maps are associations between particular concepts or terms in one system and concepts or terms in another system that have the same (or similar) meaning. Mapping is the process of defining a set of maps ...
>
> The purpose of mapping is to provide a link between one international terminology, classification and code system and another in order to obtain a number of benefits. These include:
>
> Data reuse, that is, SNOMED CT based clinical data can be reused to report statistical and management data using other terminologies, classifications and code systems
>
> Retention of the value of data when migrating to newer database formats and schemas
>
> Avoidance of entering data multiple times and the associated risk of increased cost and errors
>
> Interoperability [more about this term will be explained below] amongst international terminologies, classifications and code systems

Although SNOMED CT and CPT-4 provide clinical and procedural nomenclature, a system for health *data*, such as laboratory results and vital signs, was lacking. Further, the need to standardize the nomenclature of this data became more pressing as clinical documents were starting to be sent electronically. To that end, in 1994, Dr. Clem McDonald at the Regenstrief

---

[36] SNOMED II, 1979; SNOMED 3.0, 1993; and SNOMED RT, in collaboration with Kaiser Permanente, 2000.

[37] Australia, Canada, Denmark, Lithuania, Sweden, the Netherlands, New Zealand, the United Kingdom, and the United States.

[38] SNOMED International. Retrieved from http://www.snomed.org

Institute[39] organized a committee to develop a common language for data. Over time, the language has expanded to include not just medical laboratory code names but also nursing diagnoses, nursing interventions, outcomes classification, and patient care data sets. The project went under the name Logical Observation Identifiers Names and Codes (LOINC). This initiative is ongoing at the Regenstrief Institute, where LOINC[40] is a nonprofit activity provided free of charge. Its endorsement by the American Clinical Laboratory Association and the CAP has aided its acceptance.

Because all these diverse terminology sets address different needs, to truly be of use they have to interface with one another. To accomplish this task, SNOMED has developed ongoing cooperative relationships with both *ICD*[41] and LOINC activities.[42] The integration is exemplified in Exhibit 8.2.

EXHIBIT 8.2. SNOMED and LOINC Coding

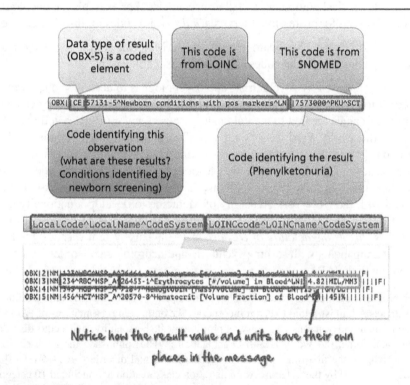

Source: LOINC: What LOINC Is. Retrieved July 11, 2018 from https://loinc.org/get-started/what-loinc-is

---

[39] The Regenstrief Institute is owned by a nonprofit foundation and is closely associated with Indiana University in Indianapolis.

[40] Available at https://loinc.org Retrieved July 11, 2018.

[41] See, for example: Position Statement: SNOMED CT to International Classification of Diseases for Mortality and Morbidity Statistics (ICD-11—MMS) Map. November 13, 2017. Retrieved July 11, 2018, from https://www.snomed.org/news-articles/position-statement-snomed-ct-to-international-classification-of-diseases-for-mortality-and-morbidity-statistics-icd11-mms-map

[42] SNOMED CT: LOINC. Retrieved July 11, 2018, from https://www.snomed.org/snomed-ct/mapping-to-other-terminologies/loinc

While the above nomenclatures cover most data requirements, there are other, important systems that meet other needs. Three will be mentioned here: Healthcare Common Procedural Coding System (HCPCS),[43] *Diagnostic and Statistical Manual of Mental Disorders (DSM)*, and National Drug Codes (NDCs).

HCPCS was established in 1983 as a coding system for gathering encounter data for Medicare and Medicaid beneficiaries and is maintained by CMS. These codes are essential for Medicare billing and are coupled with *ICD* codes.

HCPCS consists of three levels of codes:

Level I. Physician services. Most of the acceptable codes come from the AMA's CPT. Additionally, CMS designates temporary codes while making decisions on permanent designations.

Level II. Nonphysician services not covered by the CPT. Important items in this category are durable medical equipment and pharmaceuticals. For example, an oncologist might use Level I codes for professional services *and* Level II codes for in-office chemotherapy.

Level III. Used by local Medicare Intermediaries, Medicaid contractors and private insurance companies for special codes. They were discontinued in 2003.

DSM codes are used by psychiatrists and psychologists to describe behavioral and psychiatric conditions. The need for these standard descriptions and terminology came from the great variety of names applied to mental health issues at any given time and over the years. For example, the World War I term "shell shock" turned into "battle fatigue" and "combat stress reaction" before the current term "post-traumatic stress disorder" was chosen. The need also arose because of the lack of attention to or specificity of these disorders in the standard nomenclatures. To solve those problems, the American Psychiatric Association (APA) collaborated with the New York Academy of Medicine to develop a nationally acceptable psychiatric classification that would be incorporated within the first edition of the AMA's *Standard Classified Nomenclature of Disease* in 1938. This system was designed primarily for diagnosing inpatients with severe psychiatric and neurological disorders. According to the APA, a

much broader classification system was later developed by the U.S. Army (and modified by the Veterans Administration) to better incorporate the outpatient presentations of World War II servicemen and veterans (e.g., psychophysiological, personality, and acute disorders). At the same time, the World Health Organization (WHO) published the sixth edition of *ICD*, which, for the first time, included a section for mental disorders. *ICD–6* [1948] was heavily influenced by the Veterans Administration classification and included 10 categories for psychoses and psychoneuroses and seven categories for disorders of character, behavior, and intelligence. The APA Committee on Nomenclature and Statistics developed a variant

---

[43]Prior to 2001, CMS was known as The Health Care Financing Administration (HCFA); therefore, the original name for HCPCS was "Health Care Financing Administration Common Procedural Coding System."

of the *ICD*–6 that was published in 1952 as the first edition of *DSM. DSM* contained a glossary of descriptions of the diagnostic categories and was the first official manual of mental disorders to focus on clinical use.[44]

Subsequent editions have been coordinated with contemporaneous versions of the *ICD* codes. At present, *DSM-5* (2014) is being revised to address problems with *ICD*-10 CM.[45] The *DSM* criteria have been very controversial over the years. For example, homosexuality was listed as a pathology until *DSM-II* in 1973. Not all professionals have agreed with *DSM* categories. For example, recently one author stated that "*DSM 5* will likely trigger a fad of Adult Attention Deficit Disorder leading to widespread misuse of stimulant drugs for performance enhancement and recreation and contributing to the already large illegal secondary market in diverted prescription drugs."[46]

NDCs were the result of the Drug Listing Act of 1972, which amended the Federal Food, Drug, and Cosmetic Act. (Please see Chapter 7, "Healthcare Technology"). The Act required

drug establishments that are engaged in the manufacturing, preparation, propagation, compounding, or processing of a drug … to register their establishments and list all of their commercially marketed drug products with the Food and Drug Administration (FDA) … Drug products which are not properly listed are considered misbranded and may be subject to regulatory action. "Properly listed" means that all data provided to the FDA for each product is correct, including the trade name or proprietary name, if any, dosage form and route of administration, the ingredient information, package information, and the National Drug Code (NDC).[47]

Each formulation of each drug has a unique three-part, 10-digit number[48] that must be updated at least twice yearly. The first segment of 4 or 5 digits, is the "labeler code" (the "drug establishments" of the Act), which is assigned by the FDA. The second segment, 3 or

---

[44] American Psychiatric Association. *DSM history*. Retrieved July 11, 2018, from https://www.psychiatry.org/psychiatrists/practice/dsm/history-of-the-dsm

[45] For example, see Proposal #1: Correction of Selected ICD-10-CM codes for opioid withdrawal, sedative, hypnotic, or anxiolytic withdrawal, and amphetamine or other stimulant withdrawal. Retrieved July 11, 2018, from https://www.psychiatry.org/psychiatrists/practice/dsm/proposed-changes/proposal-1

[46] Frances, A. J. (2012, December 4). DSM-5 is a guide not Bible—ignore its ten worst changes: APA approval of DSM-5 is a sad day for psychiatry. *Psychiatric Times*. Retrieved July 11, 2018, from http://www.psychiatrictimes.com/blogs/dsm-5/dsm-5-guide-not-bible—simply-ignore-its-10-worst-changes Also see Wakefield, J. C. (2016). Diagnostic issues and controversies in DSM-5: Return of the false positives problem. *Annual Review of Clinical Psychology, 12*, 105–132.

[47] FDA: ANNEX B—The Drug Listing Act of 1972 Information Bulletin. Retrieved July 11, 2018, from https://www.fda.gov/Drugs/GuidanceComplianceRegulatoryInformation/DrugRegistrationandListing/ucm079592.htm The requirement also includes "establishments that repackage or otherwise change the container, wrapper, or labeling of any drug package in the distribution of the drug from the original place of manufacture to the person who makes final delivery or sale to the ultimate customer."

[48] The Health Insurance Portability and Accountability Act (HIPAA), discussed further on, requires NDAs have 11 digits. Because of this conflict, many labelers will add a zero or asterisk before the FDA-required code. This conflict is a good example of the need for harmonization among different uses for the same information.

4 digits long, is the "product code," which specifies the drug's strength, dosage form, and formulation. The third segment, the "package code," is 1 or 2 digits long and identifies package forms and sizes. The latter two segments are generated by the "labeler." "The current edition of the NDC Directory is limited to prescription drugs, OTC drugs, and insulin products that have been manufactured, prepared, propagated, compounded, or processed by registered establishments for commercial distribution."[49]

Interoperability

Introduction and Definition. Once the above elements are in place, healthcare entities must be able to easily exchange data with others. This ability to seamlessly communicate data among all authorized users is called "interoperability." Two explanatory definitions for this term are in common use. The professional health information organization (HIO) Health Information Management Specialty Society (HIMSS), defines three levels of interoperability:

1. *Foundational* interoperability allows data exchange from one information technology system to be received by another and does not require the ability for the receiving information technology system to interpret the data.

2. *Structural* interoperability ... defines the structure or format of data exchange (i.e., the message format standards) where there is uniform movement of health data from one system to another such that the clinical or operational purpose and meaning of the data is preserved and unaltered ... It ensures that data exchanges between information technology systems can be interpreted at the data field level.

3. *Semantic* interoperability ... is the ability of two or more systems or elements to exchange information and to use the information that has been exchanged ... This level of interoperability supports the electronic exchange of health-related financial data, patient-created wellness data, and patient summary information among caregivers and other authorized parties. This level of interoperability is possible via potentially disparate electronic health record (EHR) systems, business-related information systems, medical devices, mobile technologies, and other systems to improve wellness, as well as the quality, safety, cost-effectiveness, and access to healthcare delivery.[50]

The International Organization for Standardization (commonly called ISO) categorizes the components of interoperability as:

Semantic Interoperability (Content): Data Standards; Information Content Standards

Technical Interoperability (Infrastructure): Information Exchange Standards; Identifiers Standards; Privacy and Security Standards

---

[49]FDA. *National drug code database background information*. Retrieved July 11, 2018, from https://www.fda.gov/Drugs/DevelopmentApprovalProcess/UCM070829

[50]HIMSS. *What is interoperability?* Retrieved July 11, 2018, from http://www.himss.org/library/interoperability-standards/what-is

Functional Interoperability: Functional Standards (interoperability use cases, HIM practice standards); Business Standards (business rules, guidelines, practice checklists); Health Information Technology (HIT) Safety Standards[51]

The organization Health Level Seven (HL7) (a standards development organization discussed below) and the HIT association, American Health Information Management Association (AHIMA), also use this latter definition.

In order to fully deliver this capability, two elements are needed: a uniform format and agreed-upon common computer language.

In contrast to the eventual universal acceptance of medical classification systems and terminology discussed above, efforts to develop standard formats for data transmission have been contentious and, hence, fragmented. As a result, problems with interoperability in healthcare are arguably the single greatest obstacles to truly useful electronic data interchange.

To explain this issue by analogy, consider the American railroads of the 19th century.[52] Many different companies built their own tracks and set their own distances between them (the gauge) to prevent competitors from using their lines. In order to facilitate a transcontinental railroad and ensure efficient transport of war materiel and troops, Congress passed the Pacific Railway Act of 1862, which, with reference to the Central Pacific and Union Pacific Railroads, stated: "The track upon the entire line of railroad and branches shall be of uniform width, to be determined by the President of the United States so that, when completed, cars can be run from the Missouri River to the Pacific Coast."[53]

However, by 1871, the United States still had 23 different gauges, most disparities occurring in the former Southern states of the Confederacy. With the spread of transcontinental commerce, railroads found it increasingly costly to transfer goods from one set of trains to another because of different gauges. As a result, over Memorial Day weekend in 1886, after a massive conversion effort, the Southern railroads converted to the Northern standard of 4ft 8½ in.[54]

Liken this history to the current situation with a multitude of information system companies that cannot easily transfer data among themselves. One reason for this problem is the jockeying by large companies to make *their* system the standard to gain a business advantage. As was the situation with the railroads, there are two possible solutions to achieve standardization: industry-wide consensus and/or government intervention. The development of

---

[51] ISO/TC 215 Health Informatics Standards Catalog. International Standards, Technical Specifications, Technical Reports 2017. Retrieved July 7, 2018, from https://www.ahima.org/~/media/AHIMA/Files/AHIMA-and-Our-Work/ISOTC215 StandardsCatalog2017.ashx?la=en

[52] Hilton, G. W. (2006). A history of track gauge: How 4 feet, 8½ inches became the standard. *Trains*. Retrieved from http://trn.trains.com/railroads/abcs-of-railroading/2006/05/a-history-of-track-gauge

[53] "Pacific Railway Act." 1 July, 1862. Retrieved from http://www.loc.gov/rr/program/bib/ourdocs/PacificRail.html

[54] Except for large portions of the Denver and Rio Grande and the Toledo, Cincinnati, and St. Louis Railroads, by 1887 every major railroad in the country was using the standard gauge. Most of this narrow-gauge section was converted to the standard by 1900.

systems to facilitate interoperability will be presented first, followed by efforts to implement measures in the healthcare arena.

General Background. The story of interoperability begins in 1916 at the nexus of a public-private initiative. In that year, the American Institute of Electrical Engineers (now IEEE) invited the American Society of Mechanical Engineers (ASME), the American Society of Civil Engineers (ASCE), the American Institute of Mining and Metallurgical Engineers (AIME), and the American Society for Testing and Materials (now ASTM International) to form an independent, national organization to "coordinate standards development, approve national consensus standards, and halt user confusion on acceptability."[55] Subsequently, they invited the U.S. Departments of War, Navy, and Commerce to found the American Engineering Standards Committee (AESC). As an example of its activities, its first task, in 1919, was to approve the standard for pipe threads. Over the next 10 years, it also approved national standards in the fields of mining, electrical and mechanical engineering, construction and highway traffic. In 1926, AESC hosted an international conference that led to the creation of the International Standards Association (ISA). In 1928, the AESC was reorganized and renamed the American Standards Association (ASA). The ASA played an important role in World War II by developing uniform production standards for manufacturing. In 1947, a successor to the ISA was created and became the ISO. The ASA was the American representative organization to that body. As technology advanced in the 1950s and 1960s, the ASA helped industry and government organizations develop standards for such emerging fields as nuclear energy and information technology. The ASA was again reorganized in 1966 and changed its name to the United States of America Standards Institute (USASI). Importantly, in 1968, the USASI "formed a Certification Committee to oversee the licensing of its mark to manufacturers who marketed products that were judged by an independent test to comply with an approved American National Standard."[56] In 1969, USASI became the American National Standards Institute (ANSI), which retains that name today. ANSI's role in healthcare information systems is further explained below.

Interoperability first became a *computer* issue in the transportation field in the 1960s when shipping, rail, trucking, and airline companies sought to convert from paper to electronic shipping bills. In 1968, they created the nonprofit Transportation Data Coordinating Committee, which subsequently developed successful standards for data transmission among companies with different systems. At that time, large, centralized computers (mainframes) provided automated data processing. In this environment, two types of "protocols" (sets of rules that allow networked computers to talk to one another) needed to be developed, direct and indirect. Direct standards allowed an operator to use a computer remotely. Indirect standards allowed the remote operator to access information from the remote computer, process it locally, then return the information. The teletype network (Telnet) protocol (developed in 1969 and standardized in 1973) was used for direct access, and the File Transfer Protocol (FTP; published in 1971) was used for indirect access. While the basic FTP concept is still

---

[55] ANSI. *Historical overview.* Retrieved July 11, 2018, from https://www.ansi.org/about_ansi/introduction/history
[56] ANSI. *Historical overview*, op. cit.

being used,[57] more secure versions, such as SFTP (SSH File Transfer Protocol),[58] have been developed. In order to use these protocols in the same facility, networks of terminals linked to the main computer were developed and called local area networks (LANs). In the United States, the LAN concept was developed from 1973 to 1975 at Xerox PARC (Palo Alto Research Center) and was patented under the name Ethernet. In 1975, microprocessors were introduced that allowed personal computers (PCs) to be created. The introduction of PCs ushered in an era of local computing—processing could be done by individuals at their desks—as opposed to needing to communicate with the centralized processing of a mainframe computer. In 1978, the Transportation Data Coordinating Committee was renamed the Electronic Data Interchange Association. The following year, it was chartered by ANSI as the Accredited Standards Committee (ASC) X12[59] to develop and maintain electronic data interchange standards across a variety of industries, including healthcare.[60]

At the end of 1979, ISO's Technical Committee 97 approved a working draft of the Open Systems Interconnect (OSI) Reference Model for network systems. The OSI Model specified seven layers for the exchange of data between computers.[61] (For comparison, Ethernet was OSI Level 2 and the ARPANET, the Internet precursor described below and launched in 1969, was OSI Level 4.)

Parallel to the development of the networks themselves were efforts to *link networks to other networks*, which became the internet.[62] Just as LANs were being used *within* companies, the internet was to be a wide area network (WAN) covering many types of users (including LANs) over a larger geographic area. Briefly, this effort began in 1958, when President Eisenhower created the Advanced Research Projects Agency (ARPA) in the Defense Department to coordinate academic, industry, and government partners in the development of scientific projects for national defense. (ARPA was renamed Defense Advanced Research Projects Agency [DARPA] in 1972.) The concept for a computer network sponsored by ARPA was published in 1967, and in 1969, ARPANET was formed with four Interface Message Processors, or "nodes": the University of California at Los Angeles (UCLA), the Augmentation Research Center at Stanford Research Institute (now SRI International), UC Santa Barbara, and the University of Utah School of Computing.

---

[57] See Statz, P. (2010, February 15). FTP for beginners. *Wired*. Retrieved December 25, 2017, from https://www.wired .com/2010/02/ftp_for_beginners

[58] For example, see https://www.ssh.com/ssh/sftp (retrieved July 11, 2018).

[59] The standard itself is "X12" so it is called either ANSI X12 or ASC X12.

[60] For a list of document types developed for healthcare, see the insurance section at: https://www.edibasics.com/ edi-resources/document-standards/ansi. For a technical explanation of the X12 format, see https://docs.oracle.com/cd/ E19398-01/820-1275/6ncv5s178/index.html Both retrieved July 11, 2018. X12 is the standard for electronic data interchange in North America. Other standards, such as United Nations/Electronic Data Interchange for Administration, Commerce, and Transport (UN/EDIFACT), created in 1985, are used elsewhere in the world.

[61] For a good, brief explanation of these layers, see Windows network architecture and the OSI model. Retrieved July 11, 2018, from https://support.microsoft.com/en-us/help/103884/the-osi-model-s-seven-layers-defined-and-functions-explained

[62] For a short, authoritative history of the Internet, see Internet Society. *Brief history of the Internet*. Retrieved July 11, 2018, from https://www.internetsociety.org/internet/history-internet/brief-history-internet

Two items were required to make ARPANET work: one was informational and the other was operational. First, network engineers needed an authoritative publication to issue technical and organizational notes; that function was fulfilled by the Request for Comment (RFC) series, which is still an important source of information.[63] The RFC series is also the oldest online publication.

The operational requirement was a method of data delivery *through* the network. The origins of this scheme date to the late 1950s, when the military was seeking a way to secure communications in case of a first nuclear strike. If there were unique, direct links between users, a single disruption could wipe out the connections. The solution came from Paul Baran at the RAND Corporation with a scheme called "distributed adaptive message block switching." The concept involved breaking a message into blocks and delivering the component blocks to the receiver through multiple, decentralized networks. At the destination, the message would be reassembled in its original form. Donald Davies at the National Physical Laboratory in the United Kingdom had similar ideas but used the term "packet switching"; this less cumbersome terminology stuck. The description of this system for ARPANET was published in 1974 and was called the Transmission Control Program (TCP).[64] Its purpose is to collect and reassemble the data packets. It was then paired with the Internet Protocol (IP), which directs the packets to the correct recipient. Together they became known as TCP/IP, which is in the public domain. The process occurs in the following way.

At the sender, the message is formatted into packets. Each packet has a header that contains the destination address (IP address), source address, number of packets, and the number each packet has in the sequence. The body of each packet has a portion of the total message. The packets are sent through a variety of networks that can deliver the entire message most efficiently. At the receiving end, they are reassembled to duplicate the message as it was originally sent.[65] This type of packet switching, which is characteristic of the internet, is called "connectionless." The other type of packet switching is called "connection-oriented." With this latter method, packets are sent sequentially over a predefined route in the sequenced order of the message. (By analogy, think about transmission of a multipage fax.)

In 1981, while the TCP/IP system was being developed, the National Science Foundation (NSF) expanded access to the ARPANET when it created the Computer Science Network

---

[63] See RFC Editor. Retrieved July 11, 2018, from https://www.rfc-editor.org. Six categories of RFCs are Standards, Draft Standards (RFCs that are expected to become internet standards), Best Current Practice, Experimental, Informational, and Historic. Four sources ("streams") that provide RFCs are: (1) the Internet Engineering Task Force (IETF), whose mission is "to make the Internet work better by producing high quality, relevant technical documents that influence the way people design, use, and manage the Internet." It focuses on engineering and standards; (2) the Internet Research Task Force (IETF), which focuses on research areas of the internet; (3) the Internet Architecture Board (IAB), which oversees the architecture of the internet, including its protocols and other standards. It is part of the Internet Society (ISOC), which was formed in 1992 by members of the IETF who needed to create a parent nonprofit organization when NSF funding ran out. The IETF is also part of the ISOC. And (4) independent submissions.

[64] Not only was the TCP described at this time, but it is the first mention of the term *Internet*. See Cerf, V., Dalal, Y., & Sunshine, C. (1974, December). *Specification of internet transmission control program.* Network Working Group. Request for Comments (RFC), 675. Retrieved July 11, 2018, from https://tools.ietf.org/html/rfc675

[65] For an animation of the concept of packet switching, see https://en.wikipedia.org/wiki/Packet_switching - /media/File: Packet_Switching.gif (retrieved July 11, 2018).

(CSNET) to enhance universities' connectivity. At that time, data transmission used the Network Control Program (NCP), which was a direct, unilateral connection between users. The NCP was turned off on January 1, 1983, when ARPANET officially switched to using TCP/IP. That date is often called the birthday of the internet. Also in 1983, the Domain Name System (DNS)[66] was established, identifying different types of users: .edu, .gov, .com, .org, .net, and so on. In 1985, the NSF started funding five supercomputing centers: the John von Neumann Center at Princeton University; the San Diego Supercomputer Center (SDSC) on the campus of the University of California, San Diego; the National Center for Supercomputing Applications (NCSA) at the University of Illinois at Urbana-Champaign; the Cornell Theory Center at Cornell University; and the Pittsburgh Supercomputing Center, jointly sponsored by Carnegie Mellon University, the University of Pittsburgh, and Westinghouse Corporation. To allow research and educational organizations to more easily access these supercomputers, the NSF created NSFNET in 1986.

In 1989, the Federal Engineering Planning Group (FEPG) established two Federal Internet Exchange (FIX) points: Federal Internet Exchange East (FIX-E) was in College Park, Maryland, at the University of Maryland; Federal Internet Exchange West (FIX-W) was in Mountain View, California, at the NASA Ames Research Center. Their purpose was to connect existing federal networks: NSFNET, NASA Science Network (NSN), Energy Sciences Network (ESNet), and the nonclassified military network, called MILNET. The FIX structure was the precursor to the creation of the current, global system of Internet Exchange Points (IXPs), where networks can connect to other networks to exchange traffic.[67]

With the creation of these networks, ARPANET was decommissioned in 1990. Coordination of federal networking (and other scientific activities) was more permanently established in 1993 when President Clinton issued Executive Order 12881, launching the National Science and Technology Council (NSTC).[68] Its Committee on Computing, Information, and Communications (CCIC) created the Federal Networking Council (FNC), which coordinated networking activities of federal agencies, including the Department of Defense (DoD) (also incorporating DARPA), the Department of Education, the NSF, NASA, and the Department of Health and Human Services (HHS).

One of the FNC's most memorable actions was publication of the definition of the internet:

Unanimous passage of a resolution by the Federal Networking Council (FNC) on 10/24/95 supporting the following definition of "Internet":

---

[66]In 1994, the U.S. government began to privatize the internet. Four years later, it turned over the DNS function to the Internet Corporation for Assigned Names and Numbers (ICANN), a California nonprofit corporation. Numbered addresses had been assigned starting in the early 1970s. This function was assumed by the Internet Assigned Numbers Authority (IANA). In March 2003, the U.S. Department of Commerce contracted with ICANN to perform the IANA functions. The archiving function for these names and addresses was awarded to Network Solutions, Inc. in 1999.

[67]For a map of global IXPs, see https://www.internetexchangemap.com Retrieved July 11, 2018.

[68]Executive Order 12881: Establishment of the National Science and Technology Council. November 23, 1993. Retrieved July 11, 2018, from http://govinfo.library.unt.edu/npr/library/direct/orders/2252.html

RESOLUTION:

The Federal Networking Council (FNC) agrees that the following language reflects our definition of the term "Internet."

"Internet" refers to the global information system that—

i. is logically linked together by a globally unique address space based on the Internet Protocol (IP) or its subsequent extensions/follow-ons;

ii. is able to support communications using the Transmission Control Protocol/Internet Protocol (TCP/IP) suite or its subsequent extensions/follow-ons, and/or other IP-compatible protocols; and

iii. provides, uses or makes accessible, either publicly or privately, high level services layered on the communications and related infrastructure described herein.

The FNC was absorbed into several CCIC subcommittees in 1997. Today, the functions of the CCIC are managed by the Networking and Information Technology Research and Development (NITRD) Program,[69] which is a subcommittee of the Committee on Technology of the NSTC.

In 1990, at the time the ARPANET gave way to the above-mentioned networks, another innovation was emerging: the World Wide Web. While its basic concepts had been articulated for decades,[70] the most oft-cited source was a 1945 article written by Vanevar Bush (1890–1974) titled "As We May Think."[71] In the article, Bush stated a problem that still exists: "There is a growing mountain of research . . . . The difficulty seems to be, not so much that we publish unduly in view of the extent and variety of present-day interests, but rather that publication has been extended far beyond our present ability to make real use of the record." To solve this problem, he proposed a

device for individual use, which is a sort of mechanized private file and library. It . . . is a device in which an individual store [*sic*] all his books, records, and communications, and which is mechanized so that it may be consulted with exceeding speed and flexibility. It is an enlarged intimate supplement to his memory . . . If the user wishes to consult a certain book, he taps its code on the keyboard . . . Any given book of his library can thus be called

---

[69]"The Networking and Information Technology Research and Development (NITRD) Program is the Nation's primary source of federally funded work on advanced information technologies (IT) in computing, networking, and software … [It] provides a framework and mechanisms for coordination among the Federal agencies that support advanced IT R&D and report IT research budgets … " See also: The NITRD Program. Retrieved July 11, 2018, from https://www.nitrd.gov/about/about_nitrd.aspx. The NITRD was established by the High-Performance Computing Act of 1991 (P.L. 102–194) (sponsored by then Senator Albert Gore) and reauthorized by Congress in the American Innovation and Competitiveness Act of 2017 (P.L. 114–329).

[70]See Wright, A. (2014, May 22). The secret history of hypertext. The conventional history of computing leaves out some key thinkers. *The Alantic.*

[71]Bush, V. (1945, July). As we may think. *The Atlantic.* Bush had been vice president and dean of the Engineering Department at MIT and president of the Carnegie Institution in Washington prior to World War II. During the war, he was in charge of the Office of Scientific Research and Development (OSRD). Among his other duties, he was responsible for the initiation and early management of the Manhattan Project. In his position as head of the OSRD, he became, in effect, the first Presidential Science Advisor and an extremely influential thought leader in the sciences.

up and consulted with far greater facility than if it were taken from a shelf. As he has several projection positions, he can leave one item in position while he calls up another. He can add marginal notes and comments.

Bush presciently commented on the device's use in medicine: "The physician, puzzled by a patient's reactions, strikes the trail established in studying an earlier similar case, and runs rapidly through analogous case histories, with side references to the classics for the pertinent anatomy and histology."

At the end of World War II, computer engineer Douglas Engelbart read and was inspired by Bush's vision.[72] By the early 1960s, he was working at the Augmentation Research Center at the SRI. The word "Augmentation" was used as a guiding philosophy that the work on computers was to augment *human capabilities*; it was a concept contrasted to work on artificial intelligence (AI), where *computers* did the "thinking." In pursuit of this goal, by the late 1960s the SRI group had developed a complete computer hardware and software system called the oN-Line System (NLS), financed by NASA and ARPA. On December 9, 1968, Engelbart presented the system's capabilities at the fall joint meeting of the Association for Computing Machinery/Institute of Electrical and Electronic Engineers in San Francisco. This demonstration, titled "A Research Center for Augmenting Human Intellect," was so revolutionary that it came to be known as the Mother of All Demos. Engelbart and colleagues introduced capabilities that are now commonplace: windows, video conferencing, word processing, hypertext (explained further below), collaborative real-time editing (between the conference location and the SRI), command inputs, and use of a computer mouse[73] for on-screen navigation.[74] These capabilities became the model for the PC of today and technologies for accessing and navigating the World Wide Web.

While the internet was being developed, as Bush had predicted, the volume of research and other data grew dramatically. The scientific community, in particular, was having troubles easily collaborating and sharing research findings. These frustrations were especially felt by CERN (European Organization for Nuclear Research) scientist Tim Berners-Lee, who recalled: "I found it frustrating that in those days, there was different information on different computers, but you had to log on to different computers to get at it. Also, sometimes you had to learn a different program on each computer. So finding out how things worked was really difficult. Often it was just easier to go and ask people when they were having coffee."[75]

To address this problem, in March1989, Berners-Lee issued *Information Management: A Proposal*[76] for internal organizational use. Because of the importance of this document, a brief excerpt is cited below.

---

[72]Madrigal, A. (2013, July 7). The hut where the internet began. *The Atlantic.*

[73]Engelbert designed the mouse, and it was built by William English.

[74]For a recording of this presentation, see https://ww.youtube.com/watch?v=yJDv-zdhzMY It is remarkable that all the functions now taken for granted were displayed in 1968. It is also interesting to note how quickly the system worked.

[75]Interview with Tim Berners-Lee, available at https://www.w3.org/People/Berners-Lee/Kids.html Retrieved July 8, 2018.

[76]Berners-Lee, T. *Information management: A proposal.* Retrieved July 8, 2018, from https://www.w3.org/History/1989/proposal-msw.html

Many of the discussions of the future at CERN and the LHC [The Large Hadron Collider] era end with the question—"Yes, but how will we ever keep track of such a large project?" This proposal provides an answer to such questions. Firstly, it discusses the problem of information access at CERN. Then, it introduces the idea of linked information systems, and compares them with less flexible ways of finding information.

It then summarises my short experience with non-linear text systems known as "hypertext," describes what CERN needs from such a system, and what industry may provide. Finally, it suggests steps we should take to involve ourselves with hypertext now, so that individually and collectively we may understand what we are creating ... In 1980, I wrote a program for keeping track of software with which I was involved ... Called *Enquire*, it allowed one to store snippets of information, and to link related pieces together in any way. To find information, one progressed via the links from one sheet to another ... I used this for my personal record of people and modules. It was similar to the application *Hypercard* produced more recently by Apple for the Macintosh. A difference was that *Enquire*, although lacking the fancy graphics, *ran on a multiuser system* [emphasis added], and allowed many people to access the same data.

Although the concept was first greeted with skepticism, by 1981, Berners-Lee completed the documentation for four technologies that would make this system work.

First, the documents at a location (such as CERN) needed an address to which inquiries could be made. The system Berners-Lee developed is called the Uniform Resource Identifier (URI) but is commonly called a Universal Resource Locator (URL).

Second, to be accessible, the documents needed to be formatted in a standard language. The standard he developed is called HyperText Markup Language (HTML). Anticipating the need for other web languages, in 1986, the ISO published the Standard Generalized Markup Language (SGML), ISO 8879. SGML is not actually a language but defines the elements of an acceptable markup language; it is a very large and complex set of policies (specifications) for defining the elements of what is called a Document Type Definition (DTD). The DTD specifies the *types* of documents in each language (such as HTML) and the *structure* of each of those documents. For example, documents may be reports, bibliographies, and the like. The DTD also specifies use of markup code to identify how parts of the document should be interpreted, like beginning and end, paragraphs and footnotes. SGML does not describe how the elements are displayed (e.g., size type, font, or background color), merely how they fit into the structure of the specified report. In this way, when an SGML-compliant document is sent, if the receiver's system has a DTD "reader" (or "SGML compiler"), the recipient can interpret and display the document by identifying its type. HTML is a "simple" subset of SGML acceptable for use on the internet.

Third, there needed to be a method (protocol) for linking the searcher with the host of the information. The protocol must be flexible enough to handle a variety of activities through the link (if allowed by the host)—for example, document retrieval and editing activities. These functions are made possible by the Hypertext Transfer Protocol (HTTP).

Finally, once this system is in place, a tool should be available to search for sites with the desired information. To fill this need, Berners-Lee created WorldWideWeb.app, the first web browser. The term "WorldWideWeb" (with no spaces between the words) was coined at CERN in 1990 in a joint paper by Berners-Lee and colleague Robert Cailliau.[77] The following year, CERN hosted the first website: info.cern.ch. In April 1993, CERN put the codes for these systems in the public domain, meaning that they would be available and royalty-free forever. Berners-Lee moved to MIT in 1994 and founded the World Wide Web Consortium (W3C), whose mission is "to lead the World Wide Web to its full potential by developing protocols and guidelines that ensure the long-term growth of the Web."[78] It is now the standards body for the World Wide Web.

As these systems came into widespread use, their shortcomings became apparent and solutions were required. From 1990 to 1995, HTML went through a number of revisions, first at CERN, then at the IETF, and finally at W3C. By 1999, W3C decided that HTML 4.01 was to be the last version. The reason for this decision was that many users found the structure of HTML very rigid, not allowing for modification of its DTD. As Brewton et al. put it: "As websites became more widespread, the shortcomings of HTML began to be exposed. The major problem was that HTML had no means of representing structured data. Data elements that had a hierarchical relationship could not be efficiently represented in the language."[79]

To fix these problems, in 1996, the W3C created the eXtensible Markup Language (XML) Working Group to formulate a new, more flexible language: XML, which is subset of, and hence compliant with, SGML standards. To compare and contrast these two languages, Refsnes explains: "XML is **not a replacement** [emphases in original] for HTML. XML and HTML were designed with **different goals**: XML was designed to **describe data** and to focus on **what data is**. HTML was designed to **display data** and to focus on **how data looks**. HTML is about **displaying** information, XML is about **describing** information."[80]

Refsnes goes on to explain how XML achieves this benefit: "The tags used to markup HTML documents and the structure of HTML documents are **predefined**. The author of HTML documents can only use tags that are defined **in the HTML standard**. XML allows the author to **define his own tags** and his own document structure."

On a practical level, the problem is that HTML documents may display data in formats that are not compatible across different systems. With XML, the data is wrapped in *self-defined* tags that can be accessed and processed by many different applications and programming languages. This benefit also means that XML can be used not only with computers but also with other devices, like smart phones, appliances, and other programmable

[77]Berners-Lee, T., & Cailliau, R. (1990, November 12). WorldWideWeb: Proposal for a HyperText Project. Retrieved July 11, 2018, from https://www.w3.org/Proposal.html Berners-Lee discussed other names that were considered as well as his current views on the web in a 2017 WBUR interview. See Khalid, A. (2017). *What the founder of the World Wide Web thinks about the state of the web.* WBUR interview. Retrieved July 8, 2018, from http://www.wbur.org/bostonomix/2017/04/04/world-wide-web-inventor-future Cailliau went on to co-develop (with Nicola Pellow) the first web browser for the Classic Mac OS operating system.

[78]For a full explanation of the mission and vision of this organization, see https://www.w3.org/Consortium/mission Retrieved July 11, 2018.

[79]Brewton, J., Yuan, X., & Akowuah, F. (2012). *XML in health information systems.* Retrieved July 11, 2018, from https://pdfs.semanticscholar.org/496f/4c51c61935aa7ed689e9ca39b10e3a4b0409.pdf

[80]Refsnes, J. E. *XML basics—an introduction to XML.* Retrieved July 11, 2018, from https://www.xmlfiles.com/xml

equipment. Further, by specifying the tags, some data can be made inaccessible to certain users. The flexibility of XML's features also allows a greater specificity when conducting searches. For example, using XML to search for references to "car," you get car and not cartoon, carton, boxcar, carry, and so on.

In creating the language, the W3C set the following design goals for XML:

1. XML shall be straightforwardly usable over the Internet.

2. XML shall support a wide variety of applications.

3. XML shall be compatible with SGML.

4. It shall be easy to write programs which process XML documents.

5. The number of optional features in XML is to be kept to the absolute minimum, ideally zero.

6. XML documents should be human-legible and reasonably clear.

7. The XML design should be prepared quickly.

8. The design of XML shall be formal and concise.

9. XML documents shall be easy to create.

10. Terseness in XML markup is of minimal importance.[81]

In order to facilitate XML use, W3C developed the Extensible HyperText Markup Language (XHTML) as "a family of current and future document types and modules that reproduce, subset, and extend HTML, reformulated in XML."[82] Work in XHTML (which was a reformulation of HTML 4.01 in XML) was completed in 2000.[83] XML-based file formats became so popular that, in 2007, Microsoft Office began to use them with its suite of programs: Word (.doc became .docx), Excel (.xls became .xlsx), and PowerPoint (.ppt became .pptx). By 2009, the W3C had decided to cease work on XHTML 2.0 and commit to developing HTML 5. In October 2014, W3C released HTML 5 as its recommended standard to replace XHTML but included the latter's features and other enhancements. HTML 5[84] includes audio and video capabilities and is a package of three interoperable codes: HTML, described above, as the structure of the documents; Cascading Style Sheets (CSS),[85] which provide the style (e.g., fonts, colors, spacing) for the document; and JavaScript, a content-rendering language designed more specifically than XML for presentation

---

[81]W3C. (2008, November 26). Extensible Markup Language (XML) 1.0 (5th ed.) W3C Recommendation. Retrieved July 8, 2018, from https://www.w3.org/TR/xml

[82]W3C: What is XHTML? Retrieved July 11, 2018, from https://www.w3.org/TR/xhtml1/introduction.html

[83]For a more detailed history, see HTML 5.2: W3C Recommendation, 14 December 2017. Retrieved July 11, 2018, from https://www.w3
.org/TR/html52/introduction.html—background

[84]The latest version is HTML5.2 W3C Recommendation, 14 December 2017. Retrieved July 8, 2018 from https://www
.w3.org/TR/html52/introduction.html—background

[85]It is called cascading because the web designer can specify one style for all document pages instead of having to add these elements to each page individually, as was the case with the previous HTML documents.

of data.[86] Further, by wrapping these functions together, HTML 5 can run on multiple different devices (called cross-platform application development), avoiding the need for programmers to create applications for specific browsers.

Applications to Healthcare. The reason for this extensive background is to give the reader an appreciation of the length of time it took to get to the current information age and the complexity of technology and relationships among organizations involved in its genesis and continued operations. It also provides the nontechnical healthcare professional with the terminology and background for productive collaboration with IT specialists. Given this setting, we can now look at interoperability/data exchange efforts in healthcare.

Private interoperability efforts in healthcare mainly began in the hospital sector, where *intra*-organizational interoperability was needed.[87] From a commercialization standpoint, this focus made the most sense since hospitals were the revenue-generating centers of the healthcare system and they needed ways to link all their units together. As mentioned above, when microprocessors were introduced in about 1975, they made it possible for institutions to move from the centralized processing of mainframe and minicomputers to workstations in different operational units. If these workstations were merely typewriters with a screen that connected to a centralized processing unit (so-called dumb terminals), there was no interface problem. However, when the workstations started to be capable of decentralized processing (so-called smart terminals), operational units found that specialized software could help them do their jobs better. Therefore, radiology departments, laboratories, pharmacies, and the like all adopted systems tailored to their needs. In order for these systems to seamlessly transmit patient data to one another, interfaces needed to be created among them. Maintenance of these interfaces can cost hundreds of thousands of dollars, since each system needs to be modified when any of the component systems are changed. Further, it can take weeks or longer to write the code for such changes; in the meantime, the system operates suboptimally and can experience further interoperability issues while the original ones are being addressed.

---

[86] A few important points about JavaScript should be noted. (1) It is not the same as Java. (2) It does not replace XML but can work with it. (3) A subset of JavaScript, JavaScript Object Notation (JSON; pronounced JASON), is an easy-to-use, language-independent, text-based data interchange format designed for transmitting structured data. It is gaining widespread use, especially for business-to-business applications to transfer data between web applications and web servers. In its representation of data, it does not require tags, as does XML. For two explanations of the differences between XML and JSON, see w3schools.com: JSON versus XML. Retrieved July 11, 2018, from https://www.w3schools.com/js/js_json_xml.asp Strassner, T. XML vs JSON. Retrieved July 8, 2018, from http://www.cs.tufts.edu/comp/150IDS/final_papers/tstras01.1/FinalReport/FinalReport.html (4) JavaScript standard is maintained by ECMA International, an affiliate of ISO and the International Electrotechnical Commission (among other organizations), which is comprised of computer-industry members. (Its original name was European Computer Manufacturers Association.) See "ECMA International. June 2018." Retrieved July 11, 2018, from https://www.ecma-international.org/activities/General/presentingecma.pdf See also: ECMS International: The JSON Data Interchange Syntax ECMA 404. 2nd ed. December 2017. Retrieved July 11, 2018, from http://www.ecma-international.org/publications/files/ECMA-ST/ECMA-404.pdf

[87] For an excellent, detailed accounting of the early development of standards (including personal interviews), see Spronk, R. (2014, May 9). *The early history of health Level 7.* Retrieved July 11, 2018, from http://www.ringholm.com/docs/the_early_history_of_health_level_7_HL7.htm

To explain attempts at solving interoperability problems in healthcare, we will focus on four areas: technical solutions, governmental initiatives, private efforts, and Health Information Exchanges (HIEs).

Technical Solutions for Data Exchange in Healthcare. When computerized tomography (CT) scanning was emerging in the late 1970s, radiologists recognized the need for a standard format for production and exchange of images between devices. As a result, in 1983, the American College of Radiology (ACR) and the National Electrical Manufacturers Association (NEMA) formed a joint committee to develop those standards and to facilitate picture archiving and communication systems (PACSs) that could interface with other hospital information systems. This structure would also allow data queries from inside and outside the institution.

From 1985 to 1993, the ACR-NEMA Standard 300 (as it was then called) underwent substantial revisions and was replaced by a version now called Digital Imaging and Communications in Medicine (DICOM).[88] DICOM is the international standard for transmission, storage, retrieval, printing, processing, displaying, and exchanging *medical imaging information* between imaging and other devices. In addition to radiology, these applications have been expanded to other medical disciplines that use imaging, such as cardiology, pathology, gastroenterology, dermatology, dentistry, ophthalmology, and surgery.

While the imaging standards were being developed, pathologists identified a need for medical laboratory instruments to interface with other systems within and outside their institutions. The ASTM took on this task and published standards in 1988.[89] Successor versions are still in use. Of note is that Clem McDonald (see above) was a key participant in this process and proposed the original vocabulary for the standard. When he found the language insufficient, he and colleagues developed LOINC.

These two specialized systems exemplify the operational separation of information systems.

Still lacking was a protocol to bring all of them together. This effort began in 1979, when the ISO developed the OSI model and reference base for network systems that specified seven layers for the exchange of data between computers. (See above.) Starting that year, a system based on this model was introduced at University of California at San Francisco (UCSF) and was subsequently picked up by a number of vendors for hospital use. One of these vendors was Simborg Systems, which sold its own OSI Level 7 product called StatLAN. By 1985, the company was struggling, so its founder, Don Simborg, crafted a uniform standard for *all* health information systems to use that would allow them to interface with best-of-breed solutions, like DICOM and ASTM's Standard Guide for Laboratory Informatics. In March 1987,

---

[88] DICOM is the registered trademark of the National Electrical Manufacturers Association, which maintains the standard for technical details, see PS3.1 DICOM PS3.1 2017e, Introduction and Overview. Retrieved July 11, 2018, from http://dicom.nema.org/medical/dicom/current/output/pdf/part01.pdf

[89] These standards are still published as: Standard Guide for Laboratory Informatics. They are maintained by a subcommittee of ASTM Committee E31 on Healthcare Informatics. The latest edition was released in 2013. See ASTM E1578–13. Retrieved July 11, 2018 from https://www.astm.org/Standards/E1578.htm

Simborg Systems held a meeting of four hospitals[90] that were using StatLAN, vendors who had agreed to use the protocol at those hospitals, and industry leaders. By the second day of the meeting, a small group proposed that a nonprofit, independent company be established and offered to develop standards for its product. In October 1987, after two more small-committee meetings, the protocol product was published as HL7. The name was derived from the term Health, Level 7 (corresponding to the OSI designation). Most of its content was based on StatLAN.

By 1989, version 2.0 of HL7 was able to integrate patient administration messages (what HL7 calls ADT), including demographics, insurance information, status changes (such as admission, transfer, and discharge), pharmacy, laboratory, radiology, and accounting. This capability reduced the time and expense of fixing interoperability problems and was the primary marketing tool that expanded HL7 use. In June 1994, HL7 became an ANSI Accredited Standards Organization.[91]

Today, HL7 International is a not-for-profit, standards-developing organization, which, with its members, provides

a framework (and related standards) for the exchange, integration, sharing, and retrieval of electronic health information. These standards define how information is packaged and communicated from one party to another, setting the language, structure and data types required for seamless integration between systems. HL7 standards support clinical practice and the management, delivery, and evaluation of health services, and are recognized as the most commonly used in the world.[92]

The next list explains a few of the standards HL7 maintains.

Clinical Document Architecture (CDA). CDA describes the standard formats (templates) for clinical documents so that they can be shared. The code, written in XML, structures such items as admission history and physical exam; progress notes; consultation notes; operative reports; diagnostic imaging reports; and discharge summaries.

Medical Logic Modules and Arden Syntax.[93] Although identifying *types* of document structures is important, the problem of extracting usable medical information from those

[90]Moses Cone, Auburn Faith Community, Rochester General, and Hospital of the University of Pennsylvania.
[91]"ANSI X12 is a uniform standard for interindustry electronic interchange of business transactions. The structure of the X12 standard is similar to that of ASTM standards. The HL7 standard is closely modeled on the ANSI X12 Business Data Interchange standard. There are some differences that distinguish the HL7 standard from the ANSI X12 standard [HL7v1]. The ANSI X12 standards apply primarily to batch transmission of data among systems. The HL7 standard differs from ANSI X12 in that it accommodates on-line exchange of individual transactions and LAN interfacing." See The early history of health Level 7, op. cit.
[92]Introduction to HL7 Standards. This document also explains the seven reference categories that comprise the HL7 standards. Retrieved July 11, 2018, from http://www.hl7.org/implement/standards/index.cfm?ref=nav
[93]For an excellent, detailed explanation of MLMs, Arden Syntax and related topics, see De Clercq, P., Kaiser, K., & Hasman, A. (2008). Computer-interpretable guideline formalisms. *Studies in Health Technology and Informatics*, 139, 22–43. Retrieved July 11, 2018, from https://www.ncbi.nlm.nih.gov/pmc/articles/PMC2858861

documents remains. In order to be able to query them in a meaningful way, two more elements are necessary. First, information must be "packaged" in modules that, when linked with other "packages," can be used in clinical decision making. These packages are called Medical Logic Modules (MLMs) and make up clinical databases. Next, in order for institutions to share the content of the MLMs, they must have a standardized syntax (i.e., the rules for the way the sentences are structured and punctuated must be the same). To accomplish this task, MLMs are written in what is called Arden Syntax,[94] which HL7 maintains.

Clinical Context Object Workgroup (CCOW). The CCOW was originally an independent healthcare industry consortium (mainly working at Duke University) but is now part of HL7. The CCOW's task is to maintain the Context Management Specification. This standard enables a user to get a unified view of information on subjects of interest (like patients) from many different operational systems at a single point of contact, like a computer screen. Operationally, this function allows a user to log onto a computer and query a single patient's information that comes from a variety of data bases (e.g., EMR, billing, and diagnostic imaging).

Structured Product Labeling (SPL).[95] In addition to standards for providers, HL7 provides criteria for other healthcare entities. For example, the SPL Working Group specifies the format for prescription drug submissions to the FDA. Although the FDA required use of the SPL in submissions to the Center for Drug Evaluation and Research (CDER) in 2005, the importance of this format was heightened by the FDA Amendments Act of 2007 (Public Law 110-85), which specified submissions must be made electronically. Further, since 2009, the FDA required all over-the-counter (OTC) and veterinary medicine companies to use SPL.

It would seem from the above explanations that the interoperability problem is nearly solved; however, many problems still remain. The most obvious problem is that there are three HL7 versions in use: HL7 Version 2 Series (V2); HL7 Version 3 (V3); and HL7 Fast Healthcare Interoperability Resources. To further understand the problem, these versions are briefly explained below. Of note is that all use XML.

The current Version 2 Series is V2.8 (published in 2014) and is the most widespread in use; when people refer to HL7, it is usually this version. Its prevalence is due to preference by clinical interface specialists who like its ability to integrate disparate clinical systems as needs arise.

---

[94] The Arden Syntax is named after the 1989 Columbia-Presbyterian Medical Center retreat at the Arden Homestead, where sharing health knowledge bases was discussed. The content was substantively derived from HELP of LDS Hospital in Salt Lake City and CARE, the language of the Regenstrief Institute for Health Care in Indianapolis.

[95] For a list of FDA-approved SPLs, see U.S. National Library of Medicine, Dailymed. Retrieved July 8, 2018 from https://dailymed.nlm.nih.gov/dailymed/index.cfm

> The V2 standard provides 80 percent of the interface framework, plus the ability to negotiate the remaining 20 percent of needs on an interface-by-interface basis ... [One way it does so is by] providing support for local variations in data interchanges by allowing optional fields, additional messages, or additional portions of messages.[96]

This flexibility also means that this series is not a plug-and-play product; 20% of the effort must be expended integrating other systems on an ongoing basis. V2.X versions are backward-compatible, meaning newer editions can work with older ones.

The latest Version 3 (published in 2015) called HL7 Version 3 (V3)—Normative Edition. In contrast to V2, V3 has been promoted by government and medical informatics specialists who wanted a completely new and standardized format. As such, V3 is not compatible with any V2 version. In order to achieve uniformity, V3 is based on the Reference Information Model (RIM), a suite of applications that completely describe all transactions and the different "players" involved. In other words, the RIM provides a "storyboard" or "life cycle description" about each event.[97] To describe these stories, the RIM has four primary subject areas: Entity, Role, Participation, and Acts. As an example, if one were looking up a surgical procedure, the entity would be a person, the role is a patient, and the surgeon would be a participant performing the specific act, which is surgery. Within these four areas are many detailed subsidiary descriptions called classes, attributes, associations, and generalizations. For example, "an Act Relationship represents the binding of one act to another, such as the relationship between an order for an observation and the observation event as it occurs. A Role Link represents relationships between individual roles (such as patient and surgeon)."[98] Since the entire story is mapped, it is easier to get a complete picture of what happened and also to evaluate the system for conformance to standards (see below for the discussion about certification). However, because V3 cannot interface with V2, its use has been limited to those organizations that have not previously used V2 versions and to entities for which governments (many of which are international) enforce this standard.

The previous two standards were developed in an era when the interoperability needs of the user were mostly intra-organizational or between the organization and a few others outside. As the amount of data and the number of locations in which it may be found

---

[96] Corepoint Health: Versions of the HL7 Standard. Retrieved July 9, 2018, from https://corepointhealth.com/resource-center/hl7-resources/hl7-standard-versions

[97] HL7. Section 3: Clinical and Administrative Domains: HL7 Version 3 Normative Edition, 2011. Retrieved July 11, 2018, from http://www.hl7.org/implement/standards/product_brief.cfm?product_id=95

[98] HL7: HL7 Reference Information Model Version: V 01-25 (6/29/2003). Retrieved July 11, 2018, from https://www.hl7.org/documentcenter/public_temp_D7ACDC14-1C23-BA17-0C730FD004E179CD/wg/mnm/Draft-rim-std.pdf.

For a more detailed explanation of the RIM categories and schematics describing how the areas relate to one another, see Beeler, G.W. Introduction to HL7 RIM. Retrieved July 11, 2018, from http://www.hl7.org/documentcenter/public_temp_DC52FF5C-1C23-BA17-0C49D379640A4751/calendarofevents/himss/2009/presentations/Reference Information Model_Tue.pdf

have grown dramatically, and because decision-making windows are shorter, information systems now need the ability to:

1. *Achieve seamless communication among many different types of entities* (e.g., patients, hospitals, physician groups, pharmacies, skilled nursing facilities, etc.).

2. *Integrate use among many more types of linked devices* (e.g., not only desktop computers but devices such as laptops, notepads, smartphones and diagnostic devices that communicate wirelessly).

3. *Link many more types of programs with one another* (e.g., clinical and financial systems were originally separate; now there is a need to link such systems as EMRs with insurance/billing systems).

4. *Use internet and cloud-based applications for access, communication, and storage of information.*

5. *"Mine data"*[99] *more quickly to make clinical decisions for individual treatment and policies for population health.* This advantage will occur when the user can quickly find and extract only the needed data instead of whole records (as with V2 and V3).

6. *Provide a secure environment for information technology.* The previous versions do not have this capability, so organizations use virtual private networks (VPNs), which often are cumbersome and slow.

7. *Allow communication with external entities that have disparate systems.* Included in this benefit are patients' ability to access their medical records in real time.

In order to deliver these benefits and address the shortfalls of V2 and V3, starting in 2011, HL7 began developing Fast Healthcare Interoperability Resources (FHIR; pronounced "fire"),[100] which defines how health data should be structured and where it should be located so that health information can be shared over the web.[101] The local applications, such as EMRs and financial systems, are then responsible for populating this structure with actual data. The way FHIR works and differentiates itself from V2 and V3 document searches is that it allows smaller and more precise data inquiries. This capability comes from employing commonly used "Resources." A Resource is a clearly defined data packet that answers common queries. For example, "Patient" will contain a patient's name and demographic information. Other Resources include "Coverage" (insurance information), "Problem List," "Medication List," and so on. Each of these Resources contains elements in standard coding previously described. For example, a "Laboratory Results" Resource would be written

---

[99]Extracting large amounts of data for analysis in order to improve decision making.

[100]For the latest version, see https://www.hl7.org/fhir/directory.html Retrieved March 2, 2019.

[101]For technical descriptions, see FHIR's index page at: https://www.hl7.org/fhir/index.html. Like the other two HL7 versions, these descriptions can get complex and use much esoteric jargon. Two readable sources for more details are: Corepoint Health: "The Future of Interoperability: Web APIs and HL7 FHIR." (Whitepaper). Retrieved from https://corepointhealth.com/wp-content/uploads/Future-of-Interoperability-white-paper.pdf and Redox: "Here's Everything We've Learned about FHIR." Retrieved from https://try.redoxengine.com/fhir/?gclid=EAIaIQobChMI2M74l6Hy2AIVAQdpCh0hygAWEAAYASAAEgKaBPD_BwE (free registration required). All retrieved July 11, 2018.

with LOINC. Resources need not be lists of data but can also be text, which is one reason why FHIR can use both XML and JSON (see footnote 86). As is the case with V2, FHIR Resources are expected to cover about 80% of needs, with the remainder being custom designed. Most of these Resources are still being developed and are listed by "maturity level" as they come close to being ready for use. The first FHIR normative version was released December 27, 2018. Although FHIR can be used internally as well as externally, V2 and V3 are already entrenched within organizations to tie applications together. Many experts, therefore, believe that users will be operating with hybrid systems into the near future. According to IT expert Russell Leftwich, FHIR

> will be the preferred technology for new development, particularly when it involves accessing data across many servers. The existing standards are based on technology of a previous era. New areas like genomics are being tackled by FHIR, something that was never included in older versions of HL7. Other areas like clinical research which had half-baked HL7v3 versions will get more exposure. FHIR will be the lingua franca of these emerging areas.[102]

Indeed, two recent announcements speak to the private sector's endorsement of FHIR. First, in their joint insurance venture, the Cleveland Clinic and health insurer Oscar are using FHIR to allow enrollees to select a primary care physician.[103] The next module will allow appointment scheduling. Second, Apple's iPhone will use FHIR to allow owners to access their medical records, initially at about a dozen U.S. medical centers. "In addition to the iPhone Health app, Apple has developed ResearchKit, software to help researchers develop iPhone apps to conduct health studies, and HealthKit, a platform that allows consumers to share health data on their iPhone or Apple Watch with health and fitness apps."[104]

Once the structure is in place, it is necessary to be able to share data among systems. The sharing benefits of FHIR accrue from its use by web application programming interface (API) technology, which allows a variety of electronic devices, software, and applications to securely communicate with each other over the internet. An API tells a programmer how to write the application so that it can communicate with other operating systems or applications.

An analogy will illustrate how this structure works. If you are looking for hotels in a particular city, you will go to a website (the user interface) that allows you to enter the data you need to make a choice, such as dates, number of people, size of room, price range, and so on. When you are ready for the search, the site's application programming connects you with each hotel in the network and quickly returns the information you requested. Although each hotel's information system is different, the APIs act like messengers that run back and forth

---

[102] Millard, M. (2017). FHIR holds big promise for interoperability, but will need to coexist with other standards for the foreseeable future. [Interview with Russell Leftwich, MD, senior clinical advisor of interoperability at InterSystems and member of the HL7 board of directors]. *Healthcare IT News.* Retrieved July 11, 2018, from https://www.healthcareitnews .com/news/fhir-holds-big-promise-interoperability-will-need-coexist-other-standards-foreseeable-future#main-content

[103] Small, L. (2018, January 26). Oscar, Cleveland Clinic use FHIR to streamline data exchange. *FierceHealthcare.* Retrieved July 11, 2018 from https://www.fiercehealthcare.com/ehr/oscar-cleveland-clinic-use-fhir-to-streamline-data-exchange

[104] Singer, N. (2018, January 25). Apple, in sign of health ambitions, adds medical records feature for iPhone. *New York Times,* B6.

between applications, databases, and devices.[105] APIs can accomplish this task by specifying the way a programmer can write the code so that two software systems can "talk to" one another. Now consider the healthcare equivalent. You are a physician looking over a patient's EMR, and you want to get missing laboratory data from another site. The inquiry requires an API from your system to access the outside database's API. The standard to allow this communication is called SMART (Substitutable Medical Applications, Reusable Technologies), which was developed and is run by the Boston Children's Hospital Computational Health Informatics Program and the Harvard Medical School Department of Biomedical Informatics. Starting in 2010 with a $15 million federal grant, its purpose is to make customized EMRs (and other systems) interoperable. By 2013, when FHIR development was gaining industry traction, SMART decided to work with HL7 and created "SMART on FHIR," essentially becoming FHIR's API. To clarify these relationships, Redox, an IT integration company, explains: "FHIR defines the structure of where data should live and how it should look. The EHRs are responsible for filling that structure with actual patient data. SMART defines how third-party apps launch within an EHR, how to determine which EHR user is interacting with the app, and what patient's data is being accessed."[106]

While the above descriptions are admittedly technical, they make clear the reasons why the quest for interoperable healthcare systems is still ongoing and that the problems will not be resolved anytime soon by the standards organizations. We therefore need to understand the other initiatives that are trying to accomplish interoperability.

Governmental Initiatives

National Library of Medicine. The National Library of Medicine (NLM)[107] originated in 1836 with a collection of medical books housed by the U.S. Army Surgeon General. (It moved to its present location at the National Institutes of Health in 1962.) As the collection grew, the NLM assumed functions other than housing books, the most seminal of which was publication of the *Index Medicus*. From 1879 to 1964, this publication was a manually compiled (not always by the NLM), monthly, topical listing of articles published in thousands of medical and biological science journals. In 1964, after 7 years of NLM planning, a fully operational electronic storage and retrieval system was implemented named MEDLARS (Medical Literature Analysis and Retrieval System). Although the compilation and storage were automated (and became available online; see below), print copies of the *Index Medicus* continued until 2004. In late 1971, an online version of MEDLARS (called MEDLARS Online, or MEDLINE) became available for remote libraries to search MEDLARS at the NLM. However, MEDLINE had a limited set of journals it could search and it could support only 25 simultaneous users. In 1997, after web browsers and the World Wide Web made

---

[105]See Upwork: "Intro to APIs: What Are APIs and What Do They Do?" Retrieved July 11, 2018, from https://www.upwork.com/hiring/development/intro-to-apis-what-is-an-api

[106]Redox. *What is SMART on FHIR?* Retrieved July 11, 2018, from https://www.redoxengine.com/library/what-is-smart-on-fhir

[107]For a summary explanation of what the National Library of Medicine does, see National Library of Medicine Functional Statement (9/2004). Retrieved July 11, 2018, from https://www.nlm.nih.gov/about/functstatement.html

better connections possible, a free interface, called PubMed, became available that allowed the public to search MEDLINE.

In 1979, while online capabilities were being developed, the NLM contracted with the Association of American Medical Colleges (AAMC) "to study trends in biomedical information transfer and access, and to identify the implications for health sciences libraries."[108] The results of that study, published in 1982, found the same interoperability issues for academic medical centers that affected other healthcare organizations: Their information systems were: "fragmented mixtures of single function, manual, and computer-based files that can neither communicate or exchange information effectively."[109]

In response to the study, the NLM issued a request for proposals for strategic planning for information resource management within academic institutions. In September 1983, contracts were awarded to the medical centers at Columbia University, Georgetown University, the University of Maryland, and the University of Utah. One year later, the NLM held a symposium where the four universities reported their results. The success of these efforts spurred expansion of the initiative, called the Integrated Advanced Information Management System (IAIMS) program, which supported a variety of institutional information system plans. At first, the initiatives focused on the use of the library for academic information management; then the projects expanded to institution-wide information management. In a few years, the IAIMS program expanded beyond academic institutions, and the NLM recognized the need for standardized terminology among the noninteroperable systems it was supporting. In this context, we now return to the MEDLINE program. To facilitate searches, MEDLINE uses a system of Medical Subject Headings (MeSH); if you search for articles using MEDLINE, the program will provide you with similar studies with the same MeSH. The problem is that the terminology from all the articles and information systems must be compatible for a useful search. Although some healthcare sectors specify a particular syntax and vocabulary, other sectors may use different elements.

To address this standard terminology problem, in 1986, the NLM launched the Unified Medical Language System (UMLS). Its purpose was not only to facilitate locating research articles on MEDLINE but also to assist linkages among physicians, pharmacies, and payers to help with such tasks as EMR use and development, data classification, and compilation of dictionaries and language translators.[110] The UMLS consists of three parts called "Knowledge Sources:"

1. *The Specialist Lexicon and Lexical Tools*. The UMLS gathers terms into a dictionary, which is used by the other two parts, explained next. In this compilation, it supports use by a natural language processing system. (Please see Exhibit 8.3.)

[108]Stead, W. W. (1997). The evolution of the IAIMS: Lessons for the next decade. *Journal of the American Medical Informatics Association, 4*(2), s4–s9.

[109]Matheson, N., & Cooper, J. A. D. (1982). Academic information in the academic health sciences center roles for the library in information management *Journal of Medical Education, 57* (10 Part 2), 1–93.

[110]National Library of Medicine. *What is the UMLS?* Retrieved from https://www.nlm.nih.gov/research/umls/quickstart .html

EXHIBIT 8.3. **Specialist Lexicon and Lexical Tools**

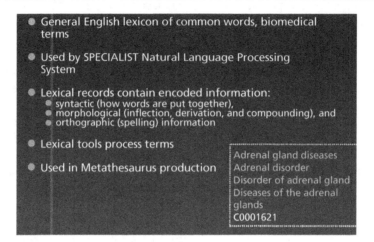

- General English lexicon of common words, biomedical terms
- Used by SPECIALIST Natural Language Processing System
- Lexical records contain encoded information:
  - syntactic (how words are put together),
  - morphological (inflection, derivation, and compounding), and
  - orthographic (spelling) information
- Lexical tools process terms
- Used in Metathesaurus production

Adrenal gland diseases
Adrenal disorder
Disorder of adrenal gland
Diseases of the adrenal glands
C0001621

Source: Kleinsorge, R., and Willis, J., from the National Library of Medicine: Unified Medical Language System. Basics. December 5, 2008. Retrieved July 9, 2018 from https://www.nlm.nih.gov/research/umls/pdf/UMLS_Basics.pdf

2. *Semantic Network.* The two functions of the Semantic Network are defining categories and specifying relationships among the terms. (Please see Exhibit 8.4.)

3. *Metathesaurus.* Uses the first two Knowledge Sources to create a unique identifier for a concept. Its terms and codes come from many vocabularies, including CPT, *ICD*-10-CM, LOINC, MeSH, SNOMED CT, and RxNorm (see below). (Please see Exhibit 8.5.)

In addition to UMLS, the NLM has other important roles in aiding interoperability:[111]

- It partners with other government agencies (particularly the Office of the National Coordinator [ONC], CMS, FDA, and VA) to further interoperability among public agencies and achieve nationwide goals.

- It supports, licenses, or develops key clinical vocabularies identified for Meaningful Use (MU) and Health Insurance Portability and Accountability Act (HIPAA)

---

[111] See NLM. *Health information technology and health data standards at NLM.* Retrieved July 11, 2018, from https://www.nlm.nih.gov/healthit/index.html; and NLM. *Supporting interoperability—terminology, subsets and other resources from NLM.* Retrieved from https://www.nlm.nih.gov/hit_interoperability.html

EXHIBIT 8.4. Semantic Network

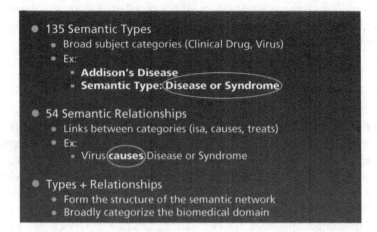

EXHIBIT 8.5. Metathesaurus

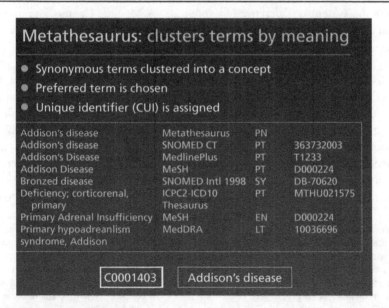

CUI = Concept Unique Identifiers

Source: Kleinsorge, R., and Willis, J., from the National Library of Medicine: Unified Medical Language System. Basics. December 5, 2008. Retrieved July 9, 2018 from https://www.nlm.nih.gov/research/umls/pdf/UMLS_Basics.pdf

transactions: SNOMED CT, LOINC, and RxNorm (a standard naming system for pharmaceuticals).[112]

- ▨ It represents the United States on matters related to the structure and content of SNOMED CT, as a member of the International Health Terminology Standards Development Organisation (IHTSDO).

- ▨ It coordinates efforts to develop mappings between HIPAA code sets and standard clinical vocabularies.

- ▨ It supports training and research/demonstrations in informatics.

***VistA* (Veterans Health Information System and Technology Architecture).** This initiative was born from a desire to create an interoperable system among federal healthcare entities that use EMRs and want to gather meaningful data to better manage the delivery of care.[113] The planning started in 1968 at the National Center for Health Services Research and Development of the U.S. Public Health Service (PHS). (This center is now the Agency for Healthcare Research and Quality [AHRQ].) The idea was to design a system that could be implemented in veterans' facilities, the DoD, the Indian Health Service, and PHS hospitals. The plan was to first introduce the system into PHS hospitals; but they were being closed, so that by 1981 none were left. The project was therefore moved to the Veterans Administration (VA), which, at that time, was part of the Department of HHS.

In 1978 the system was deployed at about 20 VA Medical Centers and 3 years later it was named the Decentralized Hospital Computer Program (DHCP). In 1994 it was renamed VistA (Veterans Health Information System and Technology Architecture). Of note is that in the early 1980s, F. Whitten Peters and Vincent Fuller of the Williams and Connolly law firm established that because this software was developed from PHS projects, it was legally in the public domain, i.e., public and private entities were able to use it without charges or restrictions on modifications. The importance of this status is that this system could have been developed quickly and inexpensively as the national interoperability standard by private as well as governmental users.[114] Also in the early 1980s, the DoD adopted a modified version of the DHCP and renamed it the Composite Health Care System (CHCS). However, the DoD's computer coding diverged from the VA's version so that starting in the mid-1980s the two were never interoperable. In 2000, Congress started to urge the two departments to make their

---

[112]"RxNorm is two things: a normalized naming system for generic and branded drugs; and a tool for supporting semantic interoperation between drug terminologies and pharmacy knowledge base systems. The National Library of Medicine (NLM) produces RxNorm. Purpose of RxNorm Hospitals, pharmacies, and other organizations use computer systems to record and process drug information. Because these systems use many different sets of drug names, it can be difficult for one system to communicate with another. To address this challenge, RxNorm provides normalized names and unique identifiers for medicines and drugs. The goal of RxNorm is to allow computer systems to communicate drug-related information efficiently and unambiguously." NLM: RxNorm Overview. Retrieved July 11, 2018, from https://www.nlm .nih.gov/research/umls/rxnorm/overview.html

[113]For a detailed history of VistA's origins and development, see World VistA. *Vista history*. Retrieved July 11, 2018, from http://worldvista.org/AboutVistA/VistA_History

[114]The ability to use the system on a national scale was subsequently confirmed when countries as different as Finland, Germany, Egypt, and Nigeria adopted it for their hospitals.

systems interoperable; however, after spending hundreds of millions of dollars, the systems were still incompatible. Finally, on June 5, 2017, VA Secretary David Shulkin announced that the VA "will adopt the same EHR system as DoD, now known as MHS GENESIS, which at its core consists of Cerner Millennium. VA's adoption of the same EHR system as DoD will ultimately result in all patient data residing in one common system and enable seamless care between the Departments without the manual and electronic exchange and reconciliation of data between two separate systems."[115] Attempts at integration are still ongoing.

Health Insurance Portability and Accountability Act. The next government effort to aid interoperability started on August 21, 1996, when Public Law 104–191, the Health Insurance Portability and Accountability Act of 1996 (HIPAA), became law.[116] Four of the five titles in this Act deal with insurance issues. Act II, described as Administrative Simplification, deals with *national standards for electronic health transactions*. It covers three topics: data standardization, privacy, and security. The first topic will be discussed here; the latter two will be considered below when security is examined.

CMS defines a transaction as "an electronic exchange of information between two parties to carry out financial or administrative activities related to health care." Such activities (augmented in 2010 by the Affordable Care Act) include:

- Claims and encounter information
- Payment and remittance advice
- Claims status
- Eligibility
- Enrollment and disenrollment
- Referrals and authorizations
- Coordination of benefits
- Premium payment

Each type of exchange must be in a uniform format using the ASCX12 standard (see above).[117] For example, each of the following transmissions will have its own ASCX12 standard format: claim submission by provider to payer; payer request to provider for additional information; requested information from provider to payer; and payer's electronic remittance to provider.

Further, within these formats, the information must be in an approved standard coding language.

---

[115]U.S. Department of Veterans Affairs, Office of Public and Intergovernmental Affairs. (2017, June 5). *VA Secretary announces decision on next-generation Electronic Health Record*. Retrieved July 11, 2018, from https://www.va.gov/opa/pressrel/pressrelease.cfm?id=2914

[116]For a full text, see Health Insurance Portability and Accountability Act of 1996 Public Law 104–191. Retrieved July 11, 2018, from https://www.gpo.gov/fdsys/pkg/PLAW-104publ191/html/PLAW-104publ191.htm

[117]Another standard, called NCPDP, is also permitted for retail pharmacies. Retrieved July 11, 2018, from https://www.ncpdp.org/Resources/HIPAA

CMS requires the following code sets for transactions:

- *Diagnoses. ICD*-10

- *Procedures. ICD*-10 (for hospital inpatient procedures); CPT 4 (for physician services, outpatient procedures, and home health services); HCPCS Level I codes for some CMS-specified temporary codes (i.e., for covered services until a permanent CPT code is assigned).

- *Diagnostic tests*. CPT 4 (These tests include laboratory and imaging examinations.)

- *Treatments*. NDCs and HCPCS Level II codes.

- *Equipment and supplies*. HCPCS Level II codes.

- *Dental services*. Code on Dental Procedures and Nomenclature (CDT).

In addition to the standard codes for the above products and services, HIPAA called for unique identification numbers for all healthcare stakeholders, such as physicians, hospitals, skilled nursing facilities, and the like. Importantly, patients were also to receive a unique identifier. Because of concerns over privacy, however, this part of the law was never implemented. In fact, Congress inserted language into the 1999 Omnibus Appropriations Act prohibiting allocation of funds to adopt a national patient identifier. Failing this public effort, in 2015, the College of Healthcare Information Management Executives (CHIME) issued a $1 million challenge to the private sector to develop a unique identifier. On November 15, 2017, CHIME suspended the initiative.[118] Since privacy of health data is still a major concern, some IT experts believe that instead of using a unique identifier, a biometric identification system should be used to help patients access their information across different information platforms.

Executive Order 13335. The next significant government intervention occurred on April 27, 2004, with President George W. Bush's Executive Order 13335—Incentives for the Use of Health Information Technology and Establishing the Position of the National Health Information Technology Coordinator.[119]

This order:

1. Established the position of National HIT Coordinator under the Secretary of HHS. The unit the Coordinator directs is known as the Office of the National Coordinator, or ONC.

2. Gave the National Coordinator the charge to "develop, maintain, and direct the implementation of a strategic plan to guide the nationwide implementation of interoperable health information technology in both the public and private health care sectors that will reduce medical errors, improve quality, and produce greater value for health care expenditures."

---

[118]Hagland, M. (2017, November 15). CHIME's leaders suspend national patient ID initiative. *Healthcare Informatics*. Retrieved July 11, 2018, from https://www.healthcare-informatics.com/article/interoperability/breaking-chime-s-leaders-suspend-national-patient-id-initiative

[119]Text retrieved March 2, 2019, from https://www.federalregister.gov/documents/2004/04/30/04-10024/incentives-for-the-use-of-health-information-technology-and-establishing-the-position-of-the

3. Required that "key technical, scientific, economic, and other issues affecting the public and private adoption of health information technology are addressed."

4. Required the ONC to evaluate "evidence on the benefits and costs of interoperable health information technology and assess to whom these benefits and costs accrue."

5. Required the ONC to "address privacy and security issues related to interoperable health information technology and recommend methods to ensure appropriate authorization, authentication, and encryption of data for transmission over the Internet."

6. Mandated eight initiatives with measurable outcome goals: Cyber Security; Innovation; Nationwide Health Information Network (NwHIN); Federal Health Architecture; Rural Health IT; State-Level Initiatives; Health IT Adoption; and Clinical Decision Support.

After David J. Brailer, MD, PhD, was appointed the first coordinator, he issued a strategic action framework in which he identified seven critical needs: "Avoid medical errors; Improve use of resources; Accelerate diffusion of knowledge; Reduce variability in access to care; Advance consumer role; Strengthen privacy and data protection; and Promote public health and preparedness."[120] The president announced the goal of having interoperable records by 2014.

Unfortunately, this governmental effort has not resulted in nationwide interoperability.

HITECH Act. Another attempt to boost to this effort came with passage of the HITECH Act (Title XIII of the American Recovery and Reinvestment Act of 2009), which called for the "development of a nationwide health information technology infrastructure that allows for the electronic use and exchange of information and that … promotes a more effective marketplace, greater competition … [and] increased consumer choice."[121] Its intent was to encourage sharing of information (including with patients) and discourage barriers based on proprietary business considerations.

As a result of this Act, in 2011, the "Centers for Medicare & Medicaid Services (CMS) established the Medicare and Medicaid Electronic Health Record (EHR) Incentive Programs to encourage Eligible Professionals (EPs), Eligible Hospitals, and Critical Access Hospitals (CAHs) to adopt, implement, upgrade (AIU), and demonstrate meaningful use of certified EHR technology (CEHRT)."[122]

Incentive payments totaled about $36 billion—up to $44,000 for Medicare-eligible providers or up to $63,750 for Medicaid-eligible providers. The funds were provided over

---

[120]Thompson, T. G., & Brailer, D. J. (2004, July 21). *The decade of health information technology: Delivering consumer-centric and information-rich healthcare*. Framework for Strategic Action. Retrieved July 11, 2018, from http:// www.providersedge.com/ehdocs/ehr_articles/the_decade_of_hit-delivering_customer-centric_and_info-rich_hc.pdf

[121]Title XIII—Health Information Technology. Public Law 111–5, February 17, 2009. 123 STAT. 227. "Subtitle A—Promotion of Health Information Technology. 'SEC. 3001. Office of the National Coordinator for Health Information Technology.'" Retrieved July 11, 2018, from https://www.hhs.gov/sites/default/files/ocr/privacy/hipaa/understanding/coveredentities/hitechact.pdf

[122]CMS.gov (2017, November 29). *Electronic Health Records (EHR) Incentive Programs* (updated). Retrieved July 11, 2018, from https://www.cms.gov/Regulations-and-Guidance/Legislation/EHRIncentivePrograms/index.html?redirect=/ehrincentiveprograms

several years and based on the number of patients who were served in these categories. They also came with some basic requirements. First, the system had to be certified by an organization approved by HHS (certification will be discussed further below). Second, the system had to have at least two elements of communicability: electronic prescribing (whereby the physician "writes" a prescription using the EMR and sends it electronically to a specific pharmacy) and a "patient portal" that gives patients the ability to communicate with their physicians and access their medical information. Third, provider-selected clinical quality measures needed to be reported to CMS. These communication capabilities and quality measures reporting constitute what CMS calls "meaningful use" of the electronic systems. According to CMS,[123] the meaningful use incentive program consists of three stages:

> *Stage 1* set the foundation for the EHR Incentive Programs by establishing requirements for the electronic capture of clinical data, including providing patients with electronic copies of health information.
>
> *Stage 2* expanded upon the Stage 1 criteria with a focus on advancing clinical processes and ensuring that the meaningful use of EHRs supported the aims and priorities of the National Quality Strategy. Stage 2 criteria encouraged the use of CEHRT [certified EHR technology] for continuous quality improvement at the point of care and the exchange of information in the most structured format possible.
>
> In October 2015, CMS released a final rule that modified Stage 2 to ease reporting requirements and align with other quality reporting programs. The final rule also established *Stage 3* in 2017 and beyond, which focuses on using CEHRT to improve health outcomes.

Recognizing that much of the care in this country is provided by solo physicians, small groups, and nonprofit community health centers that would find EHR development expensive and difficult, the HITECH Act authorized establishment of Regional Extension Centers (RECs)[124] to help them. The 62 RECs were tasked with helping these providers with: EHR implementation and project management; health IT education and training; vendor selection and financial consultation; practice/workflow redesign; compliance with privacy and security requirements; partnering with state and national HIE; and ongoing technical assistance. The RECs do not charge for their services and cannot provide aid to *private* providers other than advice.

After 2016, the meaningful use program was folded into the Merit-based Incentive Payment System (MIPS), discussed in Chapter 9, "Quality." While the incentive program did stimulate investment in IT systems, provider groups claim that the bonuses did not compensate for the implementation costs and the ongoing excessive administrative expenses. For example, the American Hospital Association has stated that "the average-sized hospital spent nearly $760,000 to meet MU administrative requirements annually. In addition, they

---

[123] Ibid.

[124] HealthIT.gov. *Regional Extension Centers (RECs)*. Retrieved July 11, 2018, from https://www.healthit.gov/providers-professionals/regional-extension-centers-recs —listing

invested \$411,000 in related upgrades to systems during the year, over 2.9 times larger than the information technology (IT) investments made for any other domain."[125]

Standards and Interoperability Framework. In 2011, the ONC created the Standards and Interoperability Framework as "a collaborative community of participants from the public and private sectors who are focused on providing the tools, services and guidance to facilitate the functional exchange of health information."[126]

The framework issues the Interoperability Standards Advisory, a document whose core purposes are:

1. To provide the industry with a single, public list of the standards and implementation specifications that can best be used to address specific clinical health information interoperability needs. Currently, the ISA is focused on interoperability for sharing information between entities and not on intra-organizational uses.

2. To reflect the results of ongoing dialogue, debate, and consensus among industry stakeholders when more than one standard or implementation specification could be used to address a specific interoperability need, discussion will take place through the ISA public comments process. The web-version of the ISA will improve upon existing processes, making comments more transparent, and allowing for threaded discussions to promote further dialogue.

3. To document known limitations, preconditions, and dependencies as well as provide suggestions for security best practices in the form of security patterns for referenced standards and implementation specifications when they are used to address a specific clinical health IT interoperability need.

    The ISA is designed to provide clarity, consistency, and predictability for the public regarding the standards and implementation specifications that could be used for a given clinical health IT interoperability purpose.[127]

Starting in 2017, the ISA's focus expanded to include public health and health research interoperability and administrative functions related to healthcare services.

The ISA is not a prescriptive governmental intervention to solve the interoperability problem. Rather, "the ISA itself is a non-binding document and meant to be advisory in nature, standards and implementation specifications listed in the ISA may be considered for rulemaking or other Federal requirements. However, those decisions would be made on a case-by-case basis by the administering organization."[128] The effectiveness of the ISA remains to be seen.

---

[125] AHA. (2017, October). *Regulatory overload: Assessing the regulatory burden on health systems, hospitals, and post-acute care providers* (p. 4). Retrieved July 11, 2018, from https://www.aha.org/system/files/content/17/regulatory-overload-report.pdf

[126] See CMS *eCQI Resource Center*. Retrieved July 11, 2018, from https://ecqi.healthit.gov/content/about-ecqi This site replaced the Clinical Quality Framework Initiative, which closed June 1, 2017.

[127] HealthIT.gov. *Introduction to the ISA*. Retrieved from https://www.healthit.gov/isa

[128] Ibid.

21st Century Cures Act. Interoperability of health information networks (HINs) is a major focus of the 21st Century Cures Act's (Section 4003), passed December 13, 2016.[129] The vision of this plan is to achieve interoperability via a single "on ramp" for all HINs so they can safely exchange data regardless of geographic location or software product. The ONC has named this effort the Trusted Exchange Framework and Common Agreement (TEFCA),[130] whose two-part format and work plan are displayed in Exhibit 8.6.

Part A lists the six principles to which all stakeholders should adhere in order to facilitate interoperability. Part B is where the work must be done in order to develop the technical and organizational standards to make the system operate properly. To accomplish this work, in the spring of 2018, the ONC issued a competitive Funding Opportunity Announcement (FOA) for private entities to bid on a single, multiyear cooperative agreement to act as a Recognized Coordinating Entity (RCE). The ONC was supposed to announce RCE choices in late 2018; as of early 2019, no decision had been made.

The organization of the TEFCA is displayed in Exhibit 8.7.

The 21st Century Cures Act established another entity to help the ONC with this project: the Health Information Technology Advisory Committee (HITAC). According to the ONC:

> The Health Information Technology Advisory Committee (HITAC) will recommend to the National Coordinator for Health Information Technology, policies, standards, implementation specifications, and certification criteria, relating to the implementation of a health information technology infrastructure, nationally and locally, that advances the electronic access, exchange, and use of health information. HITAC unifies the roles of, and replaces, the Health Information Technology Policy Committee and the Health Information Technology Standards Committee, as in existence before the date of the enactment of the 21st Century Cures Act.[131]

Its first meeting was held in January 2018.[132]

The federal government and other stakeholders have also been concerned that IT companies use blocking software to prevent users from sending and obtaining information from each other. The reason for this fear is that these companies do not want their customers to be able to easily switch to competitors' products. To address this potential problem, the 21st Century Cures Act mandates the HHS Secretary to require that a certified EHR

---

[129] An Act—To accelerate the discovery, development, and delivery of 21st century cures, and for other purposes. (21st Century Cures Act). Public Law 114–255. Passed December 13, 2016. See Title IV, Sec. 4002 and Sec.4004. Retrieved July 11, 2018, from https://www.congress.gov/114/plaws/publ255/PLAW-114publ255.pdf

[130] Office of the National Coordinator for Health Information Technology. (2018, January 5). *Draft Trusted Exchange Network (draft for public comment)*. Retrieved July 11, 2018, from https://www.healthit.gov/sites/default/files/draft-trusted-exchange-framework.pdf

[131] The Health Information Technology Advisory Committee (HITAC). Retrieved July 11, 2018, from https://www.healthit.gov/hitac

[132] Slabotkin, G. (2018, January 19). HHS sees key role for new advisory panel in achieving interoperability. *HealthData Management*. Retrieved July 11, 2018, from https://www.healthdatamanagement.com/news/hhs-sees-key-role-for-new-advisory-panel-in-achieving-interoperability

EXHIBIT 8.6. Format of the TEFCA

Part A—Principles for Trusted Exchange

General principles that provide guardrails to engender trust between Health Information Networks (HINs). Six (6) categories:

» Principle 1- Standardization: Adhere to industry and federally recognized standards, policies, best practices, and procedures.

» Principle 2 - Transparency: Conduct all exchange openly and transparently.

» Principle 3 - Cooperation and Non-Discrimination: Collaborate with stakeholders across the continuum of care to exchange electronic health information, even when a stakeholder may be a business competitor.

» Principle 4 - Security and Patient Safety: Exchange electronic health information securely and in a manner that promotes patient safety and ensures data integrity.

» Principle 5 - Access: Ensure that patients and their caregivers have easy access to their electronic health information.

» Principle 6 - Data-driven Accountability: Exchange multiple records at one time to enable identification and trending of data to lower the cost of care and improve the health of the population.

Part B—Minimum Required Terms and Conditions for Trusted Exchange

A minimum set of terms and conditions for the purpose of ensuring that common practices are in place and required of all participants who participate in the Trusted Exchange Framework, including:

» Common authentication processes of trusted health information network participants;

» A common set of rules for trusted exchange;

» A minimum core set of organizational and operational policies to enable the exchange of electronic health information among networks.

Source: ONC: A User's Guide to Understanding: The Draft Trusted Exchange Framework. Retrieved July 11, 2018 from https://www.healthit .gov/sites/default/files/draft-guide.pdf

EXHIBIT 8.7. Organization of the TEFCA

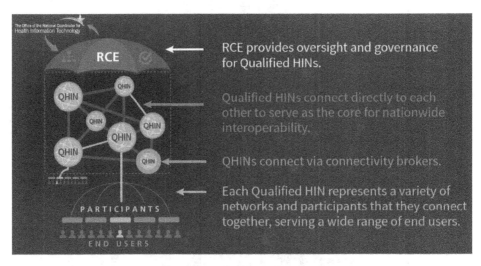

Source: ONC: A User's Guide to Understanding: The Draft Trusted Exchange Framework. Retrieved July 11, 2018 from https://www.healthit.gov/sites/default/files/draft-guide.pdf

"does not take any action that constitutes information blocking."[133] In particular, the system cannot prohibit or restrict communication regarding the usability, interoperability, security, or relevant information regarding users' experiences when using the HIT.

Starting in 2018, users were required to attest that their systems are in compliance with the antiblocking provision.[134] Many providers and other stakeholders are very concerned that terms of this attestation are vague, because each violation comes with a $1 million fine. Particular confusion exists about how the privacy and security requirements of HIPAA may conflict with this act.

Draft U.S. Core Data for Interoperability and Proposed Expansion Process. One requirement of interoperability is having a common data set. Since different systems had different sets, in 2012, the ONC adopted a "Meaningful Use Common Dataset." By 2015, the HHS Secretary issued the Health IT Certification Criteria (2015 edition) final

---

[133] An Act—To accelerate the discovery, development, and delivery of 21st century cures, and for other purposes. (21st Century Cures Act). Public Law 114–255. Passed December 13, 2016. See Title IV, Sec. 4002 and Sec. 4004. Retrieved July 11, 2018, from https://www.congress.gov/114/plaws/publ255/PLAW-114publ255.pdf

[134] CMS. (2017, October). *Advancing Care Information Prevention of Information Blocking Attestation: Making sure EHR information is shared.* Retrieved July 11, 2018, from https://www.cms.gov/Medicare/Quality-Initiatives-Patient-Assessment-Instruments/Value-Based-Programs/MACRA-MIPS-and-APMs/ACI-Information-Blocking-fact-sheet.pdf

EXHIBIT 8.8. Draft USCDI Version 1 Data Classes

1. Patient name	2. Sex (birth sex)
3. Date of birth	4. Preferred language
5. Race	6. Ethnicity
7. Smoking status	8. Laboratory tests
9. Laboratory values/results	10. Vital signs
11. Problems	12. Medications
13. Medication allergies	14. Health concerns
15. Care team members	16. Assessment and plan of treatment
17. Immunizations	18. Procedures
19. Unique device identifier(s) for a patient's implantable device(s)	20. Goals
21. Provenance	22. Clinical notes

Source: ONC: Draft U.S. Core Data for Interoperability (USCDI) and Proposed Expansion Process. January 5, 2018. Retrieved July 11, 2018 from https://www.healthit.gov/sites/default/files/draft-uscdi.pdf

rule,[135] which adopted the 2015 Edition Common Clinical Data Set (CCDS). In 2018, the ONC issued the U.S. Core Data for Interoperability (USCDI) and Proposed Expansion Process, which issued a list of data classes and established a process and timeline to make available such data classes for exchange through the TEFCA.[136] (Please see Exhibit 8.8.)

Private Initiatives. Because standard platforms (HL7) and government initiatives have not provided the interoperability capabilities the market needs, three types of private initiatives have emerged.

1. Non-healthcare companies have offered services where individuals can store their healthcare information online so that it is readily available in emergencies. Strictly speaking, this type of product is not interoperable software, but it can solve the problem of data availability. Examples include Microsoft's HealthVault[137] and Google Health (introduced in 2008 and shut down in 2011).

---

[135] 80 FR 62601, 2015 Edition Health Information Technology (Health IT) Certification Criteria, 2015 ed. Base Electronic Health Record (EHR) Definition, and ONC Health IT Certification Program Modifications. Retrieved July 11, 2018, from https://www.federalregister.gov/documents/2015/10/16/2015-25597/2015-edition-health-information- technology-health-it-certification-criteria-2015-edition- base?utm_content=previous&utm_medium=PrevNext&utm_source=Article

[136] ONC. (2018, January 5). Draft U.S. Core Data for Interoperability (USCDI) and Proposed Expansion Process. Retrieved July 11, 2018, from https://www.healthit.gov/sites/default/files/draft-uscdi.pdf

[137] Microsoft HealthVault. Retrieved July 11, 2018, from https://www.healthvault.com/en- us/healthvault-for-consumers

2. Even though same-vendor platforms are basically the same, they lacked interoperability due to customization requirements at each customer's sites. These vendors have worked hard to make their systems compatible across their customers, and this effort appears to be successful. An example is Epic's Care Everywhere product that, with relatively minimal work, will allow one Epic user to communicate seamlessly with other users. Further, Epic announced that its One Virtual System Worldwide service will "search for and collect patient records from clients and other organizations that use other EHRs and networks that work with the Epic clients, enabling outside clinicians to have a merged view of information on a patient from multiple provider organizations."[138]

3. Another private sector solution is for different companies to band together and make sure their systems can easily communicate with one another. Such an example is CommonWell Health Alliance,[139] which was formed in 2013 by Cerner, McKesson, Allscripts, athenahealth, Greenway, and RelayHealth; other firms have joined since then. Currently, the organization claims "more than 5,000 provider sites in all 50 states, D.C. and Puerto Rico have gone live with CommonWell services and have generated millions of transactions on the network."[140]

Health Information Exchanges. In addition to the projects mentioned above, HIEs have emerged as another solution to interoperability problems. Because they have taken a number of public and private sponsorship forms, they will be discussed as a separate category.

Definitions According to HIMSS, a "HIE provides the capability to electronically move clinical information among disparate healthcare information systems and maintain the meaning of the information being exchanged."[141]

The Office of the National Coordinator (ONC) for Health IT has defined three forms of HIE:[142]

Directed exchange is used by providers to easily and securely send patient information—such as laboratory orders and results, patient referrals, or discharge summaries—directly to another health care professional. This information is sent over the internet in an encrypted, secure, and reliable way amongst health care professionals who already know and trust each other and is commonly compared to sending a secured email.

Query-based exchange is used by providers to search and discover accessible clinical sources on a patient. This type of exchange is often used when delivering unplanned care [such as emergency room visits].

---

[138]Goedert, J. (2018, January 31). Epic initiative seeks to facilitate data exchange. *HealthData Management*. Retrieved July 11, 2018, from https://www.healthdatamanagement.com/news/epics-gathering-of-data-to-support-ehrs-and-hie-is-intended-to-eliminate-gaps-in-care

[139]CommonWell Health Alliance. Retrieved July 11, 2018, from http://www.commonwellalliance.org

[140]HIMSS. (2017, May 23). HIE in Practice interview with Jitin Asnaani, Executive Director of CommonWell Health Alliance. Retrieved July 11, 2018, from http://www.himss.org/library/commonwell-health-alliance

[141]Healthcare Information and Management Systems Society (HIMSS). (2017). *HIMSS dictionary of health information technology terms, acronyms, and organizations* (4th ed.). Boca Raton, FL: CRC Press, Taylor & Francis Group.

[142]Ibid.

Consumer-mediated exchange provides patients with access to their health information, allowing them to manage their health care online in a similar fashion to how they might manage their finances through online banking.

HIEs can also be classified by where data resides:

Centralized systems have all the data in one place, and users can access it with appropriate security clearance.

Decentralized systems have the data residing in user organizations, and the HIE acts as an intermediary to the three types of activities explained above.

Hybrid systems have some data centrally stored, and the rest resides with the users.

Further, there are a variety of sponsorship and financial models:

State-wide HIEs are run by the governments of their respective states or may be the State's Designated Entity (SDE). Some state-wide (and regional) HIEs use an umbrella approach and serve as the aggregator for disparate private HIEs.

Private/Proprietary HIEs concentrate on a single community or network, often based within a single organization, and include overall management, finance and governance. Examples may include hospital/IDN [Integrated Delivery Network], payer-based HIEs and disease-specific HIEs. Some software vendors have also established an HIE network for their clients across the U.S. Additionally, the industry may see other evolving entities such as Accountable Care Organizations (ACOs) supporting information exchange.

Hybrid HIEs/HIOs [Health Information Organizations] are often collaborations between organizations, such as an ACO and a vendor network, within a state or region. The Kentucky HIE is an example of a hybrid model.

Regional/Community HIOs are inter-organizational and depend on a variety of funding sources. Most are not-for-profit.[143]

Given all the possible combinations that can define an HIE, one can appreciate the difficulty in evaluating which characteristics will work best. However, an appreciation of their evolution will help one understand their pitfalls and current status.

History and Current Status   The John A. Hartford Foundation provided start-up funds in 1990 for planning and development activities in seven communities in Iowa, Washington, Minnesota, New York, Vermont, Ohio, and Memphis. These initiatives were called Community Health Management Information Systems (CHMISs).

Fundamentally, CHMISs were a community and payer-centric means to healthcare assessment. A centralized data repository that contained individual level demographic, clinical, and

---

[143]HIMSS. *FAQ: Health Information Exchange (HIE)*. Retrieved July 11, 2018, from http://www.himss.org/library/health-information-exchange/FAQ

eligibility information for a geographically defined community provided data to stakeholder organizations (e.g., local agencies, payers, employers, and researchers) who were consumers of the data for assessment activities and other purposes. A secondary component of CHMISs was a transaction system to facilitate billing and patient eligibility information retrieval in order to reduce costs.[144]

Some of the problems CHMISs encountered were due to lack of cost-effective technology. Not only were hardware, software, and integration work expensive, but connectivity required such costly expenses as the need for dedicated data-use cables between participating organizations and the exchange. As internet solutions became available and hardware costs were reduced, these problems became much less important. However, CHMISs did experience several important obstacles that have plagued subsequent HIE versions.

First, many exchanges received their initial funding from private or governmental grants. When the money runs out, users very often argue over the structure of the sustainable business model needed to continue operations. One important question is: How much does each user pay? Models might include payment based on the size of the organization; however, how does one compare sizes of different types of businesses? For example, hospitals may pay based on number of beds while insurers are measured by number of covered lives. Another payment model is charge per use; however, the relative costs would be greatest for primary care physicians whose use is greatest and whose revenue is lower than other specialties and large organizations.

Second, in order for the exchange to work properly, it requires participation from all sectors of the local market, including competitors. A major contested issue centers on these questions: Who "owns/controls" the data, who has access to the data, and how much of data can be accessed? This issue was of particular concern given the data-centric structure of the CHMISs.

Third, despite best efforts at prevention, data breeches are common. All stakeholders, particularly patients, are concerned that exchanges furnish a more easily hackable gateway to participants' data.

The next attempt at HIEs was called Community Health Information Networks (CHINs). Although they had their origins in the mid-1980s, they achieved prominence and functionality in the early 1990s. Instead of the data-centric model of CHMISs, CHINs were built around networks of different systems. Of the perhaps several hundred CHINs that existed or were in planning stages in the 1990s, only one survived as a state-wide information network, the Utah Health Information Network (UHIN).[145] Incorporated in 1993, it is "a nonprofit coalition of healthcare providers, payers, state government and other stakeholders whose mission is to

---

[144] Vest, J. R., & Gamm, L. D. (2010) Health information exchange: Persistent challenges and new strategies. *Journal of the American Medical Informatics Association, 17,* 288–294.

[145] UHIN. Retrieved July 11, 2018, from https://uhin.org. The other successful CHIN that is usually mentioned is the Wisconsin Health Information Network, formed in 1992 as a joint venture between Aurora Health System and Ameritech. When Ameritech exited that line of business, Aurora become the CHIN owner, using it for its own system. The Wisconsin *Statewide* Health Information Network (WISHIN) was formed in 2010 as the multiuser statewide information exchange.

positively impact healthcare through reduced costs, improved quality, and better results by fostering data-driven decisions." What differentiates this organization from many that failed is its broad public and private sponsorship (including funding) and clear functional goals.

Following the CHIN failures, the federal government intervened in HIE development as a result of President George W. Bush's Executive Order 13335 (see above). On July 21, 2004, HHS Secretary Thompson "released the first outline of a 10-year plan to transform the delivery of health care by building a new health information infrastructure, including electronic health records and a new network to link health records nationwide."[146] This initiative came with funding for "the formation of regional health information organizations," subsequently called RHIOs. As many as 200 RHIOs formed and had three advantages over previous attempts. The first was the political support and funding just mentioned.

The second was the gathering movement to use information systems to improve patient quality (including efficiency) and safety following the Institute of Medicine's 1999 and 2001 reports. (Please see Chapter 9 for more details.)

Third, other, contemporaneous initiatives complemented formation of RHIOs. In 2003, the Medicare Modernization Act (MMA) authorized AHRQ and the CMS to award $6 million grants to five states to test initial standards in electronic prescribing (eRx). The ability for physicians to send electronic prescriptions to any pharmacy regardless of the patient's insurance was the first truly universal interoperable function performed by exchanges. (Please see the Surescripts discussion below.) Results of this project informed e-prescribing meaningful use requirements previously described. The other program started in 2004 when

> the Agency for Healthcare Quality and Research (AHRQ) Health Information Technology Portfolio funded $166 million in grants and contracts to improve healthcare decision making, support patient-centered care and improve quality and safety. This funding included the State and Regional Demonstration (SRD) project to support state and regional level HIEs. AHRQ awarded $5 million grants to six states: Indiana, Delaware, Rhode Island, Tennessee, Colorado, and Utah. The SRDs established information exchange over large geographic areas and generated best practices for developing policy, governance, trust and technical solutions to meet the needs of broad stakeholder groups.[147]

To meet their aims, RHIOs employed a variety of data centralization models and sponsorships. Their aims stressed the priorities of cost savings and quality improvement goals. While technical costs that affected the CHMISs were no longer as important, the remaining issues, particularly the sustainable business model, still caused these plans to fail.

---

[146]HHS.gov (2004). Thompson Launches "Decade of Health Information Technology." *Strategic Report Outlines Steps to Implement Widespread Adoption of Electronic Health Records and New Nationwide Interoperable Health Information Network.* Retrieved July 11, 2018, from https://web.archive.org/web/20041015040119/http://hhs.gov/news/press/2004pres/20040721a.html

[147]Presented by NORC at the University of Chicago to The Office of the National Coordinator of Health Information Technology: Dullabh, P., Moiduddin, A., Nye, C., & Virost, L. (2011). *The evolution of the State Health Information Exchange Cooperative Agreement Program: State plans to enable robust HIE.* Retrieved July 11, 2018, from https://www.healthit.gov/sites/default/files/pdf/state-health-info-exchange-program-evolution.pdf

Current exchange programs trace their origins to the ONC's National Health Information Infrastructure (NHII), which was a result of the 2004 Executive Order mentioned above. The NHII's mission was to provide "a set of standards, services and policies that enable secure health information exchange (HIE) over the Internet";[148] in other words, it was the healthcare standardization for the RHIOs. The NHII became the National Health Information Network (NHIN) and by 2007 was called the Nationwide Health Information Network (NwHIN).[149]

The effort received a boost from passage of the HITECH Act in 2009, which allowed the ONC to issue a funding opportunity announcement (FOA) to establish partnerships with states that wished to set up their own HIEs (the State HIE Cooperative Agreement Program). By March 2010, 50 states and 6 territories received initial awards ($564 million) to begin planning for and establishing their programs. The organization of partners in this cooperative agreement was initially called the NwHIN Cooperative; the name was then changed to NwHIN Exchange. By 2010, partners' exchanges were used by thousands of public and private organizations and millions of patients. However, not all of these exchanges were successful.[150] A 2016 evaluation of the State HIE Cooperative Agreement Program revealed some important lessons about how successful initiatives can be implemented. (Please see Exhibit 8.9.)

EXHIBIT 8.9. Evaluation of the State HIE Cooperative Agreement Program

The overarching goal of the state HIE Program was to rapidly build HIE capacity by: (1) ensuring every provider has at least one option for meeting the HIE requirements of meaningful use (MU); (2) fostering creation and use of networks of exchange through which information can flow; (3) filling existing gaps in exchange capacity (e.g., overcoming technical barriers, lack of services); and (4) ensuring exchange can occur across networks. Given the program's design as a one-time investment over a four-year period, ONC recognized it would be challenging "for states to implement and operate comprehensive statewide HIE services" using HITECH funds alone. As such, states were encouraged to fill service gaps, leverage existing information exchanges, and coordinate with key stakeholders in pursuit of sustainable HIE solutions . . . .

Overall, states with a solid HIE foundation experienced greater success; these states were able to accelerate their progress with State HIE Program support. States with little foundation in HIE struggled to establish themselves in the early program years and only made measurable advances in the later years. In later program years, states with state-led HIE showed more success with HIE than true SDE [state-designated entity] or SDE-like models . . . .

[148] *What is the NHIN?* Retrieved July 11, 2018, from https://www.healthit.gov/sites/default/files/what-Is-the-nhin--2.pdf This purpose started with the NHII and continued with its successors.

[149] The exact dates for name transitions are not consistent in their history. Also, "national" and "nationwide" networks are both often called NHINs, further confusing their origins. This accounting presents an overview of their roles without needing to specify exact dates.

[150] Conn, J. (2016, September 15). Health information exchanges are coming of age and proving their worth. *Modern Healthcare.* Retrieved July 9, 2018, from http://www.modernhealthcare.com/article/20160915/NEWS/160919974

Lessons Learned

Across grantee reports, several common key drivers eased the implementation of HIE, encouraged participation by hospitals and providers, and accelerated progress:

- Involvement of diverse stakeholders was of great value to build relationships, establish trust, improve acceptance, align goals, leverage existing HIE assets, and create a sense of ownership for all those involved.

- Initial service offerings played an important role in driving momentum for HIE by building services based on provider needs and demand, rather than building a service or standard and then trying to recruit adopters.

- Governing bodies varied in their official responsibilities, legal authority, membership, and affiliation with government—all of which had implications for the design, pace of development, and sustainability of HIE.

- Starting simply, rolling out services incrementally, and layering on complexity over time in response to growing provider demand, allowed states to demonstrate immediate value and gain buy-in for HIE.

- Delivery system reform has played, and will continue to play, a role in HIE expansion. The State HIE Program has facilitated provider efforts to meet the requirements of MU, and existing HIE infrastructure will play an important role supporting delivery system reform efforts.

Challenges

- Developing and implementing HIE infrastructure and services was more resource intensive (in time, money, and effort) than grantees anticipated.

- Common standards and incentives were needed to achieve interoperability.

- Grantees encountered barriers in their relationships with EHR developers and HIE vendors, as well as lack of developer readiness to accommodate the needs of HIE stakeholders.

- Sustainability was a persistent concern among grantees.

Sustainability

The State HIE Program catalyzed HIE through a substantial, one-time infusion of funds. Many factors will contribute to the sustainability of HIE services, whether state-led or otherwise—including diverse stakeholder engagement, a flexible infrastructure, continued marketing of benefits, and clear and consistent policies and regulation. Grantees expressed concerns about the financial sustainability of their HIE efforts, wondering whether they would be able to secure the necessary financial investment to continue operating in the short term—needed to demonstrate long-term value to stakeholders. Post-program, seven grantees are no longer operational. Grantees who continue to operate reflected that they may require more examples of the value-add of HIE to motivate continued stakeholder commitment and investment. Long-term sustainability requires that grantees seek out new financial contributors (including payers, ACOs, and long-term care providers) and offer them reasonably priced services that address their needs and priorities for exchange.

Source: Dullabh, P et al. (for NORC at the University of Chicago): Evaluation of the State HIE Cooperative Agreement Program. Final Report. March 2016. Retrieved July 11, 2018 from https://www.healthit.gov/sites/default/files/reports/finalsummativereportmarch_2016.pdf

EXHIBIT 8.10. **Evaluation of the Beacon Community Cooperative Agreement Program**

The Beacon Program offers insights for policies and programs that aim to promote and invest in the use of health IT, and to foster and scale sustainable initiatives in service delivery redesign, quality improvement, and payment reform. Results from this evaluation show that Communities achieved mixed progress on broad health care use and quality measures; the extent to which Communities leveraged existing efforts and engaged providers was a facilitator of successful outcomes. Communities also found their efforts hindered in critical ways by challenges stemming from provider readiness, legal and policy constraints, and the technologies used. These findings suggest important considerations for future program design, evaluation, and policy:

- Programs intended to demonstrate meaningful impact on cost, quality, and health outcomes require sufficient time to become operational and demonstrate results.

- Support in aligning regional efforts with federal initiatives will foster continued progress and sustainability of investments made under the Beacon Program.

- Providers, health systems, and health plans would benefit from analyses that demonstrate the need and return on investment for performance measurement and electronic data exchange, as market dynamics and shifts in policy priorities affect their willingness to engage.

- The apparent inability of the private sector to achieve interoperable systems suggests the need for national leadership to support their creation.

- Claims data alone are limited in their usefulness in demonstrating the true impact of programs comprising diverse interventions that are refined over time.

Source: Singer, RF et al. (for NORC at the University of Chicago): Evaluation of the Beacon Community Cooperative Agreement Program. Final Report. November 2015. Retrieved July 11, 2018 from https://www.healthit.gov/sites/default/files/norc_beacon_evaluation_final_report_final.pdf

In 2010, the ONC also set up the Beacon Community Program and chose 17 local sites from among nationwide responses to a request for proposals. The purposes of those grants were to focus on IT solutions for narrower uses; Beacon interventions primarily targeted diabetes, cardiovascular care, asthma, and chronic obstructive pulmonary disease. An evaluation of these programs was conducted in 2015. Its lessons are summarized in Exhibit 8.10.

Exhibits 8.9 and 8.10 provide valuable advice concerning necessary elements for success of these ventures. It will be interesting to see if future efforts draw on these experiences.

By 2012, the ONC needed to fulfill a mandate in the HITECH Act to establish a governance mechanism for the NwHIN. After receiving comments from a request for information (RFI), the federal government decided to privatize this oversite in a continued public/private partnership.[151] The NwHIN Exchange was renamed the eHealth Exchange, and three of its coordinating committee members were appointed to serve on the board of

---

[151]Mostashari, F. (2012, September 7). Enabling trusted exchange: Governing the Nationwide Health Information Network. *Health IT Buzz*. Retrieved July 11, 2018, from https://www.healthit.gov/buzz-blog/electronic-health-and-medical-records/enabling-trusted-exchange-governing-nationwide-health-information-network

a new nonprofit named Healtheway. The announcement of this new nonprofit/governmental venture explained that it would "encompass at least four federal agencies (CMS, DoD, SSA, and VA) as well as 21 non-federal entities that can all share patient records for episodes of care … "; it claimed that in 2011, 500 hospitals, 30,000 clinical users, and 3,000 providers were using the system for a patient population coverage area of 65 million people and 1 million shared records.[152] An important part of this transition was a plan to go from a free governmental initiative to a sliding scale payment model based on annual user revenues and also system testing fees.[153]

In June 2015, Healtheway announced that the "organizattion's purpose has expanded dramatically"; in particular, the focus was to be on leading new operational data exchange initiatives; supporting collaboration across industry and government; and expanding education and research. With these changes, Healtheway was renamed the Sequoia Project, continuing to serve as "the neutral convener to advance health IT interoperability."[154] One year later, the Sequoia Project launched Carequality,[155] the culmination of a 3-year project to build a national "interoperability framework" (i.e., a national HIE). Less than a month after this release, IT companies athenahealth, eClinicalWorks, Epic, NextGen Healthcare, and Surescripts signed up as participants. By the end of 2017, Carequality claimed it connected more than 1,000 hospitals, 25,000 clinics, and 580,000 healthcare providers and handled more than 1.7 million clinical documents per month. While this growth is impressive, there are significant gaps in stakeholder involvement. For example, a search of the Carequality website for Cook County (IL) university hospitals reveals that Rush and Loyola University hospitals use Carequality but the University of Illinois, University of Chicago, and Northwestern-affiliated hospitals do not. Also, Advocate Health System hospitals (the largest system in the state) and Stroger (Cook County) Hospital do not use this HIE.[156]

Starting in 2010, another initiative of the NwHIN was launched—the Direct Project. In 2013, the ONC awarded development and oversight responsibility for the project to a nonprofit organization called DirectTrust. According to that organization: "The most important thing to know about Direct health information exchange is that it is just like email, but with an added layer of security and trust-in-identity operating behind the scenes."[157] Instead of relying on usual email security (such as Gmail), Direct Project

---

[152] Ahier, B. (2012, September 4). With eHealth Exchange, we are entering new era of HIE. *Healthcare IT News*. Retrieved July 11, 2018, from http://www.healthcareitnews.com/blog/ehealth-exchange-we-are-entering-new-era-hie

[153] See *eHealth Exchange Annual Participation & Testing Fees*. Retrieved July 11, 2018, from http://sequoiaproject.org/ehealth-exchange/onboarding/fees-2 As an example, annual maintenance fees for organizations with less than $1 million in revenue are $4,750 per year, while those with more than $10 million in revenue are $19,900 per year.

[154] HIMSS News. (2015, June 26). *Healtheway launches new strategy and changes corporate name to The Sequoia Project*. Retrieved July 11, 2018, from http://www.himss.org/news/healtheway-launches-new-strategy-and-changes-corporate-name-sequoia-project

[155] HealthData Answers. *Millions connected through Carequality Interoperability Framework*. Retrieved July 11, 2018, from https://www.healthdataanswers.net/millions-connected-carequality-interoperability-framework. Carequality website available at http://sequoiaproject.org/carequality

[156] The Sequoia Project (2018, July 11). *Who uses Carequality to share health data*. Retrieved July 11, 2018, from https://sequoiaproject.org/carequality/active-sites-search Of note is that some ambulatory care affiliates of those systems (such as Advocate) use Carequality, even though the hospitals do not.

[157] DirectTrust. *DirectTrust 101*. Retrieved July 11, 2018, from https://www.directtrust.org/directtrust-101

subscribers use health information service providers (HISPs), which are certified for data integrity. A variety of organizations can be HISPs, including EHR vendors and healthcare systems. In order to take advantage of this security, users have unique Direct addresses; for example, for a physician it could be: SmithMD@direct.NorthMedicalGroup.com. There are three advantages of this system: all types of attachments can be sent; the data format does not have to be compatible with the recipient's system; and "any device capable of sending an encrypted message (in one of several communication protocols) to the addressee's HISP could be an end-point for sending and receiving a Direct message, including medical devices used by patients at home."[158] During 2017, there were more than 167 million Direct message transactions between DirectTrust addresses, which numbered 1.6 million. The number of healthcare organizations served by DirectTrust accredited HISPs was more than 106,000.[159] The fees for membership are much more complex than those for Sequoia and depend on such parameters as type of member (hospital system, medical or dental practice, etc.), annual revenue, size of population served, and/or public or private status.[160]

To tie the HIE organizations together, in 2014, the Strategic Health Information Exchange Collaborative (SHIEC)[161] was organized as a trade association. Its mission is to help "members more efficiently engage with our suppliers, industry consultants and other allied organizations so that together we can create more innovative and more cost-effective solutions for the communities we serve."[162] Currently there are more than 60 members and more than 30 strategic business and technology partners (companies that provide products and services to the HIEs). In September 2015, SHIEC announced it would start a project called the Patient Centered Data Home™ (PCDH). The initiative's purpose is to allow a patient to access health data if care is needed away from its usual source. After small-scale testing, its national roll-out was announced in January 2018. Briefly, the process works as follows: When a patient presents to a SHIEC-member facility away from home, that provider sends a message to the patient's "data home" saying that the patient needs care. The receiving SHIEC member facility then acknowledges that records are available and can facilitate their transfer. When treatment is complete, updated records can be sent back to the "data home" so the patient can receive appropriate follow-up. SHIEC's goal is to enhance connectivity and sharing best practices among members with diverse IT systems; it is not aiming to increase interoperability. As the organization has stated:

---

[158] Ibid.

[159] Globe Newswire. (2018, January 18). *Direct message transactions increased 101% during 2017*. Retrieved July 11, 2018, from https://globenewswire.com/news-release/2018/01/18/1296548/0/en/DirectTrust-Reports-Strong-Growth-in-Direct-Transactions-Number-of-Direct-Exchange-Addresses-and-Users.html

[160] DirectTrust. *What are the membership fees?* Retrieved July 11, 2018, from https://www.directtrust.org/membership

[161] SHIEC. Retrieved from https://strategichie.com/initiatives/pcdh

[162] HiMSS. (2017, July 26). Strategic Health Information Exchange Collaborative (SHIEC). Interview with Dick Thompson, Executive Director and CEO of Quality Health Network and Board Chair of SHIEC. Retrieved July 11, 2018, from http://www.himss.org/library/strategic-health-information-exchange-collaborative-shiec

What we have also learned within SHIEC is that all health and healthcare markets are local markets with distinct characteristics, issues and challenges. We truly understand that any potential interoperability solutions must address the needs, characteristics and challenges of the local ecosystem. People and process are as or perhaps even more important than technology.[163]

In addition to its mandate to provide seamless interoperability to enhance quality of care, the government is also interested in potential cost savings from HIEs. Getting an exact estimate for the return on investment of any information systems has always been difficult, particularly since the technology is constantly evolving and better and less-costly systems are becoming available. Nevertheless, recent studies indicate that savings can accrue from these systems. For example, Adjerid et al.[164] found

> significant cost reductions in healthcare markets that have established operational HIEs, with an average reduction in spending of $139 (1.4% decrease) per Medicare beneficiary per year … these reductions occur disproportionately in healthcare markets where providers have financial incentives to use an HIE to reduce spending and when HIEs are more mature.

Although Surescript started earlier than the projects mentioned above, it is the best example of a truly interoperable network and worth discussing separately.[165] In 2001, three pharmaceutical benefit management (PBM) companies—Express Scripts, Medco Health (now part of Express Scripts), and Caremark (now part of CVS Caremark)—formed RxHub. This company's purpose was to allow prescribers to electronically check a patient's insurance eligibility and drug coverage (including formulary status) and then deliver a prescription to that patient's pharmacy. In a defensive reaction that same year, the National Association of Chain Drug Stores and the National Community Pharmacists Association formed Surescripts to enable physicians to electronically send prescriptions directly to pharmacies. By 2003, RxHub started to focus its efforts on the eligibility and coverage functions exclusively. Since these two companies now offered complementary functions across services for e-prescribing, they merged in 2008 to form a new company, also called Surescripts. This new company got a strong boost in 2009 from the HITECH Act's financial reward for using e-prescribing. (The program ended in 2013 and thereafter has been part of meaningful use penalties if practitioners do not use this prescribing method.)

Surescripts operates the hub that makes the system interoperable among a variety of software products. (Please see Exhibit 8.11 for how an e-prescribing scheme works.)

---

[163] Globe Newswire. (2018, January 4). *SHIEC's patient-centered data home initiative launches nationally: Nationwide expansion of PCDH lays foundation for HIEs to support better patient care by making it possible to share patient medical records across geographies*. Retrieved July 11, 2018, from https://globenewswire.com/news-release/2018/01/04/1283449/0/en/SHIEC-s-Patient-Centered-Data-Home-Initiative-Launches-Nationally.html

[164] Adjerid, I., Adler-Milstein, J., & Angst, C. M. (2016, April 14). *Reducing Medicare spending through electronic information exchange: The role of incentives and exchange maturity*. Retrieved July 11, 2018, from https://papers.ssrn.com/sol3/papers.cfm?abstract_id=2765098

[165] Surescripts. Retrieved July 11, 2018, from http://surescripts.com

EXHIBIT 8.11. Sample Scheme for e-Prescribing HIE

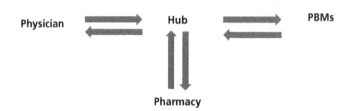

Physician writes a prescription.
The prescription is electronically cleared through the Hub and transmitted to the PBM.
The PBM checks patient eligibility and formulary status of the drug, transmitting the results back the physician through the Hub.
The physician can then continue with the prescription or change it, for example to a formulary branded drug or generic.
The physician uses the Hub to transmit the prescription to a contracted pharmacy or one the patient chooses.
The pharmacy can also check patient information as well as submit billing through the Hub.

In addition to prescriptions, the system is certified to transmit discharge and visit summaries, patient charts, referrals, lab orders, and results. The company itself certifies the e-prescribing software sold to organizations that use the network,[166] including prescribers, pharmacies, and PBMs. In addition to charges for certification and the initial system-interoperability setup, the sustaining business model is based on transaction fees paid by the pharmacies and PBMs. (Note: The system is free for prescribers.) The original companies of the merged entity still retain ownership of Surescripts; however, because these organizations are rivals, it has a freestanding governance process. Although the e-prescribing process is going well, in April 2019 the Federal Trade Commission (FTC) filed an antitrust lawsuit against Surescripts claiming it engaged in anticompetitive behavior to keep other companies from this sector.[167] Specifically, the FTC charged that Surescript requires long-term exclusivity from customers and dramatically increases fees if they buy prescriptions from another company. The case is still active at this time.

Certification

As the efforts toward universal, interoperable information systems have progressed, the products need to be reviewed for initial and ongoing compliance to standards. To that end, several months after the ONC was formed in 2004, it identified certification of health IT products as one of its key priorities. Shortly thereafter, the National Alliance for HIT (which ceased operations in 2009), HIMSS (formerly called the Health Information Management Specialty Society) and AHIMA formed the Certification Commission for Health Information Technology (CCHIT) to fulfill that function. In 2005, CCHIT was awarded a 3-year HHS contract to develop IT compliance criteria that would allow products to become certified. In 2006,

---

[166]For a listing of these organizations, see http://surescripts.com/network-connections Retrieved July 11, 2018.
[167]Bartz, D: Surescripts faces U.S. antitrust lawsuit over electronic prescription monopoly. *Reuters*, April 24, 2019 Retrieved May 24, 2019 from: https://www.reuters.com/article/us-usa-ftc-surescripts-idUSKCN1S02KO

CCHIT started to focus on office-based physicians' EHRs and in 2007 expanded activities to inpatient EHR products. In 2009, after the HITECH Act established financial incentives (and eventual penalties) tied to meaningful use, the federal government needed to know if providers (and their EHRs) were in compliance. In response to this need, in 2010, the ONC issued Health Information Technology: Initial Set of Standards, Implementation Specifications, and Certification Criteria for Electronic Health Record Technology. Its purpose was "to complete the adoption of an initial set of standards, implementation specifications, and certification criteria, and to more closely align such standards, implementation specifications, and certification criteria with final meaningful use Stage 1 objectives and measures."[168] CCHIT was the only certifying body at that time. In 2011, the ONC chose the ANSI to be its Approved Accreditor (AA) for the certification program; that is, ANSI was to accredit organizations (like CCHIT) to be certifiers. By 2012, other organizations were applying for accreditation as Authorized Certification Bodies (ACBs). In addition to CCHIT, the next ACB was the Drummond Group (https://drummondgroup.com). Other ACBs followed, and by November 2014, CCHIT ceased its certification activities.

The structure of the certification process is displayed in Exhibit 8.12. To understand this figure, a few explanations are needed:

1. The ONC derives its authority for conducting this process from CFR (Title) 45, which is referenced above.

2. The ONC derives standards from ISO/IEC documents referenced in the figure.

3. The ONC works with the following agencies and entities as part of its program operations:

   NIST (National Institute of Standards and Technology). Per the HITECH Act, NIST, a federal agency within the Department of Commerce, and ONC collaborated to establish the voluntary certification program and continue to work together to develop the necessary functional and conformance testing requirements, test cases, and test tools in support of the Program.

   NVLAP (National Voluntary Laboratory Accreditation Program). Administered by NIST, the Program specifies that only test results from a NVLAP-accredited testing laboratory could be used as the basis for a certification determination by an ONC-ACB.

   ONC-ATL (ONC-Authorized Testing Laboratory). A NVLAP-accredited testing laboratory that performs health IT testing to determine conformance with ONC's standards and certification criteria according to the ONC-approved test method.

   ONC-AA (ONC-Approved Accreditor). Selected by ONC to serve a 3-year term to accredit and oversee ONC-ACBs under the Program requirements.

---

[168]Office of the National Coordinator for Health Information Technology (ONC), Department of Health and Human Services. Final Rule: Health Information Technology: Initial Set of Standards, Implementation Specifications, and Certification Criteria for Electronic Health Record Technology. 45 CFR Part 170. Federal Register 75 (144):45590–44654. July 28, 2010. Rules and Regulations. Retrieved July 28, 2018. from https://www.gpo.gov/fdsys/pkg/FR-2010-07-28/pdf/2010-17210.pdf

EXHIBIT 8.12. **Structure of the ONC Health IT Certification Program**

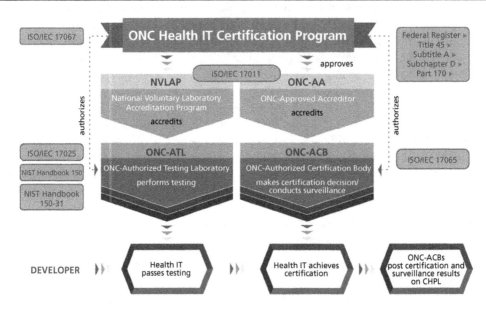

Source: About the ONC Health IT Certification Program. Retrieved July 11, 2018 from https://www.healthit.gov/policy-researchers-implementers/about-onc-health-it-certification-program

ONC-ACB (ONC-Authorized Certification Body). Certifies health IT based on test results supplied by ONC-ATLs; posts results on the Certified Health IT Product List (CHPL); and is responsible for conducting surveillance of certified health IT.

Health IT Developer. Presents health IT to be tested and certified under the Program.[169]

A current, accurate number of providers (particularly doctors and hospitals) with certified EMRs is not available, since the ONC (perhaps the best source for such information) publishes such data that is 2 or 3 years old.[170]

---

[169] *ONC Health IT Certification Program Overview, v1.2* (2016, January 30). Retrieved July 11, 2018, from https://www.healthit.gov/sites/default/files/PUBLICHealthITCertificationProgramOverview_v1.1.pdf

[170] See ONC (2017, July). *Certified health IT developers and editions reported by hospitals participating in the Medicare EHR Incentive Program.* Retrieved from https://dashboard.healthit.gov/quickstats/pages/FIG-Vendors-of-EHRs-to-Participating-Hospitals.php and *Certified health IT developers and editions reported by ambulatory primary care physicians, medical, and surgical specialists, podiatrists, optometrists, dentists, and chiropractors participating in the Medicare EHR Incentive Program.* Retrieved July 11, 2018, from https://dashboard.healthit.gov/quickstats/pages/FIG-Vendors-of-EHRs-to-Participating-Professionals.php While both were published July 2017, the Charts use 2014 and 2015 data.

Privacy and Security of Information

Even if all systems were interoperable, a significant remaining problem is ensuring the privacy and security of healthcare information. "Privacy" usually refers to confidentiality (nondisclosure) of information while "security" refers to protection of physical sources of information (such as paper charts or computers).

Attention to this issue is ancient; for example, it is a key part of the Hippocratic Oath: "What I may see or hear in the course of the treatment or even outside of the treatment in regard to the life of men, which on no account one must spread abroad, I will keep to myself, holding such things shameful to be spoken about."[171]

While such confidentiality was accepted practice for medical professionals for centuries, its establishment in the modern, English-speaking world dates from the code of medical ethics written by Dr. Thomas Percival in 1803 for use in the Manchester, England, hospital where he practiced. With regard to this topic, he wrote:

> In the large wards of an Infirmary the patients should be interrogated concerning their complaints, in a tone of voice which cannot be overheard ... Secrecy, and delicacy when required by peculiar circumstances, should be strictly observed. And the familiar and confidential intercourse, to which the faculty are admitted in their professional visits, should be used with discretion, and with the most scrupulous regard to fidelity and honour.[172]

This work is important for American medicine since it was the basis for the original AMA code of ethics,[173] first adopted in 1847. With respect to confidentiality, the AMA document quotes Percival verbatim and then continues:

> The obligation of secrecy extends beyond the period of professional services; none of the privacies of personal and domestic life, no infirmity of disposition or flaw of character observed during professional attendance, should ever be divulged by him except when he is imperatively required to do so. The force and necessity of this obligation are indeed so great, that professional men have, under certain circumstances, been protected in their observance of secrecy by courts of justice.[174]

In addition to professional codes of ethics, licensure and certification also contain provisions for confidentiality of patient information. For example, as the hospital electronic

---

[171] Translation from the Greek by Ludwig Edelstein. From *The Hippocratic Oath: Text, translation, and interpretation*, by Edelstein, L. (1943). Baltimore, MD: Johns Hopkins Press. The oath is attributed to Hippocrates (5th century BCE), but the true author is not known.

[172] Percival, T. (1803). *Medical ethics; or, a code of institutes and precepts, adapted to the professional conduct of physicians and surgeons*. Printed by S. Russel, Manchester. Retrieved July 11, 2018, from https://play.google.com/books/reader?id=tVsUAAAAQAAJ&printsec=frontcover&output=reader&hl=en&pg=GBS.PR3

[173] AMA. *History of the Code*. Retrieved July 11, 2018, from https://www.ama-assn.org/sites/default/files/media-browser/public/ethics/ama-code-ethics-history.pdf

[174] AMA. (1848). *Code of ethics of the American Medical Association. Adopted May 1847*. T. K. and P. G. Collins, Printers. Philadelphia. Retrieved July 11, 2018, from http://ethics.iit.edu/ecodes/sites/default/files/Americaan%20Medical%20Association%20Code%20of%20Medical%20Ethics%20%281847%29.pdf

information age was emerging in 1994, The Joint Commission published 10 standards relating to the management of information. With regards to its role vis-à-vis governmental regulations, The Joint Commission states: "While The Joint Commission does not survey against specific HIPAA regulations ... , the standards do require compliance with applicable law and regulation. Standard DSCT.1 requires organizations to maintain the privacy and confidentiality of information."[175]

As the electronic exchange of healthcare information expanded, new laws and regulations needed to be written to protect healthcare information. The federal protections come from these acts and rules:

- The Health Insurance Portability and Accountability Act of 1996 (HIPAA). In addition to the data standardization requirements described above, Sections 261 through 264 of HIPAA deal with the electronic exchange, privacy, and security of health information. Since Congress failed to enact specific privacy legislation within 3 years of HIPAA's passage (as the law required), HHS published a final Privacy Rule (Standards for Privacy of Individually Identifiable Health Information) on December 28, 2000; a final modification was published in August 2002. According to HHS:"A major goal of the Privacy Rule is to assure that individuals' health information is properly protected while allowing the flow of health information needed to provide and promote high quality health care and to protect the public's health and well-being."[176]

- In addition to the Privacy Rule, HIPAA also contains a Security Rule (Security Standards for the Protection of Electronic Protected Health Information), which sets requirements for protecting certain health information stored or transmitted in electronic formats, called "electronic protected health information" (e-PHI); the definition of PHI is below. By specifying administrative, technical, and physical security procedures for assuring "the confidentiality, integrity, and availability of e-PHI,"[177] the Security Rule provides operational guidance for the Privacy Rule. Unlike the Privacy Rule, the Security Rule does not apply to PHI transmitted orally or in writing. As was the case with the Privacy Rule, congressional inaction caused HHS to issue its own regulations; proposed regulations were published in August 1998, and final rule appeared in February 2003.

Because the HITECH Act of 2009 mandated improved enforcement of the Privacy and Security Rules, in August of that year responsibility for monitoring and enforcing the HIPAA

---

[175]The Joint Commission. *Medical record security*. Retrieved July 11, 2018, from https://www.jointcommission.org/standards_information/jcfaqdetails.aspx?StandardsFaqId=1212&ProgramId=46

[176]HHS.gov. *The HIPAA Privacy Rule*. Retrieved July 11, 2018, from https://www.hhs.gov/hipaa/for-professionals/privacy/index.html. See also Office of Civil Rights. *Summary of the HIPAA Privacy Rule*. Retrieved July 11, 2018, from https://www.hhs.gov/sites/default/files/privacysummary.pdf

[177]HHS.gov. *Summary of the HIPAA Security Rule*. Retrieved July 11, 2018, from https://www.hhs.gov/hipaa/for-professionals/security/laws-regulations/index.html

regulations as well as reporting compliance was transferred to the Office of Civil Rights (OCR).

In order to understand this part of HIPAA, it is instructive to answer the questions below. The reader should refer to the HHS websites[178] for more detailed information and legal advice.

■ *Who is obligated to comply with HIPAA regulations?*

The regulations recognize three types of organizations that are called "covered entities."

1. Health plans are individual and group plans that provide or pay the cost of medical care. Included in this category are private insurers, Medicare and Medicaid (including managed care plans and Medicare supplements), prescription drug insurers, long-term care insurers (excluding nursing home fixed-indemnity policies), and employer-sponsored group health plans. (See the Privacy Rule for exceptions.)

2. Healthcare providers "include all 'providers of services' (e.g., institutional providers such as hospitals) and 'providers of medical or health services' (e.g., non-institutional providers such as physicians, dentists and other practitioners) as defined by Medicare, and any other person or organization that furnishes, bills, or is paid for health care."[179]

   The healthcare provider must be engaged in electronic transmission of what HIPAA considers a standard transaction (e.g., claims, eligibility inquiries, referral authorizations, etc.) using the HIPAA-specified format. The provider is legally responsible for the privacy and security even if it contracts with a third party to perform certain services, such as billing and collections.

3. Healthcare clearinghouses "are entities that process nonstandard information they receive from another entity into a standard (i.e., standard format or data content), or vice versa ... [They] include billing services, repricing companies, community health management information systems, and value-added networks and switches if these entities perform clearinghouse functions."[180]

   For example, a physician's office's information system may not be interoperable with that of an insurance company's claims processing department. A clearinghouse translates the physician's bill into language the insurance company system can understand and also translates the reply from the insurer back to the physician.

Although individuals and organizations considered to be covered entities have strict privacy requirements, they are allowed to exchange PHI with each other without an individual's authorization. Reasons for these exchanges include facilitating treatment, verifying eligibility, and conducting billing processes.

---

[178] See, for example: HHS.gov. *Health information privacy*. Retrieved July 11, 2018, from https://www.hhs.gov/hipaa/index.html

[179] Ibid.

[180] Ibid.

▦ *What is considered private information?*

The information covered by HIPAA is called Protected Health Information (PHI). PHI is individually identifiable health information that relates to:

▦ the individual's past, present or future physical or mental health or condition,

▦ the provision of health care to the individual, or

▦ the past, present, or future payment for the provision of health care to the individual, and that identifies the individual or for which there is a reasonable basis to believe can be used to identify the individual.[181]

Such information includes demographics, unique identifiers (such as Social Security or driver's license numbers) and specific combinations such as name, address, and birthdate.

The Privacy Rule covers all ways the PHI is held and transmitted, viz. oral, print, or electronic media. Further, the individual's information must be protected no matter how it is obtained (i.e., a healthcare provider is responsible for all information generated in the course of caring for a patient including information obtained from another provider or other entity).

In order to be exempt from the Privacy Rule, the PHI can be "deidentified" by one of two methods: (a) A qualified statistician can attest that, after the PHI is modified, the individual cannot be uniquely identified; or (b) specified data are removed, resulting in the covered entity not being able to identify the individual.

▦ *How are businesses that perform services for covered entities handled?*

These types of firms are called "business associates." The Privacy Rule defines a business associate as

> a person or organization, other than a member of a covered entity's workforce, that performs certain functions or activities on behalf of, or provides certain services to, a covered entity that involve the use or disclosure of individually identifiable health information. Business associate functions or activities on behalf of a covered entity include claims processing, data analysis, utilization review, and billing. Business associate services to a covered entity are limited to legal, actuarial, accounting, consulting, data aggregation, management, administrative, accreditation, or financial services. However, persons or organizations are not considered business associates if their functions or services do not involve the use or disclosure of protected health information, and where any access to protected health information by such persons would be incidental, if at all. A covered entity can be the business associate of another covered entity.[182]

---

[181] HHS.gov: The HIPAA Privacy Rule, op. cit.

[182] Office of Civil Rights. *Summary of the HIPAA Privacy Rule*. Retrieved July 11, 2018, from https://www.hhs.gov/sites/default/files/privacysummary.pdf

The covered entity must have a business associate contract with such individuals or organizations. The contract must contain terms specified by HHS that protect PHI.[183]

■ *What are some things a covered entity or business associate must do in order to comply with the Security Rule?*

In general, the covered entity must make sure the e-PHI is kept confidential (not available or able to be accesses by unauthorized persons); its integrity is maintained (meaning data is not altered or destroyed in an unauthorized manner); and it is available (accessible and usable on demand by authorized persons).

These measures can be divided into organizational/administrative, technical, and physical safeguards.

Among the covered entity's organizational/administrative safeguards, it must:

■ Perform a risk analysis that evaluates the likelihood and impact of potential threats to the security, integrity, and impermissible uses or disclosures of e-PHI; develop and implement security measures to mitigate the risks; develop documentation about the analysis, risk reduction measures, and any violations of policies; and train staff to comply with appropriate procedures for securing data.

■ Take prompt, reasonable steps to cure a breach of a business associate's contractual responsibility to protect e-PHI.

■ Appoint a security official responsible for developing and implementing security policies and procedures. This person can also be the security and privacy officer to whom breaches are reported.

■ Implement policies and procedures that authorize who can access what parts of e-PHI (role-based access).

■ Perform a periodic assessment of how well its security policies and procedures meet the requirements of the Security Rule.

Regarding physical safeguards, the covered entity must:

■ Limit physical access to its facilities only to authorized personnel.

■ Implement policies and procedures to specify proper use of and access to workstations and electronic media.

■ Implement policies and procedures regarding the transfer, removal, disposal, and reuse of electronic media.

In regard to technical safeguards, the covered entity must:

■ Implement policies and procedures that allow only authorized persons to access e-PHI. This requirement deals with types of personnel who have access and *how* they can gain access (e.g., passwords).

---

[183]HHA.gov. *Business associate contracts.* Retrieved July 11, 2018, from https://www.hhs.gov/hipaa/for-professionals/covered-entities/sample-business-associate-agreement-provisions/index.html

- Have in place hardware, software, and/or procedures that audit information systems with respect to e-PHI access and use. For example, this audit will track who accessed what information at what time and date.

- Implement policies and procedures to ensure that e-PHI is not improperly altered or destroyed. For example, the systems must not allow alteration of medical information, although erroneous or unclear entries may be corrected by *adding* further clarifications. Also, this requirement mandates the system is backed up at appropriate intervals.

- Implement security measures that guard against unauthorized access to e-PHI that is either sent or received over an electronic network (e.g., creating firewalls and prohibiting web surfing).

- *How much PHI is a covered entity required to furnish when it receives a legitimate request?*
  "A covered entity must make reasonable efforts to use, disclose, and request only the minimum amount of protected health information needed to accomplish the intended purpose of the use, disclosure, or request."[184] For example, when a request is received for laboratory results, the sender must not send other parts of the medical record. A system using XML would be very useful in helping a covered entity comply with this requirement, since it can label specific bits of information and make them searchable.

- *What are patient rights under the Privacy and Security Rules?*[185]

  - *Right to receive privacy notice.* All providers who directly interact with the patient and all health plans must provide patients with their privacy notices upon first contact or enrollment, respectively. Any updated notices must also be provided. A patient may also request a copy of the notice at any time. Health plans must periodically furnish these notices even if no changes have occurred.

  - *Rights regarding patient record access and correctness.* Patients have the right access their medical records and correct/amend errors. (An exception is details in psychotherapy notes.) If the patient and provider differ on the correctness of the recorded information, the patient has a right to insert a statement expressing that different view.

  - *Right to request an audit of information use.* Patients have the right to know how their health information was used (i.e., what was sent to whom and when). The requested information need only be provided for a maximum of 6 years prior to the request.

    > [The] Privacy Rule does not require accounting for disclosures: (a) for treatment, payment, or health care operations; (b) to the individual or the individual's personal representative; (c) for notification of or to persons involved in an individual's health care or payment for health care, for disaster relief, or for facility directories;

---

[184]Op. cit. HHS.gov. *The HIPAA Privacy Rule*. See also: HHS.gov. *Minimum necessary requirement*. Retrieved July 11, 2018, from https://www.hhs.gov/hipaa/for-professionals/privacy/guidance/minimum-necessary-requirement/index.html
[185]For ease of reference, all quotations in this section refer to HHS language in one of the previously cited HIPAA documents.

(d) pursuant to an authorization; (e) of a limited data set; (f) for national security or intelligence purposes; (g) to correctional institutions or law enforcement officials for certain purposes regarding inmates or individuals in lawful custody; or (h) incident to otherwise permitted or required uses or disclosures. Accounting for disclosures to health oversight agencies and law enforcement officials must be temporarily suspended on their written representation that an accounting would likely impede their activities.

- *Right to restrict use of information.* Individuals have the right to request that a covered entity restrict use or disclosure of protected health information for treatment, payment, or healthcare operations; disclosure to persons involved in the individual's healthcare or payment for healthcare; or disclosure to notify family members or others about the individual's general condition, location, or death. A covered entity is under no obligation to agree to requests for restrictions. A covered entity that does agree must comply with the agreed restrictions, except for purposes of treating the individual in a medical emergency.

  Patients can also request a restriction on providing insurers with data on self-pay transactions.

  In addition to restricting health information transmission, patients have the right to restrict disclosure of their names and addresses for purposes of fundraising, marketing, or research.

  Because many organizations are particularly concerned about marketing with respect to HIPAA rules, a brief explanation will be presented about how this function can be handled. For purpose of HIPAA, HHS defines marketing as "any communication about a product or service that encourages recipients to purchase or use the product or service."

  In general, a covered entity must obtain a patient's permission to use or disclose PHI for marketing, including any direct or indirect compensation it receives from third parties who may use the PHI. However, the Privacy Rule provides the following exceptions:

  - Face-to-face marketing communications between a covered entity and an individual ...
  - A covered entity's provision of promotional gifts of nominal value;
  - Communications to describe health-related products or services, or payment for them, provided by or included in a benefit plan of the covered entity making the communication;
  - Communications about participating providers in a provider or health plan network, replacement of or enhancements to a health plan, and health-related products or services available only to a health plan's enrollees that add value to, but are not part of, the benefits plan;
  - Communications for treatment of the individual; and
  - Communications for case management or care coordination for the individual, or to direct or recommend alternative treatments, therapies, health care providers, or care settings to the individual.

■ *Right to require consent for release of PHI.* "A covered entity must obtain the individual's written authorization for any use or disclosure of protected health information that is not for treatment, payment or health care operations or otherwise permitted or required by the Privacy Rule." The reader should consult HHS websites about special provisions for release of psychotherapy information, which generally requires separate authorizations.

It should be noted that *many states have restrictions on release of PHI that are stricter than HIPAA.* For example, many special protections exist for data on HIV status and genetic testing.

> A covered entity is permitted, but not required, to use and disclose protected health information, without an individual's authorization, for the following purposes or situations: (1) To the Individual (unless required for access or accounting of disclosures); (2) Treatment, Payment, and Health Care Operations; (3) Opportunity to Agree or Object; (4) Incident to an otherwise permitted use and disclosure; (5) Public Interest and Benefit Activities; and (6) Limited Data Set for the purposes of research, public health or health care operations.

A "limited data set" contains deidentified PHI as described above.

■ *Right to obtain copies of records.* Patients have the right to a record of their medical records. The HITECH Act mandates the right to obtain electronic copies of their records when the covered entity has an EMR.

Covered entities may impose reasonable, cost-based fees for the cost of copying and postage.

Some states have fee schedules for providing such records.

■ *What are the penalties for violating HIPAA regulations?*
HHS may impose *civil* money penalties

> on a covered entity of $100 per failure to comply with a Privacy Rule requirement. That penalty may not exceed $25,000 per year for multiple violations of the identical Privacy Rule requirement in a calendar year. HHS may not impose a civil money penalty under specific circumstances, such as when a violation is due to reasonable cause and did not involve willful neglect and the covered entity corrected the violation within 30 days of when it knew or should have known of the violation.

Criminal penalties may also apply for anyone who "knowingly obtains or discloses individually identifiable health information in violation of HIPAA." The fine is $50,000 and up to 1-year imprisonment,

> with criminal penalties increasing to $100,000 and up to five years imprisonment if the wrongful conduct involves false pretenses, and to $250,000 and up to ten years imprisonment if the wrongful conduct involves the intent to sell, transfer, or use individually identifiable health information for commercial advantage, personal gain, or malicious harm.

The OCR maintains a list of violations under investigation and those that have been settled and archived.[186] However, only violations involving 500 or more people are listed on the OCR website.

Criminal sanctions are enforced by the Department of Justice.

Despite all the governmental requirements to secure PHI, many breaches still occur across industries. A recent study[187] by IBM Security and Ponemon Institute detailed the costs and reasons for these breaches. While the average global cost of data breach per lost or stolen record was $141, for healthcare organizations, the average was $380. The distribution for root causes of data breaches varied by country; in all sectors in the United States, the causes are malicious or criminal attack: 52%; system glitch: 24%; and human error: 24%. More specifically, Gabriel et al. reported that

> Approximately one-third of all healthcare data breaches occurred in hospitals, and the most individual patients were impacted when hospitals were breached compared with other types of healthcare providers, such as doctors, nurses, and social workers. Therefore, despite the high level of hospital adoption of EHRs and the federal incentives to do so, the most common type of data breach in hospitals occurred with paper records and films. These paper and film breaches occurred mostly due to theft, improper disposal, and unauthorized access. However, the overall number of patients affected by these breaches was relatively small. Conversely, network servers were found to be the least frequent location of data breaches, but these breaches impacted the most patients overall. In addition, this study found that there were large numbers of thefts of laptops, which can easily be physically removed and stolen regardless of EHR or biometric security system implementation.[188]

Teaching, pediatric, nonprofit hospitals and larger facilities were statistically more likely to have breaches. Noteworthy was that "health IT sophistication, biometric security use, health system membership, hospital region, and area characteristics were not significantly different in terms of data breach percentages."

Further insight into this problem is provided by Verizon's annual data breach report.[189] Among its findings with respect to healthcare are:

■ The actors responsible for the breaches are: 32% External (6% Partner breaches) and 68% Internal. The study notes that healthcare "is the only industry where employees are the predominant threat actors in breaches."

[186]U.S Department of Health and Human Services. Office for Civil Rights. Breach Portal. Retrieved July 11, 2018, from https://ocrportal.hhs.gov/ocr/breach/breach_report.jsf

[187]IBM Security and Ponemon Institute. (2017, June 13). 2017 Cost of Data Breach Study: United States. Retrieved July 11, 2018, from https://www.ponemon.org/blog/2017-cost-of-data-breach-study-united-states

[188]Gabriel, M. H., Noblin, A., Rutherford, A., Walden, A., & Cortelyou-Ward, K. (2018, February 14). Data breach locations, types, and associated characteristics among US hospitals. *The American Journal of Managed Care, 24*(2), 78–84. Retrieved July 11, 2018, from https://www.ajmc.com/journals/issue/2018/2018-vol24-n2/data-breach-locations-types-and-associated-characteristics-among-us-hospitals?p=2

[189]*Verizon's 2017 data breach* investigations *report*. Retrieved July 11, 2018, from https://www.ictsecuritymagazine.com/wp-content/uploads/2017-Data-Breach-Investigations-Report.pdf

▪ Privilege misuse, miscellaneous errors, and physical theft and loss represent 80% of breaches within healthcare. Of the errors, half are due to misdelivery of data (e.g., giving laboratory data to the wrong patient).

▪ The reasons for the breaches are: 64% financial, 23% "fun," and 7% grudge.

▪ The compromised data is: 69% medical, 33% personal, and 4% payment.

Another type of breach is ransomware attacks—when systems are locked down by malware (unwanted software intended to harm or destroy computer systems) and can be reopened only by the owner in exchange for payment. Ransomware reports are not always included in data breach statistics because it is unknown whether any information is stolen in these attacks. Its importance as a problem, however, is growing rapidly. The Verizon report cited above notes that in 2016, ransomware accounted for 72% of malware incidents in the healthcare sector.

One reason healthcare data breaches are so common is that they are lucrative sources of information. According to Kruse et al.: "Research suggests that an individual's medical information is 20 to 50 times more valuable to cybercriminals than personal financial information. Access to medical information enables cybercriminals to commit identity theft, medical fraud, extortion, and the ability to illegally obtain controlled substances."[190]

As these breaches have increased calls for better security measures, the pressures for interoperability have opened a new opportunity for hackers: As more systems communicate freely with each other, more portals of entry will exist to enable access to larger stores of data. One area of particular concern is medical devices: intravenous pumps, pacemakers, intensive care unit monitors, and home monitors that deposit data into an EMR.[191] As devices are integrated into larger systems, they pose an increasing hacking threat. For example, in 2017, Abbott recalled 465,000 pacemakers because they "required firmware updates to correct vulnerabilities that leave the devices open to hackers."[192]

In order to minimize these problems, in 2017, the FDA issued nonbinding recommendations it would consider in its approval process. A summary of this document is below.

As part of a comprehensive quality system under 21 CFR part 820,[193] medical device manufacturers must manage risks including those associated with an electronic

---

[190]Kruse, C. S., Frederick, B., Jacobson, T., & Monticone, D. K. (2017). Cybersecurity in healthcare: A systematic review of modern threats and trends. *Technology and Health Care*, 25(1), 1–10.

[191]Twentyman, J: Hacking medical devices is the next big security concern. *Financial Times* 2017. Retrieved July 11, 2018 from https://www.ft.com/content/75912040-98ad-11e7-8c5c-c8d8fa6961bb?desktop=true&conceptId=8d5d7bae-a5df-33f0-9acf-cc57badf805b&segmentId=7c8f09b9-9b61-4fbb-9430-9208a9e233c8 - myft:notification:daily-email:content: headline:html

[192]Arndt, R. 2017. Abbott recall signals new era in medical-device cybersecurity. *Modern Healthcare*. Retrieved July 11, 2018, from http://www.modernhealthcare.com/article/20170901/NEWS/170909986?utm_source=modernhealthcare& utm_medium=email&utm_content=20170901-NEWS-170909986&utm_campaign=hits

[193]Code of Federal Regulations Title 21—Food and Drugs Chapter I—Food and Drug Administration, Department of Health and Human Services Subchapter H—Medical Devices Part 820 Quality System Regulation. Retrieved July 11, 2018, from https://www.accessdata.fda.gov/scripts/cdrh/cfdocs/cfcfr/CFRSearch.cfm?CFRPart=820

interface that is incorporated into the medical device. The following considerations should be appropriately tailored to the selected interface technology, and the intended use and use environments for the medical device.

1. Purpose of the Electronic Interface: Device manufacturers should consider the purpose for each of the electronic interfaces. This should include the types of data exchanges taking place (e.g., sending, receiving, issue command and control).

2. The Anticipated Users: Manufacturers should determine the anticipated user(s) for each of the electronic interfaces. Examples of users include: clinical user, biomedical engineers, home healthcare user, IT (information technology) professional, system integrator, system designers, patients, researchers, and medical device designers.

3. Risk Management: Manufacturers should consider ways to mitigate risks identified in the risk analysis. This includes risks that arise from others connecting to the electronic interface.

4. Verification and Validation: Manufacturers should establish, maintain, and implement appropriate verification and validation to ensure that their devices with electronic interfaces work correctly prior to delivery, during the integration process, continue to work while in use, and through maintenance and release of software updates.

5. Labeling Considerations: Manufacturers should include information that users may need to connect predictably and safely to the interface for its intended purpose.

6. Use of Consensus Standards: Manufacturers should consider the use of consensus standards related to medical device interoperability.[194]

Management Considerations

Some managers see implementing IT as the solution to many of their operational (including clinical) and financial problems. However, as the old saying goes, if you automate your current systems, you will make the same mistakes, only faster. Further, you will also introduce new and often unanticipated problems. Therefore, it is first necessary to understand the operations as they exist *before* IT implementation, correct inadequacies, and *then* plan IT implementation. This process is discussed in Chapter 9.

The research in IT implementation consistently supports this recommendation. For example, while Carayon and Karsh's survey found only anecdotal evidence in healthcare organizations to support certain best practices, they concluded that "[a] unifying theme amongst all references is that practices must have a comprehensive understanding of how clinical and administrative work is performed in their environment and how these processes might change with the introduction of health IT."[195]

---

[194]U.S. FDA (2017, September 6). *Design considerations and pre-market submission recommendations for interoperable medical devices: Guidance for industry and food and drug administration staff document.* Retrieved July 11, 2018, from https://www.fda.gov/downloads/MedicalDevices/DeviceRegulationandGuidance/GuidanceDocuments/UCM482649.pdf

[195]Carayon, P., & Karsh, B. (2010, October). Incorporating health information technology into workflow redesign—summary report. (Prepared by the Center for Quality and Productivity Improvement, University of Wisconsin–Madison, under Contract No. HHSA 290-2008-10036C). AHRQ Publication No. 10-0098-EF. Rockville, MD: Agency for Healthcare Research and Quality. Retrieved July 11, 2018, from https://healthit.ahrq.gov/sites/default/files/docs/citation/workflowsummaryreport.pdf

In another research study about the importance of management in IT implementation, Dorgan and Dowdy[196] focused on 100 manufacturing companies in France, Germany, the United Kingdom, and the United States from 1994 to 2002. They found that "IT expenditures have little impact on productivity unless they are accompanied by first-rate management practices.... [a finding that holds] regardless of a company's location, size, sector, or historical performance." In other words: "Companies should first improve their management practices and then invest in IT." Further, Dorgan and Dowdy were able to quantify this management effect.

Improving management practices alone increased productivity by 8%. Implementing IT alone (i.e., without management practice improvement) increased productivity by only 2%; however, "companies with more powerful IT didn't do better financially ... [perhaps because] the cost of new IT investments balanced out the financial gain they generated." The good news is that companies that implemented better management practices and *then* employed IT achieved a synergistic 20% productivity improvement.

A further management consideration for IT implementation is the resistance any new initiative will face when it disrupts established routines. Deployment of appropriate change management measures will require anticipating the reasons for this opposition. Some of these reasons are listed in Exhibit 8.13. The reader is referred to the article by Lluch cited in the exhibit for a more detailed explanation of these issues.

EXHIBIT 8.13. Organizational Barriers to HIT Implementation

- Structure of healthcare organisational systems
- Hierarchy
- Team work and cooperation
- Autonomy
- Tasks
- Changes in work processes and routines
- Face-to-face interaction versus new ways of working
- People policies
- Training, IT/HIT skills
- Support
- Trust and liability
- Lack of legal framework
- Accountability to their employer and to policy makers

[196]Dorgan, S. J., & Dowdy, J. J. (2004). When IT lifts productivity. *The McKinsey Quarterly, 4*, 13–15.

- ■ Centre of gravity and autonomy
- ■ Incentives
- ■ Information and decision processes

Source: Lluch, M: Healthcare professionals' barriers to health information technologies. A literature review. *International Journal of Medical Informatics* 80: 849–862, 2011. Retrieved July 11, 2018 from https://www.sciencedirect.com/science/article/pii/S1386505611001961

Other Issues and Trends

As the capabilities of IT systems continue to mature and their potential uses expand, a number of other emerging considerations have arisen.

Telehealth/Telemedicine

Definitions. Several terms exist for the topic of using remote healthcare services. The best definitions are those used by the WHO:[197]

> *eHealth* is the cost-effective and secure use of information communication technologies (ICT) in support of health and health-related fields, including health-care services, health surveillance, health literature, and health education, knowledge and research.

> *mHealth* (also known as mobile health) [is] defined as the use of mobile devices—such as mobile phones, patient monitoring devices, personal digital assistants (PDAs) and wireless devices—for medical and public health practice.

> [*Telehealth* is defined as] the delivery of health care services, where patients and providers are separated by distance. Telehealth uses ICT for the exchange of information for the diagnosis and treatment of diseases and injuries, research and evaluation, and for the continuing education of health professionals. Telehealth can contribute to achieving universal health coverage by improving access for patients to quality, cost-effective, health services wherever they may be.

> [*Telemedicine* is the] delivery of health care services, where distance is a critical factor, by all health care professionals using information and communication technologies for the exchange of valid information for diagnosis, treatment and prevention of disease and injuries, research and evaluation, and for the continuing education of health care providers, all in the interests of advancing the health of individuals and their communities.

More specifically, four

elements are germane to telemedicine:

1. Its purpose is to provide clinical support.
2. It is intended to overcome geographical barriers, connecting users who are not in the same physical location.

---

[197] WHO (2016). *Global diffusion of eHealth: Making universal health coverage achievable. Report of the third global survey on eHealth; Global Observatory for eHealth.* Retrieved July 11, 2018, from http://apps.who.int/iris/bitstream/10665/252529/1/9789241511780-eng.pdf?ua=1

3. It involves the use of various types of ICT.

4. Its goal is to improve health outcomes.[198]

Using this definition, telemedicine is framed as a subset of telehealth, which in turn is a subset of eHealth.

Users. As defined above, the two principle users of telehealth/telemedicine are providers and patients (or their guardians/advocates/representatives). Additionally, payers, suppliers, and public stakeholders may be involved through such educational programs as disease-specific information or management, public announcements such as vaccination campaigns, and billing issues.

Providers. The reason providers are using telehealth programs has recently changed. For example, the principal reason in 2016 was satisfying current consumer demand, which was listed by 72% of organizations; by 2017, only 36% gave that response.[199] The reason for this shift was provided by Ashwood et al.,[200] who found that "12 percent of direct-to-consumer telehealth visits replaced visits to other providers, and 88 percent represented new utilization. Net annual spending on acute respiratory illness increased $45 per telehealth user." The authors concluded that although such visits may be more convenient and replace in-person care for some patients, *the result of these programs was largely to increase volume and hence costs.*

Also declining over that period was use to improve outcomes (66%–55% response). The reason given most often in 2017 for using telehealth was "expanded access/reach."[201] This research offers the opinion that *providers are shifting away from using telehealth strictly to satisfying patients to using it as a business tool to help achieve strategic objectives.*

Whatever reasons providers have for employing telehealth, there are four major barriers to conducting telehealth programs (in addition to formation costs):

1. *Licensure.* Each state has its own professional licensure laws. For purposes of telehealth, a professional must be licensed where the patient resides. Therefore, for example, physicians who provide out-of-state services must obtain another medical license.[202]

   To help with this obstacle, the Health Resources and Services Administration (HRSA) offers competitive Licensure Portability Grant Program (LPGP) awards to

---

[198]WHO. (2010). *Telemedicine: Opportunities and developments in Member States: Report on the second global survey on eHealth 2009. Global Observatory for eHealth Series, 2.* Retrieved July 11, 2018, from http://www.who.int/goe/publications/goe_telemedicine_2010.pdf

[199]Avizia. *Closing the Telehealth gap.* Retrieved July 11, 2018, from https://info.avizia.com/hubfs/assets/Resources/White%20Papers/Avizia_Research_Report_Closing_the_Telehealth_Gap_2017.pdf

[200]Ashwood, J. S., & Uscher-Pines, L. (2017). Direct-to-consumer Telehealth may increase access to care but does not decrease spending. *Health Affairs, 36*(3), 485–491.

[201]Avizia, op. cit.

[202]Telehealth Resource Centers. *Cross-state licensure.* Retrieved July 11, 2018, from https://www.telehealthresource center.org/toolbox-module/cross-state-licensure

state professional licensing boards "to develop and implement state policies that will reduce statutory and regulatory barriers to telemedicine."[203] Also, as mentioned in Chapter 5, "Healthcare Professionals" (section on physician licensure), The Interstate Medical Licensure Compact[204] is expanding its reach to allow physicians to more easily gain licensure in multiple states. For nursing, the Enhanced Nurse Licensure Compact (eNLC),[205] launched January 2018, will give nurses the ability to care for out-of-state patients (including by electronic media).

A similar issue is the ability to prescribe medications across state lines. Generally, pharmacies (especially large chains) have been willing to fill short courses of non-narcotic medications for patients traveling out of state. However, given the growing misuse of drugs, a more secure method was developed by the National Association of Boards of Pharmacy (NABP) called PMP InterConnect.[206]

In addition to licensure, some also advocate for a specialty in telemedicine. For example, Nochomovitz and Sharma have advocated for creation of "medical virtualists" who "will spend the majority or all of their time caring for patients using a virtual medium."[207]

2. *Malpractice coverage.* Since malpractice laws (such as statutes of limitation) and likelihood of successful suits are also state-specific, insurance carriers typically insure providers' activities only where they physically practice. (Exceptions are public employees, such as VA and military professionals, because the government is the insurer.) Therefore, the practitioner must be sure of insurance coverage before providing out-of-state services.

3. *Payment.* Payment varies widely by payer and may depend on the type of service as well as accessibility for the patients. For example, Medicare[208] will pay for remote professional services if the beneficiary resides in a county outside of a Metropolitan Statistical Area (MSA) or a rural Health Professional Shortage Area (HPSA) located in a rural census tract. The HRSA determines HPSAs and the Census Bureau defines the MSAs. Telehealth services not covered by payers are those rendered as follow-up to previous face-to-face visits. (For example, follow-up phone calls to discuss test results are factored into the complexity of care calculation to determine payment for the face-to-face visit.)

[203] HRSA. *Telehealth programs.* Retrieved July 11, 2018, from https://www.hrsa.gov/rural-health/telehealth/index.html

[204] *The Interstate Medical Licensure Compact.* Retrieved from http://www.licenseportability.org

[205] *Enhanced Nurse Licensure Compact (eNLC) implementation.* Retrieved July 11, 2018, from https://www.ncsbn.org/enhanced-nlc-implementation.htm

[206] NABP. *PMP InterConnect.* Retrieved July 11, 2018, from https://nabp.pharmacy/initiatives/pmp-interconnect

[207] Nochomovitz, M., & Sharma, R. (2018). Is it time for a new medical specialty? The medical virtualist. *JAMA, 319*(5), 437–438.

[208] CMS. *Telehealth services.* Retrieved July 11, 2018, from https://www.cms.gov/Outreach-and-Education/Medicare-Learning-Network-MLN/MLNProducts/downloads/TelehealthSrvcsfctsht.pdf

4. *Legal restrictions.* In addition to Medicare and Medicaid payment conditions, states vary widely in their own laws about permissible telemedicine activities within their jurisdictions.[209]

Despite these barriers, the market for telehealth services is expected to grow. For example, telemedicine company Teladoc reported an 89% revenue growth in 2017 and has contracts with Aetna and the Blue Cross Blue Shield Association for its telemedicine services.[210] In 2017, 54% of physicians responding to an AMA study said they will adopt telemedicine capabilities in the next 2 years.[211]

Since telehealth is not confined to one country, it is also interesting to look at the global potential. This market is expected to grow from $18 billion in 2016 to $38 billion in 2022, largely driven by the need to monitor the increasing number of patients with chronic diseases.[212]

Some telehealth services are relatively straightforward and have been in existence for decades: Radiology, dermatology, and pathology images have been transmitted for remote consultation since the 1960s.[213] Other services are more recent. For example, "telestroke" care is the exam, diagnosis, and treatment planning for stroke patients who are brought to a remote facility; the consultation is performed by staff at a tertiary care center using live video feeds as the patient interacts with the on-site physician.[214] The limitations are, of course, cost, technology availability, and the above-mentioned considerations.

Patients. When researching actual patient use and their willingness to engage in telehealth services, one must first be aware of the methods of the studies. Quite often they are online surveys, thus skewing the results to tech-savvy users. In a recent study of the 18% of consumers who said they had used telehealth services, the cited benefits were: "time savings and convenience (59 percent); faster service and shorter wait times to see the doctor (55 percent); and cost savings because of less travel (43 percent)."[215] For those who did not use telehealth,

---

[209] See Marks, J. D. (2018, July 10). *State telehealth laws and Medicaid policies: 50-state survey dindings.* Retrieved July 11, 2018, from https://www.manatt.com/Insights/Newsletters/Manatt-on-Health/State-Policy-Levers-for-Telehealth-50-State-Surve?utm_source=manattonhealthnewsletter&utm_medium=email&utm_campaign=manattonhealth_6.28.18

[210] Sweeney, E. (2018, February 28). With 89% revenue growth in 2017, Teladoc looks to deepen partnerships with large insurers. *FierceHealthcare.* Retrieved July 11, 2018, from https://www.fiercehealthcare.com/tech/teladoc-earning-insurer-partnerships-telehealth?mkt_tok=eyJpIjoiTUdKbFpqbG1OVEExWVRNMiIsInQiOiJUQ2w2b1wvbUxXTG5zb3R2ZWh4bzVTWHl0SzdLQ2lJM3lyTEczM2JyYkRBS0lTdzRBaTFTVnFHaFIwajFJN1pJY0pOXC9xb2NOOVWpOMXJzdjlwNU5EYjA0cVVcL1h5STI2RURrYjRTZkR6OGJIaDE0K0FBbUd4VGtHMnlcLzRUT2FIOVQifQ%3D%3D&mrkid=936233

[211] Accenture and the American Medical Association (AMA). (2017, August 15). Tackling cyber threats in healthcare. Retrieved July 11, 2018, from https://www.ama-assn.org/sites/default/files/media-browser/public/government/advocacy/medical-cybersecurity-findings.pdf

[212] Zion Market Research (2017, March 16). *Global telemedicine market set for rapid growth to reach USD$38 billion by 2022.* Retrieved July 11, 2018, from https://www.zionmarketresearch.com/news/telemedicine-market

[213] Thrall, J. H. (2007). Teleradiology part I. History and clinical applications. *Radiology, 243,* 613–617.

[214] For a recent example, see *"Telestroke" technology will expand access to emergency stroke care across Minnesota.* Retrieved July 11, 2018, from https://www.mhealth.org/blog/2018/january-2018/telestroke-technology-will-expand-access-to-emergency-stroke-care-across-minnesota

[215] Avizia, op. cit.

58% said they did not have the opportunity. However, patients still had strong feelings about barriers to using this technology, especially: preference for face-to-face visits (even when telehealth is available); security/privacy of the encounter; ambiguity about what services are available and how to access them; and uncertainty about insurance coverage.

Blockchain

Blockchain is a data storage and transaction mechanism that has existed since the early 1990s but only came into widespread recognition in the 2000s with the need for a secure, auditable financial trail for bitcoin trading. In the past several years it has garnered attention from the healthcare sector as a solution to such problems as interoperability and data security. Easily understandable explanations of how blockchain technology works can be found online in video presentations.[216] Briefly, a data "block" is first created that contains specific information and a unique address enabling an authorized user to access that block. Each subsequent addition of data creates a new block with its own data, unique address, and a link to the previous block. Such data compilations will, therefore, create a chain of blocks. Unlike an HIE or clearinghouse, the block chain is not centralized. Instead, copies of the entire chain are distributed among users. After verification of a new block to be added to the chain, all authorized users receive a copy. Each block is time-stamped and signed, using a private key, and access is encrypted. This procedure documents the data's provenance and gives users the ability to trace and verify when the block was created and by whom, how it has been used or moved among different data sources, and whether it has been modified. This process makes data alteration and hacking extremely difficult. However, this architecture also makes data access much easier and faster. Further, because patients can limit permission to use portions of the data, their privacy is enhanced. As an example, Vanderbilt University is using blockchain to share medical records.[217]

An additional feature of blockchain technology is its ability to incorporate "smart contracts"—built-in, logic-driven actions that are triggered when specified events occur. For example, if a laboratory creates a new block with test results, the smart contract can be programmed to notify the patient and the ordering physician. Another example might be automatic patient notification when a new user is added to the blockchain. (This latter action can also be used for security purposes if someone is trying to hack into the system.) (Please see Exhibit 8.14 for a schematic of how a healthcare system might use this technology.)

---

[216]For example, see *How does a blockchain work—simply explained*. Retrieved July 11, 2018, from https://www .youtube.com/watch?v=SSo_EIwHSd4; and *What is blockchain*. Retrieved from https://www.youtube.com/watch? v=93E_GzvpMA0 For more general overviews, see IBM Global Business Services Public Sector Team (2016). *Blockchain: The chain of trust and its potential to transform healthcare—our point of view*. Retrieved July 11, 2018, from https://www.healthit.gov/sites/default/files/8-31-blockchain-ibm_ideation-challenge_aug8.pdf Capgemini (2017, August 1). *Blockchain: A healthcare industry view*. Retrieved July 11, 2018, from https://www.capgemini.com/wp-content/uploads/2017/07/blockchain-a_healthcare_industry_view_2017_web.pdf and FY18 HIMSS Blockchain Work Group (2017, October 23). *Part 1: Navigating the blockchain landscape—opportunities in digital health*. Retrieved July 11, 2018, from http://www.himss.org/news/part-1-navigating-blockchain-landscape-opportunities-digital-health

[217]Slabodkin, G. (2018, July 2). Vanderbilt leverages blockchain, FHIR for secure sharing of medical records. *Health-Data Management*. Retrieved July 11, 2018, from https://www.healthdatamanagement.com/news/vanderbilt-leverages-blockchain-fhir-for-secure-sharing-of-medical-records?utm_campaign=MorningRounds-Jul%202%202018&utm_medium=email&utm_source=newsletter

EXHIBIT 8.14. **Blockchain Use in a Healthcare System**

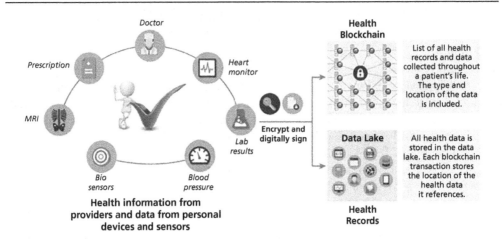

Source: Linn, L. A., &and Koo, M. B.: Blockchain for health data and its potential use in health IT and health care related research. Retrieved July 11, 2018 from https://www.healthit.gov/sites/default/files/11-74-ablockchainforhealthcare.pdf

In 2016, the ONC issued a white paper challenge for uses of blockchain in healthcare settings. The first-place winner (14 other papers were also considered winners) was "A Case Study for Blockchain in Healthcare: 'MedRec' Prototype for Electronic Health Records and Medical Research Data."[218] The authors describe a medical records system called MedRec that uses blockchain technology to manage

> authentication, confidentiality, accountability and data sharing … [Its] modular design integrates with providers' existing, local data storage solutions, facilitating interoperability and making [the] system convenient and adaptable … medical stakeholders (researchers, public health authorities, etc.) [are] incentivized to participate in the network as blockchain 'miners' … [providing] … them with access to aggregate, anonymized data as mining rewards, in return for sustaining and securing the network …

In addition to provider EMRs, blockchain applications can also be used for such health-care functions as case management, clinical research studies, and insurance transactions (e.g., enrollment, eligibility verification, and claims adjudication).

---

[218]Ekblaw, A., Azaria, A., Halamka, J. D., & Lippman, A., MIT Media Lab, & Beth Israel Deaconess Medical Center. (2016, August). A case study for blockchain in healthcare: "MedRec" prototype for electronic health records and medical research data. Retrieved July 11, 2018, from https://www.healthit.gov/sites/default/files/5-56-onc_blockchainchallenge_mitwhitepaper.pdf

Interest in blockchain applications in healthcare has spurred development of companies geared to helping users establish these platforms. Some examples are briefly discussed below.

In this arena, perhaps the best-known blockchain application is Ethereum,[219] which was started in 2014 with the crowd-funded Ethereum Foundation, a Swiss nonprofit organization. "Ethereum is a decentralized platform that runs smart contracts ... on a custom built blockchain."

Emrify[220] is a company that uses a blockchain technology with smart contract functionality (built on an Ethereum platform) to enable individuals to sell their personal health data. For example, an individual can gather data in a Personal Health Record using such tools as a Fitbit, glucometer, "smartscale," and so on. That person can then shop for the going rate for releasing such data to interested parties, arrange for sale, and then transfer the data via blockchain using what Emrify calls a Health Information Token. This system creates a more secure marketplace for better-quality, API-validated data. For those familiar with bitcoin, the analogy is that providers of the data are "miners" and the Health Information Token is the cryptocurrency.

1upHealth's[221] investor is Boston Children's Hospital. It provides "intelligent analysis" of patients' health by gathering their inpatient data and coupling it with wearable sensor data gathered as an outpatient. 1upHealth was created

> to offer a platform where patients can share their wearable device and health data with health systems in order to prepare providers for the shift to value based care. 1upHealth makes hospitals money by reducing readmissions in value payment structures such as bundled payment models, at risk organizations, and for the readmissions reduction program. We use the intelligence of machine learning to help prioritize member care through alerts that identify at-risk patients through metrics like gait length, heartrate, location, steps, coughs, and other personal attributes after patients leave the hospital.

Finally, Gem[222] developed the first blockchain product for health claims management and has partnered with the CDC to search for solutions to population health problems.

Despite these exciting innovations, blockchain is generally considered a complementary technology rather than one that replaces existing institutional information systems.[223] Several cautions are listed next.

1. Provider hospitals will still want to generate and retain their own EMR, even though it may be part of a blockchain system. These systems are, therefore, subject to privacy and security measures of these traditional products.

---

[219] *Ethereum*. Retrieved July 11, 2018, from https://www.ethereum.org

[220] Emrify, Inc. *Health Passport: A decentralized personal health record platform to deliver trusted health information to the right hands at the right time anywhere in the world.* Retrieved July 11, 2018, from https://icosbull.com/eng/ico/emrify-health-passport/whitepaper

[221] *1UpHealth*. Retrieved July 11, 2018, from https://1up.health

[222] *Gem*. Retrieved July 11, 2018, from https://gem.co/health

[223] Slabodkin, G. (2018, February 15). Blockchain not a panacea for managing health records, fed expert says. *Health Data Management*. Retrieved July 11, 2018, from https://www.healthdatamanagement.com/news/blockchain-is-not-a-panacea-technology-for-managing-health-records

2. For effective interoperability, all potential users must be on the same blockchain.

3. Use of blockchain products must comply with HIPAA and HITECH regulations.

Cloud-Based Services

For much of computer history, most software and data storage have been under direct ownership and control of the user. As the "information age" has accelerated, a number of changes have caused a rethinking of that model:

1. In order to successfully run and grow their businesses, firms are requiring an increasing number of different software programs (or suites of programs, like MS Office). These programs are expensive to purchase and maintain service agreements.

2. The software programs are undergoing rapid changes with new versions being issued frequently. Each time a key program is changed, the organization may lose time (and money) installing the update.

3. Even as locally owned hardware has dramatically increased data storage size, the needs for increased storage capacity and the ability to manage large databases have often outstripped this hardware and company expertise.

To meet those challenges, cloud computing was developed. "In the simplest terms, cloud computing means storing and accessing data and programs over the Internet instead of your computer's hard drive. The cloud is just a metaphor for the Internet."[224] In fact, the term "cloud" comes from early computer network graphics that used a cloud icon to stand for the space where networks would link together—that is, the internet. More recently, many IT companies have appended the words "as a Service" to promote their products as cloud-based. (Please see Exhibit 8.15 for some examples.) Because many of these services are not truly cloud-based products, more precise and uniformly accepted definitions are needed.

EXHIBIT 8.15. Examples of "as a Service" Offerings Marketed as Cloud-Based Products

Address verification as a Service	Encryption as a Service	Mobility backend as a Service
Anything as a Service	Enterprise resource	Monitoring as a Service
API as a Service (APIaaS)	Management as a Service	Network access control as a Service
Application delivery as a Service	Ethernet as a Service	Network as a Service
Application platform as a Service	Everything as a Service	Operations as a Service
Architecture as a Service	Firewall as a Service	Optimization as a Service

---

[224]Griffith, E. (2016, May 3). What is cloud computing? *PC Magazine*. Retrieved July 11, 2018, from https://www.pcmag.com/article2/0,2817,2372163,00.asp

Authentication as a Service	Framework as a Service	Payment as a Service
Backend as a Service	Globalization as a Service	Quality as a Service
Backup as a Service	Hadoop as a Service	Query as a Service
Big data as a Service	Hardware as a Service	Recovery as a Service
Broker as a Service	High performance computing as a Service	Remote backup as a Service
Business as a Service	Identity as a Service	Risk assessment as a Service
Business process as a Service	Infrastructure PaaS	Robot as a Service
Cloud load balancers as a Service	Insight as a Service	Security as a Service
Cloud search as a Service	Integrated development	Service desk as a Service
Collaboration as a Service	Environment as a Service	Solutions as a Service
Commerce as a Service	Integration as a Service	Storage as a Service
Communication as a Service	Integration platform as a Service	Telepresence as a service
Computing as a Service	Integration platform as a Service	Test environment as a Service
Contact center as a service	IT as a service	Testing as a Service
Conversations as a Service	Java platform as a Service	Transport as a Service
Data as a Service	Knowledge as a Service	Unified communications as a Service
Database as a Service	Light as a Service	User interface as a Service
Desktop as a Service	Logon as a Service	Video conferencing as a Service
Development as a Service	Management as a Service	Video surveillance as a Service
DevTest as a Service	Mashups as a Service	Voice as a Service
Disaster recovery as a Service	Message queuing as a Service	Website as a Service
Drupal as a Service	Metal as a Service	
Email as a Service	Mobility as a Service	

Source: Simmon, E. and the NIST Cloud Computing Cloud Services Working Group, NIST Cloud Computing Program Information Technology Laboratory: NIST Special Publication 500-322, Evaluation of Cloud Computing Services Based on NIST SP 800-145. February 2018. Retrieved July 11, 2018 from https://nvlpubs.nist.gov/nistpubs/SpecialPublications/NIST.SP.500-322.pdf

The NIST of the U.S. Department of Commerce defines cloud computing as "a model for enabling ubiquitous, convenient, on-demand network access to a shared pool of configurable computing resources (e.g., networks, servers, storage, applications, and services) that can be rapidly provisioned and released with minimal management effort or service provider inter-action."[225] In elaborating on this definition, the NIST introduces five essential characteristics, three cloud service models, and four types of cloud deployments.

Five Essential Characteristics

1. On-demand self-service
2. Broad network access
3. Resource pooling
4. Rapid elasticity
5. Measured service

Three Service Models

1. Software as a Service (SaaS)
2. Platform as a Service (PaaS)
3. Infrastructure as a Service (IaaS)

Four Deployment Models

1. Public
2. Private
3. Community
4. Hybrid

The three service models are briefly explained below in order from least to most control by the customer.

1. *Software as Service* (SaaS, pronounced "sarse"). Software is the service provided and is accessed when needed from the internet. Examples include email, like Gmail, and social networking, like Facebook. Healthcare functions include EMRs and medical office practice management systems. This option is usually used by smaller organizations that do not have the resources to run their own IT departments. Also, only internet-accessible devices are needed to run the services the organizations need.

2. *Platform as Service* (PaaS, pronounced "parse"). The major difference between SaaS and PaaS is that the latter allows more control over software development and use. For example, healthcare organizations seeking to merge may want to develop custom applications that will allow seamless data flow. They can engage a PaaS firm for all the other functions. According to Salesforce.com (whose Force.com is a PaaS):

   > At its core, platform as a service (PaaS) eliminates the expense and complexity of buying, configuring, and managing all the hardware and software needed to run

---

[225] Ibid.

applications ... Additionally, large companies often need specialized facilities to house their data centers and a team to maintain them. Enormous amounts of electricity also are needed to power the servers as well as the systems to keep them cool. Finally, a failover site is needed to mirror the data center so information can be replicated in case of a disaster.[226]

Other companies in this space are MySQL and Oracle.

3. *Infrastructure as Service* (IaaS, pronounced "I-arse"). Vendors who offer this service provide the infrastructure for the customer's IT system. This infrastructure includes actual or virtual hardware (often called virtual machine [VM] hardware),[227] firewalls, IP addresses, and data storage. Examples include Rackspace and Amazon Web Services.

Many businesses use combinations of these services. It should also be noted that these service providers are business partners and must comply with HIPAA regulations with respect to PHI.

Given the previously mentioned healthcare trends, organizations are increasingly using cloud-based services. For example, a 2017 HIMSS hospital study found that "[r]oughly 65 percent of study respondents currently utilize the cloud or cloud services within their organization. Much of the usage leans toward clinical application and data hosting, data recovery and backup, and the hosting of operational applications."[228] In line with this use, cloud services use is approximately: 88% SaaS, 54% IaaS, and 10% PaaS. In view of increasing ransomware and other attacks, as well as natural disasters, hospital chief information officers (CIOs) are increasingly concerned with post-disaster data recovery. To meet that need, in 2017, 75% of hospital CIOs said they planned to use IaaS services within the next year compared to about 15% in 2014.

Playing off healthcare organizations' willingness and need to use cloud-based services, many companies are expanding their offerings to solve client problems. Three examples of how healthcare organizations are using cloud services are described next.

1. *Interoperability.* In 2017, Google announced its Cloud Healthcare API[229] which will "extract data from electronic health records and 'other proprietary data' by using DICOM, FHIR and HL7 protocols" in order to facilitate interoperability.

---

[226]Salesforce.com. Retrieved July 11, 2018, from https://www.salesforce.com/paas/overview and *8 core services of a platform as service.* Retrieved July 11, 2018, from https://a.sfdcstatic.com/content/dam/www/ocms/assets/pdf/misc/8-Core-Services-of-a-Cloud-Platform-eBook.pdf (Free registration required.)

[227]"A virtual machine is a software computer that, like a physical computer, runs an operating system and applications. The virtual machine is comprised of a set of specification and configuration files and is backed by the physical resources of a host. Every virtual machine has virtual devices that provide the same functionality as physical hardware and have additional benefits in terms of portability, manageability, and security." *Vmware: What is a Virtual machine?* Retrieved July 11, 2018, from https://pubs.vmware.com/vsphere-50/index.jsp?topic=%2Fcom.vmware.vsphere.vm_admin.doc_50%2FGUID-CEFF6D89-8C19-4143-8C26-4B6D6734D2CB.html

[228]HIMSS. *2017 essentials brief: Cloud.* Retrieved July 11, 2018, from http://www.himssanalytics.org/research/essentials-brief-2017-cloud-study (Registration required.)

[229]Slabotkin, G. (2018, March 6). Google announces Cloud Healthcare API to unlock health data. *HealthData Management.* Retrieved July 11, 2018, from https://www.healthdatamanagement.com/news/google-announces-cloud-healthcare-api-to-unlock-health-data

2. *Enrollment.* The federal government is planning to move healthcare.gov to an Amazon-hosted cloud infrastructure by the end of the first quarter of 2019.[230]

3. *Population health management and reporting.*

> Accountable Health Partners (AHP), a clinically integrated network of hospitals and physicians in Rochester, N.Y., has successfully moved to new reimbursement models using a cloud-based data repository and analytics platform … to support its population health management initiatives … Under a three-year Accountable Cost and Quality Arrangement (ACQA) with Excellus BlueCross BlueShield, quality measures are reported via the Arcadia analytics dashboard in an effort to share responsibility for providing coordinated care to patients to improve quality indicators—such as cancer screening rates, hypertension and diabetes control—and reduce unnecessary healthcare costs.[231]

Artificial Intelligence/Voice Recognition

The term "artificial intelligence" (AI) means different things to different people. As Marr stated: "the focus of artificial intelligence shifts depending on the entity that provides the definition."[232]

In its simplest form, the term "AI" is used when referring to computer learning and reasoning that mimics human behavior. However, the real use for AI is to be able to mimic this behavior while processing larger amounts of data faster than a human. The example most widely known is IBM's Watson.[233] Two healthcare areas are of particular importance with regard to AI are clinical decision support and predictive analysis.

AI has the capacity not only to suggest differential diagnoses based on signs and symptoms but also to integrate data from various sources and devices to help with clinical decisions. For example, in 2016, the Cleveland Clinic signed a 5-year agreement with IBM Watson Health "to expand the clinic's health IT capabilities including the use of IBM's secured cloud, social, mobile and Watson cognitive computing technologies across its clinical and administrative operations."[234] As clinic CEO Dr. Tomislav Mihaljevic said: "Now, the

---

[230] Sweeney, E. (2018, March 12). Healthcare.gov is moving to the cloud; 2018 downtime was less than expected. *Fierce-Healthcare.* Retrieved July 11, 2018, from https://www.fiercehealthcare.com/tech/cms-healthcare-gov-bobby-saxon-downtime-cloud?mkt_tok=eyJpIjoiTlRVNE5UY3dZVGszTURJMyIsInQiOiJRa0xoYkpob0xQRFFvZ3ZlR29JNTVGcUZ1elh0SStlK0tJcVFcL01FOXdhM1pQZGZ1S0t2YU5xOTVWMzZkaEdTUU5WODR6QjVFK1VlT3dJTGxDU0NXWSt0UzJsUjJUS2dUZkJRZHpBWGtpY2FsUUdTFBWeU8yMFZaLXC9rRDY1TWNOIn0%3D&mrkid=936233

[231] Slabodkin, G. (2018, February 5). Providers are embracing SaaS models to meet value demands. *HealthData Management.* Retrieved July 11, 2018, from https://www.healthdatamanagement.com/news/providers-are-embracing-saas-models-to-meet-value-demands

[232] Marr, B. (2018, February 14). The key definitions of artificial intelligence (AI) that explain its importance. *Forbes.* Retrieved July 11, 2018, from https://www.forbes.com/sites/bernardmarr/2018/02/14/the-key-definitions-of-artificial-intelligence-ai-that-explain-its-importance/#707721544f5d For other related definitions, such as machine learning, see Bresnick, J. (2017, July 6). Machine learning in healthcare: Defining the most common terms. *HealthIT Analytics.* Retrieved July 11, 2018, from https://healthitanalytics.com/news/machine-learning-in-healthcare-defining-the-most-common-terms

[233] *IBM Watson Health.* Retrieved July 11, 2018, from https://www.ibm.com/watson/health

[234] Slabodkin, G. (2018, March 14). Cleveland clinic lays out its health IT strategy for future. *HealthData Management.* Retrieved July 11, 2018, from https://www.healthdatamanagement.com/news/cleveland-clinic-lays-out-its-health-it-strategy-for-future

day will come when our decisions are supported by data from wearables, imaging, implants, genetic profiling, along with insights from global health trends and published research. And care through that will become more personalized and individualized than ever."

AI-assisted clinical decision making is also being used to match patients with the most appropriate resources. For example, at the Mayo Clinic, "Watson for Clinical Trials Matching is programmed to accurately and consistently match patients to clinical trials for which they might be eligible, so that healthcare providers and patients can consider appropriate trials as part of a care plan."[235]

Despite the great promise of AI-aided and other clinical decision software, the regulations for their use are still not completely clear. At the time of this writing, the latest information is two draft guidances issued December 7, 2017, by then-FDA Commissioner Scott Gottlieb, M.D., titled "Clinical and Patient Decision Support Software" and "Changes to Existing Medical Software Policies Resulting from Section 3060 of the 21st Century Cures Act." In a press release, Gottlieb stated:

> [G]enerally, CDS [clinical decision support software] that allows for the provider to independently review the basis for the recommendations are excluded from the FDA's regulation. This type of CDS can include software that suggests a provider order liver function tests before starting statin medication, consistent with clinical guidelines and approved drug labeling. However, the FDA will continue to enforce oversight of software programs that are intended to process or analyze medical images, signals from *in vitro* diagnostic devices or patterns acquired from a processor like an electrocardiogram that use analytical functionalities to make treatment recommendations, as these remain medical devices under the Cures Act ... We're making clear that certain digital health technologies—such as mobile apps that are intended only for maintaining or encouraging a healthy lifestyle—generally fall outside the scope of the FDA's regulation. Such technologies tend to pose a low risk to patients, but can provide great value to consumers and the healthcare system.[236]

The problem with this guidance is that it does not cover hybrid models and take into account AI-based systems. Until this issue is cleared, AI-based system results will need to be reviewed and implemented by a medical professional.

A related issue is the emergence of voice-recognition technology. This know-how can be paired with AI to create opportunities for patient interaction such as appointment and medication reminders; encouragement to obtain age-, sex-, and condition-specific preventive and maintenance services; and detection of physiological fluctuations that can alert clinician to a deteriorating clinical status. Examples in the latter category include stroke and Alzheimer's disease.

---

[235] Monegain, B. (2018, March 14). Mayo Clinic boosts clinical trials with IBM Watson artificial intelligence. Supercomputer matches more patients to breast cancer clinical trial than had previously participated, the organizations say. *Healthcare IT News.* Retrieved July 11, 2018, from http://www.healthcareitnews.com/news/mayo-clinic-boosts-clinical-trials-ibm-watson-artificial-intelligence

[236] Statement from FDA Commissioner Scott Gottlieb, M.D., on advancing new digital health policies to encourage innovation, bring efficiency and modernization to regulation December 7, 2017. Retrieved July 11, 2018, from https://www.fda.gov/NewsEvents/Newsroom/PressAnnouncements/ucm587890.htm

EXHIBIT 8.16. **Top Five Healthcare IT Companies (by Installations) as of July 2017**

Hospitals	Physician Groups
Epic	Epic
Cerner	Allscripts
Meditech	eClinicalWorks
McKesson	NextGen Healthcare
Medhost	GE Healthcare

Source: Office of the National Coordinator for Health Information Technology: Health Care Professional Health IT Developers. Retrieved July 11, 2018 from https://dashboard.healthit.gov/quickstats/pages/FIG-Vendors-of-EHRs-to-Participating-Professionals .php

Industry Consolidation

As was the case with hospitals and insurance companies, there has been much consolidation and dominance of few providers in the IT market. The top five companies (particularly the top two or three) dominate their market, and the trend will undoubtedly continue. No antitrust concerns have yet been raised, however. (Please see Exhibit 8.16.)

Expanding Patients' Access to and Control of Their Data

A recent federal government initiative is geared to expanding patients' access and control of their health data. Announced on March 6, 2018, at the HIMSS 18 conference, the plan has three main parts. Currently, the goals are clear but the specifics are still lacking.

1. *MyHealthEData* initiative "aims to empower patients by ensuring that they control their healthcare data and can decide how their data is going to be used, all while keeping that information safe and secure."[237]

2. Medicare's "Blue Button 2.0" will give beneficiaries access to the most recent 4 years of claims data "in a universal and secure digital format." Medicare first launched Blue Button in 2010 as a joint effort between CMS and the VA as an API where beneficiaries could "push a website button" and get access to their claims in a downloadable PDF file.[238]

3. CMS will examine requirements for Medicare Advantage and Health Insurance Exchange plans to provide the same information as Medicare's Blue Button 2.0.

---

[237] Trump Administration Announces MyHealthEData Initiative at HIMSS18 (2018, March 3). Retrieved July 11, 2018, from https://www.cms.gov/Newsroom/MediaReleaseDatabase/Fact-sheets/2018-Fact-sheets-items/2018-03-06.html
[238] Medicare.gov. *Medicare's Blue Button & Blue Button 2.0*. Retrieved July 11, 2018, from https://www.medicare.gov/manage-your-health/blue-button/medicare-blue-button.html

Administrative Simplification

Section 4001 of the 21st Century Cures Act directs the ONC (in partnership with CMS) to reduce regulatory and administrative burdens related to the use of EHRs. The need for this relief has been documented in several research studies showing that physicians spend more time on the EHR than face-to-face with patients.[239] This administrative burden is highlighted by one study of family physicians showing that 44% of computer time is spent on clerical tasks while 32% is spent on medical care.[240] To accomplish this mandate, the federal government proposes to "streamline" the meaningful use criteria by cutting back on documentation required with evaluation and management codes. Instead, the focus will be on interoperability initiatives and preventing information blocking.

SUMMARY

HIT has great potential to make data access easier; avoid unnecessary, costly, and duplicative tests; enhance administrative and clinical decision making; and empower individuals to engage in preventive health and maintenance activities. The major obstacle that prevents these and other benefits is lack of interoperability. This problem requires two interventions. The first is agreement among governmental entities and HIT providers on uniform standards. The second is the willingness of patients to have a unique identifier that can be used to trace activities across all parts of the healthcare system. The former issue is technically feasible; the latter will require a major cultural shift, where individuals trust government and software systems to safeguard their privacy. Given the large number of data breaches in recent years, this shift is unlikely in the foreseeable future.

---

[239] See, for example: Young, R. A., Burge, S. K., Kumar, K. A., & Wilson, J. M. (2018). A time-motion study of primary care physicians' work in the electronic health record era. *Family Medicine*, *50*(2), 91–99.
[240] Arndt, B. G., Beasley, J. W., Watkinson, M. D., Temte, J. L., Tuan, W. J., Sinsky, C. A., & Gilchrist, V. J. (2017). Tethered to the EHR: Primary care physician workload assessment using EHR event log data and time-motion observations. *Annals of Family*, *15*(5), 419–426.

CHAPTER

9

QUALITY

HAMLET.

Come, give us a taste of your quality.

—William Shakespeare, *Hamlet*, Act 2, Scene 2

No one will dare to say that they can measure that which is not.

—St. Augustine: Confessions Book XI, Chapter XVI (Paragraph 21)

INTRODUCTION

The late Harvard professor L. J. Henderson, MD (1878–1942) was alleged to have said: "It was not until 1910 or so that a random patient with a random disease consulting a random doctor stood better than a 50-50 chance of being helped."[1] One hundred years later, the situation was not much changed: "Across the core report measures tracked in the NHQR [National Healthcare Quality Report], the median level of receipt of needed care was 59%"[2] This finding applied nearly equally to preventive, acute, and chronic care.[3] More recently, some improvements in care have been achieved,[4] particularly in the area of reducing Hospital Acquired Conditions (HACs), including hospital-acquired infections, patient falls, and medication errors.[5] However, consumers rate healthcare below the quality, safety, and satisfaction ratings enjoyed by other sectors. (Please see Exhibit 9.1 for examples.) Further, public dissatisfaction with quality of care has expanded into a discussion about value for money or, as former Harvard Public Health School Dean Julio Frenk noted, "There's no other sector that spends that kind of money with so little evidence of what works and what doesn't and how it should best be applied."[6]

Past chapters presented definitions at the beginning of each topic. The definition of quality, however, has changed over many centuries, and only recently has a stable, workable definition emerged. Therefore, current definitions will be presented after the discussion of historical context.

---

[1] Shalowitz, J. (2010). Implementing successful quality outcome programs in ambulatory care: Key questions and recommendations. *Journal of Ambulatory Care Management*, *33*(2), 117–123.

[2] Agency for Healthcare Research and Quality. (2009). Publication No. 090001 (p. 2). Retrieved July 12, 2018, from http://www.ahrq.gov/qual/nhqr08/nhqr08.pdf

[3] McGlynn, E. A., Asch, S. M., Adams, J., Keesey, J., Hicks, J., DeCristofaro, A., & Kerr, E. A. (2003). The quality of health care delivered to adults in the United States. *New England Journal of the Medicine*, *348*(26), 2635–2645.

[4] Agency for Healthcare Research and Quality. (2016, May 16). *2015 National healthcare quality and disparities report and 5th anniversary update on the national quality strategy*. Quality and Disparities in Quality of Health Care. Retrieved from https://www.ahrq.gov/research/findings/nhqrdr/nhqdr15/quality.html

[5] AHRQ National Scorecard on Hospital-Acquired Conditions Updated Baseline Rates and Preliminary Results 2014–2016. Retrieved June 2018 from https://www.ahrq.gov/sites/default/files/wysiwyg/professionals/quality-patient-safety/pfp/natlhacratereport-rebaselining2014-2016_0.pdf

[6] Care delivery hot topic at Mexico health summit. (2004, November 13). *The China Post*. Retrieved April 16, 2017, from www.chinapost.com.tw/news/2004/11/13/54401/Care-delivery.htm (Note: The *China Post* ceased publication in 2017 and the website is no longer available.)

EXHIBIT 9.1. American Consumer Satisfaction Index 2017 (Scores Out of 100)

Health insurance	73
Hospitals	75
Ambulatory care	77
Life insurance	78
Supermarkets	79
Internet retail	82
Soft drinks and breweries	84

Source: The American Consumer Satisfaction Index (2017). Retrieved July 12, 2018, from https://www.theacsi.org/acsi-benchmarks/benchmarks-by-industry

HISTORY OF HEALTHCARE QUALITY AND DEVELOPMENT OF KEY CONCEPTS AND INSTITUTIONS

Ancient Origins

Several thousand years ago, people lived in nomadic tribes, each with its own customs and gods. As civilizations formed and people settled together in one location, there needed to be a common set of secular rules so conflicts of tribal laws would not cause civil unrest. To legitimize these laws, rulers of diverse populations invoked their "divine connections" to enable them to enforce their provisions. The first known legal text was the Ur-Nammu Code (ca. 2100 BCE–2050 BCE). It was written in the simple style of "If (crime) . . . , then (compensation) . . . " The code listed certain capital offenses (e.g., murder, adultery, and rape), but the remainder of the penalties specified payment of monetary damages. For example, "If a man knocks out a tooth of another man, he shall pay two shekels of silver." Three hundred years later (ca. 1776 BCE), the Babylonian king Hammurabi (ca. 1810 BCE–1750 BCE) expanded previous statutes and had them engraved on a stele in the Akkadian language. This code resembles previous ones in several respects. First, the text starts with a prologue naming gods and establishing Hammurabi's legal authority; for example: "Anu and Bel [two gods] called me, Hammurabi, the exalted prince, the worshiper of the gods, to cause justice to prevail in the land."[7] Second, the legal dictates are in the traditional "If . . . , then . . . " format.

[7] Harper, R.F. (1904). *The code of Hammurabi King of Babylon about 2250 B.C.* (2nd ed.). Chicago: University of Chicago Press. *Note:* 1. This text is the source for the quotations of the cited laws. 2. The Code of Hammurabi was discovered in 1901 in Susa (in modern Iran), and the dates were not accurately determined then; hence the erroneous date in Professor Harper's title. The dates in the text are correct. The code was probably first established at Sippar (in current Iraq), where there was a temple dedicated to the god of justice, Shamash (sun god). On top of the stele is a carving depicting Shamash handing Hammurabi the authority to issue and administer the laws. It is believed that when the Elamites conquered Babylonia, they moved the code to their capital in Susa. For a more detailed discussion of this king and the historical period, see: Charpin, D. (2012). *Hammurabi of Babylon.* London: I.B. Tauris & Co.

Third, some of the penalties are similar, including fines and, particularly, death penalties for comparable infractions.

However, Hammurabi's Code differs in two principal ways from previous statutes. First, for many crimes, the penalties are not compensatory but retributive. For example, compare this decree from Hammurabi's Code with the one cited above: "If a man knock out a tooth of a man of his own rank, they shall knock out his tooth." Second, it specifically mentions medical acts: both rewards for success and penalties for failures. For example:

> 215. If a physician operates on a man for a severe wound (or make a severe wound upon a man) with a bronze lancet and saves the man's life; or if he opens an abscess (in the eye) of a man with a bronze lancet and saves that man's eye, he shall receive ten shekels of silver (as his fee).

> 218. If a physician operates on a man for a severe wound with a bronze lancet and causes the man's death; or opens an abscess (in the eye) of a man with a bronze lancet and destroys the man's eye, they shall cut off his fingers.

Thus, almost 4,000 years ago, we have published outcome goals and fee schedules.

From that time until the medieval period, laws concerning quality of care were rare. When statutes were issued, they set educational and examination requirements for the practice of medicine. (See the History of Western Medical Care section in Chapter 4, "Healthcare Professionals" for the decrees of Roger II in 1140.) Hospitals were not regulated by secular authorities for three reasons: most care was delivered at home; institutional care, when it did occur, was provided in church-run institutions; and many "hospitals" were no more than almshouses for the poor.

"Modern" attention to the quality of hospitals dates to the French Revolution and its aftermath, when formal government committees initiated numerous efforts to improve the public's health.[8] For example, in Parisian hospitals prior to that time, three patients were routinely placed together in wide beds. Architect Nicholas Etienne Clavareau (1757–1815) proudly wrote that he had reduced "all beds at the Hôtel-Dieu and St. Louis to a width of three feet"[9] so that only one patient at a time could occupy a bed.

1900–1950

Real, comprehensive quality initiatives are the product of 20th-century science and values (i.e., the ability and willingness to improve medical care). These efforts started with Ernest A. Codman, MD (1869–1940), a surgeon at Massachusetts General Hospital. For years, Codman had prodded the hospital to track patient outcomes and determine the causes of errors, a program he called the "End Result System." Colleagues considered the process radical for two reasons. First, it exposed them to public scrutiny and threatened their reputations (and, as Codman would later say, their incomes). The second reason was that the reviews were to be

---

[8] Weiner, D. B. (1993). *The citizen-patient in revolutionary and imperial Paris* (p. 3). Baltimore: Johns Hopkins University Press.

[9] Clavareau, N. E. (1805). *Mémoires sur les hôpitaux civils de Paris* (p. 51). Paris: Prault. This accomplishment is often misrepresented in the quality literature, which states that the beds were *moved* 3 feet apart.

supervised not by surgeons but by hospital administrators under direction of a member of the board of trustees. (This structure is recognizable today as the separation of those who gather and analyze the data from those affected by the process.) Because of disagreements, Codman resigned from the hospital staff and, in 1911, started his own private hospital, the Codman Hospital, in Boston. The hospital remained open until 1917, when, burdened by debt and called to service in World War I, Codman closed it. While the hospital was open, Codman applied the End Results System through rigorous tracking of patients (e.g., applying such then-novel measures as assigning each patient a unique identifier for all admissions and keeping track of lengths of stay). In 1915, he privately published the first of three reports on his findings: *A Study in Hospital Efficiency as Demonstrated by the Case Report of the Second Two Years of a Private Hospital.*[10] In that short text, he outlined the quality improvement process that is substantively followed today and explained the reasons for "Lack of Perfection" in surgical treatment. (Please see Exhibit 9.2.)

EXHIBIT 9.2. Causes of "Lack of Perfection" in Surgical Treatment

All results of surgical treatment that lack perfection may be explained by one or more of the following causes:

Errors due to lack of technical knowledge or skill	E-s
Errors due to lack of surgical judgment	E-j
Errors due to lack of care or equipment	E-c
Errors due to lack of diagnostic skill	E-d
These are partially controllable by organization.	
The patient's enfeebled condition	P-c
The patient's unconquerable disease	P-d
The patient's refusal of treatment	P-r
These are partially controllable by public education.	
The calamities of surgery or those accidents and complications over which we have no known control	C
These should be acknowledged to ourselves and to the public, and study directed to their prevention.	

Source: Codman, E. A. (1915). *A study in hospital efficiency as demonstrated by the case report of the second two years of a private hospital* (p. 7). Boston: Th. Todd Co.

---

[10]The final report on about 300 operations was presented in: Codman, E. A. (1918). *A study in hospital efficiency: As demonstrated by the case report of the first five years of a private hospital.* Boston: Thomas Todd. A reprinted edition was issued by the Joint Commission in December 1995.

[W]e want to illustrate a definite method by which the organization of a Surgical Service of a Hospital can be based on the End Result System. We believe the same general method can be applied to other branches of clinical work besides surgery. The Idea is so simple as to seem childlike, but we find it ignored in all Charitable Hospitals, and very largely in Private Hospitals. It is simply to follow the natural series of questions which anyone asks in an individual case.

What was the matter?

Did they find it out beforehand?

Did the patient get entirely well?

If not—why not?

Was it the fault of the surgeon, the disease, or the patient?

What can we do to prevent similar failures in the future?

We believe that the general acceptance of a system of hospital organization based on the truthful record of the answers to these questions means the beginning of True Clinical Science.

If his writings were all he contributed, Codman's contributions would probably have gone unheeded. Two other events solidified his influence: the formation of the American College of Surgeons (ACS) and the Progressive Movement of the early 20th century.

The formation of the ACS is a story with origins in the concern for quality of care and scientific rigor. In September 1904, prominent Chicago gynecologist Dr. Franklin Martin gathered several colleagues to start a surgical journal. The reason for this venture was the prevalence of for-profit medical publications that were not serving the scientific needs of surgeons. Recall from the discussion on physician education that this era was also the time of proprietary medical schools—before Flexner's reforms were implemented. After careful planning, *Surgery, Gynecology & Obstetrics* (*SG&O*) launched its first issue in July 1905. By 1910, the success of the journal prompted its editors to host what would be an annual meeting of a society called the Clinical Congress of Surgeons of North America. At the third annual meeting in New York in 1912, its president, Philadelphia surgeon Dr. Edward Martin (no relation to Franklin Martin), crafted a proposal to enhance clinical quality that he had a colleague introduce as a resolution. Edward Martin knew that because of progress in surgical capabilities throughout the country, there had been a rapid increase in the number of hospitals. Unfortunately, many of these facilities did not have the equipment necessary to allow proper performance of surgical operations. Further, many hospitals were poorly administered. Martin thought it possible to standardize and evaluate hospitals in such a way that the public could know which hospitals delivered safe and effective care.[11]

From this initiative came the Committee on the Standardization of Hospitals. Dr. Codman was appointed its chair, and the group included prominent surgeons such as

---

[11] Davis, L. (1960). *Fellowship of surgeons, a history of the American College of Surgeons*. Chicago: Charles C. Thomas.

Dr. William Mayo.[12] The chair's position was formalized after the ACS was incorporated in Illinois on November 25, 1912.

In its first report, the committee recommended "[t]hat each of us do what he can to induce the trustees of his own hospital to organize a followup system for all patients treated [and]...each of us do what he can to induce the fellow members of his staff to appoint efficiency committees who may look into present conditions in his own hospital in order that we may, as far as possible, do our own house cleaning."[13] In other words, implement an End Results system in their respective institutions.

Part of the recommendation was establishment of medical records that included such items as a patients' vital signs, clinical history, record of operations, and results of laboratory and radiology exams. This record keeping was needed for two reasons. First, it was essential to evaluate patient care outcomes. This benefit, Codman argued, should interest hospital administrators and trustees who would be able to assess the quality of surgeons in their institutions. Second, the ACS wanted surgeons who were applying for fellowships to submit case records for examination. Since surgeons wanted to become fellows of the college, they were strong advocates for improvement in hospital record keeping. Because of this pressure by surgeons, hospitals demanded that the ACS help them implement these activities. As a result, Codman organized subcommittees to provide template forms and advice on how to improve laboratory, pathology, and radiology departments.

This help quickly became costly, and the ACS thought a better place for a hospital standards organization was the American Medical Association (AMA) or American Hospital Association (AHA). While both of those groups were eager to cooperate in hospital improvement, the financial burden caused them to refuse assumption of the primary responsibility. The ACS was, therefore, stuck with shouldering the cost. In response, the ACS raised money by charging fellows $500, enabling it to transfer $50,000 to the endowment of the Committee on the Standardization of Hospitals. The burden was further lessened in 1916 when the Carnegie Foundation made a $30,000 gift for the standardization program.

Beyond giving help and advice, the next step for the committee was to codify the recommendations into standards. As is the case today with recommendations for quality improvement, three issues needed to be addressed: rigor, transparency, and compulsory compliance.

When starting a new quality program, any gathered information can be used both for positive and negative evaluations of the organization. Because of the threat of bad publicity, large, prestigious hospitals were reluctant to participate in quality reviews. (Recall the original resistance to Dr. Codman's suggestions at Massachusetts General Hospital.) In order to encourage participation, the quality evaluation activities were initially kept confidential.

Further, if organizations are required to participate before they have the opportunity to review their results and improve on them, they might be tempted to manipulate the data

---

[12] It was no accident that Dr. Codman was appointed chair of this committee. He had met Dr. Edward Martin in England in 1910 while riding back to London from a visit to a tuberculosis sanitarium. During that trip, Codman explained his End Results method, which impressed Martin. See: Roberts, J. S., Coale, J. G., & Redman, R. R. (1987). A history of the Joint Commission on Accreditation of Hospitals. *JAMA, 258*(7), 936–940.

[13] Report of the Committee on Standardization of Hospitals. *Surgery, Gynecology & Obstetrics, 18*, 7.

to avoid embarrassment. This concern led to making participation in the initial program voluntary.

By today's standards, a quality program that is not rigorous, transparent, and mandatory would seem to be suspect. However, many successful current programs began without these features and became more effective as greater information was available and participation grew. For example, the Physician Quality Review Initiative[14] started as a (relatively) simple, voluntary, and confidential reporting system for doctors who cared for Medicare patients. Once information was available, the reporting and standards became more extensive and complex, penalties were imposed for nonreporting or not achieving certain standards, and physician information became available on the government website: https://www.medicare .gov/physiciancompare.

Since no uniform criteria were then extant, the ACS decided that its first task was to write a set of minimum standards that applied to all aspects of hospital care, not just surgery. Once these standards were widely met, they could be expanded in breadth and complexity. (Please see Exhibit 9.3 for a copy of the original standards adopted by the ACS Board of Regents on December 20, 1919.)

As Roberts et al.[15] noted:

> With the adoption of the Minimum Standard, the accreditation process that continues today was set in motion. The following steps are included in this process: the development of reasonable standards that every organization should be expected to meet and that the health professions agree will have a positive effect on improving the quality of patient care; the voluntary request for survey and approval by a health care organization; the survey of the organization by professionals who assess compliance with the standards and provide consultation to support achievement of greater levels of compliance; and the subsequent efforts of organizations to use the standards and survey results to improve patient care.

Initially, only 89 of the 692 hospitals that had been surveyed met the standards; but as the desire to improve quality grew, by 1950, 3,290 hospitals (more than half of the hospitals in the United States) had been accredited.

While the ACS was critical to the success of accreditation, it is important to understand societal pressures at the turn of the 20th century that provided impetus for quality improvement. Recall the factors cited in the Development of Employer-Sponsored Health Insurance section of Chapter 6, "Payers," that encouraged formation of employer-sponsored coverage in the early 20th century. Remember also that the period was the era of medical education reform and public protection laws, like the Pure Food and Drugs Act of 1906. In short, "[h]ospital standardization became a watchword for American surgeons

---

[14]The program became the Physician Quality Reporting System (retrieved from https://www.cms.gov/Medicare/ Quality-Initiatives-Patient-Assessment-Instruments/PQRS/index.html) and was phased out at the end of 2016 when it was replaced by new methodologies mandated by the Medicare Access and CHIP Reauthorization Act of 2015 (MACRA). Retrieved from https://www.cms.gov/medicare/quality-initiatives-patient-assessment-instruments/value-based-programs/macra-mips-and-apms/macra-mips-and-apms.html More will be said about this newer program later in this chapter.

[15]Roberts, et al. (1987), A history of the Joint Commission on Accreditation of Hospitals. op. cit.

EXHIBIT 9.3. Original ACS 1919 Standards

The Minimum Standard

1. That physicians and surgeons privileged to practice in the hospital be organized as a definite group or staff. Such organization has nothing to do with the question as to whether the hospital is "open" or "closed," nor need it affect the various existing types of staff organization. The word STAFF is here defined as the group of doctors who practice in the hospital inclusive of all groups such as the "regular staff," "the visiting staff," and the associate staff."

2. That membership upon the staff be restricted to physicians and surgeons who are (a) full graduates of medicine: in good standing and legally licensed to practice in their respective states or provinces; (b) competent in their respective fields and (c) worthy in character and in matters of professional ethics; that in this latter connection the practice of the division of fees, under any guise whatever, be prohibited.

3. That the staff initiate and, with the approval of the governing board of the hospital, adopt rules, regulations, and policies governing the professional work of the hospital; that these rules, regulations, and policies specifically provide:

   (a) That staff meetings be held at least once each month. (In large hospitals the departments may choose to meet separately.)

   (b) That the staff review and analyze at regular intervals their clinical experience in the various departments of the hospital, such as medicine, surgery, obstetrics, and the other specialties; the clinical records of patients, free and pay, to be the basis for such review and analyses.

4. That accurate and complete records be written for all patients and filed in an accessible manner in the hospital—a complete case record being one which includes identification data; complaint; personal and family history; history of present illness; physical examination; special examinations, such as consultations, clinical laboratory, X-ray and other examinations; provisional or working diagnosis; medical or surgical treatment; gross and micro-scopical pathological findings; progress notes; final diagnosis; condition on discharge; follow-up and, in case of death, autopsy findings.

5. That diagnostic and therapeutic facilities under competent supervision be available for the study, diagnosis, and treatment of patients, these to include, at least (a) a clinical laboratory providing chemical, bacteriological, serological, and pathological services; (b) an X-ray department providing radiographic and fluoroscopic services.

Source: American College of Surgeons: The 1919 "Minimum Standard" document. Retrieved July 14, 2018, from https://www.facs.org/about-acs/archives/pasthighlights/minimumhighlight

during the Progressive Era, and Codman's reforms briefly occupied a niche within the movement."[16]

---

[16]Crenner, C. (2001). Organizational reform and professional dissent in the careers of Richard Cabot and Ernest Amory Codman, 1900–1920. *Journal of the History of Medicine and Allied Sciences, 56*(3), 211–237. In addition to his role with the Standards Committee, in 1920 Codman founded the National Registry of Bone Sarcoma, the first national disease registry According to the National Cancer Registrar's Association, the first *hospital* registry was established at Yale–New Haven Hospital in New Haven, CT, in 1926, and the first central registry was established in Connecticut in 1935. Retrieved from http://www.ncra-usa.org/About/History

1950–1970s

The ACS continued to run the hospital accreditation program until 1950 when three factors forced it to reevaluate its lone role: hospital expansion after World War II, increasing complexity of medical practice, and, as a result of those two factors, growing costs. As a result of those events, on December 15, 1951,[17] the ACS joined with the American College of Physicians, the AHA, the AMA, and the Canadian Medical Association[18] to form the Joint Commission on Accreditation of Hospitals (JCAH) as an independent, nonprofit organization. (Several years earlier, in 1945, the American Osteopathic Association established its own quality review process for osteopathic hospitals.)

The next major forces shaping quality initiatives came from two sources: the conceptual advances pioneered by University of Michigan Professor Avedis Donabedian and the passage of Medicare and Medicaid.

Donabedian divided quality assessments into outcome, structure, and process measures—a framework that is still used. His classic explanation of these features is worth reading in its original text:[19]

> Many advantages are gained by using outcome as the criterion of quality in medical care. The validity of outcome as a dimension of quality is seldom questioned ... outcomes tend to be fairly concrete and, as such, seemingly amenable to more precise measurement...
>
> Another approach to assessment is to examine the process of care itself rather than its outcomes. This is justified by the assumption that one is interested not in the power of medical technology to achieve results, but in whether what is now known to be "good" medical care has been applied ... The estimates of quality that one obtains are less stable and less final than those that derive from the measurement of outcomes. They may, however, more relevant to the question at hand: whether medicine is properly practiced...
>
> A third approach to assessment is to study not the process of itself, but the settings in which it takes place and the instrumentalities of which it is the product. This may be roughly designated as the assessment of structure, although it may include administrative and related processes that support and direct the provision of care. It is concerned with such things as the adequacy of facilities and equipment; the qualifications of medical staff and their organization; the administrative structure and operations of programs and institutions providing care; fiscal organization and the like. The assumption is made that given the proper settings and instrumentalities, good medical care will follow. This approach offers the advantage of dealing, at least in part, with fairly concrete and accessible information.

---

[17]The ACS formally turned over authority JCAH on December 6, 1952.

[18]In 1958, Canadian Council on Hospital Accreditation was incorporated, and, by 1959, it became independent of the JCAH. The Canadian Hospital Association (now HealthCareCAN), the Canadian Medical Association, the Royal College of Physicians and Surgeons, and l'Association des Médecins de Langue Française du Canada, established the Canadian Commission on Hospital Accreditation. The commission's purpose is to create a Canadian program for hospital accreditation. The American Dental Association joined the JCAH as an additional corporate member in 1978.

[19]Donabedian, A. (1966). Evaluating the quality of medical care. *The Milbank Memorial Fund Quarterly, 44*(3). Part 2: Health Services Research I. A Series of Papers Commissioned by the Health Services Research Study Section of the United States Public Health Service. Discussed at a Conference Held in Chicago (October 15–16, 1965), 166–206.

It has the major limitation that the relationship between structure and process or structure and outcome, is often not well established.

In addition to publication of Donabedian's classic paper, in 1965 Titles XVIII and XIX of the Social Security Laws (Medicare and Medicaid) were signed into law and provided a further impetus to quality review. With their passage, the federal government needed some guarantee that the care it was funding met acceptable quality standards. Further, the Medicare law specified that:

> Nothing in this title shall be construed to authorize any Federal officer or employee to exercise any supervision or control over the practice of medicine or the manner in which medical services are provided, or over the selection, tenure, or compensation of any officer or employee of any institution, agency, or person providing health services; or to exercise any supervision or control over the administration or operation of any such institution, agency, or person.[20]

The government, therefore, needed independent, nonfederal bodies to accredit hospitals (and other organizations) and monitor their quality of care; it turned to the JCAH, the American Osteopathic Association hospital accreditation,[21] and State Survey Agencies[22] for these tasks. (The term for this delegation of authority for quality review is "deemed status.") Subsequently the Centers for Medicare and Medicaid Services (CMS) set certain quality requirements for hospitals called Conditions for Coverage (CfCs) and Conditions of Participations (CoPs).[23] In 2008, CMS granted Det Norske Veritas Healthcare, Inc. (now called the DNVHC NIAHO accreditation program)[24] deemed status. In addition to reviewing hospitals, the JCAH launched accreditation programs for long-term care facilities (1966); organizations serving developmentally disabled persons (1969); psychiatric facilities, substance abuse, and community mental health programs (1970); ambulatory healthcare programs (1975); and hospices (1983). Subsequently, private sector payers also adopted accreditation requirements for these types of facilities. Thus, with payment linked to accreditation,[25] quality-related activities were effectively made mandatory.

In August 1966 (1 month after Medicare and Medicaid became operational), the JCAH board decided to change its philosophy of review. Instead of evaluations based on meeting

---

[20]Prohibition against any federal interference. Sec. 1801. [42 U.S.C. 1395]. Retrieved July 12, 2018, from https://www.ssa.gov/OP_Home/ssact/title18/1801.htm

[21]Now called the Health Facilities Accreditation Program (HFAP), it accredits more than 200 acute-care hospitals (not only osteopathic facilities) and 200 other entities including ambulatory surgical centers, ambulatory care/office-based surgery, behavioral/mental health facilities, and clinical laboratories. Retrieved July 12, 2018, from www.hfap.org

[22]For a list of State Survey Agencies authorized to accredit healthcare organizations, see: https://www.cms.gov/Medicare/Provider-Enrollment-and-Certification/SurveyCertificationGenInfo/downloads/state_agency_contacts.pdf (Current as of January, 2017). Retrieved July 12, 2018.

[23]CMS.gov: Conditions for Coverage (CfCs) & Conditions of Participations (CoPs) Retrieved July 12, 2018, from http://www.cms.gov/Regulations-and-Guidance/Legislation/CFCsAndCoPs/index.html?redirect=/CFCsAndCoPs/Accessed

[24]See: www.dnvglhealthcare.com *What distinguishes this Oslo-based company's reviews is that its criteria are derived from ISO 9001 standards.* Retrieved July 12, 2018.

[25]Accreditation is based on a review of the quality activities of the entire organization. A separate review, called "certification," may be conducted for a *program* within the organization. For example, an accredited hospital may also earn certification for such disease management programs as diabetes, asthma, stroke, heart failure, and cancer.

basic criteria, institutions had to show their efforts to attain optimal achievable standards. This change came about for two reasons. First, it was a natural evolution of the accreditation process. From the beginning of the ACS program, the plan was to impose greater rigor on the process when hospitals had, for the most part, achieved compliance with the basics. That time had come. The second reason was strategic. Since Medicare and Medicaid allowed accreditation by State Survey Agencies and other entities, many of those organizations copied JCAH criteria and were challenging the latter's industry leadership.[26] For example, in 1966, the Commission on Accreditation of Rehabilitation Facilities (CARF) was created.

Groups that are today called Quality Improvement Organizations (QIOs) also had their origins with the passage of the Medicare and Medicaid laws in 1965. As mentioned above, the federal government was concerned with the quality of care beneficiaries would receive and the appropriateness of the utilization of such care under those programs. Therefore, in addition to the hospital accreditation requirement, the law created the independent National Medical Review Committee, whose function was "to study the utilization of hospital and other medical care and services for which payment may be made under this title with a view to recommending any changes which may seem desirable in the way in which such care and services are utilized or in the administration of the programs."[27]

The committee had to report annually to the Secretary of Health, Education and Welfare (now HHS), who was required to send the report promptly to Congress.

Since this part of the law was never effectively implemented, Congress passed provisions in the Social Security Amendments of 1972 (Public Law 92–603) that strengthened the oversight. Four of these quality provisions are of note:

(1) Establishment of a peer review system through the use of organizations representing a substantial number of practicing physicians in local areas to be called Professional Standards Review' Organizations (PSRO's) (these organizations would assume responsibility for comprehensive and ongoing review of services provided under Medicare and Medicaid) [replacing the National Medical Review Committee];

(2) establishment of an Office of Inspector General for Health Administration within the Department of Health, Education, and Welfare [HEW] having the responsibility to review and audit Medicare and other health programs on a continuing and comprehensive basis and the authority to suspend any regulation, practice, or procedure employed in the administration of such programs if he determines that the suspension will promote efficiency and economy of administration or that the regulation, practice, or procedure involved is contrary to or does not carry out the objectives and purposes of applicable provisions of law;

(3) requirement that the Secretary of HEW make reports of a provider's significant deficiencies (such as staffing, fire, safety, and sanitation) a matter of public record readily available at Social Security offices if, after a reasonable lapse of time (not to exceed 90 days), such deficiencies are not corrected;

---

[26]Porterfield, J. P. (1972). From the director's office. *Bulletin of the Joint Commission on Accreditation of Hospitals*, 4, 1–2.

[27]Title XVIII (Medicare) of the Social Security Act. Section 1868 (c).

(4) requirement that the Secretary of HEW develop and employ proficiency examinations to determine whether health care personnel, not otherwise meeting specific formal criteria included in Medicare regulations, have sufficient professional competence to be considered qualified personnel for Medicare purposes.[28]

The PSROs were tasked with determining whether the care was appropriate, whether inpatient care could have been effectively delivered at other sites, and whether the quality of services met "professionally recognized standards of health care ... If a PSRO determines that a physician or other supplier of health care goods or services is guilty of abuse against the Medicare or Medicaid programs, it is required to report this to the Centers for Medicare & Medicaid Services (CMS) for the imposition of whatever sanctions are appropriate."[29]

Despite the terms of the new law, PSROs did not succeed in their intended purpose. For example, according to Ginsburg: "PSRO Medicare review generates a small net savings to the federal government while producing a net loss to society as a whole because some of the savings to the government are costs that have been transferred to private patients."[30] He said that data was inadequate to evaluate PSROs' activities on hospital lengths of stay or what effect it had on the Medicaid program.

The reasons for PSRO failure are instructive when one considers developing quality improvement programs today. According to Hart:

> Several interrelated factors have impeded implementation of the PSRO program: deficiencies in HEW's program administration; physician opposition [particularly by the AMA and state medical societies]; and internal PSRO problems in organizing, developing program plans, converting to conditional states, developing working relationships with State Medicaid and Maternal and Child Health agencies, obtaining support from some hospitals, developing long-term care facility review programs, and coordinating with Health Systems Agencies. HEW failed to promptly effectively organize and adequately Staff the PSRO program and obtain or direct cohesive, vigorous efforts among participating branch agencies.[31]

Further, since the job of the PSRO was only to "report and recommend," there was no linkage between findings and the ability to improve care.

---

[28] Ball, R. M. (1973, March). Social Security amendments of 1972: Summary and legislative history. *Social Security Bulletin*. 1973. pages 3–25. Retrieved July 12, 2018, from https://www.ssa.gov/policy/docs/ssb/v36n3/v36n3p3.pdf

[29] Social Security Administration. Program Operations Manual System: HI 00208.080 Role of Professional Standards Review Organizations (PSRO's). Retrieved July 12, 2018, from https://secure.ssa.gov/poms.nsf/lnx/0600208080

[30] Statement of Paul B. Ginsburg, Chief, Income Security and Health Unit, Congressional Budget Office (1981, March 24). Before the Subcommittee on Oversight and the Subcommittee on Health Committee on Ways and Means United States House of Representatives. Retrieved July 12, 2018, from https://www.cbo.gov/sites/default/files/97th-congress-1981-1982/reports/81doc16.pdf

[31] Hart, G. J. (2018, July 12). Implementation of the Professional Standards Review Organization Program. Testimony before the House Committee on Ways and Means: Oversight Subcommittee. April 4, 1977. Retrieved July 12, 2018, from http://www.gao.gov/assets/100/98419.pdf

Because of these failures, Congress included language in the Tax Equity and Fiscal Responsibility Act of 1982 (TEFRA)[32] to replace the PSRO program with utilization and quality control peer review organizations, called Peer Review Organizations (PROs). These organizations were independent bodies with which HEW contracted to assess utilization and quality of care for the Medicare program. These functions became even more important since TEFRA also mandated implementation of a prospective payment system (Diagnosis Related Groups [DRG]s) that gave hospitals financial incentives to admit healthier patients, skimp on inpatient care, and reduce lengths of stay. (Recall the section on hospital payment mechanisms in Chapter 4, "Hospitals and Healthcare Systems.") In carrying out its mandate, PROs were empowered to deny payment to providers that did not comply with standards. This authority gave PROs more leverage than PSROs had to carry out its directives.

What followed the enabling of PROs was a series of scope of work cycles that still exist today.

Each cycle had its own themes to advance implementation of quality improvement.[33] For example, the first cycle (1984–1986) focused on retrospective case reviews while the second cycle (1986–1989) directed more attention to analyzing and improving processes of care. In 1990, the Institute of Medicine (IOM) issued a report evaluating PROs and offered the following critique:

Medicare Utilization and Quality Review Peer Review Organizations (PROs) constitute a potentially valuable infrastructure for quality assurance. Nevertheless, it is the perception of the committee that Medicare PROs

- give primary attention to utilization rather than quality,

- focus on outliers rather than the average provider,

- concentrate on inpatient care,

- impose excessive burdens on providers,

- do not use positive incentives to alter performance,

- are perceived as adversarial and punitive,

- use a sanctioning process that is largely ineffective,

- are rendered relatively inflexible by program funding arrangements,

- use methods that are redundant with other public and internal quality assurance programs, and

- have not been evaluated with respect to their effect on quality.[34]

As a result of this report, major changes were made to PRO activities in the third cycle (1989–1993), under the name Health Care Quality Improvement Initiative (HCQII).

---

[32]Peer Review Improvement Act of 1982 (Title I, Subtitle C of the Tax Equity and Fiscal Responsibility Act of 1982) (Public Law 97-248).

[33]Bhatia, A. J., Blackstock, S., Nelson, R., & Ng, T. S. (2000). Evolution of quality review programs for Medicare: Quality assurance to quality improvement. *Health Care Financing Review, 22*(1), 69–74.

[34]Lohr, K. N. (Ed.). (1990). *Medicare: A strategy for quality assurance: Volume I. Committee to design a strategy for quality review and assurance in Medicare Division of Health Care Services* (p. 3). Washington, DC: Institute of Medicine. National Academy Press.

Although the HCQII built on previous efforts to move the quality focus from individual clinical errors to studying systemic patterns of care and their outcomes, two features advanced this capability. First, prior reviews had been conducted using ad hoc reviewer opinions about care. HCQII implemented "explicit, more nationally uniform criteria to examine patterns of care and patterns of outcomes."[35] Second, using these explicit criteria, PROs developed specific initiatives geared at improving processes of care. For example, the first such program was the Cooperative Cardiovascular Project (CCP), whose purpose was to improve the care for patients with acute myocardial infarction. Its success at improving care[36] encouraged the development of further disease-focused projects, such as for diabetes and other cardiovascular illnesses. The HCQII evolved into the Health Care Quality Improvement Program (HCQIP) program as more attention was paid to continuous quality improvement methods.

Since healthcare organizations were becoming more integrated and more care was being delivered in out-of-hospital settings, there was a need to enlarge the purview of PROs to nursing homes, home health agencies, and physician offices. Further, improvement in information systems and databases were making systemic evaluations more feasible. As a result of such changes, during the sixth Scope of Work (1989–2002), PROs were renamed Quality Improvement Organizations. The QIOs continued state-specific programs but also expanded their activities to the national stage using partnerships with such organizations as the Joint Commission and the AHA. These national programs focused on heart attacks, heart failure, breast cancer, stroke, diabetes, and pneumonia.

In 2011, the QIO activities were aligned with the National Quality Strategy (NQS) established by the Patient Protection and Affordable Care Act (ACA). Further, the Trade Adjustment Assistance Extension Act of 2011 (Section 261) gave the CMS contracting authority to restructure the QIO program and consolidate contracts with state-by-state organizations into regional ones. As a result, in 2014 the QIO functions were split into two programs. The first is the Beneficiary and Family Centered Care-Quality Improvement Organizations (BFCC-QIOs).

> BFCC-QIOs address all beneficiary concerns and appeals, quality of care reviews, cases of suspected "patient dumping" covered by the Emergency Medical Treatment and Labor Act (EMTALA), and other types of case review. The two new BFCC-QIOs, Livanta and KEPRO,[37] serve all 50 states and three territories, which are grouped into the five regions.

The second program is carried out nationally by 14 firms, which are called Quality Innovation Network-Quality Improvement Organizations (QIN-QIOs); they perform the traditional quality-specific work of the QIOs: "The work of QIN-QIOs is grounded in foundational principles that align with the goals of the CMS Quality Strategy: (a) eliminating disparities; (b) strengthening infrastructure and data systems; (c) enabling local

---

[35] Jencks, S. F., & Wilensky, G. R. (1992). The health care quality improvement initiative: A new approach to quality assurance in Medicare. *JAMA*, 268(7), 900–903.

[36] Marciniak, T. A., Ellerbeck, E. F., Radford, M. J., Kresowik, T. F., Gold, J. A., Krumholz, H. M.... Vogel, R. A. (1998). Improving the quality of care for Medicare patients with acute myocardial infarction: Results from the Cooperative Cardiovascular Project. *JAMA*, 279, (17), 1351–1357.

[37] Livanta: http://www.livanta.com; Kepro: https://www.kepro.com. Both retrieved July 12, 2018.

innovation; and (d) fostering learning organizations."[38] The current major goals of the program are: promoting effective prevention and treatment of chronic disease; making care safer and reducing harm caused in the delivery of care; promoting effective communication and coordination of care; and making care more affordable. Each of these goals has specific initiatives. For example, community programs to combat antibiotic resistance and reduce healthcare-acquired illnesses in nursing homes support the safety goal.

The QIO programs will undergo more changes in the future as healthcare priorities change. The current scope of work is due to expire in 2019, and results of current efforts are being reviewed.[39]

1980s and Total Quality Management

The next major change in healthcare quality assessment was a by-product of adoption of continuous quality improvement (often called Total Quality Management [TQM]) in manufacturing in the United States in the 1980s. To fully understand this movement, one must first understand its historical context. In the early 20th century, the process for improving manufactured goods and labor processes largely followed the teachings of Frederick Winslow Taylor (1856–1915), who espoused the principle of scientific management. Taylor believed that "[i]n the past . . . the theory has been that if one could get the right man, methods could be safely left to him . . . In the past, man has been first; in the future, the system must be first."[40] Although Taylor is criticized for a system favoring the manager over the laborer, his intent was for a mutually beneficial relationship:

> The majority . . . believe that the fundamental interests of employés [*sic*] and employers are necessarily antagonistic. Scientific management, on the contrary, has for its very foundation the firm conviction that the true interests of the two are one and the same; that prosperity for the employer cannot exist through a long term of years unless it is accompanied by prosperity for the employé and vice versa; and that it is possible to give the workman what he most wants, high wages, and the employer what he wants, a lower labor cost, for his manufactures.[41]

Improving the system consisted of breaking down a process into component tasks, finding the best way to perform each task, and redesigning the job for maximum efficiency. The human element in performing these jobs would be optimized by rewarding workers to produce their maximum possible output; benchmarks were determined by time-motion studies.

Despite good intentions about shared benefits, managers took to heart Taylor's admonition that "[i]t is only through enforced standardization of methods, *enforced* adoption of the best implements and working conditions, and *enforced* cooperation that this faster work

---

[38] QIO Program: Quality Innovation Network-Quality Improvement Organizations. Retrieved July 12, 2018, from http://qioprogram.org/sites/default/files/resources/documents/QIN-QIO_Fact_Sheet_June2017_508.pdf

[39] See: CMS. Current Work. QIO Program 11th SOW (2014–2016). [The 11th Scope of Work cycle ends July 31, 2019.] Retrieved July 12, 2018, from https://www.cms.gov/Medicare/Quality-Initiatives-Patient-Assessment-Instruments/QualityImprovementOrgs/Current.html

[40] Taylor, F. W. (1919). *The principles of scientific management* (pp. 6–7). New York: Harper & Brothers.

[41] Taylor, F. W., op. cit., p. 10.

can be assured. And the duty of enforcing the adoption of standards and of enforcing this cooperation rests with the *management* alone"[42] (emphases in original).

Further, Taylor's approach to achieving efficiency ingrained into management the concept of *quality assurance*, that is, with the proper task design and worker motivation, the output can be perfected. From these dogmas came the widespread belief that lack of perfection is due to worker laziness or ignorance of the task.

The initial break in this latter view came in 1924, when Walter Shewhart (1891–1967) produced the first control chart, which graphs variations in process outputs over time. Although the technique was developed to monitor the manufacturing of telephone equipment at Western Electric,[43] healthcare examples include documentation of how many wound infections or medication errors occur each month over the course of several years. From the introduction of this chart came additional understanding of process variation. First, any process, whether in manufacturing or delivering a service, has normal, statistically measurable variations in how well it works. Shewhart called these variations "common causes." Common cause variations are the inevitable result of the process design and are due to random chance events. Second, the process may occasionally fall out of statistical control, due to what Shewhart called "special causes." These causes deserve attention because something happened that made the system deviate from the way it was intended to function. For example, a piece of equipment may be reaching the end of its useful life and produce defective products or a new worker was not trained properly on a task.

Understanding these concepts leads to several important management implications. First, unlike Taylor, Shewhart recognized that perfection is not possible; managers can, at best, design a process to keep the quality of its output within statistical variation control. In other words, *quality assurance* must be replaced by *continuous quality assessment*. Second, since common causes are a function of the process design, workers should not be blamed for errors when variation is under statistical control. Workers *do* need to be assessed, however, when special causes occur. Finally, the only way to improve the process is by redesigning the way the work gets done—not by exhorting workers to do better in order to achieve perfection.

The latter concept led to another of Shewhart's innovations—the process of continuous improvement, called the Shewhart Cycle. In this process, a plan is first developed to address the problem. Next, the plan is implemented. The results of implementation are assessed once enough data is available. The successful parts of the plan are then set in place. Further improvements restart the process. The method is called Plan-Do-Check-Act or just PDCA.[44]

---

[42]Taylor, F. W., op. cit., p. 83.

[43]The successor to the Western Electric facility was Bell Labs, an institution responsible for such inventions as microwave appliances and the silicon chip. For an excellent source of the accomplishments of this institution, see: Gertner, J. G. (2012). *The idea factory. Bell Labs and the great age of American innovation.* New York: Penguin.

[44]More recently, some authors refer to the process as Plan-Do-Study-Act, or PDSA. Dr. Paul Batalden augmented the process in the 1980s when he was in charge of quality improvement at HCA (then called the Hospital Corporation of America). He used the acronym FOCUS-PDCA: Find a process to improve; Organize to improve the process; Clarify current knowledge of the process; Understand the source of process variation; and Select the process improvement. Then apply PDCA processes.

The programs of quality control that Shewhart started were continued by his followers, who included W. Edwards Deming (1900–1993) and Joseph M. Juran (1904–2008). Their contributions to quality in manufacturing were first appreciated in Japan after World War II when industry needed to be physically and managerially rebuilt. As Gitlow[45] pointed out:

> W.E. Deming, J. Juran, and others went to Japan after World War II and taught the Japanese much about quality. Deming taught the Japanese about the Shewhart cycle, the concept of special and common causes of variation, the realization that statistics could be used on the shop floor, and an appreciation of a system. Juran taught the Japanese management principles and practices . . . From these teachings and more, the Japanese developed their own schools of thought on quality.

The result was production of globally competitive, high-quality products, of which Toyota autos are perhaps the best-known example.

By the 1980s, as Japanese manufactured goods (particularly autos and electronics) began competing with American products on both cost and quality, U.S. companies decided to embrace the quality control methods and re-import them. One of the first American companies to totally adopt a culture of quality was Motorola,[46] which adopted these activities not only in manufacturing but also in such business processes as billing, collections, and inventory management. In 1986, Motorola started its well-known quality improvement program known as "Six Sigma." The term refers to performance that reduces defects to 6 standard deviations from the norm, or 3.4 defects per million opportunities for error.

In recognition of the importance of quality improvement for U.S. businesses, Congress established an award to encourage companies to engage in this practice. Named the Baldrige Award[47] (in memory of former commerce secretary and quality proponent Malcolm Baldrige), it first bestowed prizes in 1988, but only to manufacturing firms. Subsequently, service companies, small businesses, educational institutions, nonprofits, and healthcare organizations were added as separate categories.[48]

As might be inferred from the above history, the research on the effectiveness of quality improvement processes for manufacturing was well established by the time these methods were reintroduced into the United States. However, only in the late 1980s and early 1990s were the first studies conducted that examined the application of these principles to the

---

[45] Gitlow, H. S. (1994). A comparison of Japanese total quality control and Deming's theory of management. *The American Statistician, 48*(3), 197–203.

[46] Shalowitz, J. (1995). Total quality management at Motorola: A successful blueprint for manufacturing and service organizations. *The Journal of Health Administration Education, 13,* 15–23.

[47] ASQ. *Malcolm Baldrige National Quality Award.* Retrieved July 12, 2018, from http://asq.org/learn-about-quality/malcolm-baldrige-award/overview/overview.html

[48] It wasn't until 2002 that the first Baldrige award was given to a healthcare organization (SSM Health Care).

delivery of health services. The results of those investigations not only demonstrated proof of concept for the same quality improvement tools that worked in manufacturing but also highlighted the importance of organizational factors in this effort. Typical of such findings at that time were studies such as one looking at intensive care unit performance: "managerial process variables related to the quality of caregiver interaction [culture, leadership, communication, coordination and problem-solving/conflict management] is the strongest correlate of unit efficiency, evaluated technical quality of care, the ability to meet family member needs, and nursing turnover."[49] The authors concluded that management *does* make a difference in quality performance.

In the fall of 1987, 21 healthcare organizations agreed to participate in an 8-month study of the applicability of industrial quality improvement methods in healthcare, called the National Demonstration Project (NDP) in Quality Improvement in Health Care. Twenty-one other companies[50] that had successfully implemented quality improvement agreed to advise and support these participants. When the first reports were presented in June 1988, many of the healthcare organizations showed marked improvement in their targeted quality projects.

As Godfrey noted:

> One of the first striking findings for many of the health-care organizations was the critical importance of looking at care as a process. Health care traditionally had been very doctor-focused. The physician was responsible for the clinical outcome. Health-care organizations soon discovered how complex their processes were; the large number of people involved; the importance of correct, timely and available information; and the many, unmanaged hand-offs in each process.[51]

Because of its success, the NDP was extended 3 more years. In 1991, as a direct outgrowth of the NDP, the nonprofit Institute for Health Improvement (IHI) was founded, with Donald Berwick, MD, MPP, as its first chief executive officer.[52] According to the IHI:

> In our first decade, we focused on the identification and subsequent spread of best practices. This work reduced defects and errors in microsystems such as the emergency department or the intensive care unit.
>
> In our second decade, we established a defining focus on innovation, R&D [research and development], and the bold creation of new solutions to old problems. We reinvented multidimensional systems of care and began transforming entire systems. This work manifested in

---

[49] Shortell, S. M., Zimmerman, J. E., Rousseau, D. M., Gillies, R. R., Wagner, D. P., Draper, E. ... Duffy, J. (1994, May). The performance of intensive care units: Does good management make a difference? *Medical Care, 32*, 508–525.

[50] Companies included AT&T, Corning, Ford, Hewlett-Packard, IBM, and Xerox.

[51] Godfrey, A. B. (1996, September). Quality Health Care. *Quality Digest.* Retrieved July 12, 2018, from https://www.qualitydigest.com/sep96/health.html

[52] For a classic article on quality improvement in healthcare that is still relevant, see: Berwick, D. M. (1989). Continuous improvement as an ideal in health care. *New England Journal of Medicine, 320*, 53–56.

the renowned 100,000 Lives Campaign[53] and 5 Million Lives Campaign,[54] spreading best practice changes to thousands of US hospitals and creating a vibrant worldwide improvement community.

As we entered our third decade, we recognized a new need for health care as a complete social, geopolitical enterprise. To accelerate the path to the health and care we need, IHI created the Triple Aim, a framework for optimizing health system performance by simultaneously focusing on the health of a population, the experience of care for individuals within that population, and the per capita cost of providing that care.[55]

In May 2017, the IHI and another healthcare quality organization, the National Patient Safety Foundation (NPSF),[56] began working together.

One other trend of note influenced healthcare quality improvement efforts at this time—hospital/health system consolidation.[57] Quality improvement activities expanded to cover not only larger but also more diverse healthcare entities.

As a result of all these activities, accreditation needed to change as well. In 1987, the Joint Commission on Accreditation of Hospitals changed its name to the Joint Commission on Accreditation of Healthcare Organizations (JCAHO) to reflect its larger role in accreditation of diverse types of healthcare units.[58] In that same year, the JCAHO also issued its next generation of accreditation methods: "The Agenda for Change." Building on previous standards, this initiative added two new principles: First, the organization being accredited had to show it had in-place processes for continuous quality improvement; no longer were attainment of basic or optimal achievable standards sufficient for accreditation. Second, in view of research findings about the importance of management and governance to quality improvement, those functions were now held responsible for organization-wide quality results and had to demonstrate their involvement.

While these methods of quality improvement and their assessment were evolving, four other concerns became apparent: the method of analysis of medical practice, the interpretation of results, benchmarking, and efficiency. The first difficulty concerned the way healthcare professionals thought about medical problems. In 1964, Dr. Alvan R. Feinstein published a series of articles in *Annals of Internal Medicine*, each title leading with the phrase: "Scientific Methodology in Clinical Medicine." The subjects of these articles

---

[53] Institute for Health Improvement. *Overview of the 100,000 Lives Campaign*. Retrieved July 12, 2018, from https://www.ihi.org/Engage/Initiatives/Completed/5MillionLivesCampaign/Documents/Overview of the 100K Campaign.pdf This initiative and the following one were a result of efforts started with the publication of *To Err Is Human* in 1999 (see text further on).

[54] Institute for Health Improvement: Protecting 5 Million Lives from Harm. Overview. Retrieved July 12, 2018, from http://www.ihi.org/Engage/Initiatives/Completed/5MillionLivesCampaign/Pages/default.aspx

[55] Institute for Healthcare Improvement. *History*. Retrieved July 12, 2018, from http://www.ihi.org/about/pages/history.aspx

[56] National Patient Safety Foundation. *History and timeline*. Retrieved July 12, 2018, from http://www.npsf.org/?page=historyandtimeline

[57] See Chapter 4, "Hospitals," for further details as well as: Dor, A., & Friedman, B. (1994). Mergers of not-for-profit hospitals in the 1980s: Who were the most likely targets? *Review of Industrial Organization, 9*(4), 393–407.

[58] On January 7, 2007, JCAHO changed its name to the Joint Commission.

were the basis of his influential book, *Clinical Judgment*.[59] Feinstein explained that each act of patient care had an experimental structure: A sick patient was treated and an outcome was observed. "The 'experiments' needed substantial scientific improvement, however, in quality of basic data, taxonomic classification of phenomena, and specifications of clinical reasoning."[60] (Recall similar needs mentioned in Chapter 8, "Information Technology.")

Second, in addition to the requirement to apply scientific methodology to clinical decision making, the *way* results were interpreted also came under scrutiny. For example, in their classic paper "Judgment under Uncertainty,"[61] Tversky and Kahneman point to the availability bias: "There are situations in which people assess the frequency of a class or the probability of an event by the ease with which instances or occurrences can be brought to mind. For example, one may assess the risk of a heart attack among middle-age people by recalling such occurrences among one's acquaintances."

In other words, physicians can make clinical judgment errors based on their past experiences as well as the last similar case they encountered.

The third major problem concerned benchmarking. Organizations wanted to know: Who is doing the best job now? *and* What is the best achievable result? But, as pointed out later in this chapter, benchmarks change. To illustrate this issue, as late as the 1970s, many physicians still believed that high blood pressure (hypertension) was a normal consequence of aging; except in the most extreme cases, any attempt to lower it in the elderly would result in serious harm. It was only in 1977 that, based on scientific evidence, the medical community started to recommend treatment of hypertension to certain levels.[62] These recommendations have continued to evolve to the present day.[63]

Finally, organizations came to realize that quality was not *only* about achieving "best" results but *also* accomplishing goals while using the minimum resources necessary. In addition, tasks should be accomplished as quickly as possible. In other words, *efficiency* became part of the quality improvement equation. Since healthcare resources (including funding) have usually been plentiful in the United States, this part of the equation had not received as much attention. However, other countries with national healthcare systems face budgetary pressures and scrutinize costs more closely. The person who had the earliest and most profound influence in this regard was Dr. Archibald ("Archie") Leman Cochrane (1909–1988), who was concerned with both effectiveness and efficiency—particularly of the British National Health System. In respect to evidence-based effectiveness, he wrote: "Two of the most striking changes in word usage in the last twenty years are the upgrading

[59] Feinstein A. R. (1967). *Clinical judgment*. Baltimore: Williams and Wilkins.

[60] Feinstein, A. R. (1994). Clinical judgment revisited: The distraction of quantitative models. *Annals of Internal Medicine*, *120*, 799–805.

[61] Tversky, A., & Kahneman, D. (1974). Judgment under uncertainty: heuristics and biases. *Science*, New Series, *185*(4157), 1124–1131.

[62] Report of the Joint National Committee on detection, evaluation, and treatment of high blood pressure. A cooperative study. *JAMA*, *237*, 255–261.

[63] Whelton, P. K., & Carey, R. M. (2017, November 20). The 2017 clinical practice guideline for high blood pressure. *JAMA*, *318*(21), 2073–2074. Retrieved July 12, 2018, from https://jamanetwork.com/journals/jama/fullarticle/ 2664351?utm_source=silverchair&utm_medium=email&utm_campaign=article_alert-jama&utm_content=olf&utm_ term=112017

of 'opinion' in comparison with other types of evidence, and the downgrading of the word 'experiment.'" Concerning efficiency, he noted: "There is a strong suggestion that the increase in input since the start of the NHS has not been matched by any marked increase in output in the 'cure' section."[64] Cochrane called for more evidence-based medical practice, with recommendations based on randomized clinical trials. (Please see Chapter 3, "Introduction to Managerial Epidemiology.") To honor his pioneering work, the Cochrane Collaboration was formed in 1993 as a global source of evidence-based practice recommendations.[65]

In the late 1970s, private-sector, payer-focused quality assessment activities started as the result of the emergence of managed care plans. Recall that managed care was a solution that health plans offered employers to lower their insurance costs. When these plans started to grow, employers and the government became concerned that the financial incentives might affect the quality of care. In response to this fear, in 1979 the federal Office for Health Maintenance Organizations (HMOs) encouraged formation of what was to become the National Committee for Quality Assurance (NCQA).[66] The NCQA was cosponsored by the principal managed care trade associations: the American Managed Care and Review Association (AMCRA) and the Group Health Association of America (GHAA).[67] As Iglehart[68] noted:

> Initially, the NCQA made little headway in developing a rigorous quality-review system. Managed—care plans were reluctant to participate, since their competitors in fee-for-service medicine faced no similar challenge. But as enrollment grew and pressure to ensure quality increased, executives and medical directors of health maintenance organizations (HMOs) conceded in the late 1980s, often grudgingly, that the NCQA had to become an independent body if it was ever to be credible.

Initial problem-focused reviews and corrective action processes were conducted using methods that Kaiser-Permanente employed in its California plans.[69] Bowing to the need for sustainable financial support as well as the growing pressure for an independent review

---

[64]Cochrane, A. L. (1972). *Effectiveness and efficiency. Random reflections on health services* (pp. 20, 67). Abington, Berkshire: Burgess & Son, Ltd. Printed for the Nuffield Provincial Hospitals Trust.

[65]*Cochrane*, AL. Retrieved from www.cochrane.org

[66]The HMO Act of 1973 (PL93-222) required employers who provided health insurance to their employees to offer a federally qualified HMO when one was available in their area. In addition to this mandate, federally qualified plans also got development grants. Since the federal government was encouraging (and funding) these new payment mechanisms, it had an interest in making sure their quality was appropriate. Recall an analogous situation with respect to hospital care after the Medicare and Medicaid laws were passed in 1965.

[67]AMCRA and GHAA merged in 1995 to become the American Association of Health Plans (AAHP). In 2003, AAHP merged with the Health Insurance Association of America (HIAA) to become the America's Health Insurance Plans (AHIP), which represents many of the major health insurance companies in the United States.

[68]Iglehart, J. K. (1996). The National Committee for quality assurance. *The New England Journal of Medicine, 335*, 995–999.

[69]McPartland, G. (2012, March 21). Birth of the National Committee for Quality Assurance. Retrieved July 12, 2018, from http://kaiserpermanentehistory.org/latest/birth-of-the-national-committee-for-quality-assurance

organization, in 1990 the NCQA was able to secure a $308,000 grant from the Robert Wood Johnson Foundation and reorganized as a private, 501(c)(3) (not-for-profit) organization. Its sponsorship changed to include large employers (as purchasers of care), provider organizations, and consumer groups. The NCQA subsequently expanded its purview from HMOs to other types of managed care plans,[70] as well as other organizations, such as patient-centered medical homes (PCMHs).

With the reorganization, the NCQA changed its health plan evaluation to include two types of assessments. The first type of evaluation determined whether or not a plan's *operational characteristics* warranted accreditation; a plan can be rated: Excellent, Commendable, Accredited, Provisional, Interim, or Denied. The second, and perhaps better-known, measure calculated a *quality score for the care* that contracted providers delivered to plan members. This set of measures was originally called the HMO Employer Data and Information Set (HEDIS). NCQA released its initial HEDIS quality measures in 1991, measuring the performance of about 330 health plans, and reported the results to employers. In 1993, Version 2.0 of HEDIS was renamed the Health Plan Employer Data and Information Set. In July 2007, the name was again changed to Healthcare Effectiveness Data and Information Set, which is what it is called today.

Each year, the NCQA publishes accreditation standards and updates to its current version of HEDIS.[71] It also publishes information about these assessments.[72]

Direct governmental efforts to implement quality recommendations in the United States began in 1984, when Congress authorized the formation of the U.S. Preventive Services Task Force (USPSTF) as an independent, volunteer panel of primary care and public health experts whose task is to issue evidence-based recommendations on screening and prevention services. The Department of Health and Human Services (DHHS) was directed to support its activities. In 1989, the USPSTF published its first evidence-based guidelines.[73] The importance of this publication was not only the guidelines themselves but the codification of the recommendations based on supporting evidence. (Please see Exhibit 9.4 for the current form of these recommendations.)

In addition to publication of the USPSTF recommendations, 1989 saw the birth of the Agency for Health Care Policy and Research (AHCPR), which was authorized by the Omnibus Budget Reconciliation Act of 1989 as a Public Health Service Agency in the DHHS. The agency was formed because health service researchers and policy makers thought certain conditions were being treated inappropriately and inefficiently, leading to cost and quality problems, particularly for Medicare patients. Unlike the USPSTF's mandate for *prevention and screening* recommendations, AHCPR was tasked with the development of evidence-based *treatment* reports developed by Patient Outcome Research Teams

---

[70]The first PPO was accredited in 2001. See: http://www.ncqa.org/top-25-moments-in-health-care-quality-timeline Retrieved July 12, 2018.

[71]See: *HEDIS 2018*. Retrieved July 12, 2018, from http://www.ncqa.org/hedis-quality-measurement/hedis-measures/hedis-2018

[72]NCQA list of health plan report cards. Retrieved July 12, 2018, from https://reportcards.ncqa.org/#/health-plans/list

[73]U.S. Preventive Services Task Force. (1989). *Guide to clinical preventive services: An assessment of the effectiveness of 169 preventive interventions*. Baltimore, MD: Williams & Wilkins.

EXHIBIT 9.4. **Recommendation Grade Explanations**

Grade	Definition	Suggestions for Practice
A	The USPSTF recommends the service. There is high certainty that the net benefit is substantial.	Offer or provide this service.
B	The USPSTF recommends the service. There is high certainty that the net benefit is moderate or there is moderate certainty that the net benefit is moderate to substantial.	Offer or provide this service.
C	The USPSTF recommends selectively offering or providing this service to individual patients based on professional judgment and patient preferences. There is at least moderate certainty that the net benefit is small.	Offer or provide this service for selected patients depending on individual circumstances.
D	The USPSTF recommends against the service. There is moderate or high certainty that the service has no net benefit or that the harms outweigh the benefits.	Discourage the use of this service.
I Statement	The USPSTF concludes that the current evidence is insufficient to assess the balance of benefits and harms of the service. Evidence is lacking, of poor quality, or conflicting, and the balance of benefits and harms cannot be determined.	Read the clinical considerations section of USPSTF Recommendation Statement. If the service is offered, patients should understand the uncertainty about the balance of benefits and harms.

Source: U.S. Preventive Services Task Force. *Grade definitions*. Retrieved July 12, 2018, from https://www.uspreventiveservices taskforce.org/Page/Name/grade-definitions

(PORTs). For example, two prominent PORTs dealt with cataract surgery and treatment of benign prostatic enlargement. The recommendation that caused the most controversy, however, concerned spinal fusion for low back pain. The PORT that researched this topic reported its findings in *JAMA* in 1992, concluding that "for several low back disorders no advantage has been demonstrated for fusion over surgery without fusion, and complications of fusions are common. Randomized controlled trials are needed to compare fusion, surgery without fusion, and nonsurgical treatments in rigorously defined patient groups."[74]

The findings caused a number of politically connected spine surgeons to lobby their (Republican) members of Congress to eliminate the agency when reappropriations were

---

[74] Turner, J. A., Herron, E. M., Kaselkorn, J., Kent, D., Ciol, M. A., & Deyo, R. (1992). Patient outcomes after lumbar spinal fusions. *JAMA, 268*(7), 907–911.

being discussed in 1995. Fortunately, due to bipartisan support, AHCPR survived, though with less funding.[75] In order to lessen the appearance of intervening in medical practice, the Healthcare Research and Quality Act of 1999 renamed the agency the Agency for Healthcare Research and Quality (AHRQ). Among its other tasks, AHRQ is responsible for convening and providing administrative, research, technical, and communication support for the USPSTF.[76]

1990s

In 1993, nursing quality took a large step forward with the establishment of the hospital Magnet Recognition Program under the aegis of the American Nurses Credentialing Center (ANCC), part of the American Nurses Association (ANA). The origins of this program were in the early 1980s when the country faced yet another nursing shortage: 100,000 vacant positions and inadequate staffing at 80% of hospitals. ANA research had identified organizational characteristics that facilitated nursing retention, calling it a "magnet effect." The original 14 features that fostered retention were called "Forces of Magnetism." In 1994, the University of Washington Medical Center was the first institution to receive magnet status. The goals for the program are to: identify excellence in the delivery of nursing services to patients, promote quality in a milieu that supports professional clinical practice, and provide a mechanism for disseminating best practices in nursing services. In 2008, a new model consolidated the 14 forces into five components:

1. *Transformational Leadership* (Strategic Planning; Advocacy and Influence; and Visibility, Accessibility, and Communication)

2. *Structural Empowerment* (Professional Engagement; Commitment to Professional Development; Teaching and Role Development; Commitment to Community Involvement; and Recognition of Nursing)

3. *Exemplary Professional Practice* (Professional Practice Model; Care Delivery System(s); Staffing, Scheduling, and Budgeting Processes; Interdisciplinary Care; Accountability, Competence, and Autonomy; Ethics, Privacy, and Confidentiality; Diversity and Workplace Advocacy; Culture of Safety; and Quality Care Monitoring and Improvement)

4. *New Knowledge, Innovations, and Improvements* (Research; Evidence-Based Practice; and Innovation)

5. *Empirical Outcomes* (shift from structure and process to a greater focus on outcomes for the patient, community, workforce, and organization)[77]

---

[75]This story provides an excellent example of the political power of constituencies who are affected by quality improvement initiatives. For a more detailed account, see: Gray, B. H., Gusmano M. K., & Collins, S. R. (2003). AHCPR and the changing politics of health services research. *Health Affairs* (Supplement) Web Exclusives W3:283–307. Retrieved July 12, 2018, from https://www.healthaffairs.org/doi/full/10.1377/hlthaff.W3.283

[76]*AHRQ*. Retrieved July 12, 2018, from https://www.ahrq.gov/

[77]American Nurses Credentialing Center. *Magnet Recognition Program*. Retrieved July 12, 2018, from https://www.nursingworld.org/organizational-programs/magnet

There are currently 468 Magnet facilities (including 7 international ones).[78] Achieving Magnet status requires significant organization commitment: "On average, the process of attaining Magnet status takes 4.25 years to complete with an average total investment of $2,125,000."[79] However, the effort appears to be worth the investment: "On average, MHs [Magnet hospitals] receive an adjusted net increase in patient income of $104.22–$127.05 per discharge after becoming a Magnet which translates to an additional $1,229,770–$1,263,926 per year."[80]

Recognizing that not every hospital has the resources to apply for Magnet status, the ANCC created another pathway for hospitals to recognize a supportive environment for quality nursing practice, the Pathway to Excellence. The program began with rural hospitals in Texas in 2003 under the name "Nurse-Friendly award." The ANCC took over its management in 2007 and expanded it to all categories of hospitals nationwide. The Pathway to Excellence program has its own compliance standards[81] and, unlike the Magnet program, is conducted as a "self-study" with verification by a confidential survey of the applicant's nursing staff.

In 1999, three milestones occurred in American quality improvement: the start of the National Quality Forum (NQF), publication of *To Err Is Human*, and the beginning of the Joint Commission's Oryx initiative. Because of their lasting importance, each will be discussed below.

The case for establishing the NQF came from three sources in 1998: the RAND Corporation,[82] the President's Advisory Commission on Consumer Protection and Quality in the Health Care Industry,[83] and the IOM National Roundtable on Health Care Quality.[84] According to the NQF's first president, Kenneth Kizer:

> The concept of the National Quality Forum arose in response to the strong American sentiment against government regulation and control of health care quality... I see the mission of the Forum, quite simply, as being to improve health care quality; that is, to promote delivery of care known to be effective; to achieve better health outcomes, greater

---

[78]For an up-to-date list of hospitals in the Magnet Recognition Program, see: https://www.nursingworld.org/organizational-programs/magnet/find-a-magnet-facility/ Retrieved July 12, 2018.

[79]Jayawardhana, J., Welton, J. M., & Lindrooth, R. C. (2014). Is there a business case for magnet hospitals? Estimates of the cost and revenue implications of becoming a magnet. *Medical Care*, *53*(5), 400–406. The data in this article is still cited in more recent publications.

[80]Ibid.

[81]Dans, M., Pabico C., Tate M., & Hume L. (2017). Understanding the New Pathway to Excellence® standards. *Nurse Leader*, *15*(1), 49–52.

[82]Schuster, A., McGlynn, E. A., & Brook, R. H. (1998). How good is the quality of health care in the United States? *The Milbank Quarterly*, *76*(4), 517–563.

[83]President's Advisory Commission on Consumer Protection and Quality in the Health Care Industry. (1998). Quality First: Better Health Care for All Americans. Final Report to the President of the United States. Washington, DC. See: https://archive.ahrq.gov/hcqual/final/ Retrieved July 12, 2018.

[84]Institute of Medicine National Roundtable on Health Care Quality; Donaldson M. S., (Ed.). (1998). *Statement on quality of care*. Institute of Medicine (U.S.) National Roundtable on Health Care Quality Washington, DC: National Academies Press (U.S.). The Urgent Need to Improve Health Care Quality: Consensus Statement. Retrieved July 12, 2018, from https://www.ncbi.nlm.nih.gov/books/NBK223995/

patient functionality, and a higher level of patient safety; and to make health care easier to access and a more satisfying experience. The primary strategy that we will employ to accomplish this mission is to standardize the means by which health care quality is measured and reported and to make health care quality data widely available. To actualize our agenda we have identified five key strategic goals: (1) developing and implementing a national agenda for measuring and reporting health care quality; (2) standardizing the measures used to report health care quality so that data collection is less arduous for health care providers, and so that the reported data are of greater value; (3) building consumer competence for making choices based on quality-of-care data; (4) enhancing the capability of health care providers to use quality-related data; and (5) increasing the overall demand for health care quality data.[85]

True to its origins, the NQF contracts with the federal government to create a National Quality Strategy, which includes recommendations for quality evaluation measures for purposes of bonus payments and penalties to providers under Medicare. The NQF does not research and develop criteria itself but evaluates existing and emerging measures through a rigorous, consensus-driven process.[86] In addition to its quality activities, the NQF has also had a major impact on patient safety through its program of Serious Reportable Events (SREs, or "never events"), launched in 2009.[87] Among the most well known of these events are surgery on the wrong patient, surgery on the wrong part of the right patient, and foreign objects left in patients at the time of surgery.

The American public was largely unaware of the previously mentioned studies and the launch of the NQF. What brought the issue of healthcare safety to prominence was the second major quality event of 1999, publication of *To Err Is Human: Building a Safer Health System*.[88]

The day after its publication on November 28, 1999, its major findings were prominently featured in the *New York Times, Washington Post, Los Angeles Times, USA Today*, and many other news publications and broadcasts. In this first of two scheduled reports, the main message was that, based on extrapolations from safety studies in three states, between 44,000 and 98,000 people a year were dying in the United States from medical errors. To highlight the significance of these numbers, the report noted: "More people die in a given year as a result of medical errors than from motor vehicle accidents (43,458), breast cancer (42,297), or AIDS (16,516)." In other words, medicine in this country was unsafe, and

---

[85] Kizer, K. W. (2000). The National Quality Forum. *Academic Medicine, 75*(4), 320–321.

[86] NQF (2017, August). Measure Evaluation Criteria and Guidance for Evaluating Measures for Endorsement Effective. Retrieved July 12, 2018, from https://www.google.com/url?sa=t&rct=j&q=&esrc=s&source=web&cd=4&ved=0ahUKE wjYkKbd75zcAhUY84MKHarWCowQFghHMAM&url=http%3A%2F%2Fwww.qualityforum.org%2FMeasuring_ Performance%2FSubmitting_Standards%2F2017_Measure_Evaluation_Criteria.aspx&usg=AOvVaw3g7h498wIE-7n WDgs6i5cp

[87] NQF. *Serious reportable events*. Retrieved July 12, 2018, from http://www.qualityforum.org/topics/sres/serious_ reportable_events.aspx

[88] Kohn, T., Corrigan, J. M., & Donaldson, M. S. (Eds.). (2000). *To err is human: Building a safer health system*. Washington, DC: Committee on Quality of Health Care in America, Institute of Medicine National Academy Press. [The report was issued November 29, 2009]. Retrieved July 12, 2018, from https://www.nap.edu/login.php?record_id=9728& page=https%3A%2F%2Fwww.nap.edu%2Fdownload%2F9728 (Free login required.)

something needed to be done about it.[89] The publication went into great detail analyzing the nature of the problem of unsafe care and made recommendations to address it, including the designation of "the National Forum for Health Care Quality Measurement and Reporting as the entity responsible for promulgating and maintaining a core set of reporting standards to be used by states."

The JCAHO's ORYX Performance Measurement Initiative[90] was the third major quality innovation of 1999. Starting in the first quarter of that year, hospitals were required to report choices of "outcomes for at least two clinical areas that, together, cover at least 20 percent of a hospital's patient base."[91] Hospitals could choose up to five performance measures; if they chose five, they did not have to cover the 20%. This initiative meant that quality assessment was finally using *outcomes* for accreditation, not just structure and process.

2000–2010

In 2000, another organization that was formed by businesses concerned about healthcare quality launched its first survey. Sixty large employers, with funding from the Business Roundtable,[92] the Robert Wood Johnson Foundation, and the Commonwealth Fund created The Leapfrog Group. Its name reflected the desire to jump ahead and overcome obstacles that prevented rapid improvements in quality in the U.S. healthcare system. In 2001, it issued its first hospital survey by asking three simple questions:

1. Did they have Computerized Physician Order Entry (CPOE)?
2. Were their intensive care units staffed appropriately with intensivists?
3. Did they have enough surgical volume to safely perform certain high-risk procedures?

Unlike previous quality efforts, results were to be immediately available to the public. Participation, however, was voluntary and only 200 hospitals responded in the first year. Today, membership includes Fortune 100 companies, consumer advocacy groups, and more than 30 regional business coalitions on health. Its methodology is used by organizations such as Consumer Reports[93] to rate healthcare services. The survey content has also expanded to include such items as infection rates, cesarean section rates, and medication safety.[94]

---

[89] The report defined safety as "freedom from accidental injury." "Error is defined as the failure of a planned action to be completed as intended or the use of a wrong plan to achieve an aim."

[90] Joint Commission. (2017, February 1). Facts about ORYX® for Hospitals (National Hospital Quality Measures). Retrieved July 12, 2018, from https://www.jointcommission.org/facts_about_oryx_for_hospitals/

[91] Lawrence, J. (1998, February). JCAHO's Oryx initiative links outcomes with accreditation. *Managed Care*. Retrieved July 12, 2018, from https://www.managedcaremag.com/archives/1998/2/jcahos-oryx-initiative-links-outcomes-accreditation

[92] The Business Roundtable membership is comprised of CEOs of companies "with more than 16 million employees and more than $7 trillion in annual revenues." Retrieved July 12, 2018, from http://businessroundtable.org/about

[93] Consumer Reports. *How we test health care products and services*. Retrieved July 12, 2018, from https://www.consumerreports.org/cro/2012/09/how-we-rate-health-care-products-and-services/index.htm

[94] The Leapfrog Group. *Survey content*. Retrieved July 12, 2018, from http://www.leapfroggroup.org/ratings-reports/survey-content

In 2004, anticipating the value-based purchasing movement, many Leapfrog Group members formed the Health Plan Users Group.[95] This group started to persuade health plans with which its members contracted to preferentially use hospitals that scored highly on the Hospital Survey and other reports. Each health plan submits a dashboard on how well it is steering admissions to these facilities.

In 2007, the Leapfrog Group added questions about SREs (or Never Events) to its survey after the NQF developed a list of such problems (see the section on the NQF above); however, in 2017, the group took the process further.

A hospital "fully meets standards" if they agree to all of the following if a Never Event occurs within their facility:

1. Apologize to the patient and family

2. Waive all costs related to the event and follow-up care

3. Report the event to an external agency

4. Conduct a root-cause analysis of how and why the event occurred

5. Interview patients and families, who are willing and able, to gather evidence for the root cause analysis

6. Inform the patient and family of the action(s) that the hospital will take to prevent future recurrences of similar events based on the findings from the root cause analysis

7. Have a protocol in place to provide support for caregivers involved in Never Events, and make that protocol known to all caregivers and affiliated clinicians

8. Perform an annual review to ensure compliance with each element of Leapfrog's Never Events Policy for each never event that occurred

9. Make a copy of this policy available to patients upon request[96]

As an example of a successful initiative, in 2011 the Leapfrog Group called attention to the high rate of early, elective deliveries. By highlighting this problem and working with other organizations, such as the March of Dimes and Childbirth Connection, the rate decreased from 17% in 2010 to 4.6% in 2013.

To complement the Hospital Survey, the Leapfrog Hospital Safety Grade program was launched in 2012. Compiling numerous measures twice a year, the program gives hospitals a grade ranging from A to F. The general categories used are infections, problems with surgery, practices to prevent errors, safety problems, and "doctors, nurses & hospital staff." Patients can look up more than 2,600 hospitals' grades and the details behind the scores.[97]

---

[95]The Leapfrog Group. *Health Plan Users Group*. Retrieved July 12, 2018, from http://www.leapfroggroup.org/employers-purchasers/health-plan-users-group

[96]The Leapfrog Group. *When hospitals say "I'm sorry."* Retrieved July 12, 2018, from http://www.leapfroggroup.org/influencing/never-events

[97]*Leapfrog Hospital Safety Grade*. Retrieved July 12, 2018, from http://www.hospitalsafetygrade.org/

In addition to the Hospital Survey and Hospital Safety Grade programs, the Leapfrog Group has also developed a Value-Based Purchasing (VBP) Platform; standards come from the Leapfrog Hospital Survey. The VBP compares an individual institution's score to others using state and national averages. The scores range from (low to high) 0–100 in five domains (Medication Safety, Inpatient Care Management, High-Risk Surgeries, Maternity Care, and Hospital-Acquired Conditions) and are then combined into an overall composite score referred to as the Value Score.[98]

One final program of note is the Leapfrog Group's Hidden Surcharge Calculator, which was launched in 2013.[99] The calculator takes information from the Hospital Safety Grade scores and translates it into how much more it costs to use a low-performing hospital compared to a higher-performing one using hospital-specific data.[100]

In 2001, the successor of *To Err Is Human* was published under the title *Crossing the Quality Chasm: A New Health System for the 21st Century*.[101] This study called for *systemic redesign* (not just improvement) of the U.S. healthcare system to deliver quality care. Because of its profound impact on subsequent quality initiatives, some of its 13 recommendations are highlighted next.

All health care constituencies, including policymakers, purchasers, regulators, health professionals, health care trustees and management, and consumers, commit to a national statement of purpose for the health care system as a whole and to a shared agenda of six aims for improvement... Health care should be:

- *Safe*. Avoiding injuries to patients from the care that is intended to help them.

- *Effective*. Providing services based on scientific knowledge to all who could benefit and refraining from providing services to those not likely to benefit (avoiding underuse and overuse, respectively).

- *Patient-centered*. Providing care that is respectful of and responsive to individual patient preferences, needs, and values and ensuring that patient values guide all clinical decisions.

- *Timely*. Reducing waits and sometimes harmful delays for both those who receive and those who give care.

- *Efficient*. Avoiding waste, including waste of equipment, supplies, ideas, and energy.

- *Equitable*. Providing care that does not vary in quality because of personal characteristics such as gender, ethnicity, geographic location, and socioeconomic status.

---

[98]Leapfrog Value-based Purchasing Platform. *2016 scoring methodology*. Retrieved July 12, 2018, from http://www.leapfroggroup.org/sites/default/files/Files/2016LVBPP_ScoringMethodology_Final.pdf

[99]The Leapfrog Group. (2013, October 28). *The hidden surcharge Americans pay for hospital errors*. (Updated). Retrieved July 12, 2018, from http://www.leapfroggroup.org/sites/default/files/Files/Hidden-Surcharge-White-Paper-Updated102813.pdf

[100]The Leapfrog Group. *Lives & Dollars Lost Calculator*. Retrieved July 12, 2018, from http://www.leapfroggroup.org/employers-purchasers/lives-dollars-lost-calculator

[101]Committee on Quality of Health Care in America. *Crossing the quality chasm: A new health system for the 21st century*. Washington, DC: Institute of Medicine National Academy Press. Retrieve July 12, 2018, from https://www.nap.edu/download/10027 (Free registration required.) Note: Quotations that reference this publication will refer to this citation.

These aims that define quality and safe healthcare are the best-known recommendations from this report. From this time onward, almost all publications and lectures about healthcare quality mention these six features. More will be discussed later about these characteristics.

- The quality of care should be measured and followed using acceptable metrics and the results published. The report states:

  > The committee applauds Congress and the Administration for their current efforts to establish a National Quality Report [now called the National Healthcare Quality & Disparities Reports][102] for tracking the quality of care.

- Payment methods should:

  - Provide fair payment for good clinical management of the types of patients seen. Clinicians should be adequately compensated for taking good care of all types of patients, neither gaining nor losing financially for caring for sicker patients or those with more complicated conditions.

  - Provide an opportunity for providers to share in the benefits of quality improvement.

  - Provide the opportunity for consumers and purchasers to recognize quality differences in health care and direct their decisions accordingly. In particular, consumers need to have good information on quality and the ability to use that information as they see fit to meet their needs.

  - Align financial incentives with the implementation of care processes based on best practices and the achievement of better patient outcomes.

  - Reduce fragmentation of care. Payment methods should not pose a barrier to providers' ability to coordinate care for patients across settings and over time.

These recommendations underlie the pay-for-performance arrangements now common among public and private healthcare insurers.

Private and public purchasers, health care organizations, clinicians, and patients should work together to redesign health care processes in accordance with the following rules:

1. *Care based on continuous healing relationships.* Patients should receive care whenever they need it and in many forms, not just face-to-face visits . . .

2. *Customization based on patient needs and values . . .*

3. *The patient as the source of control.* Patients should be given the necessary information and the opportunity to exercise the degree of control they choose over health care decisions that affect them. The health system should be able to accommodate differences in patient preferences and encourage shared decision making.

---

[102] Agency for Healthcare Research and Quality. *National Healthcare Quality & Disparities Reports.* Retrieved July 12, 2018, from https://www.ahrq.gov/research/findings/nhqrdr/index.html A previous version of this report is referenced in the first paragraph of this chapter.

4. *Shared knowledge and the free flow of information.* Patients should have unfettered access to their own medical information and to clinical knowledge. Clinicians and patients should communicate effectively and share information.

5. *Evidence-based decision making.* Patients should receive care based on the best available scientific knowledge.

6. *Safety as a system property.* Patients should be safe from injury caused by the care system.

7. *The need for transparency.* The health care system should make information available to patients and their families that allows them to make informed decisions when selecting a health plan, hospital, or clinical practice, or choosing among alternative treatments. This should include information describing the system's performance on safety, evidence-based practice, and patient satisfaction.

8. *Anticipation of needs.* The health system should anticipate patient needs, rather than simply reacting to events.

9. *Continuous decrease in waste.* The health system should not waste resources or patient time.

10. *Cooperation among clinicians.* Clinicians and institutions should actively collaborate and communicate to ensure an appropriate exchange of information and coordination of care . . .

Congress, the executive branch, leaders of health care organizations, public and private purchasers, and health informatics associations and vendors should make a renewed national commitment to building an information infrastructure to support health care delivery, consumer health, quality measurement and improvement, public accountability, clinical and health services research, and clinical education. This commitment should lead to the elimination of most handwritten clinical data by the end of the decade.

Three important initiatives began in the year after publication of *Crossing the Quality Chasm*. First, in December 2002, the Hospital Quality Alliance (HQA) was formed when the AHA, the Association of American Medical Colleges, and the Federation of American Hospitals invited government agencies, professional organizations, purchaser alliances, consumer organizations, and others to develop a national strategy to make quality hospital care available and transparent to the public.[103] The HQA is still responsible for a number of ongoing quality initiatives including the Hospital Consumer Assessment of Healthcare Providers and Systems (HCAHPS) survey and Hospital Compare website (both explained below).

Initially, 10 measures were developed that hospitals would voluntarily share with the public. (Please see Exhibit 9.5.) Two important activities resulted from this simple start.

---

[103]Participants in the HQA are: *Provider Organizations*: American Hospital Association; Federation of American Hospitals; Association of American Medical Colleges; National Association of Children's Hospitals and Related Institutions; National Association of Public Hospitals; American Medical Association; and American Nurses Association. *Government*: Centers for Medicare and Medicaid Services and Agency for Healthcare Research and Quality. *Employers/Consumers/Purchasers*: AARP; AFL-CIO; Consumer/Purchaser Disclosure Project; U.S. Chamber of Commerce; General Electric; Blue Cross/Blue Shield Association; National Business Coalition on Health; and America's Health Insurance Plans. *Quality Groups*: The Joint Commission and National Quality Forum.

EXHIBIT 9.5. **Initial 10 Quality Measures of the HQA**

Performance measures	Measure description—for additional information including inclusions and exclusions click on the performance measure
AMI—aspirin at arrival	Acute myocardial infarction (AMI) patients without aspirin contraindications who received aspirin within 24 hr before or after hospital arrival.
AMI—aspirin prescribed at discharge	Acute myocardial infarction (AMI) patients without aspirin contraindications who are prescribed aspirin at hospital discharge.
AMI—ACEI or ARB for LVSD	Acute myocardial infarction (AMI) patients with left ventricular systolic dysfunction (LVSD) and without angiotensin converting enzyme inhibitor (ACEI) and angiotensin receptor blocker (ARB) contraindications who are prescribed either an ACEI or ARB at hospital discharge.[a]
AMI—beta blocker at arrival	Acute myocardial infarction (AMI) patients without beta blocker contraindications who received a beta blocker within 24 hr after hospital arrival.
AMI—beta blocker at discharge	Acute myocardial infarction (AMI) patients without beta blocker contraindications who are prescribed a beta blocker at hospital discharge.
HF-LVF assessment	Heart failure patients with documentation in the hospital record that left ventricular function (LVF) were assessed before arrival, during hospitalization, or planned for after discharge.
HF-ACEI or ARB for LVSD	Heart failure patients with left ventricular systolic dysfunction (LVSD) and without angiotensin converting enzyme inhibitor (ACEI) and angiotensin receptor blocker (ARB) contraindications who are prescribed either an ACEI or ARB at hospital discharge.[a]
PNE-initial antibiotic timing	Pneumonia patients who receive their first dose of antibiotics within 4 hr after arrival at the hospital.
PNE—pneumococcal vaccination	Pneumonia patients age 65 and older who were screened for pneumococcal vaccine status and were administered the vaccine prior to discharge, if indicated.
PNE-oxygenation assessment	Pneumonia patients who had an assessment of arterial oxygenation by arterial blood gas measurement or pulse oximetry within 24 hr prior to or after arrival at the hospital.

[a] Measure revised to incorporate ARBs, per *joint agreement* of the Centers for Medicare and Medicaid Services (CMS) and the Joint Commission on Accreditation of Health Care Organizations (JCAHO) issued on November 15, 2004.

Source: *The Hospital Quality Alliance (HQA) ten-measure "Starter Set."* Retrieved July 13, 2018, from https://www.cms.gov/Medicare/Quality-Initiatives-Patient-Assessment-Instruments/HospitalQualityInits/Downloads/HospitalStarterSet200512.pdf

First, on April 1, 2005, the government-run Hospital Compare website (http://www.medicare .gov/hospitalcompare) was launched to provide patients with readily available tools to help them evaluate their hospital choices. According to CMS:[104]

> Hospital Compare allows consumers to select multiple hospitals and directly compare performance measure information related to heart attack, heart failure, pneumonia, surgery and other conditions. These results are organized by:

- General information
- Survey of patients' experiences
- Timely & effective care
- Complications
- Readmissions & deaths
- Use of medical imaging
- Payment & value of care

Second, the Deficit Reduction Act of 2005 required that, starting October 1, 2006, Medicare payments be linked to performance of quality measures. Specifically, "[h]ospitals that report the required set of quality measures to the Secretary will receive the full market basket. Hospitals that do not report quality measures will receive the market basket minus 2 percentage points."[105]

That same year, another important, and related, action occurred: passage of the Patient Safety and Quality Improvement Act of 2005 (PSQIA),[106] which legislated the strongest language ever passed to protect quality and safety improvement activities. The Act gave responsibility to AHRQ to create lists of Patient Safety Organizations (PSOs) and a network of patient safety databases. The mission of the PSOs, which must be independent of insurers and providers, is to conduct activities "to improve patient safety and the quality of health care delivery" by "collection, management, or analysis of information" and provide "feedback to participants in a patient safety evaluation system." The unique part of this law is the strong language that protects the patient safety work product from being used in any civil, criminal, disciplinary, or administrative proceedings. In particular, this work

---

[104]CMS.gov. *Hospital Compare*. Retrieved July 13, 2018, from https://www.cms.gov/medicare/quality-initiatives-patient-assessment-instruments/hospitalqualityinits/hospitalcompare.html

[105]Deficit Reduction Act of 2005. All CMS Provisions. Section 5001 (a2). Retrieved July 13, 2018, from https://www .cms.gov/Regulations-and-Guidance/Legislation/LegislativeUpdate/Downloads/DRA0307.pdf

[106]Title 42—The Public Health and Welfare: Chapter 6A—Public Health Service, Subchapter VII—Agency for Healthcare Research and Quality, Part C—Patient Safety Improvement Sec. 299b-22—Privilege and confidentiality protections. Amends the Public Health Service Act (42 U.S.C. 299 et. seq.; P.L. 109-41) by inserting sections 921 through 926, 42 U.S.C. 299b-21 through 299b-26. Section available at: https://www.gpo.gov/fdsys/pkg/USCODE-2010-title42/pdf/ USCODE-2010-title42-chap6A-subchapVII-partC.pdf Retrieved July 13, 2018. Rules for implementation of this law were published in the Patient Safety Rule of 2008. Retrieved July 13, 2018, from https://www.ecfr.gov/cgi-bin/text-idx? SID=42192f8b6c83ddc436beeab06ef0ab90&mc=true&node=pt42.1.3&rgn=div5

product is not subject to disclosure under the Freedom of Information Act. Further, the Act protects providers from punitive actions (including loss of accreditation or termination of employment) based on "good faith participation...in the collection, development, reporting, or maintenance of patient safety work product." In an age when transparency is so highly valued, it is noteworthy that such confidentiality still has a useful role.

Starting in 2008, major changes were made to the original quality list to include additional and different types of measures. These changes were added to the Hospital Compare website and used by CMS in its hospital payment calculations. Two changes are of particular importance.

First, note that the original measures evaluated only the *processes* of care. The new measures added the assessment of *outcomes* (viz. mortality rates for heart attack, heart failure, and pneumonia).

Second, in addition to clinical outcomes reporting, the *public perception about the care experience* was reported on the Hospital Compare website and used by CMS to pay hospitals. The tool, called the Hospital Consumer Assessment of Healthcare Providers and Systems (HCAHPS)[107] survey, was developed with three goals in mind: standardizing data to allow meaningful comparisons among institutions, publicly reporting results to encourage hospitals to improve the quality of care, and enhancing public accountability by making the information more available.[108]

CMS rolled out the survey in October 2006 and by July 2007 started to include the measure in payment calculations for hospitals subject to the Inpatient Prospective Payment System (those hospitals paid on the basis of DRGs). More recently, the Affordable Care Act (2010) included the HCAHPS score in the incentive payments of the Hospital Value-Based Purchasing program, starting with October 2012 discharges. (See below for an explanation of this program.)

The HCAHPS Survey[109] has 32 questions. Twenty-one questions ask "how often" or whether patients received a critical aspect of hospital care (rather than whether they were "satisfied"). These questions cover nine key topics:

1. Communication with doctors

2. Communication with nurses

3. Responsiveness of hospital staff

4. Pain management

5. Communication about medicines

6. Discharge information

---

[107] It is also called CAHPS, which is a registered trademark of the Agency for Healthcare Research and Quality (AHRQ).
[108] The HCAHPS was developed and implemented over a number of years. Starting in 2002, CMS and AHRQ conducted research and piloted tests on the instrument. After validation and a period of public comment, in 2005 it was endorsed by the NQF and approved by the Office of Management and Budget for implementation.
[109] *HCAPS Survey*. Retrieved July 13, 2018, from http://www.hcahpsonline.org/globalassets/hcahps/survey-instruments/mail/july-1-2018-and-forward-discharges/2018_survey-instruments_english_mail.pdf

7. Cleanliness of the hospital environment

8. Quietness of the hospital environment

9. Transition of care

The survey also includes four screener questions, five items to adjust for the mix of patients across hospitals, and two items that support congressionally mandated reports. Hospitals may add their own questions to the questionnaire.

The HCAHPS is administered monthly by a hospital-picked, CMS-approved vendor (or the hospital itself, if CMS approves it) to a random sample of adult inpatients between 48 hours and 6 weeks after discharge. These patients include those who have received medical, surgical, and maternity care but need not be Medicare beneficiaries. The data must be collected by one of four methods: mail, telephone, mail with telephone follow-up, or active interactive voice recognition (IVR). Multiple attempts must be made to contact the chosen patients, and hospitals are required to achieve at least 300 completed surveys over 4 calendar quarters. Results based on the most recent 4 consecutive quarters are reported on the Hospital Compare website. In April 2015, the website initiated "Star Ratings" to make the survey's results more understandable to the public.

> HCAHPS Star Ratings summarize the results for each HCAHPS measure and present it in a format that is increasingly familiar to consumers, making it easier to use the information and spotlight excellence in healthcare quality. Twelve HCAHPS Star Ratings appear on Hospital Compare: one for each of the 11 publicly reported HCAHPS measures, plus a Summary Star Rating that combines all the HCAHPS Star Ratings.[110]

After 2008, the frequency of modifications to the evaluation criteria for the Hospital Compare website accelerated to reflect changes in healthcare delivery and quality priorities. Some of these changes included:

2009   In line with shifts from inpatient to outpatient care, CMS added data on hospital outpatient facilities, including outpatient imaging and emergency department care.

2010   Recall that in 2008, inpatient mortality rates for heart attack, heart failure, and pneumonia were added to the evaluation criteria. Now, to avoid early discharges for inadequately treated patients, CMS added a measure of 30-day readmission rates for these conditions.

2011   In order to reflect increasing public health concern over Hospital Acquired Infections (HAIs), measures were implemented to assess this problem.

---

[110]*HCAHPS Star Ratings*. Retrieved July 13, 2018, from http://www.hcahpsonline.org/en/hcahps-star-ratings/

2013   Data from the hospital Value-Based Purchasing (VBP) program was added to the website.[111] The VBP program seeks to encourage hospitals to improve the quality and safety of care that all patients receive during acute-care inpatient stays by:

- Eliminating or reducing the occurrence of adverse events (healthcare errors resulting in patient harm).
- Adopting evidence-based care standards and protocols that result in the best outcomes for the most patients.
- Re-engineering hospital processes that improve patients' experience of care.
- Increasing the transparency of care for consumers.
- Recognizing hospitals that are involved in the provision of high-quality care at a lower cost to Medicare.[112]

Metrics that are used to accomplish these goals for the VBP are part of four domains:[113]

- Clinical Care
- Patient- and Caregiver-Centered Experience of Care/Care Coordination
- Safety
- Efficiency and Cost Reduction

Starting in fiscal year 2018, each of these domains is weighed equally to arrive at a Total Performance Score (TPS). Hospitals are evaluated on both *achievement* (how they performed compared to other hospitals) and *improvement* in its own performance; CMS uses the greater of either achievement or improvement scores on each measure and dimension to calculate the hospital's overall total performance. The TPS determines the financial incentive payment the hospital receives. Funding comes from a 2% reduction in DRG payments.[114]

A particularly instructive example of evolving criteria and counterproductive incentives is measurement of pain control.[115] The issue started with James N. Campbell's presidential address to the American Pain Society in 1995:

---

[111]This program was authorized by Section 3001(a) of the ACA and uses the quality data reporting infrastructure developed for the Hospital Inpatient Quality Reporting Program in Section 501(b) of the Medicare Prescription Drug, Improvement, and Modernization Act of 2003.

[112]CMS. *The Hospital Value-Based Purchasing (VBP) Program*. Retrieved July 13, 2018, from https://www.cms.gov/Medicare/Quality-Initiatives-Patient-Assessment-Instruments/Value-Based-Programs/HVBP/Hospital-Value-Based-Purchasing.html

[113]CMS.gov. *Hospital Value*. Retrieved July 13, 2018, from https://www.cms.gov/Medicare/Quality-Initiatives-Patient-Assessment-Instruments/HospitalQualityInits/Hospital-Value-Based-Purchasing-.html.

[114]For more details, see: QualityNet, available at http://www.qualitynet.org/; select the Hospitals-Inpatient tab. Retrieved July 13, 2018.

[115]For an excellent review of this issue, see: Baker, D. W. (2017). *The Joint Commission's pain standards: Origins and evolution*. Oakbrook Terrace, IL: The Joint Commission. Retrieved July 13, 2018, from https://www.jointcommission.org/assets/1/6/Pain_Std_History_Web_Version_05122017.pdf

Today, nurses and physicians routinely assess the vital signs of pulse, blood pressure, core temperature, and respirations in evaluating patients. We should consider pain the *fifth vital sign*... We need to train doctors and nurses to treat pain as a vital sign. *Quality care* means that pain is measured. *Quality of care* means that pain is treated.[116]

This call to action set off a national campaign to aggressively control pain, which resulted in markedly increased opioid use. For example, in October 2000, the Veterans Administration published *Pain as the 5th Vital Sign Toolkit* in order to "offer guidelines for the completion of comprehensive pain assessments."[117] Further, the Joint Commission launched its new pain assessment and management standards on January 1, 2001. While attention to pain control is laudable, by 2015, more than 33,000 Americans had died as a result of an opioid overdose and about 2 million people had substance use disorders related to prescription opioid pain relievers.[118] As a result, in November 2016, CMS announced that it was "finalizing the removal of the pain management dimension of the Hospital Consumer Assessment of Healthcare Providers and Systems (HCAHPS) Survey for purposes of the Hospital Value-Based Purchasing Program to eliminate any financial pressure clinicians may feel to overprescribe medications."[119]

In August 2017, CMS announced that effective January 1, 2018, it would replace the previous HCAPS pain questions with three new questions that comprise a new composite measure called "Communication About Pain."[120] Also, effective January 1, 2018, new and revised pain assessment and management standards applied to all Joint Commission–accredited hospitals.[121]

In addition to formation of the Hospital Quality Alliance (HQA), the other two major innovations of 2002 were significant programmatic changes at the JCAHO. First was establishment of the National Patient Safety Goals (NPSGs) program. The Patient Safety Advisory Group, which includes nurses, physicians, pharmacists, risk managers,

---

[116]Campbell, J. N. (1996). Presidential address, American Pain Society, November 12, 1995. Reproduced in: *Journal of Pain*, 5(1), 85–88.

[117]Geriatrics and Extended Care Strategic Healthcare Group, National Pain Management Coordinating Committee, Veterans Health Administration (2000). *Pain as the 5th Vital Sign Toolkit* (Rev.) Retrieved July 13, 2018, from https://www.va.gov/PAINMANAGEMENT/docs/Pain_As_the_5th_Vital_Sign_Toolkit.pdf

[118]National Institute on Drug Abuse. (2018, March). *Opioid crisis* (Rev.). Retrieved July 13, 2018, from https://www.drugabuse.gov/drugs-abuse/opioids/opioid-crisis

[119]CMS finalizes hospital outpatient prospective payment system changes to better support hospitals and physicians and improve patient care (2016, November 1). Retrieved July 13, 2018, from http://www.cms.gov/Newsroom/MediaReleaseDatabase/Press-releases/2016-Press-releases-items/2016-11-01.html

[120]The new questions on the written form are: During this hospital stay, did you have any pain? During this hospital stay, how often did hospital staff talk with you about how much *pain* you had? During this hospital stay, how often did hospital staff talk with you about how to treat your pain? See: *Hospital Inpatient Prospective Payment Final Rule*. Retrieved July 13, 2018, from https://s3.amazonaws.com/public-inspection.federalregister.gov/2017-16434.pdf

[121]The Joint Commission Report Requirement, Rationale, Reference (2017, August 29). *Pain assessment and management standards for hospital* (11). Retrieved July 13, 2018, from https://www.jointcommission.org/assets/1/18/R3_Report_Issue_11_Pain_Assessment_8_25_17_FINAL.pdf

and other experienced professionals, is tasked with formulating such content as Sentinel Event[122] Alerts, measurable safety standards, and survey processes. The program was initiated January 1, 2003, and its standards now apply to ambulatory healthcare, behavioral healthcare, critical access hospitals, home care, hospitals, laboratory services, long-term care (including Medicare- and Medicaid-funded services), and office-based surgery.[123]

Some examples of safety standards are listed in Exhibit 9.6.

EXHIBIT 9.6. Sample National Patient Safety Goals

Identify Patients Correctly

NPSG.01.01.01: Use at least two ways to identify patients. For example, use the patient's name and date of birth. This is done to make sure that each patient gets the correct medicine and treatment.

Improve Staff Communication

NPSG.02.03.01: Get important test results to the right staff person on time.

Use Medicines Safely

NPSG.03.04.01: Before a procedure, label medicines that are not labeled. For example, medicines in syringes, cups and basins. Do this in the area where medicines and supplies are set up.

NPSG.03.06.01: Record and pass along correct information about a patient's medicines. Find out what medicines the patient is taking. Compare those medicines to new medicines given to the patient. Make sure the patient knows which medicines to take when they are at home. Tell the patient it is important to bring their up-to-date list of medicines every time they visit a doctor.

Use Alarms Safely

NPSG.06.01.01: Make improvements to ensure that alarms on medical equipment are heard and responded to on time.

Prevent Infection

NPSG.07.01.01: Use the hand cleaning guidelines from the Centers for Disease Control and Prevention or the World Health Organization. Set goals for improving hand cleaning. Use the goals to improve hand cleaning.

NPSG.07.06.01: Use proven guidelines to prevent infections of the urinary tract that are caused by catheters.

---

[122] The Joint Commission defines and explains a sentinel event as "an unexpected occurrence involving death or serious physical or psychological injury, or the risk thereof. Serious injury specifically includes loss of limb or function. The phrase 'or the risk thereof' includes any process variation for which a recurrence would carry a significant chance of a serious adverse outcome. Such events are called 'sentinel' because they signal the need for immediate investigation and response. The terms 'sentinel event' and 'error' are not synonymous; not all sentinel events occur because of an error, and not all errors result in sentinel events." Retrieved July 13, 2018, from https://www.jointcommission.org/assets/1/6/CAMH_2012_Update2_24_SE.pdf

[123] For site-specific criteria, see: 2018 National Patient Safety Goals. Retrieved July 13, 2018, from https://www.jointcommission.org/standards_information/npsgs.aspx

Prevent Mistakes in Surgery

UP.01.01.0: Make sure that the correct surgery is done on the correct patient and at the correct place on the patient's body.

> *UP.01.02.01*: Mark the correct place on the patient's body where the surgery is to be done.

> *UP.01.03.01*: Pause before the surgery to make sure that a mistake is not being made.

Source: Joint Commission. *The Joint Commission's National Patient Safety Goals 2018*. Retrieved July 13, 2018, from https://www .jointcommission.org/assets/1/6/NPSG_Chapter_HAP_Jan2018.pdf

The second major JCAHO initiative of 2002 was a new approach to quality assessment: "Shared Visions-New Pathways." The "Shared Visions" reflected consensus opinions among healthcare organizations about the need to close the quality and safety gaps highlighted by the IOM studies described above. The "New Pathways" distinguished the differences between the past and planned accreditation processes. While the old outcomes assessments remained, "Shared Visions" called for a number of significant changes[124] starting in 2004:

- *Timing of review*. The JCAHO started to perform unannounced surveys in January 2006. Prior to that time, hospitals "geared up" especially for those visits. To enhance the credibility of the accreditation process, unannounced reviews were instituted to make sure the day-to-day operations adhered to quality and safety standards.

- *Timing of criteria assessment*. Before this initiative, the site visits surveyed hospital performance since the last appraisal; in other words, it was a *retrospective* evaluation. The new method (see below) is a *concurrent* review (i.e., a review of ongoing care at the time of the onsite survey). It is interesting to note that this timing change occurred as society was demanding more "online/real-time" information, largely as the result of advances in the internet.

- *Shortening and consolidation of redundancies*. As might be inferred from the previous discussions, many of the JCAHO's criteria were layered on one another as new initiatives were developed. The Shared Visions-New Pathways program included a major rewrite directed at correcting those problems.

- *Customization of measurements (change in what is measured)*. The traditional survey process used uniform criteria across like institutions. The new method is called the priority focus process (PFP): Through an online portal, the institution supplies organization-specific information, such as ORYX core measure data, sentinel event

---

[124]Katzfey, R. P. (2004). JCAHO's Shared Visions–New Pathways: The new hospital survey and accreditation process for 2004. *American Journal of Health-System Pharmacy*, *61*, 1358–1364. American Hospital Association: Questions Concerning the JCAHO Accreditation Survey Process. Retrieved August 4, 2017, from http://www.aha.org/advocacy-issues/quality/accreditation-faq.shtml

information, and MedPar[125] data. Using this information, the surveyors can customize the process to the institution being reviewed.

- *Use of concurrent "tracer methods."* As mentioned above, in the past, accreditation surveyors reviewed documents retrospectively. The new process started to use tracer methods for reviews. In this method, surveyors select patients who are currently being treated at the time of the review and evaluate their care pathways. For hospitals, this activity means identifying current inpatients. Likewise, surveyors evaluate operational systems that directly impact patient quality and safety (e.g., infection control and medication management). The tracer targets (such as types of patients) are determined from the PFP.

- *Grading/reporting.* Starting in January 2004, the new accreditation decision categories were simplified to: Accredited; Provisional Accreditation; Conditional Accreditation; Preliminary Denial of Accreditation; Denial of Accreditation; and Preliminary Accreditation (under the Early Survey Option). Of more importance, however, in July 2004, the new quality reports were made available to the general public at: https://www .qualitycheck.org.[126]

2010–Present

All of the above programs have continued to evolve and spread throughout the healthcare system. More recently, two significant quality initiatives have been implemented by the federal government: those specifically mandated by the ACA and hospital-specific quality payment programs (QPPs) included in the Medicare Access and CHIP Reauthorization Act of 2015 (MACRA).

ACA Quality Improvement Initiatives. The ACA has increased access to healthcare by making insurance available and more affordable to millions of Americans. This availability alone has contributed to increased quality of care. However, the law mandates three specific quality-related programs. The ACA requires the HHS Secretary to establish two aligned initiatives: a National Strategy for Quality Improvement in Health Care (the NQS)[127] whose

---

[125] "The Medicare Provider and Analysis Review (MedPAR) Files contain inpatient hospital and/or skilled nursing facility (SNF) final action stay records for all Medicare beneficiaries. MedPAR files contain the following information: procedures, diagnoses, and DRGs; length of stay; beneficiary and Medicare payment amounts; and summarized revenue center charge amounts." CMSResearch Data Assistance Center. Retrieved July 13, 2018, from https://www.resdac.org/cms-data/file-family/MedPAR

[126] These reports are only summaries of the surveys and do not provide details. At the time of this writing, CMS has issued, for comment, proposed regulation changes that would require accrediting organizations to have their final accreditation survey reports and acceptable plans of corrections available on their websites. Retrieved from https://www.federalregister .gov/documents/2017/04/28/2017-07800/medicare-program-hospital-inpatient-prospective-payment-systems-for-acute-care-hospitals-and-the

[127] Agency for Healthcare Research and Quality. (2017, March). *About the national quality strategy*. Retrieved August 23, 2017, from https://www.ahrq.gov/workingforquality/about/index.html

purpose is to set national quality priorities and develop a strategy to implement them; and a National Prevention and Health Promotion Strategy,[128] geared more to providing improvement in population health. A third requirement is the hospital-initiated community health benefit program. All three are discussed below.

The NQS is run by the AHRQ and seeks to include opinions from across the industry in order to garner wide acceptance. More than 300 diverse groups participated in the original design and content when the program was started in 2011. An important ongoing participant is the National Priorities Partners, an assembly convened under the aegis of the NQF that includes the AARP, AFL-CIO, America's Health Insurance Plans, AMA, ANA, Consumers Union, Institute for Health Improvement, Joint Commission, Leapfrog Group, National Business Group on Health, NCQA, NQF, and U.S. Chambers of Commerce. The group's purpose is to:

- Identify national goals that correspond to the priorities put forth in the National Quality Strategy;
- Provide input on measures for tracking national progress toward the goals; and
- Offer guidance on strategic opportunities to accelerate improvement.[129]

As a result of this participation, the NQS developed three "Aims," supported by six "Priorities." To implement the program, it is expected that stakeholders will employ nine "Levers," representing a core business function, resource, and/or action. (Please see Exhibit 9.7 for an explanation of these features, Exhibit 9.8 for linkage of these

EXHIBIT 9.7. **Aims and Priorities of the NQS**

Aims

1. Better Care: Improve the overall quality, by making health care more patient-centered, reliable, accessible, and safe.

2. Healthy People/Healthy Communities: Improve the health of the U.S. population by supporting proven interventions to address behavioral, social and, environmental determinants of health in addition to delivering higher-quality care.

3. Affordable Care: Reduce the cost of quality health care for individuals, families, employers, and government.

Priorities

1. Making care safer by reducing harm caused in the delivery of care.

2. Ensuring that each person and family is engaged as partners in their care.

3. Promoting effective communication and coordination of care.

---

[128]U.S. Department of Health and Human Services; Surgeon General. *National prevention strategy*. Retrieved July 13, 2018, from https://www.surgeongeneral.gov/priorities/prevention/strategy/

[129]National Quality Forum. *National priorities partnership*. Retrieved July 13, 2018, from http://www.qualityforum.org/Setting_Priorities/NPP/National_Priorities_Partnership.aspx

4. Promoting the most effective prevention and treatment practices for the leading causes of mortality, starting with cardiovascular disease.

5. Working with communities to promote wide use of best practices to enable healthy living.

6. Making quality care more affordable for individuals, families, employers, and governments by developing and spreading new health care delivery models. This priority will be accomplished by:

   ■ Establishing Health Insurance Exchanges;

   ■ Fostering Innovations to Promote Quality and Reduce Cost (Through the Center for Medicare and Medicaid Innovation [CMMI]); and

   ■ Administrative Simplification

Levers

1. Measurement and Feedback: Provide performance feedback to plans and providers to improve care

2. Public Reporting: Compare treatment results, costs and patient experience for consumers

3. Learning and Technical Assistance: Foster learning environments that offer training, resources, tools, and guidance to help organizations achieve quality improvement goals

4. Certification, Accreditation, and Regulation: Adopt or adhere to approaches to meet safety and quality standards

5. Consumer Incentives and Benefit Designs: Help consumers adopt healthy behaviors and make informed decisions

6. Payment: Reward and incentivize providers to deliver high-quality, patient-centered care

7. Health Information Technology: Improve communication, transparency, and efficiency for better coordinated health and health care

8. Innovation and Diffusion: Foster innovation in health care quality improvement, and facilitate rapid adoption within and across organizations and communities

9. Workforce Development: Investing in people to prepare the next generation of health care professionals and support lifelong learning for providers

Source: Agency for Healthcare Research and Quality (2017, March). *About the national quality strategy*. Retrieved July 13, 2018, from https://www.ahrq.gov/workingforquality/about/index.html

components, and Exhibit 9.9 for examples of priority goals.) Each year, the NQS's progress is published in the National Healthcare Quality and Disparities Report,[130] which evaluates more than 250 measures.

Also, in 2011 CMS established the Quality Improvement Council (QIC) "to guide quality improvement and promote continual learning and dissemination of quality improvement activities." The QIC brings together affinity groups from different agencies with specific, themed objectives. In 2016, CMS expanded the affinity groups to support the implementation of the CMS Quality Strategy. (Please see Exhibit 9.10 for the structure of the QIC and its affinity groups.)

---

[130]For the latest report, see: AHRQ: National Healthcare Quality & Disparities Reports. June, 2018. Retrieved July 13, 2018, from https://www.ahrq.gov/research/findings/nhqrdr/index.html

EXHIBIT 9.8. **Relationship of Aims, Priorities, and Levers**

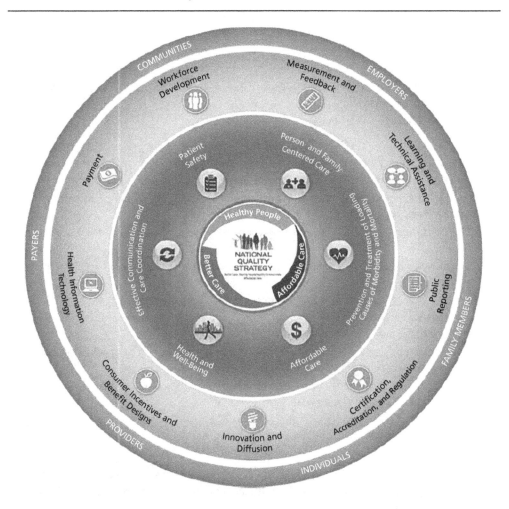

Source: Wilson, N. (2016, July 21). *The National Quality Strategy and the Public Sector: Federal Agency Alignment to the Six Priorities.* Retrieved July 13, 2018, from https://www.ahrq.gov/sites/default/files/wysiwyg/workingforquality/reports/webinar072116.pdf

Closely linked with the NQS is the National Prevention Strategy.[131] Its vision is to move "the nation from a focus on sickness and disease to one based on prevention and wellness"; its goal is to: "Increase the number of Americans who are healthy at every stage of life."

---

[131] Department of HHS. Surgeon General.gov: National Prevention Strategy. Retrieved July 13, 2018, from https://www.surgeongeneral.gov/priorities/prevention/strategy/

EXHIBIT 9.9. **National Quality Strategy Priorities and Goals, with Illustrative Measures**

Priority	Initial Goals, Opportunities for Success, and Illustrative Measures
#1 **Safer Care**	**Goal:** Eliminate preventable health care–acquired conditions **Opportunities for success:** Eliminate hospital-acquired infections Reduce the number of serious adverse medication events **Illustrative measures:** Standardized infection ratio for central line–associated blood stream infection as reported by CDC's National Healthcare Safety Network Incidence of serious adverse medication events
#2 **Effective Care Coordination**	**Goal:** Create a delivery system that is less fragmented and more coordinated, where handoffs are clear, and patients and clinicians have the information they need to optimize the patient-clinician partnership **Opportunities for success:** Reduce preventable hospital admissions and readmissions Prevent and manage chronic illness and disability Ensure secure information exchange to facilitate efficient care delivery **Illustrative measures:** All-cause readmissions within 30 days of discharge Percentage of providers who provide a summary record of care for transitions and referrals
#3 **Person- and Family-Centered Care**	**Goal:** Build a system that has the capacity to capture and act on patient-reported information, including preferences, desired outcomes, and experiences with health care **Opportunities for success:** Integrate patient feedback on preferences, functional outcomes, and experiences of care into all care settings and care delivery Increase use of EHRs that capture the voice of the patient by integrating patient-generated data in EHRs Routinely measure patient engagement and self-management, shared decision-making, and patient-reported outcomes **Illustrative measures:** Percentage of patients asked for feedback

Priority	Initial Goals, Opportunities for Success, and Illustrative Measures
#4 **Prevention and Treatment of Leading Causes of Mortality**	**Goal:** Prevent and reduce the harm caused by cardiovascular disease **Opportunities for success:** Increase blood pressure control in adults Reduce high cholesterol levels in adults Increase the use of aspirin to prevent cardiovascular disease Decrease smoking among adults and adolescents **Illustrative measures:** Percentage of patients ages 18 years and older with ischemic vascular disease whose most recent blood pressure during the measurement year is <140/90 mmHg Percentage of patients with ischemic vascular disease whose most recent low-density cholesterol is <100 Percentage of patients with ischemic vascular disease who have documentation of use of aspirin or other antithrombotic during the 12-month measurement period Percentage of patients who received evidence-based smoking cessation services (e.g., medications)
#5 **Supporting Better Health in Communities**	**Goal:** Support every U.S. community as it pursues its local health priorities **Opportunities for success:** Increase the provision of clinical preventive services for children and adults Increase the adoption of evidence-based interventions to improve health **Illustrative measures:** Percentage of children and adults screened for depression and receiving a documented follow-up plan Percentage of adults screened for risky alcohol use and if positive, received brief counseling Percentage of children and adults who use the oral health care system each year Proportion of U.S. population served by community water systems with optimally fluoridated water
#6 **Making Care More Affordable**	**Goal:** Identify and apply measures that can serve as effective indicators of progress in reducing costs **Opportunities for success:** Build cost and resource use measurement into payment reforms Establish common measures to assess the cost impacts of new programs and payment systems

Priority	Initial Goals, Opportunities for Success, and Illustrative Measures
	Reduce amount of health care spending that goes to administrative burden
	Make costs and quality more transparent to consumers
	Illustrative measures:
	To be developed

Source: The Center for Consumer Information & Insurance Oversight (2011, March). *Report to Congress: National Strategy for Quality Improvement in Health Care*. Retrieved July 13, 2018, from https://www.cms.gov/CCIIO/Resources/Forms-Reports-and-Other-Resources/quality03212011a.html

EXHIBIT 9.10. **Quality Improvement Council Affinity Groups**

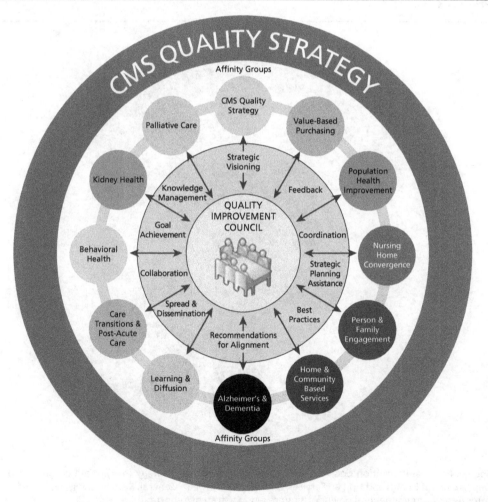

Source: Center for Clinical Standards and Quality Centers for Medicare & Medicaid Services (CMS) [Prepared by: Health Services Advisory Group, Inc.] (2017, June 2). *CMS Quality Measure Development Plan: Supporting the transition to the Quality Payment Program 2017. Annual Report*. Retrieved July 13, 2018, from https://www.cms.gov/Medicare/Quality-Initiatives-Patient-Assessment-Instruments/Value-Based-Programs/MACRA-MIPS-and-APMs/2017-CMS-MDP-Annual-Report.pdf

This goal along with strategic directions and priorities are summarized in Exhibit 9.11. This initiative draws on measures and indicators from a number of sources, most importantly *Healthy People 2020* (discussed below).

ACA Population Health Requirements. As mentioned above, the third quality-related program established by the ACA requires hospitals to actively pursue population health in their communities. The law adds Section 501(r) to the Internal Revenue Code of 1986, which requires 501(c)(3) organizations that operate one or more hospital facilities to

EXHIBIT 9.11. **National Prevention Strategy Goal, Strategic Directions, and Priorities**

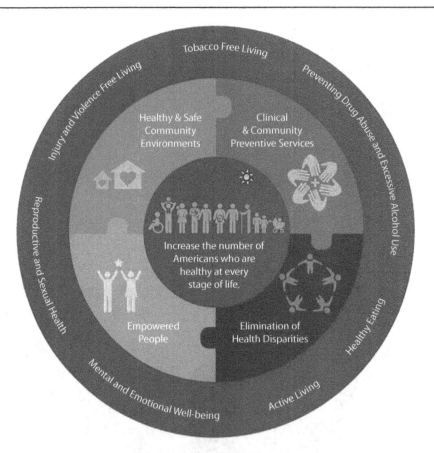

Source: National Prevention Council (2011). *National Prevention Strategy* (p. 7). Washington, DC: U.S. Department of Health and Human Services, Office of the Surgeon General. Retrieved July 13, 2018, from https://www.surgeongeneral.gov/priorities/prevention/strategy/report.pdf

conduct a community health needs assessment at least every 3 years. This evaluation must include "an implementation strategy to meet the community health needs identified through such assessment." The assessment must also take "into account input from persons who represent the broad interests of the community served by the hospital facility, including those with special knowledge of or expertise in public health" and make the report "widely available to the public."[132] The written report must be acceptable to the Secretary of HHS. Failure to comply can result in a $50,000 excise tax penalty and possible loss of tax-exempt status. Since the penalty is a tax and compliance could affect an organization's tax status, responsibility for the extensive and detailed regulations falls under the Internal Revenue Service.[133] Briefly, such reports must include not only community disease patterns but also assessment of barriers to care (including financial issues); prevention services; nutrition; and the social, behavioral, and environmental factors that affect the community's health.[134]

A related outcome of the Affordable Care Act is the Choosing Wisely program. Its origins can be traced to Dr. Howard Brody's call in 2010 for physicians to take a greater role in reducing the costs of care. He stated:

> I would propose that each specialty society commit itself immediately to appointing a blue-ribbon study panel to report, as soon as possible, that specialty's "Top Five" list... The Top Five list would consist of five diagnostic tests or treatments that are very commonly ordered by members of that specialty, that are among the most expensive services provided, and that have been shown by the currently available evidence not to provide any meaningful benefits to at least to some major categories of patients for whom they are commonly ordered.[135]

Subsequently, the Good Stewardship Working Group of the National Physicians Alliance (NPA) conducted surveys of physicians in family medicine, internal medicine and pediatrics to get consensus on non-value-added services. Their results were published in 2011:

> Physicians can adhere to the principles of professionalism by practicing high-quality, evidence-based care and advocating for just and cost-effective distribution of finite clinical resources. To promote these principles, the National Physicians Alliance (NPA) initiated a project titled "Promoting Good Stewardship in Clinical Practice" that aimed to develop a

---

[132]Compilation of the Patient Protection and Affordable Care Act [as Amended through May 1, 2010]. Public Law 111–148. Title IX—Revenue Provisions. Subtitle A—Revenue Offset Provisions Sec. 9007. Additional requirements for charitable hospitals. P. 802.

[133]*Federal Register* Vol. 79 No. 250 Part II. Pages 78954–79016. December 31, 2014. Department of the Treasury, Internal Revenue Service 26 CFR Parts 1, 53, and 602: Additional Requirements for Charitable Hospitals; Community Health Needs Assessments for Charitable Hospitals; Requirement of a Section 4959 Excise Tax Return and Time for Filing the Return; Final Rule. Retrieved July 13, 2018, from https://www.gpo.gov/fdsys/pkg/FR-2014-12-31/pdf/2014-30525.pdf

[134]James, J. (2016, February 25). Nonprofit hospitals' community benefit requirements. Under the Affordable Care Act, many nonprofit hospitals must meet new requirements to retain their tax-exempt status. *Health Affairs, Health Policy Brief*. Retrieved July 13, 2018, from http://healthaffairs.org/healthpolicybriefs/brief_pdfs/healthpolicybrief_153.pdf

[135]Brody, H. (2010). Medicine's ethical responsibility for health care reform—The top five list. *The New England Journal of Medicine, 362*, 283–285.

list of the top 5 activities in family medicine, internal medicine, and pediatrics where the quality of care could be improved.[136]

In that article, specific recommendations were made for the three surveyed specialties. For example, for family medicine: "Don't order annual ECGs or any other cardiac screening for asymptomatic, low-risk patients" and "Don't perform Pap tests on patients younger than 21 years or in women status post [after] hysterectomy for benign disease"; for internal medicine: "Don't obtain blood chemistry panels... or urinalyses for screening in asymptomatic, healthy adults" and "Use only generic statins when initiating lipid-lowering drug therapy"; and for pediatrics: "Advise patients not to use cough and cold medications" and "Use inhaled corticosteroids to control asthma appropriately."

As a result of these publications, in April 2012, the American Board of Internal Medicine Foundation (which sponsored the Working Group Study) and *Consumer Reports*

> formally launched the *Choosing Wisely* campaign with the release of "Top Five" lists from nine specialty societies... The widespread media coverage from nearly every top-tier outlet, along with positive reaction from the health care community, inspired 17 additional societies to join the campaign and release lists in February 2013.[137]

At present, more than 80 specialty societies have joined the campaign, which has expanded from physician organizations to nursing, dentistry, physical therapy, and pharmacy groups. To highlight the benefits of this initiative and recognize clinicians who led important programmatic changes, the Choosing Wisely Champions program was launched in March 2016. Three champions highlight the types of initiatives of this program:

- Radiologist Jeffrey P. Kanne helped create appropriateness criteria, which reduced routine ordering of daily chest radiographs for patients in intensive care and routine preoperative chest radiographs for asymptomatic, low-risk patients.

- Geriatrician Heidi A. Courtney's work resulted in more than 1,000 drug adjustments for elderly patients, including an effort aimed at delirium prevention that decreased incidence from 20.8% to 15.1% in the first year.

- Clinical pathologist Dana Altenburger decreased inpatient blood product usage by 46% over 3 years.

Medicare Access and CHIP Reauthorization Act of 2015. For many years, the federal government has been concerned that Medicare, Medicaid, and CHIP (formerly SCHIP) payments are largely volume-based (i.e., the more providers do, the more they are paid) rather than value-based (i.e., payments linked to quality performance). The first attempt to fix this

---

[136]The Good Stewardship Working Group. (2011). The "Top 5" lists in primary care: Meeting the responsibility of professionalism. *Archives of Internal Medicine* [now *JAMA Medicine*], *171*(15), 1385–1390.

[137]Choosing Wisely. (2017). *A special report on the first five years*. Retrieved July 13, 2018, from http://www .choosingwisely.org/wp-content/uploads/2017/10/Choosing-Wisely-at-Five.pdf For more extensive information, see the main website, http://www.choosingwisely.org/

problem occurred with passage of the Tax Relief and Health Care Act of 2006, which created the Physician Quality Reporting System (PQRS). Under that system, "eligible providers" (those who furnish services to Medicare beneficiaries) could choose specialty-specific quality measures to report to Medicare. Options existed for providers to report as individuals or, if appropriate, as a group (Group Practice Reporting Option). Initially, reporting was voluntary, without penalties or bonuses. The program was extended in the Medicare, Medicaid, and SCHIP Extension Act of 2007, the Medicare Improvements for Patients and Providers Act (MIPPA) of 2008, and the ACA of 2010. MIPPA made the program permanent; the ACA extended the PQRS incentive payments to 2014 and established penalties for non- or inadequate reporting to be applied in 2015. The quality measures used for the evaluations were issued by the NQF.

In addition to the PQRS provisions, MIPPA (Section 131) amended Section 1848 of the Social Security Act requiring the HHS Secretary to

> establish a Physician Feedback Program ... under which the Secretary shall use claims data under this title (and may use other data) to provide confidential reports to physicians ... that *measure the resources involved in furnishing care* to individuals under this title. If determined appropriate by the Secretary, the Secretary *may include information on the quality of care* furnished to individuals under this title by the physician (or group of physicians) in such reports. [Emphases added.]

The ACA (Section 3003) further extended this provision to require the HHS Secretary to

> develop an episode grouper that combines separate but clinically related items and services into an episode of care for an individual, as appropriate ...

> Effective beginning with 2012, the Secretary shall provide reports to physicians that compare ... patterns of resource use of the individual physician to such patterns of other physicians ...

> The Secretary shall, for purposes of preparing reports under this paragraph, establish methodologies as appropriate, such as to—

> (i)   attribute episodes of care, in whole or in part, to physicians;

> (ii) identify appropriate physicians for purposes of comparison ... ; and

> (iii) aggregate episodes of care attributed to a physician ... into a composite measure per individual ...

> In preparing reports under this paragraph, the Secretary shall make appropriate adjustments, including adjustments—

> (i)   to account for differences in socioeconomic and demographic characteristics, ethnicity, and health status of individuals (such as to recognize that less healthy individuals may require more intensive interventions); and

> (ii) to eliminate the effect of geographic adjustments in payment rates.

Results are to be made available to the public.

The purpose of these provisions was to create a Value-Based Payment Modifier (VBPM) that would be used to alter physician payments based on adjusted, comparative resource utilization for episodes of care. For example, based on 2016 reporting, 2018 VBPM penalties could range from −4% of Medicare payments (for groups of more than 10 physicians) to −2% for smaller reporting entities.

While these previous laws and regulations set the stage for future activities, the provisions changed in 2015 with passage of the Medicare Access and CHIP Reauthorization Act (MACRA). This law was passed for several reasons:

1. The CHIP needed to be reauthorized so it would not lose funding. MACRA extended this program to 2017. (It is now funded to 2027.)

2. The federal government needed a "fix" for the Sustainable Growth Rate (SGR) formula used for Medicare payments. (See the Medicare Part B section in Chapter 6.) This methodology was causing ever-increasing payment deficits that had never been corrected and perpetuated Medicare's payment-by-volume methodology. In repealing the SGR process, MACRA substituted a modest, fixed-fee escalator[138] and, more importantly, a value-based payment system with rewards and penalties called the Quality Payment Program.

3. The quality incentives were fragmented and getting complicated to administer. To fix these problems, the PQRS and Value-Based Modifier programs were consolidated into one plan along with the "Meaningful Use" payments and penalties concerning employment of information systems. (See Chapter 8, "Information Technology," for more details about Meaningful Use.)

4. Because of increasing fraudulent use of Medicare numbers (which mirrored Social Security numbers), MACRA mandated existing numbers would be replaced by new Medicare Beneficiary Identifiers (MBIs) in 2019. (For newly enrolled beneficiaries, the MBIs started in 2018.)

Although the exact terms of MACRA's quality assessments continue to evolve, the overall plan is described below.

The program applies to a category of providers called "Eligible Clinicians" (ECs), who include physicians, physician assistants, nurse practitioners, clinical nurse specialists, and certified registered nurse anesthetists. The EC list may be expanded by HHS in 2019 to include physical or occupational therapists, speech-language pathologists, audiologists, clinical social workers, and clinical psychologists.

ECs may participate in one of two QPPs. The first, the Merit-based Incentive Payment System (MIPS), is intended for solo practitioners and those in small groups. It contains four performance categories[139] that are combined into a weighted Composite Performance Score to adjust EC's payments:

---

[138] From July 1, 2015, to December 31, 2019, Medicare physician reimbursement rates will increase by 0.5% annually. Thereafter, through December 31, 2025, payment rates are frozen.

[139] CMS Quality Payment Program, available at https://qpp.cms.gov/ July 13, 2018. This site has a comprehensive list of the quality reporting measures in each Performance category.

1. *Quality Metrics* (replaces PQRS/Group Practice Reporting Option). Began as 60% of the composite measure in 2017 and will be reduced to 50% by 2020.

    Examples: High Priority category for Internal Medicine that can be submitted via electronic health record (EHR) or claims submission:

    Controlling High Blood Pressure: Percentage of patients 18–85 years of age who had a diagnosis of hypertension and whose blood pressure was adequately controlled (<140/90 mmHg) during the measurement period.

    Diabetes: Hemoglobin A1c Poor Control (>9): Percentage of patients 18–75 years of age with diabetes who had hemoglobin A1c > 9.0% during the measurement period

2. *Advancing Care Information* (replaces Meaningful Use). Will remain at 25% of the composite measure from 2017 to 2020. Under this category, ECs have two options:

    Option 1: Advancing Care Information Objectives and Measures (19) or

    Option 2: 2017 Advancing Care Information Transition Objectives and Measures (11).

    Compliance involves participation in: e-prescribing; health information exchanges; immunization registry reporting; medication reconciliation; patient-specific education; providing patient access; secure messaging; security risk analysis; specialized registry reporting; syndromic surveillance reporting; and having at least one patient view, download, or transmit health information to a third party.

3. *Cost* (replaces Value-Based modifier). Was not counted in 2017 but will be 10% of the composite by 2020. (Originally the intent was for this component to be 30%, but industry lobbying caused CMS to reduce the figure.) No reporting is needed since CMS will calculate this score using claims and base it on: total per capita Parts A and B costs for all beneficiaries attributed to an EC, Medicare spending per beneficiary, and episode-based measures.

4. *Clinical Practice Improvement Activities*. This category was new and remains at 15% of the composite from 2017 to 2020.

    Measures in this category include: achieving health equity; behavioral and mental health; beneficiary engagement; care coordination; emergency response and preparedness; expanded practice in access; patient safety and practice assessments; and population management.
    Example: In the "achieving health equity" measure:

    Engagement of new Medicaid patients and follow-up:
    Seeing new and follow-up Medicaid patients in a timely manner, including individuals dually eligible for Medicaid and Medicare.

As mentioned above, reporting started in 2017 to determine payment adjustments starting in 2019. After that date, depending on the Composite Performance Score, Medicare payment penalties are capped at 4% in 2019, 5% in 2020, 7% in 2021, and 9% in 2022 and in subsequent years. Bonuses can be as much as three times the annual penalty cap. Overriding payment of these bonuses, however, is the mandate for budget neutrality before mandatory fee updates have been applied. Each year's penalty or bonus has no effect on subsequent years.

Three conditions for exemption from MIPS participation are:

1. Low-volume Medicare participation ($90,000 in Medicare Part B charges during specified periods or 200 or fewer Medicare patients)[140]

2. Billing Medicare for the first year

3. Significant participation in an Advanced Alternative Payment Model (APM) program, which is the *second* QPP option

The APM option engaged a significant number of ECs (approximately 185,000–250,000 providers in 2018) and is explained below.

While the MIPS option has strong quality requirements, one purpose of MACRA is to encourage innovation by establishing value-added care programs whereby providers bear financial risk. These programs can be directed at a specific condition, care episode, or population. By implementing such plans, MACRA hopes that APMs will "contribute to better care and smarter spending by allowing physicians and other clinicians to deliver coordinated, customized, high-quality care to their patients within a streamlined payment system." In return for participating in this higher risk APM, ECs:

- Are excluded from MIPS requirements.
- Will receive annual bonuses (for 2019–2024) equal to 5% of the previous year's Part B payments, regardless of their performance scores.
- Will receive a Physician Fee Schedule update of 0.75% instead of 0.25% for the MIPS model (starting in 2026).[141]

In order to qualify for payment (and MIPS exemption) under the APM option, ECs must:

- Use a certified EHR.
- Be paid quality incentives based on quality measures comparable to those in MIPS.
- Bear more than nominal financial risk for their participation in the program or be part of a medical home. The risk is two-sided, i.e., based on what Medicare considers a target

---

[140]The exemptions allow 934,000 providers to opt out of MIPS, leaving only 39% of the 1.5 million clinicians billing under Medicare required to comply. The exclusions were updated November 2, 2017: Medicare Program; Revisions to Payment Policies under the Physician Fee Schedule and Other Revisions to Part B for CY 2018; Medicare Shared Savings Program Requirements; and Medicare Diabetes Prevention Program. Retrieved July 13, 2018, from https://s3.amazonaws.com/public-inspection.federalregister.gov/2017-23953.pdf?utm_campaign=government-affairs& utm_medium=email&utm_source=11.1.17 Special Alert Washington Connection %281%29&elqEmailId=6101

[141]From July 1, 2015 to December 31, 2019, physicians will receive a 0.5% annual Medicare reimbursement rate increase; from January 1, 2020 through December 31, 2025, payment rates are frozen.

rate for payment to the APM, ECs will be rewarded for program savings but also be responsible for a portion of any losses.[142]

■ Meet revenue or volume-based requirements. Initially, the organization of ECs must receive at least 25% of its Medicare payments through the APM activity or have 20% of its Medicare patients receiving care through the APM. Those numbers will increase to 75% and 50%, respectively, by 2021 and apply to all subsequent years.

The five types of organizations that qualify for the APM option are:

1. *Accountable Care Organizations (ACOs).* (See Chapter 4, "Hospitals and Health Systems," and Chapter 6, "Payers," for an explanation of this model.)

   ■ Medicare Shared Savings Program (MSSP) Track 2

   ■ MSSP Track 3

   ■ Next Generation ACO Model (including the Vermont All-Payer ACO Model[143])

   ■ Comprehensive End-Stage Renal Disease (ESRD) Care Two-Sided Risk Model

   ■ MSSP Track 1+ (New for 2018. The traditional Track 1 does not have enough downside risk to qualify as an APM. This new version will have a 50% shared savings rate and a fixed 30% shared losses rate.)

2. *Bundled Payment Models*

   ■ *Oncology care.* This bundle includes fee-for-service (FFS) payments, per-beneficiary Monthly Enhanced Oncology Services payments, and performance-based payments for a 6-month episode of chemotherapy. ECs must be part of the two-sided financial risk track to be considered a qualifying participant. If the episode's costs exceed the target price, providers will have to pay some of the difference back.

   ■ *Comprehensive care for joint replacement models.* Providers are at risk for the cost and quality of care starting with a hospital admission and lasting for 90 days after discharge. Penalties increase to 20% of the target cost by year 3.

   ■ Additional bundled payment models authorized as APMs for 2018. (All will start on hospital admission, include the 90-day post-discharge period and have the same shared savings rates: 5% of target price in the first 3 performance years; 10% of

---

[142] The downside risk is defined by three conditions: The financial responsibility for losses must start at no higher than 4% above the target payment rate; if the APM goes over spending targets, it must be at financial risk for at least 30% of the excess. While the APM can buy stop-loss insurance, the maximum amount of losses must be at least 4% of the spending target. For example, regardless of the exact terms of its scheme, if the target spending is $1 million and the APM exceeds that amount by $100,000, it must be responsible for payment of at least $40,000 (even after reinsurance pays). For a more detailed explanation with examples, see Atlas, R. F., Tatge, D. B., & Yeung, L. R. (2016). *All about APMs: What will it take for physicians to earn the APM bonus under MACRA?* Epstein, Becker, Green Client Alert. Retrieved July 13, 2018, from http://www.ebglaw.com/content/uploads/2016/06/HCLS-Client-Alert-All-About-APMs.pdf

[143] See CMS.gov. Vermont All-Payer ACO Model. Retrieved July 14, 2018, from https://innovation.cms.gov/initiatives/vermont-all-payer-aco-model/

target price in the fourth performance year; and 20% of target price in the fifth performance year.) These programs are for acute myocardial infarctions, coronary artery bypass grafts (CABGs), and surgical hip and femur fracture treatments.

3. *Primary Care Models*

a) *CPC+ Model.* This model is open to primary care practitioners (physicians, nurse practitioners, physician assistants, and clinical nurse specialists) who have their principal specialty designations in family medicine, geriatrics, or internal medicine. The practice can be independently owned; hospital/health system owned; within an Independent Practice Association (IPA); or participating in a commercial ACO or commercial Clinically Integrated Network. Excluded are Federally Qualified Health Centers (FQHCs), Rural Health Clinics (RHCs), concierge practices (or any practice that charges patients a retainer fee), and pediatric practices. While multispecialty practices can also qualify, for purposes of eligibility, CMS will only "count" beneficiaries who are in treatment relationships with primary care clinicians (at least 150 Medicare beneficiaries and approximately 50% or more of their current revenue generated by payer partners and Medicare).

Further, to participate, eligible CPC+ practices must perform five comprehensive primary care functions:[144] access and continuity; care management; comprehensiveness and coordination; patient and caregiver engagement; and planned care and population health.

Eligible CPC+ primary care providers can join one of two payment tracks (Track 1 and Track 2), which include three payment elements:[145]

(i) *Care Management Fee (CMF).* Both Tracks 1 and 2 will receive a set CMF paid per-beneficiary-per month (PBPM). The amount is risk-adjusted for each beneficiary using the Medicare hierarchical condition category (HCC) score. (See Chapter 6: this adjuster is the same one used by CMS to adjust Medicare Advantage payments.)

(ii) *Performance-Based Incentive Payment.* Under the CPC+, CMS will prospectively pay and retrospectively reconcile a performance-based incentive based on how well the practice performs on:

Clinical quality/patient experience measures based on performance metrics on electronic clinical quality measures (eCQM) and Consumer Assessment of Healthcare Providers and Systems (CAHPS)—a measure of patient satisfaction.

Utilization measures created from practice-level, claims-based data gathered at the practice level, including inpatient admissions and emergency department visits as well as office visits.

---

[144]For a detailed description of these five elements, see CPC+ Practice Care Delivery Requirements. Retrieved July 14, 2018, from https://innovation.cms.gov/Files/x/cpcplus-practicecaredlvreqs.pdf

[145]*Comprehensive Primary Care Plus (CPC+) Round 2* (2017, July 10). Retrieved July 14, 2018, from https://innovation.cms.gov/Files/x/cpcplus-practiceapplicationfaq.pdf

(iii) *Payment under the Medicare Physician Fee Schedule.* Track 1 continues to bill and receive FFS Medicare payments. Track 2 practices also continue to bill as usual, but the FFS payment will be reduced to account for CMS shifting a portion of Medicare FFS payments into Comprehensive Primary Care Payments (CPCPs), which will be paid in a lump sum on a quarterly basis absent a claim. The CPCP amounts are expected to be greater than the FFS payment amounts they are intended to replace.

In addition to CPCPs, CMFs and performance-based payments are higher for Track 2 than Track 1, but the downside risk (return of advanced payments) is also greater.[146] Further, over the next several years, the Medicare FFS payments will decrease as the other payments increase on a cost-neutral basis. CMS hopes this shift will give practices the flexibility and incentive to deliver care with more cost-effective and flexible approaches (e.g., electronic and alternate site visits).

b) *Medical Home Model Expanded.* The "Medical Home" category under MACRA can be quite confusing. The three different organizational classifications have different payment methods. In the first category are EC or groups who have received certification or accreditation as a PCMH by a national accrediting body. These organizations will be paid according to MIPS and receive full credit in the category of Clinical Practice Improvement Activities. The CPC+ models described above are in a second category often described as medical homes. As already mentioned, these organizations must bear some financial risk and are paid as previously described. The third category is a Medical Home Model with expanded status. To achieve this status, the group must meet criteria set by the Center for Medicare and Medicaid Innovation (CMMI) demonstration expansion authority under Section 1115A(C) of MACRA.[147] The advantage of having this qualification is that practitioners are exempt from the financial risks required of APMs. Although no models have yet been deemed eligible (and thus financial terms are not clear), if an organization is to qualify, the HHS Secretary must determine that the Medical Home expansion:

- Is expected to reduce spending without reducing the quality of care; or improve the quality of care without increasing spending (as determined by CMMI);

- Will not result in any increase in net program spending (as certified by CMS' Chief Actuary); and

- Will not deny or limit the coverage or provision of benefits for applicable individuals.

---

[146] *CPC+ Payment Methodologies: Beneficiary Attribution, Care Management Fee, Performance-Based Incentive Payment, and Payment Under the Medicare Physician Fee Schedule for Program Year 2018* (2017, December). Retrieved July 14, 2018, from https://innovation.cms.gov/Files/x/cpcplus-methodology.pdf

[147] MACRA. Center for Medicare and Medicaid Innovation, Sec. 1115A. [42 U.S.C. 1315a] Retrieved July 14, 2018, from https://www.ssa.gov/OP_Home/ssact/title11/1115A.htm

Operationally, this expanded Medical Home must:[148]

- Be composed of primary care practices or multispecialty practices that include primary care physicians and practitioners and offer primary care services. ECs include: General Practitioners; Family Physicians; Internists; Pediatricians; Geriatricians; and Primary Care Nurse Practitioners, Clinical Nurse Specialists, and Physician Assistants *and*

- Assign ("empanel") each patient to a primary clinician. (This provision is very important since many managed care plans and governmental programs only assign patients to a group.)

Further, this model must participate in at least four of the following activities:

- Planned coordination of chronic and preventive care

- Patient access and continuity of care

- Risk-stratified care management

- Coordination of care across the medical neighborhood

- Patient and caregiver engagement

- Shared decision-making

- Payment arrangements in addition to, or substituting for, FFS payments (e.g., shared savings, population-based payments)

4. *Specialty Care Models.* APMs can be specialty care-based as long as they fulfill basic APM criteria. The two currently approved models for this category are Comprehensive ESRD (End Stage Renal Dialysis) Care (CEC)[149] and the Oncology Care Model (OCM),[150] which is risk-based as opposed to the bundled payment oncology model described above.

5. *Newer Models.* In addition to the models just described, CMS has a mechanism for approving new APMs.[151] The applicant must submit its request to the CMMI for review and approval and substantively address the following questions:

- What type(s) of APM(s) would your design be?

- How will your APM result in clinical practice transformation?

---

[148] A Rule by the Centers for Medicare & Medicaid Services. (2016, November 4). Medicare program; Merit-Based Incentive Payment System (MIPS), and Alternative Payment Model (APM) incentive under the physician fee schedule, and criteria for physician-focused payment models. *Federal Register*, 77008–77831. Retrieved July 14, 2018, from https://www.federalregister.gov/documents/2016/11/04/2016-25240/medicare-program-merit-based-incentive-payment-system-mips-and-alternative-payment-model-apm For an update, see: Centers for Medicare & Medicaid Services. (2017). Medicare program; CY 2018 updates to the quality payment program. *Federal Register*, 82(125), 30010–30500. Retrieved July 14, 2018, from https://www.gpo.gov/fdsys/pkg/FR-2017-06-30/pdf/2017-13010.pdf

[149] Comprehensive ESRD Care Model. Retrieved July 14, 2018, from https://innovation.cms.gov/initiatives/comprehensive-esrd-care/

[150] Oncology Care Model. Retrieved July 14, 2018, from https://innovation.cms.gov/initiatives/oncology-care/

[151] For an overview of this process, see Alternative Payment Model Design Toolkit. Retrieved July 14, 2018, from https://innovation.cms.gov/Files/x/apm-toolkit.pdf

■ What is the rationale for your APM?

■ What is the scale of your APM?

■ How does your APM align with other payers and CMS programs?

■ How is improved clinical quality or better patient experience of care measured under your APM?

■ How easy would it be for participants to implement your APM?

Since MACRA started in 2017 and the financial changes will not start until 2019, the overall impact has yet to be seen. In the meantime, the RAND Corporation's Health Care Payment and Delivery Simulation Model estimates that "MACRA will decrease Medicare spending on physician services by −$35 to −$106 billion (−2.3 percent to −7.1 percent) and change spending on hospital services by −$32 to −$250 billion (0.7 percent to −5.1 percent) in 2015–30."[152]

At this point, it is useful to reflect on the complexity of the quality assessment environment and the burden it places on healthcare institutions. Exhibit 9.12 displays many of the health and safety regulatory reporting requirements hospitals face. Some additional requirements include Centers for Disease Control and Prevention (CDC) reporting and compliance with local toxic waste disposal laws. Other healthcare providers, such as skilled nursing facilities, may face similarly complex requirements.

QUALITY OF CARE AND THE PUBLIC'S HEALTH

Most of the initiatives mentioned in this chapter have been directed at improving the quality of care of *individuals*. At a public health level, one organization and a related initiative must be considered with respect to population-based quality of care: the Centers for Disease Control and Prevention and the Healthy People programs.

The Centers for Disease Control and Prevention

The CDC began in Atlanta during World War II as the Malaria Control in War Areas program, tasked with keeping the country safe from that disease. On July 1, 1946, it became the Communicable Disease Center[153] with a broader national mission to "support state and local health units in investigating and controlling communicable disease outbreaks"[154] and maintain the nation's health through local measures.

---

[152]Hussey, P. S., Liu, J. L., & White, C. (2017). The Medicare access and CHIP Reauthorization Act: Effects on Medicare payment policy and spending. *Health Affairs, 36* (4): 697–705.

[153]The Communicable Disease Center was renamed the Center for Disease Control in 1970. The word "Center" was changed to "Centers" in 1981. The name was again changed in 1992 to Centers for Disease Control and Prevention. By law, it retained its designation: "CDC."

[154]CDC. *Our History—Our Story*. Retrieved July 14, 2018, from https://www.cdc.gov/about/history/ourstory.htm Although the CDC was supposed to act as coordinator for all communicable diseases, venereal diseases and tuberculosis were managed by the Public Health Service. Responsibility for those conditions was transferred in 1957 and 1960, respectively.

EXHIBIT 9.12. Complexity of Quality-Related Activities Confronting Hospitals

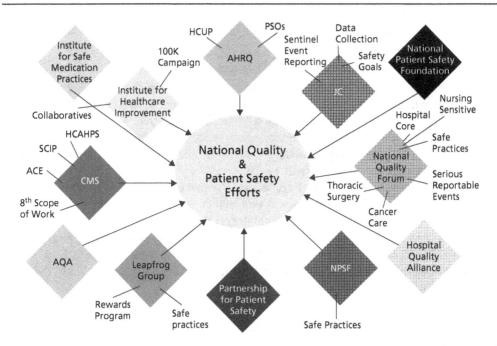

Source: National Committee on Vital Health Statistics (NCVHS) Ad Hoc Work Group on Secondary Uses of Health Data. Retrieved July 14, 2018, from www.ncvhs.hhs.gov/wp-content/uploads/2014/08/070719p2 .pdf

The CDC's national security role began during the Korean War, when the Epidemic Intelligence Service (EIS) was created to monitor the threat of biological warfare. The center's investigative capabilities were tested in 1955 when children who had received the Salk polio vaccine came down with that illness. The problem was successfully traced to manufacturing contamination at Cutter Laboratories; it was corrected, and the suspended national immunization program was resumed.[155] Two years later, CDC surveillance methods tracked the course of a massive influenza epidemic; this process guided subsequent annual, national influenza vaccine development.

---

[155]Offitt, P. A. (2005). *The cutter incident: How America's first polio vaccine led to the growing vaccine risis.* New Haven: Yale University Press.

In 1961, the CDC assumed responsibility[156] for publishing the *Morbidity and Mortality Weekly Report (MMWR)*,[157] the nation's most important source of timely public health information and recommendations. For example, the *MMWR* publishes weekly incidences of infectious diseases and recommendations for immunizations. To complement this activity, in 1981, the National Center for Health Statistics was moved to the CDC.

Subsequently, other public health responsibilities were added to the CDC's communicable disease portfolio: the National Institute for Occupational Safety and Health; Office of Noncommunicable Diseases, Injury, and Environmental Health; National Center on Birth Defects and Developmental Disabilities; National Center for Chronic Disease Prevention and Health Promotion; National Center for Environmental Health/Agency for Toxic Substances and Disease Registry; and National Center for Injury Prevention and Control.[158]

Currently, the CDC sees its roles as:

- Detecting and responding to new and emerging health threats
- Tackling the biggest health problems causing death and disability for Americans
- Putting science and advanced technology into action to prevent disease
- Promoting healthy and safe behaviors, communities and environment
- Developing leaders and training the public health workforce, including disease detectives
- Taking the health pulse of our nation[159]

It aims to fulfill these roles through three Strategic Priorities:[160]

Strategic Priority #1. By working at home and in more than 60 countries, the CDC seeks to improve global health security by detecting, tracking, diagnosing, and responding to new (e.g., Zika) and existing (e.g., influenza) diseases. Examples of past successes have included helping achieve global eradication of smallpox (1977) and naming and tracking what came to be known as acquired immunodeficiency syndrome (AIDS)—first mentioned in the *MMWR* on June 5, 1981.

---

[156]The publication's "history began on April 29, 1878, when Congress passed the National Quarantine Act. The Act required the Surgeon General of the U.S. Marine-Hospital Service (later to become the U.S. Public Health Service [PHS]) to collect reports from U.S. consular officers on the sanitary condition of vessels departing for the United States and to give notice of these vessels to federal and state officers through weekly abstracts. This mandate resulted in *The Bulletin of the Public Health*, the first precursor of *MMWR*." Shaw, F. E., Goodman, R. A., Lindegren, M. L., & Ward, J. W. (2011). A history of MMWR. *MMWR Supplements*, *60*(4), 7–14.

[157]Reports are free and can be found at https://www.cdc.gov/mmwr/index.html Retrieved July 14, 2018.

[158]For the organizational chart of the CDC, see https://www.cdc.gov/about/pdf/organization/cdc-photo-org-chart.pdf Retrieved July 14, 2018.

[159]CDC. *Mission, role and pledge.* Retrieved July 14, 2018, from https://www.cdc.gov/about/organization/mission.htm

[160]*Centers for Disease Control and Prevention's Strategic Framework, FY 2016–FY 2020.* Retrieved July 14, 2018, from https://www.cdc.gov/about/pdf/cdc-strategic-framework.pdf

Strategic Priority #2. Prevent and monitor the leading causes of illness, injury, disability, and death by providing timely, quality data on priority health and healthcare issues at the national, state, and local levels to improve the health of Americans. For example, reporting and tracking vaccination patterns have led to historically low incidences of vaccine-preventable illnesses.

Strategic Priority #3. Strengthening public health and healthcare collaboration by leveraging partnerships. For example, the CDC has worked with clinicians and healthcare organizations to decrease antibiotic-resistant infections, issue the Guideline for Prescribing Opioids for Chronic Pain to reduce overdoses and deaths, and recommend preventive screening to reduce mortality from cancers.

Healthy People

Prior to about 1980, the United States lacked an overarching plan for the nation's health and disease prevention. This situation began to change in 1979, when Dr. Julius B. Richmond issued *The Surgeon General's Report on Health Promotion and Disease Prevention.*[161] In its introduction, Richmond stated: "It is the thesis of this report that further improvements in the health of the American people can and will be achieved—not alone through increased medical care and greater health expenditures—but through a renewed national commitment to efforts designed to prevent disease and to promote health."

The report identified measurable goals for improving the health of five demographic groups: infants, children, adolescents and young adults, adults, and older adults. The following year, Richmond issued a more extensive companion document: *Promoting Health/Preventing Disease: Objectives for the Nation.*[162] The plan in this document set out specific and quantifiable objectives for controlling and promoting understanding of: (1) high blood pressure; (2) family planning; (3) pregnancy and infant health; (4) immunization; (5) sexually transmitted diseases; (6) fluoridation and dental health; (7) surveillance and control of infectious diseases; (8) smoking; (9) misuse of alcohol and drugs; (10) physical fitness and exercise; (11) control of stress and violent behavior; (12) toxic agents; (13) occupational safety and health; (14) accident prevention and injury; and (15) nutrition. These objectives were to be achieved by 1990 and act as a blueprint for health improvement activities run by federal, state, and local governmental agencies as well as individuals, families, and community-based organizations.

By 1987, some of the objective areas showed improvement (hypertension, childhood infectious diseases, and injury prevention); but because other conditions still needed work, and public health priorities had evolved and changed (such as the emergence of the human immunodeficiency virus [HIV] infection), the Public Health Service began plans for the next

---

[161] Public Health Service. (1979). *The Surgeon General's report on health promotion and disease prevention.* [Healthy People 1979]. Washington, DC: U.S. Department of Health, Education, and Welfare, Public Health Service; DHEW publication no. (PHS)79-55071. Retrieved July 14, 2018, from https://profiles.nlm.nih.gov/ps/access/NNBBGK.pdf

[162] Public Health Service. (1980). *Promoting health/preventing disease: Objectives for the nation.* [Healthy People 1980]. Washington, DC: U.S. Department of Health and Human Services, Public Health Service. Retrieved July 14, 2018, from http://files.eric.ed.gov/fulltext/ED209206.pdf

10 years. In 1990, *Healthy People 2000: National Health Promotion and Disease Prevention Objectives* was published and expanded the previous priorities to these areas:

1. Physical activity and fitness
2. Nutrition
3. Tobacco
4. Substance abuse: alcohol and other drugs
5. Family planning
6. Mental health and mental disorders
7. Violent and abusive behavior
8. Educational and community-based programs
9. Unintentional injuries
10. Occupational safety and health
11. Environmental health
12. Food and drug safety
13. Oral health
14. Maternal and infant health
15. Heart disease and stroke
16. Cancer
17. Diabetes and chronic disabling conditions
18. HIV infection
19. Sexually transmitted diseases
20. Immunization and infectious diseases
21. Clinical preventive services
22. Surveillance and data systems

In 2001, the Healthy People 2000 Final Review[163] reported that:

[P]rogress was achieved on over 60 percent of the objectives. Some of the major accomplishments include surpassing the target for reducing deaths from coronary heart disease and cancer. The Nation also met its targets for AIDS incidence, primary and secondary syphilis cases, mammography exams, and violent (homicide, suicide, and firearm-related) deaths. The tobacco-related mortality targets were also met. Both infant mortality and the number of children with elevated blood lead levels nearly met their targets as well. The Nation also made progress toward the goal of reducing health disparities for more than one-half of the special population objectives identified to be at increased risk.

---

[163]Department of Health and Human Services. Centers for Disease Control and Prevention National Center for Health Statistics Hyattsville, MD. October 2001 DHHS Publication No. 01-0256. Retrieved July 14, 2018, from https://www .cdc.gov/nchs/data/hp2000/hp2k01.pdf

By that time, Healthy People 2010 was under way and added these focus areas:

1.   Access to quality health services
2.   Arthritis, osteoporosis, and chronic back conditions
3.   Chronic kidney disease
4.   Disability and secondary conditions
5.   Health communication
6.   Medical product safety
7.   Overweight (added to the Nutrition section to reflect the growing obesity problem)
8.   Public health infrastructure
9.   Respiratory diseases
10. Vision and hearing

While the results overall were inconsistent in eight Focus Areas—educational and community-based programs, environmental health, health communication, heart disease and stroke, immunization and infectious diseases, mental health and mental disorders, occupational safety and health, and tobacco use—more than 75% of the objectives moved toward or achieved their targets.[164]

In December 2010, DHHS launched Health People 2020. It is interesting to note how the addition of priority areas reflects the changes in epidemiology and social trends. The new categories were:

1.   Adolescent health
2.   Blood disorders and blood safety
3.   Dementias, including Alzheimer's disease
4.   Early and middle childhood
5.   Educational and community-based programs
6.   Genomics
7.   Global health
8.   Healthcare-associated infections
9.   Health information technology (added to health communication)
10. Health-related quality of life and well-being
11. Lesbian, gay, bisexual, and transgender health
12. Older adults
13. Preparedness
14. Sleep health
15. Social determinants of health

---

[164]National Center for Health Statistics. (2012). *Healthy people 2010 final review*. Hyattsville, MD: U.S. Department of Health and Human Services. Retrieved July 14, 2018, from https://www.cdc.gov/nchs/data/hpdata2010/hp2010_final_review.pdf

Interim reports of the progress of the Healthy People programs have become more complex and difficult to summarize as the topic areas (now 42) and measurable objectives (now about 1,200) have greatly increased.[165] Exhibit 9.13 summarizes the changes in these programs over the past few decades.

EXHIBIT 9.13. Evolution of the Healthy People Program

Target Year	1990	2000	2010	2020
Overarching Goals	Decrease mortality: infants–adults	Increase span of healthy life	Increase quality and years of healthy life	Attain high-quality, longer lives free of preventable disease
		Reduce health disparities	Eliminate health disparities	Achieve health equity and eliminate disparities
	Increase independence among older adults	Achieve access to preventive services for all		Create social and physical environments that promote good health
				Promote quality of life, healthy development; healthy behaviors across life stages
Number of Topic Areas	15	22	28	42
Number of Objectives	226	312	969	Approximately 1,200

Source: Health Promotion Statistics Branch. Office of Analysis and Epidemiology, National Center for Health Statistics. *Healthy People 2010 final review: Overview and selected findings*. Retrieved July 14, 2018, from https://www.cdc.gov/nchs/data/hpdata2010/hp2010_final_review_slide_deck.pdf

---

[165]National Center for Health Statistics. (2016). Chapter III: Overview of Midcourse progress and health disparities. In *Healthy people 2020 Midcourse review*. Hyattsville, MD: U.S. Department of Health and Human Services. (Corrected April 20, 2017.) Page III-4. Retrieved July 14, 2018, from https://www.cdc.gov/nchs/data/hpdata2020/HP2020MCR-B03-Overview.pdf

Plans for Healthy People 2030 are already under way.[166]

DEFINITION OF QUALITY

The definitions of quality care are always evolving, given advances in medical science, quality improvement research, and society's demands. In the United States, serious attempts at providing a definition started in 1974 with the Institute of Medicine (IOM) statement about quality assurance: "The primary goal of a quality assurance system should be to make health care more effective in bettering the health status and satisfaction of a population, within the resources which society and individuals have chosen to spend for that care."[167]

In 1990, the IOM recognized that this explanation did not define quality; therefore, it offered the following modification: "Quality of care is the degree to which health services for individuals and populations increase the likelihood of desired health outcomes and are consistent with current professional knowledge."[168] The IOM arrived at this statement after reviewing more than 100 definitions in the literature and considering 18 dimensions it considered essential to describing quality of care. (Please see Exhibit 9.14 for a list of these dimensions.)

In reflecting on this definition, note that consideration of resources was eliminated. Further, this definition is still not actionable, i.e., it does not guide actions to improve the quality of care. The IOM further explained that, "[i]n contrast to other common definitions that refer to medical or patient care, our definition of quality refers to health services."

As mentioned above, the next major change in the definition of quality occurred in 2001with publication of *Crossing the Quality Chasm*. The IOM referred to the previous definition but stated that "[a]ll health care organizations, professional groups, and private and public purchasers should pursue six major [quality] aims; specifically, health care should be safe, effective, patient-centered, timely, efficient, and equitable."[169]

To these characteristics, this author adds the following definition with an explanation of its terms:

Quality healthcare is the provision of measurably safe, efficient, and effective care to appropriately selected patients at the right time and in an expert manner, consistent with the current state of medical knowledge and patient. preferences.

Measurable. If one cannot assess quality by validated, commonly accepted measures, it is not worth evaluating. The approach that "I know it when I see it" will never work because of differences of opinion. Further, without these metrics, the effects of improvement efforts cannot be accurately assessed and improvements will never be implemented.

---

[166]Office of Disease Prevention and Health Promotion. *Development of the National Health Promotion and Disease Prevention Objectives for 2030*. Retrieved July 14, 2018, from https://www.healthypeople.gov/2020/About-Healthy-People/Development-Healthy-People-2030

[167]Institute of Medicine. (1974). *Advancing the quality of health care. A policy statement by a Committee of the Institute of Medicine* (pp. 1–2). Washington, DC.: National Academy of Sciences.

[168]Lohr, K. N. (Ed.). (1990). *Medicare: A strategy for quality assurance*, Volume I, op. cit., p. 4.

[169]Committee on Quality of Health Care in America. (2001). *Crossing the quality chasm*, op. cit., p. 6.

EXHIBIT 9.14. **Dimensions in Definitions of Quality**

1. Scale of quality
2. Nature of entity being evaluated
3. Goal-oriented
4. Aspects of outcomes specified
5. Acceptability
6. Type of recipient identified
7. Role and responsibility of recipient asserted
8. Continuity, management, coordination
9. Professional standards
10. Technical competency of provider
11. Interpersonal skills of provider
12. Acceptability
13. Statements about use
14. Constrained by resources
15. Constrained by consumer and patient circumstances
16. Constrained by technology and state of scientific knowledge
17. Risk versus benefit trade-offs
18. Documentation required

Note: The first eight dimensions are explicitly incorporated in the committee's definition.

Source: Lohr, K. N. (Ed.) (1990). *Medicare: A strategy for quality assurance: Volume I. Committee to design a strategy for quality review and assurance in Medicare Division of Health Care Services* (p. 22). Washington, DC: Institute of Medicine. National Academy Press.

Safe. Properly designed systems should minimize errors. The definition starts with this term because properly designed systems should minimize errors. A prominent example is the use of checklists[170] in operating rooms to make sure that, among other things, the correct type of surgery will be performed on the right body part of the right patient and that all preoperative procedures (like antibiotic administration) were performed.

Efficient. This term has two dimensions, time and money. Quality care should be delivered in the shortest possible time and at the lowest cost.

Effective. Quality care should be founded on evidence-based medicine that works in practice. (Recall from Chapter 7, "Healthcare Technology," the difference between efficacy and effectiveness.) More will be said about this characteristic below.

---

[170]For example, see World Health Organization. *Surgical safety checklist* (1st ed.) Retrieved July 14, 2018, from http://www.who.int/patientsafety/safesurgery/tools_resources/SSSL_Checklist_finalJun08.pdf

Appropriately selected patients. This term not only emphasizes the importance of evidence-based medicine but also stresses the individuality of patients' clinical circumstances. For example, it is easiest to demonstrate good clinical outcomes for patients who did not need the care in the first place.

Right time. American medicine's culture encourages testing and treatment as soon as possible. However, science has called such practice into question. For example, the practice of "watchful waiting" has become the standard of care for many men with prostate cancer. Timing is also important in such fields as oncology; with three major available treatments—surgery, chemotherapy, and radiation—their sequencing can make a difference in outcomes. Further, even time of day of the treatment can affect the body's response.[171]

Expert manner. This phrase refers to the technical expertise of the delivered care. For example, a patient's condition might warrant surgical intervention but that procedure must be performed with technical skill.

Consistent with the current state of medical knowledge. This concept is the same as in the 1990 IOM definition and reflects the changing state of clinical knowledge. (Recall from Chapter 7, "Healthcare Technology," the interventions that were once standards and are now known to be useless or harmful.)

Patient preferences. This last requirement is perhaps the most important. Care should not proceed if the patient prefers a different plan (including no treatment). Again, the case of watchful waiting for prostate cancer considers patient preferences for potential complications in light of possible benefits.[172]

KEY QUESTIONS FOR SUCCESSFUL EVALUATION AND IMPLEMENTATION OF QUALITY MEASURES

Because of the complexity and difficulty of choosing appropriate quality measures, this section will present some key questions that must be addressed (and hopefully answered) before successful quality improvement programs can exist. The three areas of concern are: choosing the right standards, monitoring adherence to the standards, and evaluating the results of their implementation.[173] This approach is akin to the PDCA approach described above.

---

[171] "A drug's pharmacokinetics can be modified according to the time of drug administration. In fact, the circadian changes of >100 different compounds have been documented. The results obtained have led several scientific societies to provide guidelines concerning the timing of drug dosing for anticancer, cardiovascular, respiratory, antiulcer, anti-inflammatory, immunosuppressive and antiepileptic drugs." Baraldo, M. (2008). The influence of circadian rhythms on the kinetics of drugs in humans. *Expert Opinion on Drug Metabolism & Toxicology, 4*(2), 175–192.

[172] Watchful waiting in prostate cancer was perhaps the first major medical condition to account for patient preferences. See, for example: Fleming, C., Wasson, J. H., Albertsen, P. C., Barry, M. J., & Wennberg, J. E. (1993). A decision analysis of alternative treatment strategies for clinically localized prostate cancer. *JAMA, 269*(20), 2650–2658.

[173] Shalowitz, J. (2010). Implementing successful quality outcome programs in ambulatory care: Key questions and recommendations. *Journal of Ambulatory Care Management, 33*(2), 117–123.

Choosing Standards

▪ *Which/whose standards do we use?*

Numerous organizations have developed their own criteria for assessing quality. For example, as mentioned above, in designing its quality programs, CMS accepts recommendations of the NQF criteria. However, as also noted, the NQF does not develop its own criteria but recommends standards from other groups. How does an organization choose whose standards to adopt? Exhibit 9.15 lists some prominent international organizations that produce their own quality metrics.

EXHIBIT 9.15. **Examples of International Quality Improvement Organizations**

Agency for Healthcare Research and Quality-AHRQ (www.ahrq.gov)

AHRQ (formerly AHCPR) (www.ahrq.gov)

Australian Patient Safety Foundation (www.apsf.net.au)

Canadian Task Force on Preventive Health Care/Groupe D'Etude Canadien Sur Les Soins De Sante Preventifs (www.ctfphc.org)

Choosing Wisely program (http://www.choosingwisely.org/doctor-patient-lists)

The Cochrane Collaboration (www.cochrane.org)

Consumer Assessment of Healthcare Providers and Systems (CAHPS) (www.cahps.ahrq.gov)

FACCT (absorbed into the Markle Foundation): Prevention, Staying Healthy, Treating Acute Illness (Getting Better), Living with Chronic Illness, End of Life Issues (www.markle.org)

Leapfrog Group: CPOE, High Volume, Intensivists (www.leapfroggroup.org)

National Guideline Clearinghouse (www.guideline.gov)[174]

National Institute for Clinical Excellence-NICE (www.nice.org.uk)

National Patient Safety Foundation (www.npsf.org)

National Quality Forum (NQF) http://www.qualityforum.org/

NCQA: Accreditation of MCOs and HEDIS (Healthcare Effectiveness Data and Information Set) (www.ncqa .org)

---

[174]While information from this valuable website will be archived, on July 16, 2018, the site was closed because of lack of funding from the federal government. See Minemeyer, P: HHS shutters clinical guideline resource; ECRI Institute says it will launch a replacement. *FierceHealthcare,* July 19, 2018. Retrieved July 19, 2018, from https://www.fiercehealthcare .com/regulatory/hhs-ahrq-clinical-guidance-resource-ecri-institute?mkt_tok=eyJpIjoiWmprNVpHSTNNMkZrWVdKb CIsInQiOiJITVF2Z0ppcDJqZ2sxalEzV0pKNG1kQ0lHTUppK0JpQXd2ZWlWdWxjaTVWNk94eEtsd0pBSjc5cERZZ FwvdHRvWE5kb3g3UDUzT2pZczZIT2ljTjBobzd4NXJGR29WMWswZzhBdmdKTTRqa0VzeFFKbmtDZ1o1eECtoe VFuVE1FMEoifQ%3D%3D&mrkid=936233

Scottish Intercollegiate Guidelines Network-SIGN (www.sign.ac.uk)

Zentralstelle der Deutchen Artzeschraft zur Qualitatssicherung in der Medizin, GbR (http://aezq.de)

Locally developed programs (e.g., by physician groups, hospitals/health systems, health plans, or government)

While sometimes the recommendations agree, different standards can have dramatically different clinical consequences. For example, persons with chronic kidney disease become anemic, in part, because they do not produce enough erythropoietin (a hormone produced in the kidney that stimulates red blood cell production). In 2006, the National Kidney Foundation published hemoglobin values of ≥ 13.5 g/dL for male adults and ≥ 12.0 g/dL for female adults as "normal," in order to guide administration of synthesized erythropoietin for those patients.[175] Clinical studies at that time, however, indicated that giving patients that hormone to achieve target levels of hemoglobin caused cardiovascular complications, initiating an FDA warning about such treatments.[176] These problems would not have occurred if either English[177] (Hb ≤ 11 g/dL) or Japanese[178] (Hb 10–11 g/dL) targets had been adopted.

A further problem is that many practitioners and institutions deal with multiple health plans and regulatory bodies that may use different sources for their quality program criteria. It is often difficult to keep track, much less satisfy, the requirements of each. The choice and consistency of standards are therefore critical.

■ *What definition do we use?*

At least two important reasons exist for having consistent definitions for events that drive the standards. The first reason is data gathering. How do we know an event actually occurred? For example, a safety issue that concerns both inpatient and ambulatory settings is falls in older persons. Drawing on Cochrane Collaboration reviews, Gatti[179] noted that the "authors acknowledge...the wide variability in the definition of 'fall' (resulting in some patients being included in some trials and not in others)." It is therefore important that common definitions be created and used consistently.

The second reason concerns how the definition helps frame the problem and points to useful solutions. A particularly relevant example concerns medication errors. The *operational* question is: When does a medication error actually occur? All would agree that if a patient consumes an incorrectly prescribed medicine, then an error has taken place.

---

[175]Clinical practice guidelines and clinical practice recommendations for anemia in chronic kidney disease in adults (2006). *American Journal of Kidney Diseases*, 47(3), S54–S57; and *American Journal of Kidney Diseases* erratum (2006), 48(3), 518.

[176]FDA Drug Safety Communication: Erythropoiesis-Stimulating Agents (ESAs): Procrit, Epogen and Aranesp. Retrieved July 14, 2018, from https://www.fda.gov/Drugs/DrugSafety/ucm200297.htm#SA

[177]National Institute for Clinical Excellence (2006). *CG: 39 Anæmia Management in Chronic Kidney Disease* (This recommendation has been updated at: www.nice.org.uk/guidance/ng8/chapter/Key-priorities-for-implementation) Accessed July 14, 2018.

[178]Gejyo, F., Saito, A., Akizawa, T., Sakai, T., Suzuki, M., Nishi, S., ... Bessho, M. (2004). Japanese Society for Dialysis Therapy: Guidelines for renal anemia in chronic hemodialysis patients. *Therapy Apheresis Dialysis*, 8(6), 443–459.

[179]Gatti, J. C. (2002). Cochrane for clinicians: Putting evidence into practice. *American Family Physician*, 65(11), 2259.

What if, however, there were errors in the ordering, transcription, and/or dispensing of the medication that are discovered *before* the patient actually consumes it? Do those problems constitute errors? The reason we must ask these questions is that answers will help us uncover the root causes for problems. To continue this example, if we define medication errors as only those when a mistake in *administration* occurs, we will miss the fact that the large majority of mistakes occur in ordering.[180] Programs to correct medication errors will thus differ greatly, depending on problem definition and identification. In the former case, attention will be exclusively focused on bedside measures, such as identity checks and second-person confirmation of dosage. In the latter case, resources will also be devoted to such measures as implementing accurate computerized order entry and monitoring any problems that might arise from its use.

■ *For what purpose will the standards be used? What outcome is measured?*

One must ask why the standards are being established. For example, are they to be used for regulation (licensure/certification), payment guidelines (whether or how much insurers will pay providers), end points for clinical studies, or benchmarks for patients to help them choose providers or health plans? Depending on the answer to the question of use, different outcomes may be used to measure the quality for the same episode of care. For example, these metrics are all acceptable assessments of quality depending on their use: functional status; psychological status; complications (morbidity); death (mortality); patient/family judgments; appropriate/efficient use of services. Actions to optimize one outcome may have adverse effects on another outcome. For example, in a study of FFS Medicare beneficiaries discharged after heart failure hospitalizations, "implementation of the HRRP [Hospital Readmissions Reduction Program] was temporally associated with a reduction in 30-day and 1-year readmissions but an increase in 30-day and 1-year mortality."[181]

Further, knowing the reason for setting these metrics will determine who should participate in their establishment. In addition, transparency about their ultimate use will enhance the likelihood that those being reviewed will accept these standards.

■ *Who chooses the outcome? Who is the "customer"?*

This question is closely related to the previous one. From the same healthcare encounter, different stakeholders value different outcomes. For example, consider the following report:

A cancer drug's effectiveness has long been measured in 2 important ways: whether it shrinks the tumor and whether it extends patients' lives. But researchers and regulators

---

[180]Nebeker, J. R., Joffman, J. M., Weir, C. R., Bennett, C. L., & Hurdle, J. F. (2006). High rates of adverse drug events in a highly computerized hospital. *Archives of Internal Medicine* [Now *JAMA Internal Medicine*] *165*, 1111–1116.

[181]Gupta, A., Allen, L. A., Bhatt, D. L., Cox, M., DeVore, A. D., Hedienreich, P. A. ... Fonarow, G. C. (2017, November). Association of the hospital readmissions reduction program implementation with readmission and mortality outcomes in heart failure. *JAMA Cardiology*. Retrieved July 14, 2018, from https://jamanetwork.com/journals/jamacardiology/article-abstract/2663213?utm_source=BHClistID&utm_medium=BulletinHealthCare&utm_term=111317&utm_content=MorningRounds&utm_campaign=BHCMessageID

are paying increasing attention to another criterion: how a patient feels while taking the medicine. In an important change, cancer patients' own assessment of how the drug is working, called patient-reported outcomes or PROs, are increasingly part of the drug-approval process at the Food and Drug Administration.[182]

This view on quality improvement highlights its patient-centered characteristic, which differs from the usual clinical measures of effectiveness. One could also apply this question to metrics evaluating quality that are based on timeliness, efficiency, and cost-effectiveness.

■ *How often do we reevaluate standards?*

One of the criticisms physicians often level at standards is that they change so often that by the time they are implemented they do not reflect best practices. Again, see Chapter 7 for a list of treatments once thought to be standards of care but subsequently were found to be harmful. Any program of quality improvement must, therefore, include timely, periodic reevaluations of quality standards to maintain credibility among users.

■ *Do we account for factors other than medical care?*

Many physicians believe that they are being evaluated on outcomes over which they have no control. Such factors include socioeconomic conditions (such as the availability and affordability of health insurance) and patient compliance. Sponsors of pay-for-performance programs have dealt with these issues in two ways. First, they offer the opportunity to remove from the evaluation equations those patients who, after multiple efforts by the provider, do not comply with treatment recommendations. This technique has been used in England for many years; for example, family practitioners are allowed to exclude patients from quality calculations if they are noncompliant with return requests, have had allergic or other adverse reactions to recommended treatments, or have diagnoses or registrations with the practice that are very recent.[183]

The other technique, not as accurate or desirable as the first, is lowering the target that providers must achieve, recognizing that these other problems exist.

■ *Does intervention alter the outcome?*

To set appropriate standards, we need to know that what we are doing will have a positive effect on the outcomes we seek to produce. The natural histories of these conditions must, therefore, be known before evaluating outcomes of the intervention. For example, as previously mentioned, consider options for screening and treatment of prostate cancer in older men. While routine screening was the standard of care for many

---

[182]Marcus, A. D. (2007, February 13). Cancer patients gain say in drug approvals FDA and drug makers had reports from trial participants to traditional measures such as survival, tumor shrinkage. *The Wall Street Journal*, D1.

[183]Doran, T., Fullwood, C., Gravelle, H., Reeves, D., Kontopantelis, E., Hiroeh, U., & Roland, M. (2006). Pay-for-performance programs in family practices in the United Kingdom. *New England Journal of Medicine, 355*(4), 375–384.

years, after 2000, it was found that such measures did not prolong life. Further, treatment often produced worse outcomes than watchful waiting.[184]

■ *Who or what is being evaluated?*

Even if all the above questions are satisfactorily addressed, it still remains to be decided what the target of analysis will be. For example, are we evaluating individual physicians or medical groups? Are we evaluating the performance of providers or payers? A further consideration in deciding the target of analysis is whether there is enough data to make quality decisions that have statistical significance.[185]

Monitoring Standards

After the above questions are addressed and the standards are chosen, they still need to be monitored. This process raises another series of questions, which are presented and explained below.

■ *Can the standards be audited accurately and easily?*

The initial concern, particularly in the ambulatory setting, is whether standards can be accurately audited. The first aspect of this worry is the validity and reliability of the gathered data. Numerous studies call into question the accuracy of encounter data entered into information systems, particularly billing data. For example, the DHHS reported that, overall, 11% of bills for Medicare Parts A and B are "improper," resulting in $40 billion of overpayments and $1 billion in underpayments.[186] The improper billing rates run much higher for durable medical equipment (46%) and home health services (42%). While this problem is significant, it is not new. For instance, in 1997, Iezzoni reported:

> Questions about data quality forced California to conduct a special study of data accuracy, which found striking variations across hospitals in the validity and reliability of coding certain risk factors ... overcoding (coding conditions not supported by medical record documentation) rates ranged from 10% at a putatively high-mortality hospital to 74% at a facility considered low mortality.[187]

The second aspect of this concern is data retrieval. While great strides have been made in recent years to integrate ambulatory and inpatient data, the great fragmentation

[184]Chodak, G. W., & Warren, K. S. (2006). Watchful waiting for prostate cancer: A review article. *Prostate Cancer and Prostatic Diseases 9*, 25–29.

[185]See, for example, AHRQ. The challenges of measuring physician quality. Retrieved July 15, 2018, from https://www .ahrq.gov/professionals/quality-patient-safety/talkingquality/create/physician/challenges.html

[186]DHHS. *The supplementary appendices for the Medicare Fee-for-Service 2016 Improper Payments Report.* Retrieved July 14, 2018, from https://www.cms.gov/Research-Statistics-Data-and-Systems/Monitoring-Programs/Medicare-FFS-Compliance-Programs/CERT/Downloads/AppendicesMedicareFee-for-Service2016ImproperPaymentsReport.pdf

[187]Iezzoni, L. I. (1997). The risks of risk adjustment. *JAMA, 278*, 1600–1607.

among different software products makes compatible retrieval difficult. Further, difficulties in retrieval cause the findings of many research studies to be based on outdated information.

■   *Are the data adjusted for severity of illness?*

When criticized for their outcomes, the most common excuse practitioners offer is that their patients are sicker than those of their peers. While many evaluations use some type of severity adjustment, they are not always applied appropriately or consistently.[188] Furthermore, different measures do not always produce consistent quality rankings. For example, with respect to two long-available risk adjustment tools, the Acute Physiology and Chronic Health Evaluation (APACHE)[189] measure applies to individual patients, while Medis-Groups[190] are designed to measure the severity of illness at the hospital level. In another instance, Mendez et al. reported that "[c]ase mix index (CMI) has become a standard indicator of hospital disease severity in the United States and internationally. However, CMI was designed to calculate hospital payments, not to track disease severity, and is highly dependent on documentation and coding accuracy."[191] Mendez et al. cautioned use of the adjuster since it did not provide accurate results when applied to public hospitals.

Adjusting for severity is also important for effective and fair pay-for-performance programs. Such schemes must adjust their payments not only to pay appropriate amounts to providers but also to remove provider incentives for cherry picking the healthiest patients.

■   *Have we controlled for the vigilance effect?*

When quality improvement activities are implemented, more examples of errors are discovered, sometimes as many as 30-fold from baseline.[192] It is therefore important not to place blame or penalize healthcare providers at the initial stages of quality improvement activities.

■   *When are the outcomes measured?*

If the outcomes are measured too quickly after the intervention, its benefits might not yet have occurred. Yet, if the evaluation occurs too late, the benefits or complications that are observed may not have anything to do with the intervention.

---

[188]For a comprehensive analysis of this topic, see: Iezzoni, L. I. (Ed.). (2012). *Risk adjustment for measuring healthcare outcomes* (4th ed.). Chicago: Health Administration Press.

[189]Knaus, W. A., Wagner, D. P., Draper, E. A., Zimmerman, J. E., Bergner, M., Bastos, P. G., ... Damiano, A. (1991). The APACHE III prognostic system: Risk prediction of hospital mortality for critically ill hospitalized adults. *Chest, 100*(6), 1619–1636.

[190]Originally owned by MediQual, it is part of Quantros. Retrieved July 14, 2018, from https://www.quantros.com/

[191]Mendez, C. M., Harrington, D. W., Christenson, P., & Spellberg, B. (2014). Impact of hospital variables on case mix index as a marker of disease severity. *Population Health Management, 17*(1), 28–34.

[192]Barraclough, B. (2006). The role of safety and quality councils in improving the quality of healthcare: An Australian Perspective. *Healthcare Papers, 6*, 24–32.

■ *What is the threshold for an outcome to register?*

Asked another way, what is the frequency for outcomes to occur that would indicate either success or problems? For example, an adverse outcome at a frequency of 1 in 1,000 may be acceptable for one intervention but may be considered too frequent for another.

Evaluating Results

If the metrics can be appropriately chosen and effectively monitored, the process should be subjected to five additional questions:

■ *Is this process worth the cost—for both the evaluator and those being evaluated?*

The costs of compliance with quality measures are substantial and growing. Two examples illustrate this problem. *Consumer Reports* noted in 2011 that:

> Three large hospital systems—Cleveland Clinic, Henry Ford in Detroit, and Parkview Health in Fort Wayne, Ind.—have stopped reporting data on hospital-acquired infections to the Leapfrog Group, a nonprofit organization in Washington, D.C., according to our updated hospital Ratings ... "It's a simple resource issue," says William Conway, M.D., senior vice president and chief quality officer at Henry Ford. "Since we now have an increasing volume of reporting to CMS, I can't afford duplicate reporting."[193]

Further, the situation is not better for physicians. Casalino et al. found that "[e]ach year US physician practices in four common specialties spend, on average, 785 hours per physician and more than \$15.4 billion dealing with the reporting of quality measures. While much is to be gained from quality measurement, the current system is unnecessarily costly, and greater effort is needed to standardize measures and make them easier to report."[194]

Schuster et al. summarized this situation:

> Although quality measurement activities are motivated, at least in part, by a desire to improve care, the current approach has produced an explosion of measures and a measurement system characterized by inefficiency and imbalance, with measures that are duplicative (e.g., multiple measures of follow-up care for the same condition that use different periods), that are overlapping (e.g., a diabetes composite measure and a separate hemoglobin A1c measure), or that over-represent some areas of care (e.g., there are many measures covering childhood immunizations and relatively few covering chronic

---

[193]Consumer Reports (2011, October 24). Three big-name hospitals stop publicly reporting some infection data. Retrieved July 14, 2018, from https://www.consumerreports.org/cro/news/2011/10/three-big-name-hospitals-stop-publicly-reporting-some-infection-data/index.htm

[194]Casalino, L. P., Gans, D., Weber, R., Cea, M., Tuchovsky, A., Bishop, T. F., ... Evenson, T. B. (2016). US physician practices spend more than \$15.4 billion annually to report quality measures. *Health Affairs, 35*(3), 401–406.

care for children)... The cost of specific measures has received limited attention in discussions about global costs of quality measurement and is not formally considered when evaluating and selecting measures, in no small part because that cost is usually unknown. *Without understanding the cost of a specific measure, assessing its value cannot be fully determined.* [Emphasis added.][195]

■ *Is the information actionable?*

Another way of asking this question is: When all the results of the evaluations have been obtained and presented to providers, can they use this information to effect meaningful change in outcomes? For example, one managed care health plan in the Midwest gave its physician groups a quarterly report that indicated performance on such features as timeliness of referrals, patient complaints about quality of care, and billing issues. The groups were expected to furnish a response and, if necessary, a corrective action plan. Unfortunately, the only data available were the number of complaints in each category; no details were furnished that would help the groups improve the quality of their services. When the health plan was asked for additional information, it refused, stating that the details were confidential.

■ *Are the incentives aligned?*

Because the best-quality healthcare requires coordination among all providers and institutions, incentives for all participants should be aligned. A perfect example of this process is aspirin administration for acute myocardial infarction in the emergency room. This metric is used by the CMS not only for evaluating physician performance but also in quality and bonus evaluations for hospitals. Other such opportunities must be consistently sought and implemented.

■ *Is the behavioral change sustainable?*

One of the aims of outcomes evaluations is that physicians will use the information to permanently change and improve the quality of their care. Even if the information were easily obtained, cheap, transparent, and actionable, implementing sustainable behavioral change is complex and must be an organization-wide effort. For example, Grimshaw et al. (2001) found: "In general, passive approaches are generally ineffective and unlikely to result in behavior change... Multifaceted interventions targeting different barriers to change are more likely to be effective than single interventions."[196]

■ *Does making quality scores available improve decision making?*

Finally, one of the current important themes in outcomes research is transparency—making the results of studies known to relevant stakeholders so that they can make more informed decisions about obtaining or delivering healthcare. While achieving this goal is laudatory, there is much evidence that this information is not consistently being used by

---

[195] Schuster, M. A., Onorato, S. E., & Meltzer, D. O. (2017). Measuring the cost of quality: A missing link in quality strategy. *JAMA, 318*(13),1219–122.

[196] Grimshaw, J. M., Shirran, L., Thomas, R., Mowatt, G., Fraser, C., Bero, L., ... O'Brien, M. A. (2001). Changing provider behavior: An overview of systematic reviews of interventions. *Medical Care, 39*(8, Suppl II), II2–II45.

EXHIBIT 9.16. How People Make Decisions About Hospital Choice

Suppose you had to choose between two different hospitals. The first one is the hospital you and your family have used for many years without any problems, but the second hospital is rated much higher in quality by the experts. Which hospital would you be more likely to choose?

	Hospital you and your family have used for many years	Hospital rated much higher in quality by experts	Don't know/ refused
2011 RWJF/HSPH[a]	57	38	5
Trend data:			
2008[b]	59	35	6
2004[c]	61	33	6
2000[d]	62	32	6
1996[e]	72	25	3

[a] RWJF: Robert Wood Johnson Foundation; HSPH: Harvard School of Public Health
[b] Kaiser Family Foundation Poll, July 29–August 6, 2008.
[c] Kaiser Family Foundation/Agency for Healthcare Research and Quality/Harvard School of Public Health Poll, July 7–September 5, 2004.
[d] Kaiser Family Foundation/Agency for Healthcare Research and Quality Poll, July 31–October 9, 2000.
[e] Kaiser Family Foundation/Agency for Health Care Policy and Research Poll, July 26–September 5, 1996.

Source: Kaiser Family Foundation: Trends in the Use of Hospital and Provider Quality Ratings. Retrieved July 14, 2018, from https://Kaiserfamilyfoundation.files.wordpress.com/2013/01/8184.pdf

many different types of stakeholders, particularly patients. Several examples illustrate this point. First, many people still make healthcare decisions based on word of mouth rather than on objective criteria. (Please see Exhibit 9.16 for an example.)

Second, the information from easily accessible sources is frequently inaccurate. For example, Daskivich et al. "assessed the association of consumer ratings with specialty-specific performance scores (metrics including adherence to Choosing Wisely measures, 30-day readmissions, length of stay, and adjusted cost of care), primary care physician peer-review scores, and administrator peer-review scores" and found that "[o]nline consumer ratings should not be used in isolation to select physicians, given their poor association with clinical performance."[197]

Third, patients are not the only stakeholders who ignore objective data to make decisions. An example is professional use of quality data about cardiovascular surgeons in New York State. As Brown et al. discovered: "After 20 years of public reporting and

[197] Daskivich, T. J., Houman, J., Fuller, G., Black, J.T., Kim, H.L., & Spiegel, B.. Online physician ratings fail to predict actual performance on measures of quality, value, and peer review. *Journal of the American Medical Informatics Association*, 25(4), 401–407.

almost universal awareness of cardiac surgeon report cards, in 2011, cardiologists in New York State made little use of this information and rarely discussed it with patients at the time of referral for cardiac surgery."[198]

■ *If we improve care, is it reflected in the public's (i.e., patients') satisfaction? Alternatively: If we improve patient satisfaction, are we improving the quality of care?*

For several reasons, the answers to these questions are, at best, unknown. First, the definitions of patient satisfaction are varied and often depend on the specialty assessing it. In a review of 109 peer-reviewed articles about the determinants of patient satisfaction from 1980 to 2014, Batbaatar et al. found that "study results were varied due to no globally accepted formulation of patient satisfaction and measurement system."[199]

Second, patients often judge quality based on factors having nothing to do with the services and products that can actually improve health. Recall from Chapter 1, "Understanding and Managing Complex Healthcare Systems," that we can divide quality into the technical component (the actual delivery of medical care), the service component (services that aid the delivery of care but are not essential for clinical improvement), and the amenities (items and services that are unrelated to the health of the patient). Inpatient examples might include, respectively, surgery and postoperative nursing care, housekeeping, and the gift shop. Numerous studies have shown a poor correlation between patient satisfaction scores and technical measures of quality.[200] Further, in general, patients value action over inaction. For example, in a study by Hoffmann and Del Mar looking at patient preferences for treatment, screening, and testing: "The majority of participants overestimated intervention benefit and underestimated harm."[201]

Third, satisfaction is based on certain social and demographic characteristics that are not related to the quality of care. For example, the region of the country and speaking English as a first language can independently influence patient satisfaction scores.[202]

Fourth, relying only on patient satisfaction scores to improve quality can be counterproductive.[203] For example, as Fenton et al. found:

> Adjusting for sociodemographics, insurance status, availability of a usual source of care, chronic disease burden, health status, and year 1 utilization and expenditures,

[198]Brown, D. L., Epstein, A. M., & Schneider, E. C. (2013). Influence of cardiac surgeon report cards on patient referral by cardiologists in New York state after 20 years of public reporting. *Circulation: Cardiovascular Quality and Outcomes*, *6*, 643–648.

[199]Batbaatar, E., Dorjdagva, J., Luvsannyam, A., Savino, M. M., & Amenta, P. (2017). Determinants of patient satisfaction: A systematic review. *Perspectives in Public Health*, *137*(2), 89–101.

[200]For example, see Junewicz, A., & Youngner, S. J. (2015). "Patient-satisfaction surveys on a scale of 0 to 10: Improving health care, or leading it astray?" *Hastings Center Report*, *45*(3), 43–51.

[201]Hoffmann, T. C., & Del Mar, C. (2015). Patients' expectations of the benefits and harms of treatments, screening, and tests: A systematic review. *JAMA Internal Medicine*, *175*(2), 274–286.

[202]Clark, C. (2011, January 18). Patient experience scores skew by region, providers say. *HealthLeaders Media*. Retrieved July 14, 2018, from http://www.healthleadersmedia.com/physician-leaders/patient-experience-scores-skew-region-providers-say

[203]Robbins, A. (2017, April 15). The problem with satisfied patients: A misguided attempt to improve healthcare has led some hospitals to focus on making people happy, rather than making them well. *The Atlantic*. Retrieved July 14, 2018, from https://www.theatlantic.com/health/archive/2015/04/the-problem-with-satisfied-patients/390684/

respondents in the highest patient satisfaction quartile (relative to the lowest patient satisfaction quartile) had lower odds of any emergency department visit..., higher odds of any inpatient admission..., greater total expenditures..., greater prescription drug expenditures, and higher mortality. [204]

Despite these problems, research studies show that patient satisfaction is associated with the overall quality of care and thus should be an important *part* of the total assessment of quality patient care. Consider these examples:

- "[W]e found marked variation in patient satisfaction across U.S. hospitals performing major surgery. While our results do not imply causality between patient experience and quality and efficiency of care, patient satisfaction was associated with both the quality and efficiency of surgical care, with high patient satisfaction hospitals having higher process quality, lower readmission rates, lower mortality rates, and shorter length of stay. Incentives designed at improving patient satisfaction and at improving surgical quality would not force hospitals to choose between better care and more responsive care.[205]

- [E]vidence from 55 studies... demonstrates positive associations between patient experience and self-rated and objectively measured health outcomes; adherence to recommended clinical practice and medication; preventive care (such as health-promoting behavior, use of screening services and immunization); and resource use (such as hospitalization, length of stay and primary-care visits). There is some evidence of positive associations between patient experience and measures of the technical quality of care and adverse events... The data presented... support the case for the inclusion of patient experience as one of the central pillars of quality in healthcare. It supports the argument that the three dimensions of quality should be looked at as a group and not in isolation.[206]

- Patient satisfaction was positively correlated with 13 of 14 acute myocardial infarction performance measures. After controlling for a hospital's overall guideline adherence score, higher patient satisfaction scores were associated with lower risk-adjusted inpatient mortality Satisfaction with nursing care was the most important determinant of overall patient satisfaction.[207]

In concluding this section, it is important to note that the above questions should not be viewed as reasons against implementing quality improvement activities. Instead, the author hopes those brief discussions will serve as a guide through potential problems that can impair the betterment of healthcare.

---

[204]Fenton, J. J., Jerant, A. F., Bertakis, K. D., & Franks, P. (2012). The cost of satisfaction: A national study of patient satisfaction, health care utilization, expenditures, and mortality. *Archives of Internal Medicine* (now *JAMA Internal Medicine*), *172*(5), 405–411.

[205]Tsai, T. C., Oray, E. J., & Jha, A. K. (2015). Patient satisfaction and quality of surgical care in U.S. hospitals. *Annals of Surgery*, *261*(1), 2–8.

[206]Doyle, C., Lennox, L., & Bell, D. (2013). A systematic review of evidence on the links between patient experience and clinical safety and effectiveness. *BMJ Open*, *3*(1), e001570. http://bmjopen.bmj.com/content/3/1/e001570

[207]Glickman, S. W., Boulding, W., Manary, M., Staelin, R., Roe, M. T., Wolosin, R. J., ... Schulman, K. A. (2010). Patient satisfaction and its relationship with clinical quality and inpatient mortality in acute myocardial infarction. *Circulation Cardiovascular Quality Outcomes*, *3*(2), 188–195.

VOLUME/QUALITY RELATIONSHIP

It has long been known that, for many types of treatment, providers who perform more of them have better success rates. Recall that the Leapfrog Group recommended using hospitals whose high surgical volume would lead to better outcomes.

Before wholly embracing this association, however, one must ask a number of questions to clarify the nature of the connection.

- *What is the volume at which quality starts to improve?*

    The answer to this question must be determined for each service, as there is no uniformity across treatments. Further, the type and setting of the service must also be determined. For example, while an inverse association between severity-adjusted CABG surgery volume and mortality rates had been long known, Showstack et al.[208] showed that the greatest effect is for "non-scheduled"—emergency—cases.

- *Why is there a volume/quality relationship?*

    Two hypotheses can be offered. The first is the most obvious—it results from a "learning curve"; in other words, practice makes perfect. However, this explanation is not always supported. As Luft et al. pointed out:

    > Learning by doing is commonly observed and is the basis for much of medical education. Accordingly, the relation should be between mortality and experience, rather than volume, but the two are difficult to separate. More importantly, our data do not allow an investigation of whether the relevant experience is that of specific surgeons, the operating-room team, or perhaps the whole hospital staff.[209]

    More will be said about this last statement below.

    The second hypothesis is that providers with good results attract more patients; thus, the putative causation is in the direction opposite to the first explanation. This explanation has been called the "selective referral hypothesis."

    It is important to distinguish which hypothesis is correct and in what circumstances, since public policy decisions will be quite different between the two. For example, in the first case, giving extra volume to the lowest-cost provider will result in higher quality and a better value proposition. This outcome would not occur if the selective referral explanation is true.

---

[208] Showstack, J. A., Rosenfeld, K. E., Garnick, D. W., Luft, H. S., Schaffarzick, R. M, & Fowles, J. (1987). Association of volume with outcome of coronary artery bypass graft surgery scheduled vs. nonscheduled operations. *JAMA*, 257(6), 785–789.

[209] Luft, H. S., Bunker, J. P., & Enthoven, A. C. (1979). Should operations be regionalized?—The empirical relation between surgical volume and mortality. *New England Journal of Medicine*, 301, 1364–1369 See also Luft, H. S. (1980). The relation between surgical volume and mortality: An exploration of causal factors and alternative models. *Medical Care, 18*(9), 940–959.

■ *Is there a volume quality relationship for all treatments?*

The clear answer is no.[210] Further, different treatments display different patterns with respect to increasing volumes. For a number of treatments, such as CABG surgery, it appears that increasing volumes over a large range correlates with lower mortality rates. For other interventions, such as hernia repair, after a certain volume is achieved, there is no further improvement. Some procedures, such as cardiac catheterizations, initially show a decrease in problems as volume increases but there is a deterioration in quality when volumes increase to high levels.

This finding of reduced quality also applies to the outpatient sector. For example, Cheung et al. found that "[p]rimary care physicians with busier ambulatory patient practices delivered lower-quality diabetes care, but those with greater diabetes-specific experience delivered higher-quality care. These findings show that relationships between physician volume and quality can be extended from acute care to outpatient chronic disease care."[211]

Finally, for some problems, such as treatment of a strep throat infection, outcomes of treatments should not be expected to display any relationship to volumes.

The policy implications for these different patterns are very important. If there are large and increasing improvements in quality with volume, a case can be made for centralizing care for those conditions and closing those programs at low-volume facilities. However, if there is a volume after which quality improvements cannot be demonstrated, then such centralization may be sacrificing access. Of course, other arguments can be made for further centralization, such as lowered costs. This situation is a perfect example of cost/quality/access trade-offs.

■ *When a volume/quality relationship exists, is it due to the physician or the facility?*

Again, the answer depends on the treatment being studied. This question was first substantively addressed by Hanan et al., who found that:

> For total cholecystectomies [gall bladder removals], hospital volume is the more significant volume measure, but physician volume is marginally related to mortality rate. For coronary artery bypass surgeries, resection of abdominal aortic aneurysms, partial gastrectomies [removals of part of the stomach], and colectomies [colon removal], physician volume is more significant than hospital volume, but hospital volume is marginally significant.[212]

---

[210]See examples and a further explanation in Luft, H. S., Hunt, S. S., & Maerki, S. C. (1987). The volume-outcome relationship: Practice-makes-perfect or selective-referral patterns? *Health Services Research, 22*(2), 157–182. While this research is dated, the concepts about patterns are still useful.

[211]Cheung, A., Stukei, T. A., Alter, D. A., Glazier, R. H., Ling, V., Wang, X., & Shah, B. R. (2017). Primary care physician volume and quality of diabetes care: A population-based cohort study. *Annals of Internal Medicine, 166*(4), 240–247.

[212]Hanan, E. L., O'Donnell, J. F., Kilburn Jr., H., Bernard, H. R., & Yazici, A. (1989). Investigation of the relationship between volume and mortality for surgical procedures performed in New York state hospitals. *JAMA, 262*(4), 503–510.

Other more recent investigations have tried to make this distinction in order to focus quality activities. For example, based on their research, Martin et al. recommended that "[t]o improve the safety of lumbar spinal fusion surgery, quality improvement efforts that focus on surgeons' discretionary use of operative techniques may be more effective than those that target hospitals."[213]

The above research invites the question: How can the hospital contribute to the quality of care? Ghaferi and colleagues provide an explanation:

> Hospitals with either very high mortality or very low mortality had similar rates of overall complications (24.6% and 26.9%, respectively) and of major complications (18.2% and 16.2%, respectively)... In contrast, mortality in patients with major complications was almost twice as high in hospitals with very high overall mortality as in those with very low overall mortality (21.4% vs. 12.5%, $P < 0.001$). Differences in rates of death among patients with major complications were also the primary determinant of variation in overall mortality with individual operations.[214]

In other words, complications are inevitable, even with the best technical quality of care; however, how the institution handles those complications can make a significant difference in outcomes such as mortality.

MANAGING QUALITY IMPROVEMENT

In addition to understanding the information discussed above, the successful practitioner of quality improvement needs to master such management skills as leadership, managing change, operations, teams organizational design, and negotiations/conflict resolution. All of these topics are best learned in formal training programs.[215] However, a few principles[216] should be discussed that can guide attitudes and actions in the transformation from quality assurance to quality improvement. (Please see Exhibit 9.17.)

VALUE PROPOSITIONS

After gaining an understanding of the issues related to quality, we can return to the initial discussion of trade-offs in healthcare with which we started this book. Recall that in

---

[213] Martin, B. I. (2013). Hospital and surgeon variation in complications and repeat surgery following incident lumbar fusion for common degenerative diagnoses. *Health Services Research, 48*(1), 1–25.

[214] Ghaferi, A. A., Birkmeyer, J. D., & Dimick, J. B. (2009). Variation in hospital mortality associated with inpatient surgery *The New England Journal of Medicine, 361*, 1368–1375.

[215] See, for example: Graduate Programs in Healthcare Quality and Patient Safety, Feinberg School of Medicine, Northwestern University. Retrieved July 14, 2018, from http://www.feinberg.northwestern.edu/sites/cehs/masters-programs/healthcare-quality-patient-safety/index.html

[216] The author is indebted to James Roberts, MD, for presentation of these topics as a guest lecturer in the author's class "Healthcare Systems" at the Kellogg School of Management in the late 1980s to early 1990s when Dr. Roberts was Vice President for Accreditation at the Joint Commission on Accreditation of Hospitals (now the Joint Commission).

EXHIBIT 9.17. **Transformation from Quality Assurance to Quality Improvement**

Quality Assurance	Quality Improvement
1. Externally driven	1. Internally driven
2. Follows organizational structure	2. Follows patient care
3. Focused on individuals	3. Focused on process
4. Delegated to a few	4. Embraced by all
5. Works toward end points	5. Has no end points
6. "Assures quality" (perfection)	6. "Improves" quality
7. Divides analysis of effectiveness/efficiency	7. Integrates analysis

1. *Quality Assurance* is externally driven. The organizational culture is reactive and quality-related activities are geared only to satisfying external licensure or accreditation requirements. It is akin to an educational system that is structured only to teach students to perform well on standardized tests.

   Quality Improvement is internally driven. An organization that embraces quality improvement will proactively incorporate quality activities as the way it conducts business. Licensure and accreditation requirements are only part of its overall quality activities.

2. *Quality Assurance* follows organizational structure. Traditional patient care entities are organized along functional lines, and hence quality-related activities tend to be located in silos. For example, while they work together, departments of surgery, radiology, pathology, nursing, and pharmacy probably are administered separately and have their own standards for performance review.

   Quality Improvement follows patient care processes. For example, instead of the various departments working independently with their own standards, organizations that adopt quality improvement will assess the patient care process as a whole; the departments involved in that care will share in the same metrics.

3. *Quality Assurance* focuses on individuals. Each person involved in the patient care process is solely responsible for his or her actions.

   Quality Improvement recognizes that the *system of care* accounts for most of the opportunities for improvement (and errors). The focus is, therefore, on the process of care rather than on individuals.

4. *Quality Assurance* is delegated to a few. Organizations pursuing this strategy give the responsibility for quality activities to clearly identifiable people and parts of the organization. In line with item 3, when something goes wrong, those people are the ones who are blamed.

   Quality Improvement is embraced by all. While management of the quality improvement process must be coordinated by certain skilled individuals, all people in organizations that operate in this fashion recognize *their personal* responsibility for these activities. Of further importance, quality improvement must be a top-down process. In the 1980s, some organizations even went as far as adding the title "chief quality officer" to that of the CEO.

5. *Quality Assurance* works toward end points. Once certain benchmarks are attained, the organization is "done" with quality activities; the remaining task is maintenance of the achievements.

> *Quality Improvement* has no end points. The process is geared to continuously improving accomplishments, whether they are process, outcome, or safety measures.

6. *Quality Assurance* assumes systems can be perfected to achieve a zero error rate.

> *Quality Improvement* acknowledges that processes have intrinsic errors and need to be continually improved.

7. *Quality Assurance* divides the analysis of effectiveness and efficiency. It sees quality activities as separate from those that may lower cost and/or deliver care faster (including enhancing access).

> *Quality Improvement* integrates analysis of effectiveness and efficiency. It recognizes that an important part of quality activities is lowering cost and/or improving the speed and access to care.

a Pareto-optimal state, one must make trade-offs among cost, quality, and access if a change in one of these elements occurs. The only exception is a truly innovative intervention that takes these relationships to a new and better equilibrium. (Please see Chapter 7.)

In considering these trade-offs, it becomes apparent that different and conflicting definitions of value emerge. These definitions are best explained by examining the different trade-off dyads.

Cost–Quality Trade-off

While it is true that sometimes quality improvement can lower costs, more often it takes money to eventually save money. In this context, one can ask about value preferences by choosing between two statements:

> I have a budget and want to get the best quality I can for the amount of money I am willing to spend.
>
> *or*
>
> I have abundant resources to get the "best" quality, but I don't want to overpay.

The former statement is the value proposition for most of the world's healthcare systems. The latter statement reflects America's value proposition for healthcare. It should be obvious that these two statements are fundamentally very different, and they elucidate one reason why the United States cannot (and does not want to) fully adopt the healthcare systems of other countries.

Cost–Access Trade-off

The competing value definitions for this trade-off are:

> I have a budget and want the fastest and closest care I can afford.
>
> *or*
>
> I want the fastest care at a facility close to me at the lowest possible cost.

Again, the definitions exemplify the differences between other healthcare systems and that of the United States. For example, in the vaunted British and Canadian systems, there are accepted (though not always desired) queues for care that are necessary to keep the budgets intact. The American culture does not accept any delays. As a result, we have many unnecessary, duplicated facilities.[217]

Quality–Access Trade-off

This value decision does not involve money, but in the public's eye is no less controversial. Recall that, for many conditions, increased volume is associated with higher-quality care. The trade-off here comes from directing patients from lower-volume facilities to higher-volume sites.

The value propositions are therefore:

I want to maximize my quality of care while minimizing my loss of access.

or

I want to maximize my access while minimizing my loss of quality.

This trade-off choice is less of a distinction between other healthcare systems and our own, since Americans have somewhat embraced the idea of obtaining care from distant centers of excellence or high-quality, branded care such as the Mayo Clinic and Cleveland Clinic. Still, many of our rural areas lack adequately accessible resources, such as obstetrical care.

By understanding these three trade-offs, one can appreciate the difficulties in achieving consensus among the many stakeholders of the healthcare system and their value desires.

SUMMARY

On August 15, 2017, a blog post from AHRQ was titled: "The Data Are In: Health Care Quality Continues to Improve, But Disparities Persist."[218] While this statement seems to be the final word (or at least the most current one at the time of this writing), striving for healthcare quality improvement is a never-ending process. Problems in continuous improvement derive from such issues as evolving scientific definitions of quality care; measuring quality; and different stakeholder value preferences in trade-offs among cost, quality, and access.

These problems should not be used as an excuse for avoiding improvement activities but should be recognized prospectively so that objections can be addressed and the quality of care can continue to improve.

---

[217] For an excellent piece of investigative journalism, see Schorsch, K. (2015). Empty beds plague state's hospitals. *Crain's Chicago Business*, 14. Retrieved July 14, 2018, from http://www.chicagobusiness.com/article/20150124/ISSUE01/301249988/hospitals-full-of-empty-beds?utm_source=ISSUE01&utm_medium=rss&utm_campaign=chicagobusiness This article not only details the range of empty beds among Illinois hospitals, but also displays the closeness between underutilized facilities to highlight the costly redundancies.

[218] Arnold, S. (2017). *The data are in: Health care quality continues to improve, but disparities persist*. AHRQ Views. Retrieved July 14, 2018, from https://www.ahrq.gov/news/blog/ahrqviews/data-are-in.html

INDEX